The Herpesviruses

CONTRIBUTORS

Tamar Ben-Porat
P. M. Biggs
Robert W. Darlington
Friedrich Deinhardt
Glenn A. Gentry
Eli Gold
Barry Goz
Allan Granoff
Berge Hampar
Robert N. Hull
Ernest Jawetz
Mary Ann Jerkofsky
Albert S. Kaplan
George Klein
R. Z. Lockart, Jr.
Delbert G. McKercher
Lidia M. Martos
George A. Nankervis
William H. Prusoff
Charles C. Randall
Fred Rapp
William E. Rawls
D. H. Watson
Peter Wildy
Ken Wolf
Harry T. Wright, Jr.

THE HERPESVIRUSES

Edited by

Albert S. Kaplan

Department of Microbiology
School of Medicine
Vanderbilt University
Nashville, Tennessee

ACADEMIC PRESS New York San Francisco London
A Subsidiary of Harcourt Brace Jovanovich, Publishers

ACADEMIC PRESS, INC.
111 Fifth Avenue, New York, New York 10003

United Kingdom Edition published by
ACADEMIC PRESS, INC. (LONDON) LTD.
24/28 Oval Road, London NW1

Library of Congress Cataloging in Publication Data

Kaplan, Albert S. DATE
The herpesviruses.

Includes bibliographies.
1. Herpesviruses. 2. Oncogenic viruses.
I. Title. [DNLM: 1. Herpesvirus. QW160.H6 K17h 1973]
QR400.K36 576'.6484 73-2064
ISBN 0-12-397050-4

PRINTED IN THE UNITED STATES OF AMERICA

Contents

Chapter 4 Replication—Biological Aspects

Robert W. Darlington and Allan Granoff

Chapter 5 Replication of the Viruses—Morphological Aspects

D. H. Watson

Chapter 6 Replication—Biochemical Aspects

Tamar Ben-Porat and Albert S. Kaplan

Chapter 7 Immunological Relationships

Berge Hampar and Lidia M. Martos

Chapter 8 Interference and Interferon with Respect to Herpesviruses

R. Z. Lockart, Jr.

Chapter 9 Persistent and Latent Infections

Fred Rapp and Mary Ann Jerkofsky

Chapter 10 Herpes Simplex Virus

William E. Rawls

Chapter 11 Varicella—Zoster Viruses

Eli Gold and George A. Nankervis

Chapter 12 Cytomegaloviruses

Harry T. Wright, Jr.

Chapter 13 The Simian Herpesviruses

Robert N. Hull

Chapter 14 Viruses of Other Vertebrates

Delbert G. McKercher

Chapter 19 The Lucké Renal Carcinoma of the Frog

Allan Granoff

Chapter 20 Chemotherapy—Molecular Aspects

William H. Prusoff and Barry Goz

Chapter 21 Chemotherapy of Herpesviruses—Clinical Aspects

Ernest Jawetz

List of Contributors

Numbers in parentheses indicate the pages on which the authors' contributions begin.

TAMAR BEN-PORAT (163), Department of Microbiology, School of Medicine, Vanderbilt University, Nashville, Tennessee.

P. M. BIGGS (557), Houghton Poultry Research Station, Houghton, Huntingdon, England

ROBERT W. DARLINGTON (93), Laboratories of Virology and Immunology, St. Jude Children's Research Hospital, Memphis, Tennessee

FRIEDRICH DEINHARDT (595), Department of Microbiology, Rush-Presbyterian-St. Luke's and University of Illinois Medical Centers, Chicago, Illinois

GLENN A. GENTRY (45), Department of Microbiology, University of Mississippi, School of Medicine, Jackson, Mississippi

ELI GOLD (327), Department of Pediatrics, Case Western Reserve University, School of Medicine, Cleveland Metropolitan General Hospital, Cleveland, Ohio

BARRY GOZ (641), Department of Pharmacology, Yale University, School of Medicine, New Haven, Connecticut

ALLAN GRANOFF (93, 627), Laboratories of Virology and Immunology, St. Jude Children's Research Hospital, Memphis, Tennessee

BERGE HAMPAR (221), National Cancer Institute, National Institutes of Health, Bethesda, Maryland

ROBERT N. HULL (389), Lilly Research Laboratories, Eli Lilly and Company, Indianapolis, Indiana

ERNEST JAWETZ (665), Department of Microbiology, School of Medicine, University of California, School of Medicine, San Francisco, California.

Mary Ann Jerkofsky (271), Department of Microbiology, College of Medicine, The Milton S. Hershey Medical Center of the Pennsylvania State University, Hershey, Pennsylvania

Albert S. Kaplan (163), Department of Microbiology, School of Medicine, Vanderbilt University, Nashville, Tennessee

George Klein (521), Department of Tumor Biology, Karolinska Institute, Stockholm, Sweden

R. Z. Lockart, Jr. (261), Central Research Department, Experimental Station, E. I. du Pont de Nemours and Company, Wilmington, Delaware

Delbert G. McKercher (427), School of Veterinary Medicine, University of California, Davis, California

Lidia M. Martos (221), Flow Laboratories, Inc., Rockville, Maryland

George A. Nankervis (327), Department of Pediatrics, Case Western Reserve University, School of Medicine, Cleveland Metropolitan General Hospital, Cleveland, Ohio

William H. Prusoff (641), Department of Pharmacology, Yale University, School of Medicine, New Haven, Connecticut

Charles C. Randall (45), Department of Microbiology, University of Mississippi, School of Medicine, Jackson, Mississippi

Fred Rapp (271), Department of Microbiology, College of Medicine, The Milton S. Hershey Medical Center of the Pennsylvania State University, Hershey, Pennsylvania

William E. Rawls (291), Department of Virology and Epidemiology, Baylor College of Medicine, Houston, Texas

D. H. Watson (27, 133), Department of Microbiology, School of Medicine, University of Leeds, Leeds, England

Peter Wildy (1), Department of Virology, The Medical School, Birmingham, England

Ken Wolf (495), Eastern Fish Disease Laboratory, Bureau of Sport Fisheries and Wildlife, Kearneysville, West Virginia

Harry T. Wright, Jr. (353), Department of Pediatrics, University of Southern California, School of Medicine, and Department of Medicine, Childrens Hospital of Los Angeles, Los Angeles, California

Preface

Ever since their discovery, the herpesviruses have engaged the attention of virologists. This attention not only stems from the diseases these viruses cause but also from a most interesting characteristic: the propensity of the herpesviruses to enter into a latent state in hosts who have recovered from clinically apparent disease and later to cause recurrent infection.

With the development of cell culture methods and of quantitative animal virology, there has been a rapid accumulation of knowledge about the interaction of the herpesviruses with their hosts at the cellular and molecular levels. Although the early studies of the herpesviruses provided much useful information, they suffered, as did similar studies of other viruses, from the limitations inherent in the technology of the period preceding the advent of cell culture techniques. The more recent advances in our understanding of the replication of the herpesviruses, as well as the considerable interest in these viruses that has developed recently as a result of the discovery that some members of this group have oncogenic potential, make the time propitious for the publication of a comprehensive work on this group of viruses.

The purpose of this book is to collect into one volume the currently available information on *all* the herpesviruses. The first part of the work is concerned with basic aspects of the viruses, and consists of chapters dealing with the classification, morphology, physical-chemical properties, replication, and immunological relationships of all the herpesviruses. This part also includes chapters on interference and interferon as well as on persistent and latent infections. The second part is concerned with the more clinical aspects of the viruses; it deals primarily with specific diseases of man and animals and includes descriptions of the essential clinical features, pathogenesis, immunity, and epidemiology. Four of these chapters are devoted specifically to those herpesviruses which are associated with carcinogenesis. In the last two chapters the molecular and clinical aspects of antiviral chemotherapy are discussed.

The various topics presented in this volume are directed to virologists, molecular biologists, physicians, and veterinarians, as well as to teachers and graduate students who may be interested in the herpesviruses from either a basic or clinical viewpoint. It would clearly be imprudent and probably impossible for one individual to attempt to write authoritatively about all aspects of the herpesviruses. It was essential therefore to solicit the help of experts in the various areas of herpes virology, and I was quite fortunate in obtaining contributions from outstanding virologists from the United States and Europe.

While the material included in this book covers most of the available data, an effort has been made to develop a proper synthesis and interpretation of these facts so that this volume would not be a mere annotated bibliography. One of the chief difficulties of an editor is to avoid duplication of material among the different chapters. I have tried to eliminate repetition of facts although it was not always possible to do so. In some instances, repetition was considered desirable because it permitted the expression of more than one viewpoint on still unsettled issues.

Albert S. Kaplan

The Herpesviruses

Chapter 1
Herpes: History and Classification

Peter Wildy

I. Introduction

I have been asked to consider, in this chapter, the classification of the herpesviruses, to give some historical perspective, and to speculate on the origins and phylogeny of the herpesviruses. I have attempted the task in two parts. First, I shall deal with the history of herpes, going back well before any concept of virus, as we know it, had evolved. It is amusing to note that classifications of "herpes" antedated the elucidation of its etiology by many centuries. These classifications were originally nosological, but I suspect that, with the reverence of the medieval scholar for classical writings, some of these nosologies were lists of antiquated names rather than of diseases and provide good examples of the potency and danger of nomenclature. From classical classifications, I shall trace the successive classifications of the herpes group, based on histopathological appearances, virological properties, serological affinities, morphological patterns, and chemical structure. Finally, I shall deal with the methods of classifying genetical patterns in molecular terms.

The second part will deal with subclassification of herpesviruses, and since there seem to be good reasons for supposing that at least some viruses within the group may have common ancestry, I shall deal with the phylogeny of the herpesviruses and sound a warning note on nomenclature.

II. Development of the Concept of the Herpes Group of Viruses, 500 B.C. to 1972 A.D.

A. *Origin of the Word "Herpes": Nomenclature, Nosology, and Etiology*

"The word 'herpes' has been used in medicine for at least 25 centuries. However, its meaning has changed considerably during that time. . . . Possibly none of the conditions, which we designate herpes today would have been called by that name in the time of Hippocrates" (Beswick, 1962). The word ερπησ (= the creep) was evidently used in ancient times for conditions as diverse as eczema and cancer of the skin. Indeed, although Hippocrates (Littré, 1839–1861) was familiar with both herpes febrilis and shingles (from *cingulus* = a girdle; Onions, 1956), he seems only to have called the latter herpes. Galen apparently used the term inconstantly but, according to Beswick, he and subsequent medical writers until comparatively recently were consistent in their views on the pathogenesis of "herpes"; it was the excretion (or attempted excretion) of acrid waste matter by the skin. The material being excreted was supposed to be bile alone (herpes miliaris) or bile mixed with other humors (herpes exedens). Though this may have been the orthodox medical view of the etiology, folklore obviously had other explanations; the carriage of Queen Mab, the midwife of the fairies, galloped:

> O'er ladies lips, who straight on kisses dream
> Which oft the angry Mab with blisters plagues,
> Because their breaths with sweetmeats tainted are.
>
> Shakespeare, "Romeo and Juliet," Act I, Scene IV

The word herpes continued to include a miscellany of skin conditions up until the late nineteenth century. Throughout this time, it seems to have been used for zoster. The first reference to herpes febrilis as herpes was that of Morton (1694). From the beginning, writers recognized different types of herpes. Sometimes the descriptions are clear and recognizable but often they seem confused, and it is evident that names such as herpes miliaris, herpes exedens, and herpes esthiomenos were applied by different writers to different conditions. In one of the clearer accounts, Turner (1714) wrote: "The herpes is a choleric pustule breaking forth of the skin diversely, and accordingly receiving a diverse denomination." He distinguished facial herpes (simplex), herpes miliaris (shingles), serpigo (ringworm), and esthiomenos or exedens which he dismissed as a surgical condition "more properly belonging to a discourse on ulcers."

In the latter part of the eighteenth century, classification and systematization became popular, and nosologies (clinical classifications) were developed; this pastime even claimed the attention of Linnaeus (1763). A part of Plenck's (1783) system is shown in Table I. He listed 14 classes of skin disease. *Zona seu Zoster* was one of three genera in Class I. *Varicella seu Variolae spuriae* was one of five genera in Class II, nestling together with *Variola* and *Scabies.* Fever blisters or *Miliaria febrilia* belonged in a quite different class, *Vesiculae seu Phlyctenae.* Finally, *Herpes seu Serpigo*, which seems unlikely to have included any form of herpes we now recognize, was one of eight genera in Class V; it had strange companions, e.g., *Lepra*, *Elephantiasis*, and *Cutis anserina.*

The modern notion of herpes probably began with the definitions of Willan and Bateman (Bateman, 1814). The term was restricted to conditions characterized by the appearance of localized groups of vesicles, a short self-limiting course, and the absence of more than mild constitutional symptoms. Healing could not be accelerated by treatment. The species of herpes included zoster, labial herpes, and genital herpes; also included were ringworm (*H. circinatus*) and erythema multiforme (*H. iris*). These latter conditions were still classified as species of herpes until as late as 1880 and appear at least as late as 1938 in the "American Illustrated Medical Dictionary" (Dorland, 1938) where Galen's definition of herpes is given: "An inflammatory skin disease characterized by the formation of small vesicles in clusters," and 22 varieties of herpes are listed.

Herpes simplex was shown by human inoculation to be infectious by Vidal (1873). Similarly, herpes zoster was shown to be infectious by von Bokay (1909), whose observations led him to suggest as early as 1888 that zoster and chickenpox were related. Curiously, chickenpox which, according to Weller (1965), is derived from *cicer* = a chick-pea, was considered a mild form of smallpox until 1767 when Heberden distinguished it as a

TABLE I

PART OF A CLASSIFICATION OF DISEASES OF THE SKIN[a]

Class	Genus	Species	Subspecies
I Maculae	*Zona seu Zoster* (33 others)	—	—
II Pustulae	*Varicella seu Variola spuriae* (4 others)	*V. lymphaticae* *V. verrucosae* *V. duraeovales* *V. emphysematosae*	
III Vesiculae seu Phlyctenae	*Miliaria* (4 others)	*M. febrilia* *M. lactea* *M. chronica*	
V Papulae	*Herpes seu Serpigo* (7 others)	*H. simplex* (Prurigo) *H. exedens* (Lupus) *H. miliaris* (Acne) *H. pustulosus* (Impetigo) *H. syphiliticus*	
		H. spurius (Artificial eczema)	a. *H. periscelis* b. *H. collaris* c. *H. cerdonum* d. *H. a tactu toxicodendri*

[a]From Plenck (1783). The explanations in parentheses are due to Hebra (1886).

separate clinical entity (Gordon, 1962). The infectious nature of both conditions was established by the direct inoculation of volunteers (Steiner, 1875; Kundratitz, 1925).

In summary, the word herpes was applied variously to a variety of clinical skin conditions until recent times. Numerous nosologies were published; these are now of no scientific value but are historically very interesting. The idea that any form of herpes is infectious is recent.

B. Tropisms and Histopathological Patterns

At the turn of the century, much attention was devoted to histopathological appearances and these, together with clinical and epidemiological data, strongly influenced ideas on classification.

The first obvious effect of such studies was to focus attention on the sites of lesions. This led to the concept of tropisms and its use in classification.

Levaditi (1929) included herpesvirus among the *Ectodermoses neurotropes*; the system was later elaborated (Levaditi and Voet, 1935; Levaditi and Lépine, 1937). An example of such a classification is given in Table II. It is interesting that herpes genitalis and herpes febrilis belong in different groups, as do herpes zoster and varicella. The concept of tropisms became unfashionable in the 1940's (cf., for example, Olitsky and Casals, 1948); however, host tissue and cell tropisms continued in use as major taxonomic criteria much later (Holmes, 1948).

The detailed study of lesions provided a more enduring influence in classification. Thus, Unna (1896) was able to distinguish herpesvirus infections from poxvirus infections by cellular patterns, and, at about the same time, intracellular inclusions were noticed in a number of virus infections. To begin with, these bodies were interpreted as protozoal parasites (cf. Guarnieri, 1892); indeed, Ribbert (1904) discussed the inclusions seen in cytomegalic cells in these terms, and Smith and Weidman (1910–1911) even went so far as to classify them as *Entamoeba mortinatalium* (nov. sp.). Such views did not persist long, although the nature of inclusion bodies could not be resolved for some time. From our present viewpoint, the importance of inclusions is simply that they were regarded as hallmarks of virus infections and that they came to be used as criteria in virus classifications. Thus, Lipschütz (1921) equated the intranuclear inclusions of herpes simplex with those seen in zoster.

Further refinements in interpretation were introduced by Cowdry who reported the results of his labors in a series of papers. These he critically

TABLE II
PART OF LIPSCHÜTZ'S CLASSIFICATION
SHOWING THE DISTRIBUTION OF VARIOUS HERPESVIRUS DISEASES[a]

I	Lokalisierte epidermale oder epitheliale Vira:
	Herpes venereus (7 others)
II	Dermatrope Vira:
	Varicellen (8 others)
III	Dermoneurotrope Vira:
	Zoster
	Herpes febrilis
IV	Neurotrope Vira:
	(4 viruses)
V	Organotrope Vira:
	(5 viruses)
VI	Akute allgemeine Infektionkrankheiten:
	(3 examples)

[a] From Lipschütz (1930), copyright 1930, by American Medical Association.

reviewed in the paper (Cowdry, 1934) which has proved to be a milestone in the history of herpes classification. He distinguished two types of intranuclear inclusion, A and B. "The type A inclusions are pleomorphic, resistant to organic solvents and contain little or no thymonucleic acid or mineral. The nuclear involvement is total and proceeds to complete destruction and the inclusion is separated by a clear halo from the chromatin which eventually marginates" (Cowdry, 1934). He was cautious about interpreting the nature of inclusions, refused to admit that they necessarily indicated virus action, and hotly contested the view that they were composed of virus particles for several good reasons. However, he is definite that type A intranuclear inclusions are "the finger prints of a special and limited group of viruses which is small in comparison with that hodge-podge of agents to which the term 'virus' is usually applied." He lists the situations in which type A intranuclear inclusions had been found (Table III). Some two-thirds of the items listed are recognizably the herpes group we now know. Even today, Cowdry's definition of a type A inclusion stands, after slight modification by Pereira (1961).

TABLE III

COWDRY'S LIST OF CONDITIONS GIVING TYPE A INTRANUCLEAR INCLUSIONS[a]

Herpes
Yellow Fever
Chickenpox
Virus III infection
Salivary gland disease of guinea pigs
Salivary glands of moles
Kidneys of Guatemalan amazons
Fox encephalitis (from R. G. Green)
Whooping cough (from H. A. McCordock)
Salivary glands of rats (from Juanita Thompson)
Salivary glands of children (from S. B. Wolbach)
Infectious tracheitis of chickens (from Oskar Seifried)
A disease of parrots and parrakeets (from J. R. Meyer)
Kidneys of frogs (from Baldwin Lucké)
Brain of mouse with louping ill (from L. T. Webster)
Mad itch in dogs (from E. W. Hurst)
A disease of owls (from R. G. Green)
Many species in the absence of disease

[a]From E. V. Cowdry (1934). *Arch. Path.* **18**, 527, Copyright 1934, American Medical Association.

C. *Infectious Virus and Mode of Multiplication*

Herpes simplex virus was successfully transferred to rabbits (Grüter, 1920) as early as 1911 and was shown to be filterable (Luger and Lauda, 1921) and associated with a moderately specific histopathological pattern. However, the 1930's found microbiologists in conceptual difficulties regarding what a virus could be. Cowdry (1934) stated the general quandary thus: "Viruses are carried by substances whose general nature has not been proved. As soon as any virus is found to be a microorganism, it is no longer considered a member of the group." He goes on, later, to say: "No proof is forthcoming that the particles (i.e., elementary bodies) are anything other than tiny masses of nucleoprotein." He goes on to question whether viruses are minute microorganisms, autocatalytic ferments, or a new kind of living thing. The ensuing controversy on the nature of viruses had a paralyzing effect on would-be taxonomists. F. W. Andrewes (1930) wrote: "Judgment must be suspended . . . in the case of the invisible viruses or so-called 'filter-passing' organisms. Here our ignorance is almost complete: they are possibly a heterogeneous group but in the case of creatures which we cannot see and whose very existence is, in many cases, a matter of inference only, it is idle to talk of classification in the usual sense." In the face of such difficulties, it is scarcely surprising that virus classification had to await conceptual advances.

At this time, a puzzling feature of herpes simplex became known. Andrewes and Carmichael (1930) found that a large proportion of adults had herpesvirus neutralizing antibody and that recurrent herpes occurred only in such people, a finding that contrasted starkly with the general behavior of infectious diseases. This, coupled with the observation that labial herpes was not evidently infectious but provoked by nonspecific stimuli, led Doerr (1938) to suggest that herpes might be endogenously generated in the host. The puzzlement evaporated when Burnet and Williams (1939) elucidated the nature of primary herpes.

The first virological evidence for the existence of a biologically and serologically related group of herpesviruses was provided by the papers of Sabin (1934). He showed that herpesvirus, B virus, and pseudorabies virus were (1) neurotropic in the rabbit; (2) able to attack all three embryonal layers; (3) histologically indistinguishable, all producing type A intranuclear inclusions; and (4) serologically related but distinct by neutralization tests. He postulated that these three viruses might be subtypes of a species which he considered analogous to certain polytypic bacterial species: "an instance which has no exact parallel among the so-called classical viruses." A similar conclusion was later reached by Burnet *et al.* (1939). Thus, when Holmes (1948) published his universal classification, most of which now seems absurd, we find herpes simplex, pseudorabies, and B virus nestling cheek-by-jowl in the genus *Scelus* (= a rascal), although they share the nest with others such as ectromelia virus. The principal effect of Holmes's work was to stimulate interest in virus taxonomy. A vast amount of information had become available and several clusters of viruses were recognized. The record shows that a serious attempt at classification was made and an international body was set up to look after it. At the international congress at Rio de Janeiro in 1950, the following eight criteria were agreed upon: (1) morphology and methods of reproduction; (2) chemical composition and physical properties; (3) immunological properties; (4) susceptibility to chemical and physical agents; (5) natural methods of transmission; (6) host, tissue, and cell tropisms; (7) pathology, including inclusion body formation; and (8) symptomatology (purposely placed last as of minor importance) (Andrewes, 1952). It is interesting that the earliest criteria for classification had, by that time, become the least important. The herpes group now consisted of a triad (herpes simplex, B, and pseudorabies) of viruses with the tentative addition of varicella and zoster (Andrewes, 1952). At the Rome Congress, the herpes group was enlarged to five certain members, dignified by "non-Linnaean" binomials. In addition to the classical triad, varicella–zoster and virus III had been added, and the viruses of equine abortion and Pacheco's parrot disease were considered as possible members (Burnet, 1955).

During the 1950's, animal virologists were once again seriously trying to define what they meant by a virus. The position was summarized by Burnet's (1955) tentative definition of viruses in terms of small, obligate intracellular parasites which "undergo conversion into a noninfective form as a necessary step in their multiplication." That this was true of herpes simplex virus was demonstrated by infective center experiments using slips of chorioallantoic membrane or cells (Wildy, 1954; Stoker and Ross, 1958).

Great interest in the modes of multiplication of viruses developed in this period, extending to biologists, biochemists, and electron microscopists. Thin-section electron micrographs of infected cells revealed the intranuclear location of single-ring particles (Morgan *et al.*, 1954) and the cytoplasmic accumulation of two-ring particles. It soon became clear that the four available members of the herpes group had a characteristic growth pattern (see Chapters 5 and 6).

The 1950's saw the first really satisfactory definition of a virus. Lwoff's (1957) definition crystallized the concept of virus that virologists had sought so long. It has lasted well; with minor modifications it is still applicable today.

D. Morphology: The Impact of Negative Staining

The introduction of negative staining (Brenner and Horne, 1959) marks one of the turning points of virus classification. Because of this technique virus particles could be characterized in unpurified material in a way not previously imagined, thus aiding their characterization not only at the research level but in the diagnostic laboratory. It had three immediate effects: (1) particles could be characterized with respect to size, shape, surface structure, and sometimes symmetry; (2) these properties could be determined for viruses of all kinds (plant, animal, and bacteriophage); (3) large numbers of virus strains could be examined.

By chance, herpes simplex virus was the first animal virus to be examined by this technique. Its characteristic "hollow capsomeres" and envelope were immediately obvious. However, several hundred micrographs were required before the icosahedral symmetry of the nucleocapsid and the number of capsomeres could be deduced (Wildy *et al.*, 1960). Within a short time, similar morphological features had been reported for a number of viruses although few of these micrographs have demonstrated all the features the authors claim (cf. Chapter 2).

Horne and Wildy (1961) and Wildy (1962) discussed the use of morphological criteria for virus taxonomy and emphasized that the symmetry of the capsid might be a more reliable criterion than the shape of the virus particle. They also thought that other morphological criteria might be useful, e.g., number of capsomeres and presence of an envelope. It seemed obvious that such criteria would have general applicability to viruses of all kinds and illustrated how the limited knowledge of that time might be applied to a general classification of viruses. The notion was extended by Lwoff *et al.* (1962) in the form of a hierarchical system.

The effect of the introduction of negative staining on taxonomy was immediate. Andrewes *et al.* (1961) summarized the taxonomic position of viruses of vertebrates, making use of seven criteria; four of these criteria related to properties of the virus particle (type of nucleic acid, size, number of capsomeres, and possession of envelope), two related to mode of multiplication (site of formation and site of maturation) and one (ether-sensitivity) related to the functional virion. They delineated six major groups of which one was nitavirus, including the herpesviruses, cytomegaloviruses, and the viruses of infectious bovine rhinotracheitis, equine rhinopneumonitis, and avian laryngotracheitis and related diseases.

In the following year, Andrewes (1962) reviewed the classification of viruses of vertebrates. He reduced the main criteria to (1) nucleic acid component, (2) size and morphology, (3) mode of replication, and (4) resistance to ether and bile salts. Among the nitaviruses (a name which was rejected subsequently), he listed, in addition to the previously recognized herpesviruses, cytomegaloviruses of 16 species, four avian viruses, and a miscellany including infectious bovine rhinotracheitis, equine rhinopneumonitis, feline rhinotracheitis, and lumpy skin disease. It is interesting to note that measles was, at this time, a candidate for inclusion. Since 1962, other viruses have been added to the herpes group, using morphology as the principal criterion.

E. The Virus DNA

In the 1950's, the nucleic acids gained a central place in virological thinking (cf. Lwoff, 1957). The possession of RNA or DNA in the virion quickly became accepted as a cardinal criterion for classification (Cooper, 1961; Andrewes, 1962). There was indirect evidence that herpesvirus particles might contain DNA, but it was not until the early 1960's that this was demonstrated unequivocally for herpes simplex virus (Russell, 1962) and pseudorabies virus (Ben-Porat and Kaplan, 1962). It has subsequently been demonstrated for about 20 members of the herpes group (cf. Wildy, 1971). The herpesvirus DNA's are two-stranded and between 3×10^7 and 1.2×10^8 MW. Some of these published values are unreliable; for example, the estimate for herpes simplex DNA have progressively increased through the years and it seems that the higher values are more likely to be correct. In most instances, the base compositions of these DNA's have been determined by indirect means such as buoyant density determination under standard conditions. The original expectation that herpesvirus DNA's would prove to have rather high molar proportions of guanine and cytosine (G + C) was very soon shattered; in fact, they probably range more widely than for any other biological group (Fig. 1). Base composition cannot therefore be used as a determinative criterion for the herpes group which we, at present, recognize. Although the published molecular weights and base compositions of DNA's from different herpesviruses seem heterogeneous, Bellett (1967) found that six herpesviruses (infectious bovine rhinotracheitis, pseudorabies, herpes simplex, human cytomegalovirus, and equine herpesviruses 1 and 2) clustered distinctly among the 68 animal viruses compared.

A peculiar feature of herpes simplex and Marek's disease virus DNA's is that they fragment into several pieces of definite size when centrifuged on alkaline sucrose gradients. This has been attributed by Lee *et al.* (1971) to nicking in one strand only of the DNA duplex. It will be interesting to see whether this is a common attribute of the herpesviruses.

Subak-Sharpe and his colleagues have examined the DNA's of a number of viruses by nearest-neighbor analysis (summarized by Subak-Sharpe, 1967). The normalized doublet frequences (expressed as deviations from random

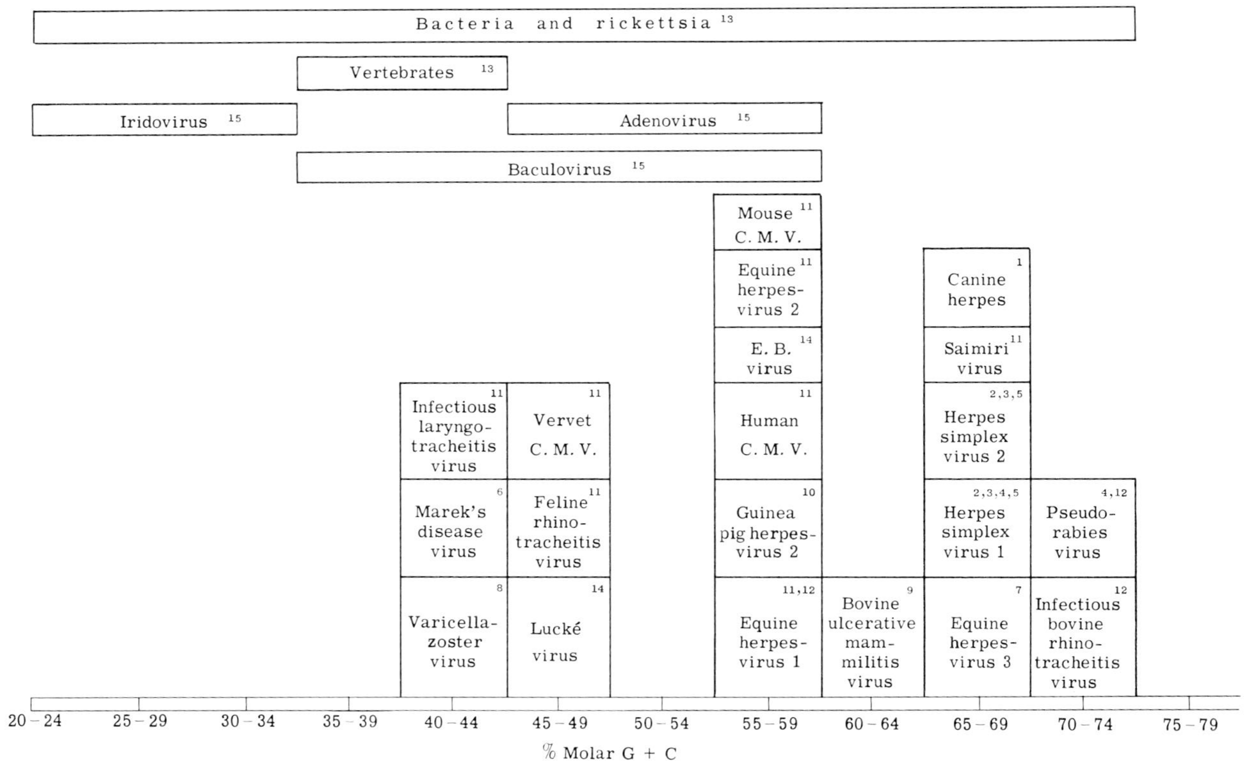

FIG. 1. Distribution of some published values for molar proportions of guanine and cytosine in the DNA's of some herpes viruses and other organisms. (1) Aurelian (1969), (2) Goodheart *et al.* (1968), (3) Halliburton *et al.* (1971), (4) Kaplan and Ben-Porat (1964), (5) Kieff *et al.* (1971), (6) Lee *et al.* (1971), (7) Ludwig *et al.* (1971), (8) Ludwig *et al.* (1972), (9) Martin *et al.* (1966), (10) Nayak (1971), (11) Plummer *et al.* (1969b), (12) Russell and Crawford (1964), (13) Sueoka (1961), (14) Wagner *et al.* (1970), (15) Wildy (1971).

expectation for a DNA of the particular base composition) show widely differing patterns. The DNA's of four papovaviruses generally resemble human DNA but those of pseudorabies, vaccinia, herpes simplex, adenovirus type 2, and equine rhinopneumonitis virus differ markedly from this pattern and between themselves. There is no clustering of the three herpesviruses.

F. Virus Proteins

Since Sabin (1934) demonstrated serological relationships between three herpesviruses, serology has become the preeminent determinative tool in recognizing viruses, and for other virus groups, serology has formed the basis for taxonomy. I am aware of no systematic serological assault on the herpes group of viruses. This is sorely needed: the available data are scarce and come from a large number of restricted comparisons made in different laboratories, using different techniques; some are shown in Fig. 2. Since the herpes viruses have a large genome, we might expect about 100 virus-specified proteins to be made. In fact, for herpes simplex, about 15 have been recognized serologically (Wildy, 1972). These proteins are made in large quantity in the infected cell and can be recognized as diffusible antigens, membrane-associated antigens, or as a part of the virion. Some herpes antigens have a nonimmunological affinity for γ-globulins of certain species (Watkins, 1964), and, for this reason, serological reactions of the herpes group must be carefully controlled. Undoubted serological crosses between certain virus species do occur, notably between herpes simplex type 1 and type 2 and B virus and between turkey herpesvirus and Marek's disease virus (see Fig. 2). These cross reactions are shown using immunodiffusion tests, where some diffusible antigens give lines of identity between strains while others do not (Buchan *et al.*, 1970; Thouless, 1972). There is no thoroughly satisfactory evidence of a group-specific antigen that is possessed by all the herpesviruses, although Kirkwood *et al.* (1972) have demonstrated lines of precipitate between widely different herpesviruses, and Ross *et al.* (1972) have shown common reactions by immunofluorescence. Thus, serological methods are of considerable use in distinguishing herpesviruses but, as yet, have no place in the definition of the group.

The modern techniques of polypeptide analysis indicate that herpes simplex virus specifies at least 12 structural polypeptides (Spear and Roizman, 1968; Olshevsky and Becker, 1970), of which 10 are probably contained in the nucleocapsid (Robinson and Watson, 1971). Similar numbers are found with pseudorabies virus (Shimono *et al.*, 1969; Stevens *et al.*, 1969), and Nazerian (1972) describes 9 polypeptides in Marek's disease virus.

Abodeely *et al.* (1971) have reported some 20 structural proteins in equine rhinopneumonitis virus, and, recently, Spear and Roizman (1972) report

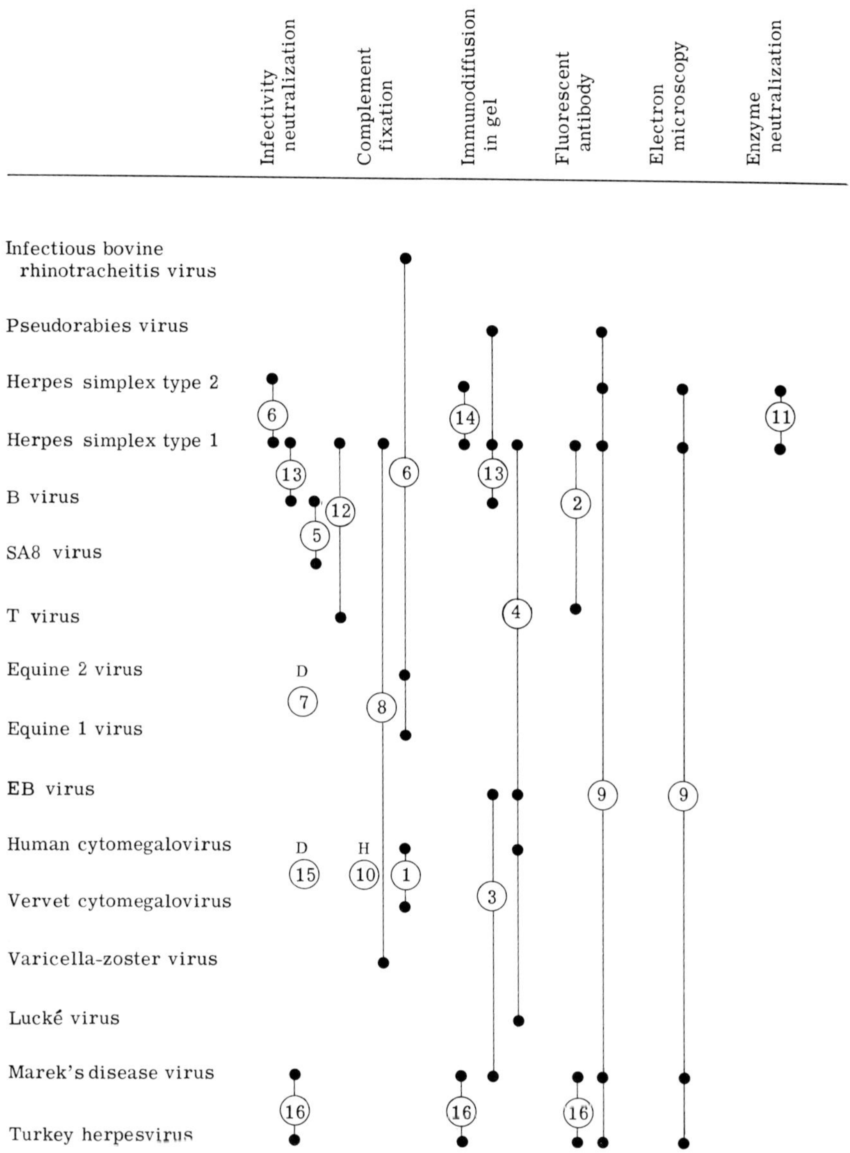

FIG. 2. Some antigenic relationships between herpesviruses, D, diverse; H, homogeneous. (1) Black *et al.* (1963), (2) Holmes *et al.* (1964), (3) Kato *et al.* (1972), (4) Kirkwood *et al.* (1972), (5) Malherbe *et al.* (1963), (6) Plummer (1964), (7) Plummer *et al.* (1969a), (8) Ross *et al.* (1965), (9) Ross *et al.* (1972), (10) Stern and Elek (1965), (11) Thouless (1972), (12) Tischendorf (1969), (13) Watson *et al.* (1967), (14) Wildy (1972), (15) Weller *et al.* (1960), (16) Witter *et al.* (1970).

24 polypeptides in the virion of herpes simplex, ranging from 28,000 to 278,000 MW. These would account for some 47% of the genetic potential of the virus. A proper comparison of these polypeptides requires critical purification of large amounts of virus protein; adequate analysis is, therefore, extremely tedious. However, so much work is going on in this direction that we can expect rapid progress.

G. Modern Definition of the Herpes Group

In 1970, the International Committee on Nomenclature of Viruses agreed that the herpes group should be given the taxonomic rank of genus and named *Herpesvirus* (cryptogram = [D/2:54–92/7:S/S:V/O]) (Wildy, 1971). The group definitive description was as follows:

> Contain double-stranded DNA, molecular weight 54 to 92 × 10^6. G + C content 57 to 74%. Virus particle about 100 to 150 nm diameter. Capsid icosahedral with 162 hollow capsomeres, 100 nm diameter, with a lipid-containing membrane and therefore sensitive to lipid solvents. The DNA is about 7% of the particle weight. BD (CsCl) 1.27 to 1.29 g/cm^3. Development begins in the nucleus and is completed by the addition of protein membranes as the virus passes into the cytoplasm. Intranuclear inclusion bodies formed. Separate subgroups have been proposed for viruses which are not readily separable from the cell and for the cytomegaloviruses. There are, however, such gradations in the properties that neither proposal is practical.

The type species given was herpes simplex virus.

Probably all interested virologists would agree with this broad description. The majority would now agree with the name *Herpesvirus* which has been used increasingly since 1953. I doubt whether many would approve of the taxonomic rank given, and I believe that this decision was unwise and premature. If a hierarchical system of classification is to be used for viruses we must formulate some guidelines as to what constitutes a family, a genus, and so on. However, the Committee wisely refrained from any attempt to subclassify the members of the group. This question poses a number of problems which are dealt with in Section III.

III. Subclassification of the Herpesviruses

In Section II, I have discussed the emergence of the herpes group of viruses in terms of evolving virological and taxonomic concepts. I will now consider the relationships of viruses within the group.

A. Attempts to Subclassify Herpesviruses

Andrewes (1962) tentatively divided the herpesviruses into four subgroups on the basis of host range and cytopathology. Group 1 comprised the original pentad of mammalian herpesviruses; group 2, the cytomegaloviruses; group 3, avian herpesviruses; and group 4, a miscellany including infectious bovine rhinotracheitis and equine rhinopneumonitis virus. Two years later, we find Melnick *et al.* (1964) noting two patterns of behavior among herpesviruses in tissue culture, i.e., viruses of group A, such as herpes simplex, from which infective virus may readily be recovered in tissue culture fluids, and others (group B) from which it may not be recovered. The group B viruses tend to have restricted host cell range. Plummer (1967) pointed out that this distinction was difficult to apply since he discerned a spectrum of "efficiency in tissue culture" rather than two behavioral groupings. Since 1967, the distinction has become increasingly blurred. The behavior of any virus in culture depends largely on the host cell and experimental conditions. Nevertheless, there is a loose association between this classification and the base composition of the DNA's of the different viruses. The frequency distribution of G + C content is very wide and fairly symmetrical. Although superficial examination suggests three peaks in the distribution, the total numbers are too small for statistical evaluation.

From the above we see a glimpse of what may, some day, become part of the subclassification of herpesviruses. At the same time, it is clear that we have no systematic factual comparisons upon which classification can be made. It is no longer sufficient to classify on the basis of woolly ideas of likenesses. Accurate quantitative, factual comparisons can be made by direct experiment, and this must be done before similarities are estimated. The basis upon which subclassification might be made is discussed in Section III, B.

B. A Basis for the Comparison of Herpesviruses

Classification must be based on factual comparisons. To be valid, these should be made under the same conditions, preferably in one laboratory, and should be quantitatively determined when possible. The most promising comparisons concern the properties of proteins (i.e., serology, polypeptide analysis, peptide mapping, amino acid sequence analysis, and complementation tests *in vivo*) and the properties of the DNA (i.e., base composition, doublet analysis, *in vitro* hybridization studies, and genetic recombination *in vivo*). By such means, degrees of similarity between pairs of viruses may be estimated, and these, in turn, should define clusters which may also be compared.

1. The Comparison of Virus Proteins

The most universally applicable tests of similarity among virus proteins are serological. The strength of this type of analysis for the herpes group was already apparent to Sabin (1934). Yet, in spite of many contributions, we have no systematic serological comparisons between large numbers of viruses. Before any record of antigenic affinity is appraised, it is necessary to state what other antigens fail to react under comparable conditions. All we can do, at present, is to note what cross reactions have been reported, as shown, for example, in Fig. 2. Thus, we see evidence of affinities between herpes simplex types 1 and 2, B virus, and pseudorabies virus. But we cannot estimate their intensity in the absence of other comparisons.

It is worthwhile to consider the techniques now available for the antigenic analysis of the herpesviruses. Virus antigenic determinants can be detected on diffusible proteins extracted from infected cells (Hayward, 1949), on the surface of the virion (Sabin, 1934), and in cell membranes (Roizman and Spear, 1971), including those represented at the surface of infected cells (Geder and Skinner, 1971).

Complement fixation tests can, therefore, be used as "sweep" tests for common antigens and can be related to molecules, membranes, or virus particles by use of appropriately fractionated antigens or antisera produced against them. However, they are unsuited to making detailed quantitative comparisons unless the reacting antigens are very precisely characterized. Immunofluorescence tests provide "sweep" identification of common reactions. They are extremely difficult to quantify and require very careful checks on specificity, since some herpes-specified proteins react unspecifically with certain γ-globulins (Watkins, 1964). They are, of course, useful in localizing the site of particular antigens and, together with immune cytolytic tests, can be used to recognize cell surface antigens. Neutralization tests provide comparisons of antigenic determinants, presumably at the surface of the virion. Although these can be quantified satisfactorily, we have to rely on the use of precisely characterized sera (e.g., the antiband II serum of Watson and Wildy, 1969) if the best comparisons are to be made. Immunodiffusion tests have the advantage that different diffusible proteins bearing antigenic determinants can be identified and that "lines of identity" provide information about which of these proteins carry common antigenic determinants. However, these tests are difficult to quantify and provide no information about the proportion of antigenic determinants that are shared between analogous proteins.

Finally, mention should be made of enzyme neutralization tests. Buchan and Watson (1969) showed that the thymidine kinases of herpes simplex type 1 and pseudorabies viruses were serologically distinct. Subsequently, Thouless (1972) has shown that the enzymes induced by type 1 and type 2 herpes simplex are serologically different, although related. This type of test deserves fuller attention, since the enzyme function introduces added specificity.

Plainly, the task of critically determining serological similarities between the herpesviruses would be vast. It would require the preparation of many defined reagents and antisera against them. It would then require quantitative measurement of reactivity between these reagents.

There have been many studies on the polypeptides of herpesviruses (see Section II, F). Analysis of virus-specified polypeptides by polyacrylamide gel electrophoresis under conditions of complete protein denaturation have revealed some similarities of pattern. But here the only valid comparison that can be made is by the coelectrophoresis of polypeptides of different viruses. This has been done on the acid-extractible proteins of herpes simplex virus types 1 and 2 (Halliburton and Hill, 1971), and it is, therefore, possible to define the similarity of pattern in quantitative terms. Useful comparative information could be made by extension of this type of study, and I see no particular reason why the information should not now be sought. More sophisticated studies on peptide mapping and sequencing are probably impracticable for use in large-scale comparisons at present. Genetic complementation indicates that virus proteins can substitute for one another functionally and in this sense implies similarity. Though the test is simple to apply to single-step mutants of a particular virus, there are complications when comparisons are tried between different viruses.

2. Comparisons of Virus DNA

The gross properties of virus DNA have proved useful in comparing strains (see Section II, E). To be satisfactory, comparisons must be done critically, using a number of different strains of the different viruses; the closer the similarity of the DNA's of any pair of strains, the more stringent these requirements become. Thus, the cosedimentation of DNA's from herpes simplex and Marek's disease virus reveal minor differences in velocity of sedimentation on sucrose gradients (Lee *et al.*, 1971). Similarly, minor differences in the buoyant density of herpes simplex virus types 1 and 2 DNA's are clearly revealed by fully orthogonal, doubly labeled, cosedimentation experiments (Halliburton *et al.*, 1971).

The base compositions are the most prominent differential characteristic of DNA's of different herpesviruses. Figure 1 clearly shows that the range of base compositions (generally determined by buoyant density of DNA) for herpesviruses is greater than that of all other viruses put together; it is far greater, for example, than the range for vertebrate DNA's. No significance may be attached to the three clusters of values (referred to previously), but possibly improved comparisons will show them to be real.

More detailed analysis of herpesvirus DNA's would contribute usefully to the subclassification of these viruses. As many have pointed out, completely defined base sequences should alone be sufficient to assess similarities accurately and directly. Unfortunately, at the present stage of technical competence, this still appears out of the question. However, indirect and less definitive means are available for comparing DNA's. I have already referred to the normalized doublet patterns of virus DNA's. Pseudorabies, herpes simplex, and equine rhinopneumonitis viruses show no similarity in doublet pattern or in general design of their DNA's (Subak-Sharpe, 1967); herpes simplex virus types 1 and 2, however, show no obvious differences (Subak-Sharpe, 1969). Nearest-neighbor analysis is laborious, and the amount of comparative information provided by it would not repay its systematic use.

The third method of comparing DNA's is by use of various sorts of hybridization procedure. These have not been much used for comparing herpesvirus DNA's. Bachenheimer *et al.* (1972) reported some homology between the DNA's of the two types of herpes simplex virus but none between these and the DNA of Marek's disease virus. Recent technical developments have magnified the potency of hybridization for taxonomic use. The most powerful of these is the electron-microscopical examination of heteroduplexes produced under controlled conditions. Using it, Davis and Hyman (1972) compared the DNA's of bacteriophages T3 and T7, showing the extent, the location, and the T_ms of homologous regions on the molecules. These they were able to relate to the genetic map. This versatile and precise technique is well suited to the quantitative comparisons of herpesvirus DNA's that are now needed; furthermore, it would be valuable in the genetic analysis of the herpesviruses.

Finally, genetic recombination remains an acid test of the relatedness of viruses. Strains of herpes simplex virus readily recombine (Wildy, 1955; Subak-Sharpe, 1968; Timbury, 1971). It will be interesting to see how far the ability to recombine extends among the different pairs of viruses in this group.

3. Other Comparisons

The general structure and biological interdependence of nucleic acids and proteins are now well understood. Thus, once he has valid comparisons of the properties of these molecules, the taxonomist can make immediate and predictable use of them. This is not the case with most other characters. For example, with herpes simplex virus strains, the pock size, ceiling temperature, and relative ability to infect chick embryo cells, all serve to distinguish the two subtypes (Ratcliffe, 1971; Parker and Banatvala, 1967; Figueroa and Rawls, 1969). Such characters are useful empirical determinants but their usefulness for comparing strains of virus is minimal unless and until their mechanisms are understood. In general, it is not worth the effort of systematically comparing large numbers of herpesviruses to elucidate biological characters such as host range, "cell-associatedness," behavior in different tissue culture systems, ceiling temperature, cytopathology, etc., if we are setting out to subclassify the herpesviruses, since simpler and more direct methods are now within our grasp.

C. Origin and Evolution of the Herpesviruses

So far, I have dealt with degrees of similarity among the herpesviruses and have discussed what kind of evidence is required to estimate these. The similarities are matters of natural fact, mostly awaiting discovery. The classification that will follow should reflect the facts but is necessarily artifactual. Any phylogenetic scheme which derives from the classification will be interpretations of that artifact.

It is premature to discuss phylogeny seriously in the absence of a firm classification, but the epidemiological peculiarities of these viruses encourage the belief that it will be possible to set up a brand of paleovirology by which the evolution of the herpesviruses may be traced and even dated. The first peculiarity is that herpesviruses are very host-dependent. Some, such as cytomegaloviruses, appear to be host-specific. A few can cross host-species barriers but probably seldom do. The second peculiarity is that in their own hosts, herpesviruses tend to give latent infections which can be reactivated sometimes many years after the primary infection. Thus, a virus may remain with its host for the host animal's lifetime (Burnet, 1955; Hope-Simpson, 1965; Andrewes, 1967). The third peculiarity is that herpesviruses usually give rise to little or no general disturbance in their specific host species, indicating by the Theobald Smith (1934) doctrine that they are all ancient, well-adapted parasites. If, on the contrary, they successfully cross host-species barriers, a fulminating and commonly fatal disease results. McCarthy (1969) lists seven such examples.

These peculiarities suggest that the herpesviruses have evolved with their host. On the basis of standard ideas of the evolution of vertebrates, Burnet (1955) suggested that B virus and herpes simplex virus must have begun separating at least 25×10^6 years ago. If all the herpesviruses have a common ancestor, their widespread occurrence in vertebrates would indicate that they have taken something like 400×10^6 years to evolve. As Nahmias (1972) has suggested, a search should be made for herpesviruses in primitive vertebrates such as cyclostomes.

Microbial taxonomists have repeatedly mourned the absence of a microbial fossil record. But, as Mandel (1969) points out, we can now trace a new kind of fossil record inscribed in the form of molecular patterns. Phylogenetic interpretations may be placed on classifications of these patterns, provided that we assume the universality of the genetic code and that analogy is valid among, say, vertebrates, bacteria, and viruses. It is probably wise to have some reservations over the second assumption.

The wide variation in base compositions of the herpesviruses invites speculation on its phylogenetic significance. Sueoka (1961) drew attention to the phylogenetic significance of base compositions in general. He has extended his theme to consider the kinetics of evolutionary change, assuming a series of single-step mutations (Sueoka, 1962; also Freese, 1962). In these terms, the distribution of values in Fig. 1 would imply either an extraordinarily effective conversion rate or a very large number of generations (assuming common ancestry). There seems every reason to be confident that difference in base composition indicates phylogenetic distance in organisms with more than 10^7 base pairs in the genome (Mandel, 1969; Stanier, 1971). It remains to be shown that this is so in genomes with as few as 10^5 base pairs, but even here it is difficult to imagine viable deletion mutations of A + T rich regions which would give rise to a shift of more than a few percent of the overall base ratio. Another reservation concerning all DNA viruses is that they come into contact with a much larger genetic system in the microenvironment of the cell. There is the opportunity for exchange of part of the virus genome with a piece of host DNA. Such an event would be necessarily exceedingly rare but, if we are considering geological time scales, the possibility cannot be ignored. Subak-Sharpe (1967) discussed doublet patterns in evolutionary terms. The profound differences in general design of the DNA's of pseudorabies, herpes simplex, and equine rhinopneumonitis viruses support the idea that these are phylogenetically rather remote from each other.

When a soundly based classification has been made, the question of the origins and evolution of the herpesviruses can be profitably considered. The most interesting point will be whether the group is mono- or polyphyletic. Convergent evolution must not at this stage be ruled out even though it is difficult to conceive a complicated virion such as that of the herpesviruses evolving independently many times over.

D. A Note on Nomenclature

Few would disagree with the notion that nomenclature should reflect classification which should be phylogenetic, if possible. Equally, in the absence of a solid classification, we need specific labels for viruses. I drew attention earlier to the potency of nomenclature and the dangers of bad nomenclature. This will be appreciated by all who have spent much time teaching. Until classification is reasonably secure and generally accepted, we require a temporary nomenclature that provides specific labels without taxonomic commitment. The trivial names we now use perform this function admirably; Aujesky's virus, Marek's virus, B virus, EB virus, T virus, etc., all specify but do not indicate relationships between viruses. It was this sort of consideration that caused Gibbs *et al.* (1966) to revolt against the hierarchical system developed by Lwoff *et al.* (1962) and the binomial nomenclature devised from it by the Provisional Committee on Nomen-

Weller, T. H., Han
Wildy, P. (1954). *A*
Wildy, P. (1955). *J.*
Wildy, P. (1962). *S*
Wildy, P. (1971). *M*
Wildy, P. (1972).
Payne, eds.), p
Wildy, P., Russell,
Witter, R. L., Na
Res. **31**, 525.

clature of Viruses. These systems are confusing to those biologists who come, for the first time, into virology. The proposals of Gibbs *et al.* (1966) were to continue with trivial names but to add a cryptogram of encoded information to indicate the general characteristics of the virus named.

Although the cryptogram certainly does nothing to prejudice future classification, its apparent precision is its undoing since the rate of accumulation of information is so great that the chances are that it will often be outdated and wrong. Furthermore, it is not strictly a name but an encoded description. The only other serious contender in nomenclature at present is the latinized binomial to which the International Committee on Nomenclature of Viruses is committed (cf. Wildy, 1971). Such names are evocative of an accepted underlying classification and I believe had better not be used until subclassification has been agreed.

Recently, Roizman *et al.* (1970) have drawn attention to other difficulties introduced by previously suggested binomials. For example, *Herpesvirus hominis* is applied to herpes simplex virus, yet we can list four other viruses of man. B. Roizman and G. de Thé (personal communication) suggest that such binomials should include numerals to denote each virus of any natural host, e.g., *Herpesvirus primatis 1 : 1* is herpes simplex virus type 1 and *Herpesvirus primatis 4* is EB virus. This unfortunately, would lead the uninitiated to suppose that the two viruses should be more closely allied than, for example, herpes simplex is to *Herpesvirus suis 1*, i.e., pseudorabies virus. It seems clear that we shall eventually be in a position to construct an informative binomial nomenclature, but before doing so, we require a satisfactory subclassification of the herpesviruses and before doing that we require many factual comparisons between virus strains. Until that time, let us continue with the arbitrary names that the herpesvirus workers, at least, know.

IV. Summary and Conclusions

I have traced the conceptual evolution of the herpes group of viruses and indicated the factors molding this concept. Prejudice, observation, and experiment mingled to form the group, and, as usual, the strongest contributions had to await technical advance.

Few disagree with the present grouping, although the official description of the group made in 1970 is already outdated and inaccurate.

The subclassification of the herpesviruses is very unsettled. I have indicated some approaches which may be worthwhile now and in the future.

In view of the power of nomenclature, I strongly believe that it would be a mistake to introduce a new set of names until there is general agreement on a classification and until the phylogenetic relationships between viruses are understood.

Plummer, G
Plummer, G
Plummer, G
Plummer, G
Ratcliffe, H.
Ribbert, H.
Robinson, D
Roizman, B
Roizman, B
Nature
Ross, C. A.
Ross, L. J.
Biggs,
Cancer
Russell, W.
Russell, W
Sabin, A. B
Shimono, I
Smith, A.
Smith, T. (
Spear, P. C
Spear, P. C
Stanier, R
Peláez
Steiner (18
Stern, H.,
Stevens, J
Stoker, M
Subak-Sh
Subak-Sh
Subak-Sh
Nort
Sueoka, N
Sueoka, N
Thouless
Timbury
Tischend
Turner, I
Unna, P
W.
Vidal, J.
von Bok
Wagner,
D.
Watkins
Watson
Watson
139
Weller,
eds

Chapter 2
Morphology

D. H. Watson

I. Introduction

The earliest electron microscopic studies on the morphology of herpesviruses using shadowcast preparations of herpes zoster virus (Ruska, 1943; Nagler and Rake, 1948) and of herpes simplex virus (Evans and Melnick, 1949) served only to confirm the size (1000–1500 Å) deduced by ultrafiltration (Elford *et al.*, 1933). More detailed information came from thin-section studies (Morgan *et al.*, 1954), and still later the negative staining method of Brenner and Horne (1959) revealed the morphological detail which has become so characteristic of the group.

II. Morphology of Particles of Herpes Simplex Virus

A. Naked and Enveloped Particles

Wildy *et al.* (1960) used the negative staining method to study herpes simplex virus. They described two basic types of particles, distinguished by the presence or absence of an outer coat or envelope. The naked particle or capsid (Fig. 1A) has an overall diameter of 1050 Å and corresponds to the single ringed particles described in thin sections (Figs. 2A and 2B) by Morgan *et al.* (1954). In negative stain, the capsids show varying degrees of angularity, some being hexagonal and others almost spherical. The capsid is composed of capsomeres which are icosahedrally arrayed with five capsomeres along each edge of the triangular facets of the icosahedron and thus 162 $[10(n-1)^2+2$ where $n=5]$ in the whole structure (Horne and Wildy, 1961). The icosahedral lattice may alternatively be described in the notation of Caspar and Klug (1962) as having a triangular number (T) of 4. Full satisfaction of the requirements of symmetry would demand that the capsomeres on the fivefold axes themselves possess fivefold symmetry. The general model of virus architecture of Caspar and Klug (1962) would describe the 162 capsomeres of herpes virus as resulting from hexamer and pentamer clustering of structure units. Wildy *et al.* (1960) noted occasional pentagonal capsomeres although most of the capsomeres which appeared angular were hexagonal. Polygonal capsomeres can be seen on high-magni-

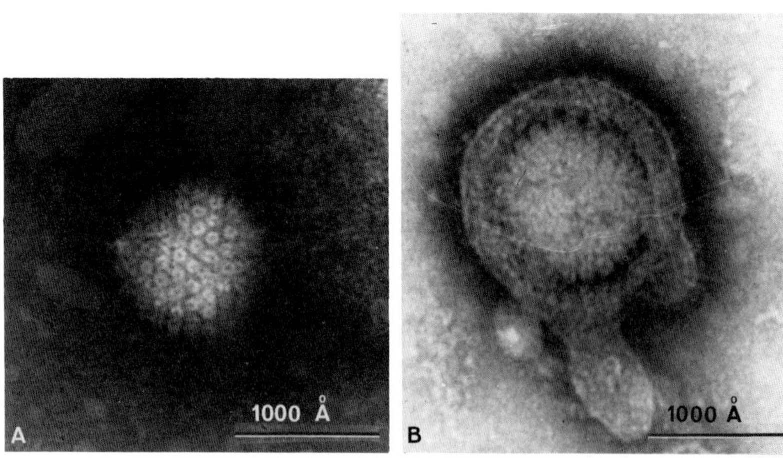

FIG. 1. (A) Naked and (B) enveloped particle of herpes simplex virus in negatively stained preparations.

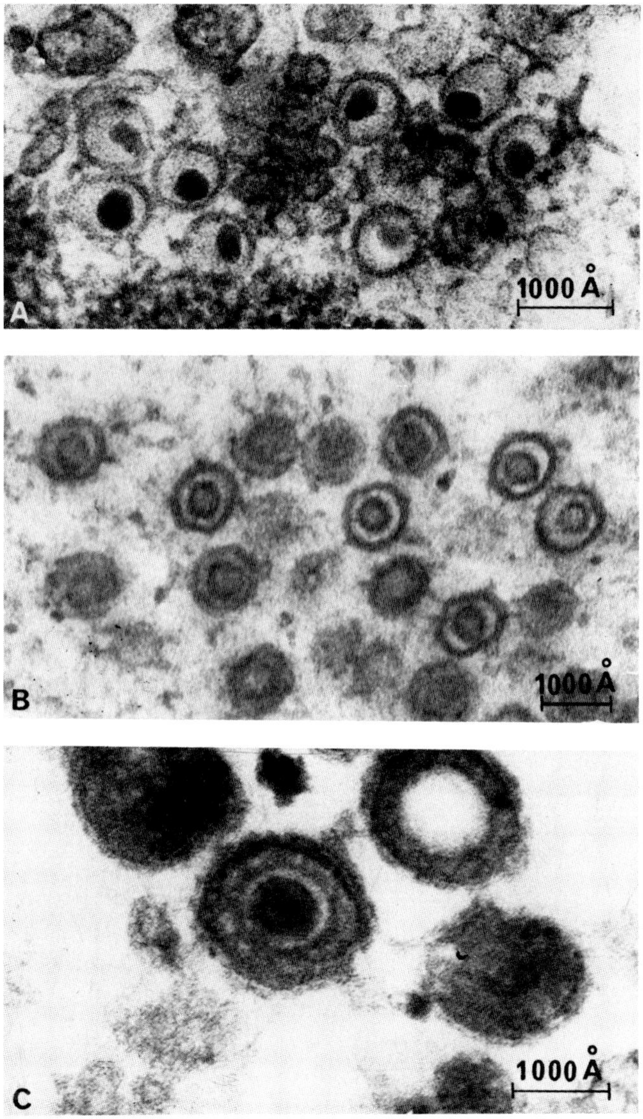

FIG. 2. Herpes simplex virus particles in thin sectioned preparations. (A) Hollow core form of naked particles, (B) dense core form of naked particle, (C) enveloped particle.

fication micrographs (Fig. 3), but it is usually not possible to equate the pentagonal ones with positions on the fivefold axes. The capsomeres are almost 100 Å in diameter and are noteworthy for the apparent axial hole which is about 40 Å in diameter and thus much larger than the "holes" described in the capsomeres of other viruses. This feature of the capsomeres gives the capsid a highly characteristic appearance.

The particles are made all the more distinctive by the fact that some are enveloped (Fig. 1B). In negatively stained preparations, the envelope is frequently distorted and hence has a very variable shape and size. Diameters

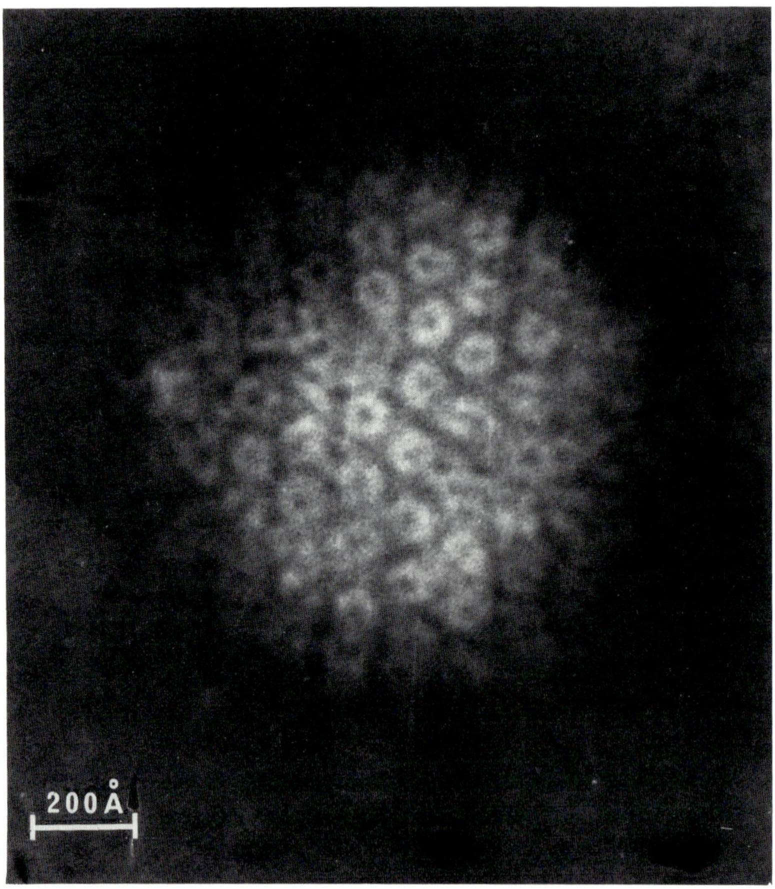

FIG. 3. High-magnification micrograph of negatively stained particle of herpes simplex virus showing polygonal shape of capsomeres.

vary from almost 1500 Å to over 2000 Å. Most envelopes contain only one capsid, but occasionally two or more capsids are seen inside one envelope.

Some preparations of herpesvirus contain particles which have the appearance of enveloped particles which have not been penetrated by negative stain (Fig. 4), and, consequently, the internal capsid cannot be clearly seen in these particles. However, it has been shown that they can be quantitatively converted to penetrated particles with a clearly visible capsid by dehydration of the particles on the grid before application of the negative stain (Watson and Wildy, 1963). In thin sections, the enveloped particles correspond to the double-ringed particles (Fig. 2C) described by Morgan *et al.* (1954). In these preparations, the shape is better preserved and the size is more uniform, about 1200–1500 Å.

Epstein (1962a) has described the envelope as a triple-layered, membranous structure indistinguishable from host cell membrane. Cytochemical evidence has shown that the envelope of particles grown in HeLa cells contains adenosine triphosphatase as does the host cell membrane (Epstein and Holt, 1963). Watson and Wildy (1963) showed that enveloped particles could be specifically agglutinated by antiserum to the host cell in which the virus

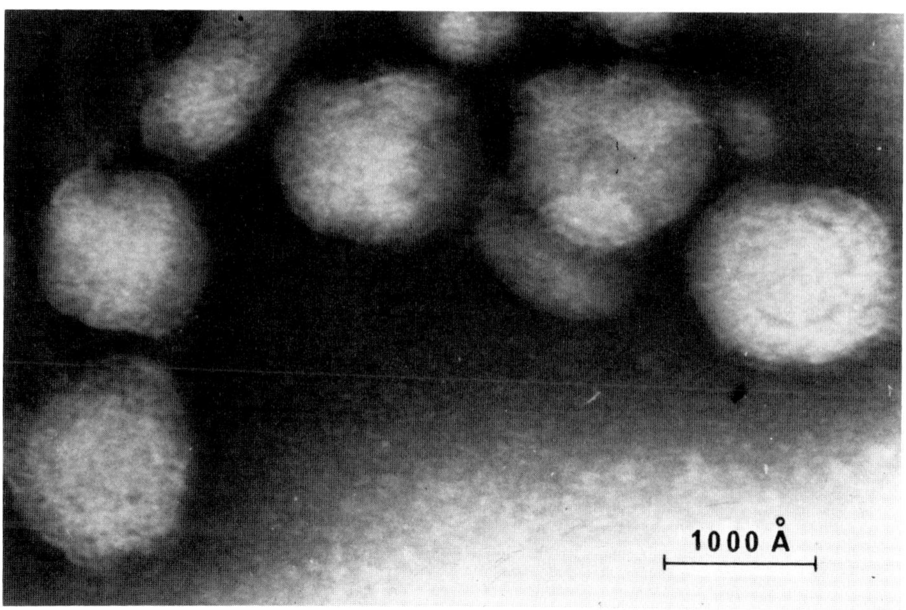

FIG. 4. Enveloped particles of herpes simplex virus which have not been fully penetrated by negative stain although outline of capsid can be discerned in some of the particles.

was grown. This observation and that of Epstein (1962a) are consistent with observations on the development of enveloped particles in the infected cell (see Chapter 5). The outer layer of the envelope in thin sections frequently shows a periodic structure which may correspond to the periodic projections or spikes seen on enveloped particles in negative stain. These spikes are about 80–100 Å long and are about 50 Å apart on the surface of the envelope. Their significance has yet to be established: it is, for example, not yet known whether they represent specific virus components such as the glycoproteins of the virus envelope, as appears to be the case for spikes of the myxoviruses and paramyxoviruses and of the alpha viruses, such as Semliki Forest virus. To describe the spikes as a specific virus structure would seem to be at variance with Epstein's conclusion that the envelope structure does not differ from that of host cell membrane, and it is therefore interesting to note that Benedetti and Emmelot (1965) and Prezbindowski *et al.* (1968) have described "spiky" layers on membranes isolated from rat liver cells that closely resemble the surface projections on enveloped herpesvirus particles.

B. "Full" and "Empty" Particles

The capsids of both naked and enveloped particles are frequently penetrated by negative stain (Fig. 5). The central region filled with negative stain

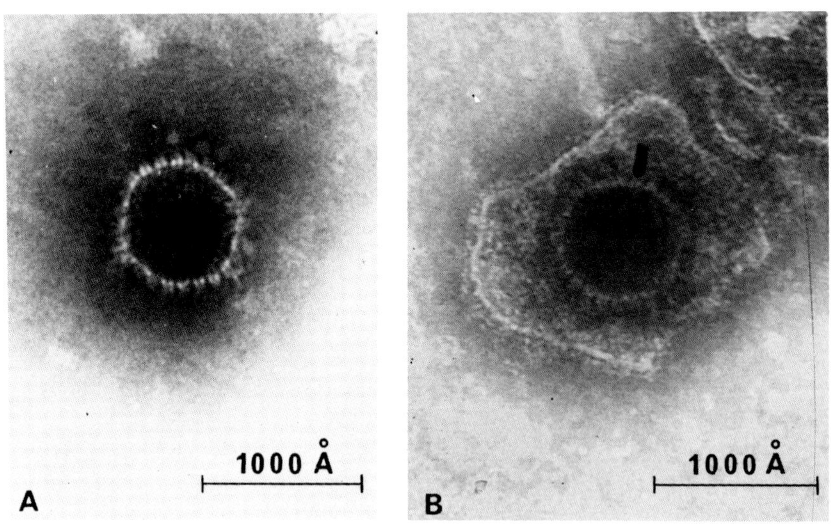

FIG. 5. (A) Naked and (B) enveloped particles of herpes simplex virus in which the capsids have been fully penetrated by phototungstate giving the appearance of "empty" particles.

is just under 800 Å across. It is known that "top component" particles (i.e., noninfective particles lacking nucleic acid; Markham and Smith, 1949) are usually completely penetrated by phosphotungstate, although this is not always true if care is not taken with the specimen preparation (Crawford *et al.*, 1962). However, although it is frequently assumed that the penetrated particles of herpesvirus are coreless, this has yet to be proved conclusively. The condition of specimen preparation may frequently cause penetration of particles (Watson, 1968), and until a population of particles which is completely penetrated can be shown to be coreless by both biochemical and biological criteria, it is safest to assume that penetration of the negative stain is artifactual. Apparently coreless particles can also be seen in sectioned preparations, but here again careful interpretation is necessary. Some "coreless" particles may show cores in adjacent serial sections (Watson *et al.*, 1964) and others may have been damaged in sectioning. A coreless appearance in thin sections does not seem to correlate with penetration in negatively stained preparations. Nevertheless, observations such as those of Miyamoto and Morgan (1971) where progressively increasing proportions of coreless particles are seen in cells sectioned at varying intervals after infection, would suggest that in some cases, at least, a coreless appearance in thin sections is real.

C. *The Core*

Although some negatively stained particles apparently contain structures within the capsid (Fig. 6) which may represent cores, a similar appearance could be caused by partial penetration. Accordingly, the best data on cores come from thin-section studies. In enveloped particles (Fig. 2C) the core appears as a densely stained region about 300 Å in diameter. Sometimes, the inner region of the core stains more densely (Morgan *et al.*, 1959). The cores of naked particles are usually less densely stained and hollow (Fig. 2A), although some naked particles do have dense cores such as those of enveloped particles (Fig. 2B). Miyamoto (1971), using negative staining of thin sections, reports finding capsids containing four granules and suggests that these may later fuse to form the hollow doughnut type of core.

Epstein (1962b) showed by enzyme digestion that the dense core region contained DNA. He further showed that the type of fixation and embedding affected core morphology. The core was rod shaped and often eccentrically placed after permanganate fixation and Aquon embedding, whereas formalin fixation and methacrylate embedding produced ellipsoidal or spherical cores (Morgan *et al.*, 1959).

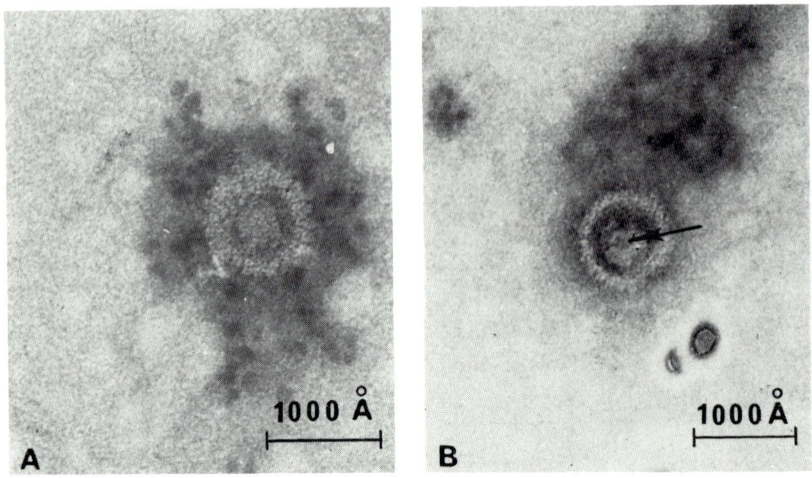

FIG. 6. Naked particles of herpes simplex virus showing apparent internal components which may, however, be penetration artifacts.

D. Other Components of the Particle

Both the envelope and capsid are shell structures, and it, therefore, follows that they account for only a small fraction of the total volume of the particles. It is not surprising that there has been much speculation on other structural components of the virus particle. These have not been conclusively demonstrated morphologically but their existence has often been inferred from other evidence. Thus Roizman *et al.* (1969) have proposed that some morphologically naked particles are surrounded by an inner envelope which is permeable to phosphotungstate and, therefore, not resolved in the electron microscope. This inner envelope would explain why the outer envelope, which is resolved in the electron microscope, is always maintained at a fixed distance from the capsid. They support this idea by their evidence that nuclear virus particles (presumably without the outer envelope) are infective, but the infectivity is sensitive to phospholipase. The infective nuclear particles differ from the infective cytoplasmic particles (presumably fully enveloped) in their sedimentation properties in sucrose gradients and in their lability in cesium chloride gradients.

Roizman *et al.* (1969) have described a small particle 250 Å in diameter containing DNA which was observed in CsCl density gradients of formaldehyde-stabilized lysates from cells infected with herpes simplex virus. A somewhat larger body was also observed: this was 450 Å in diameter and consisted of beadlike projections surrounding a central core 250 Å in diameter, presumably corresponding to the smaller body described above. The whole structure is regarded by Roizman *et al.* (1969) as an inner capsid surrounding a central core and has been correlated by them with structures appearing in thin sections of the nuclei of infected cells. Sydiskis (1969) has described similar structures for pseudorabies virus.

Roizman *et al.* (1969) have also postulated the existence of a middle capsid to which the capsomeres of the outer capsid adhere. This they envisage as having a diameter of 700–800 Å, and they believe that it corresponds to structures of this size seen in disrupted particles by Wildy *et al.* (1960) and Spring *et al.* (1968).

The existence of all these additional components must be regarded as highly speculative at the moment. Thin sections of virus particles definitely show material between the envelope and the capsid and also within the capsid; thus there is nothing inherently unlikely about the existence of additional structural components. However, to classify these components into discrete structures may be somewhat premature until they can be revealed by controlled degradation of herpesvirus particles. Attempts to achieve such degradations have so far been conspicuously unsuccessful.

III. Other Herpesviruses

In recent years, there have been increasing numbers of reports on the structure of herpesviruses, and it is plainly beyond the scope of this chapter to deal with these in any detail. Andrewes and Pereira (1967) listed 22 herpesviruses. They give references to morphological studies on 16 of these which have been shown to possess the characteristic herpesvirus structure, either by negative staining, or thin sectioning, or both. These 16 viruses are listed in Table I. The appropriate references are quoted in Andrewes and Pereira (1967) and will not be repeated here.

Table II lists a number of herpesviruses whose morphology has been studied in the years since Andrewes and Pereira's (1967) list was compiled. This table does not claim to be complete (and even if it were so at the time of writing, would be unlikely to be so at the time of publication) in view of the accelerating rate at which morphological studies are being made on new herpesviruses. A further complication is that many of the newly isolated viruses whose morphology is described are not biologically well characterized, and it is often difficult to show whether or not they differ from viruses described earlier. For this reason, I have not listed a number of possibly new herpesviruses whose structure has been described.

All these viruses exhibit some, or all, of the structural features described earlier for herpes simplex virus. Some micrographs of herpesviruses are shown in Fig. 7.

TABLE I
HERPESVIRUSES SHOWN IN ANDREWES AND PEREIRA AS EXHIBITING THE CHARACTERISTIC GROUP MORPHOLOGY[a]

Herpes simplex
Herpes B
Pseudorabies
Varicella–zoster
Infectious bovine rhinotracheitis
Malignant catarrh
Bovine ulcerative mamillitis (Allerton)
Equine abortion
Feline rhinotracheitis
Canine herpes
EB
Avian infectious laryngotracheitis
Lucké
Human cytomegalovirus
Murine cytomegalovirus
Inclusion body rhinitis

[a]See Andrewes and Pereira (1967) for references to descriptions of the morphology of these viruses.

One or two herpesviruses have been observed to contain structural elements not usually described for herpes simplex virus. Watrach *et al.* (1968) described granules 240–400 Å in diameter inside the capsid of avian infectious laryngotracheitis virus. There were usually about four granules in each capsid, although the number varied from one to six. Similar structures have been described for turkey herpesvirus (Nazerian *et al.*, 1971) and for equine abortion virus grown in cells treated with fluorodeoxyuridine (O'Callaghan *et al.*, 1968). However, these structures appear very similar to the granules found more recently by Miyamoto (1971) and suggested by him as a precursor of the hollow core of herpes simplex virus (see Section II, D). The tree shrew herpesvirus described by McCombs *et al.* (1971) also shows granules inside the capsid but these are smaller (about 130 Å in diameter). Six to eight granules were usually arranged around one central granule to form what the authors term a "pin wheel core."

Electron-microscopic measurements of virus particle size may be very unreliable, particularly in the absence of internal calibration with, for example, catalase crystals. Accordingly, despite the wide range of values quoted for the actual size of herpesviruses, it is likely that they all have the same size. Mention should, however, be made of one apparent exception; the envelope of tree shrew herpesvirus is consistently larger than that of herpes simplex virus, not only in negative stain but also in thin section.

TABLE II
VIRUSES WITH HERPES-TYPE MORPHOLOGY (OTHER THAN THOSE IN TABLE I)

Host	Name	Reference
Squirrel monkey	Herpesvirus saimiri	Morgan *et al.* (1970)
Spider monkey	Herpesvirus ateles	Melendez *et al.* (1972)
Vervet monkey	Liverpool vervet monkey virus	Clarkson *et al.* (1967)
Owl monkey	Herpesvirus aotus	Daniel *et al.* (1971)
Patas monkey	Patas monkey herpesvirus	McCarthy *et al.* (1968)
Marmoset monkey	Marmoset herpesvirus (Herpesvirus tamarinus)	Melnick *et al.* (1964)
Baboon	"SA15-like herpesvirus"	Malherbe and Strickland-Cholmley (1970)
Horse	Equine herpes 2	Plummer and Waterson (1963)
Horse	Equine herpes 3	Ludwig *et al.* (1971)
Horse	Equine cytomegalovirus (Equine herpes 4)	Hsiung *et al.* (1969)
Sheep	Pulmonary adenomatosis (Jaagsiekte)	Smith and Mackay (1969)
Rabbit	Herpesvirus cunicili (Virus III)	Nesburn (1969)
Cottontail rabbit	Herpesvirus sylvilagus	Hinze (1971)
Tree shrew	?	McCombs *et al.* (1971)
Guinea pig	Guinea pig herpesvirus 1	Middelkamp *et al.* (1967)
Guinea pig	Guinea pig herpesvirus 2	Bhatt *et al.* (1971)
Rat	Rat cytomegalovirus	Berezesky *et al.* (1971)
Snake	?	Monroe *et al.* (1968)
Iguana	Iguana virus	Clark *et al.* (1968)
Chicken	Marek's disease virus	Nazerian and Burmester (1968)
Turkey	Turkey herpesvirus	Nazerian *et al.* (1971)
Duck	Duck plague virus	Breese and Dardiri (1968)
Owl	Owl herpes	Burtscher and Schumacher (1966)
Cormorant	Lake Victoria cormorant	French *et al.* (1972)
Pigeon	Pigeon virus	Cornwell *et al.* (1967)
Catfish	Channel catfish virus	Wolf and Darlington (1971)
Erog	Frog virus 4	Gravell *et al.* (1968)

The difference is consistent and independent of the cell used to grow the virus. Furthermore, the difference is large: the herpes simplex envelopes have diameter ranging from 1220 to 2570 Å in thin section, while tree shrew herpesvirus envelopes have diameters between 2140 and 5240 Å. Furthermore, the matrix structures between the envelope and the capsid of

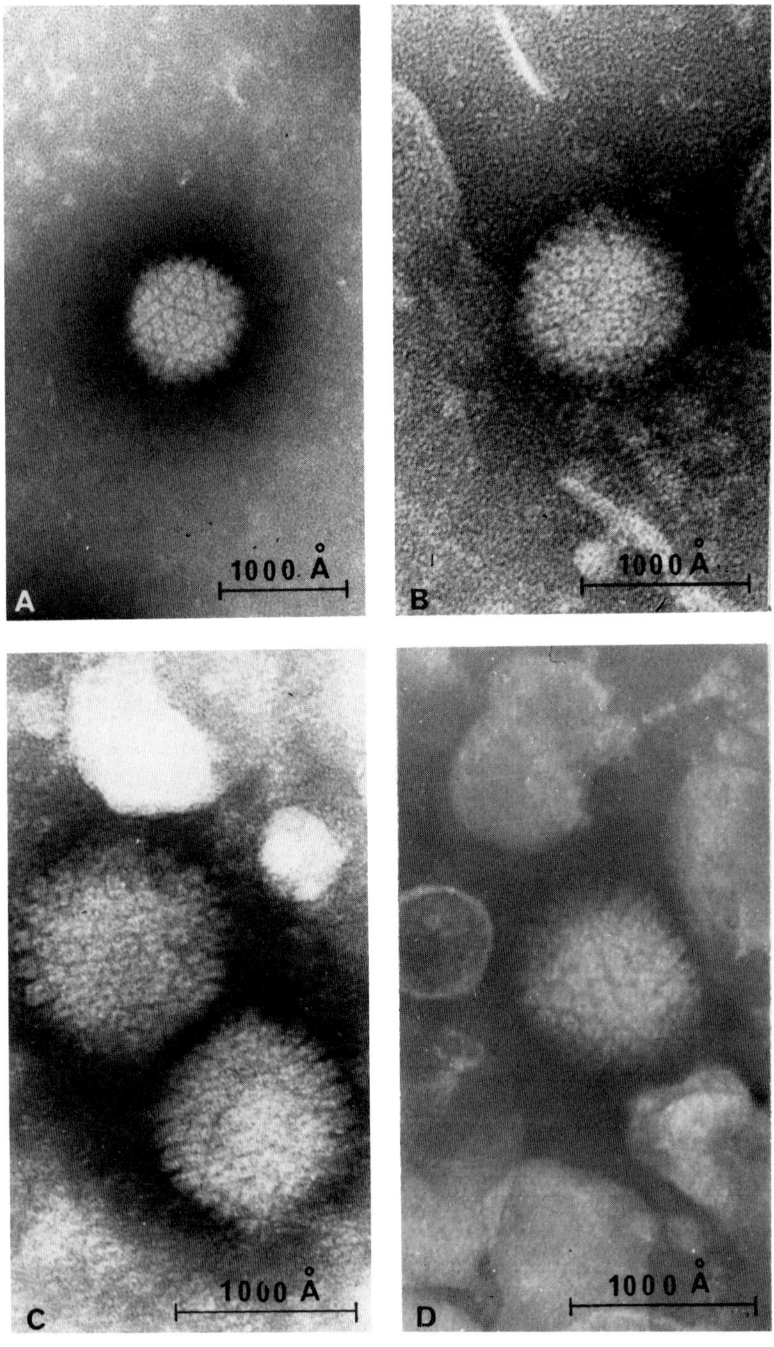
1000 Å
A
1000 Å
B
1000 Å
C
1000 Å
D

the tree shrew herpesvirus is more densely stained than the corresponding region of herpes simplex virus particles (McCombs *et al.*, 1971).

The particles of EB virus were reported as being smaller than those of herpes simplex virus by about 20% (Epstein *et al.*, 1964), although this has been contradicted by Dalton and Zeve (1967). There has been no confirmation of the difference using accurate control of magnification calibration with catalase crystals and examination of mixtures of the two viruses, and it would, therefore, appear safest to assume that the viruses do not differ in size until conclusive evidence is presented.

IV. Morphology and Clinical Diagnosis

The characteristic morphology of herpesviruses has led to an increasing use of electron microscopy in clinical diagnosis. The most important application is, of course, in the differential diagnosis of smallpox and varicella that in the early stages is often difficult on clinical grounds alone. The characteristic morphology of varicella particles clearly distinguishes them from smallpox particles (Fig. 8), and there are usually large numbers of particles in the skin lesions. Speed is obviously of great importance, and electron-microscopic examination of vesicular material by negative staining can be done very rapidly.

In the alastrim outbreak of 1966 in the English Midlands, only two false negatives were found by electron microscopy of 32 specimens from cases later confirmed by egg culture which only give a result after 2 days (Cruickshank *et al.*, 1966). Both of the false negatives concerned specimens taken early in the illness, and it seems likely that repeated tests on negative cases would allow 100% successful diagnosis. Electron microscopy proved more sensitive than the other rapid test—gel diffusion. Similarly, electron microscopy has proved to be very successful in identifying herpesvirus particles in specimens taken from cases of varicella (Cruickshank *et al.*, 1966; Macrae *et al.*, 1969). Since varicella is always well represented in any series of specimens from smallpox suspects, a positive identification of herpesvirus particles is perhaps the best evidence for absence of smallpox. Electron microscopy has proved more sensitive for detection of varicella virus than either gel diffusion or isolation in tissue culture (Macrae *et al.*, 1969). Furthermore, the lability of varicella virus means that it is usually worthless

---

FIG. 7. Particles of several viruses of the herpes group. (A) Marek's disease virus (kindly provided by Dr. D. G. Rootes and Dr. P. M. Biggs), (B) EB virus (kindly provided by Dr. K. Hummeler), (C) canine herps (kindly provided by Dr. E. A. C. Follett), and (D) pigeon herpes (kindly provided by Dr. E. A. C. Follett).

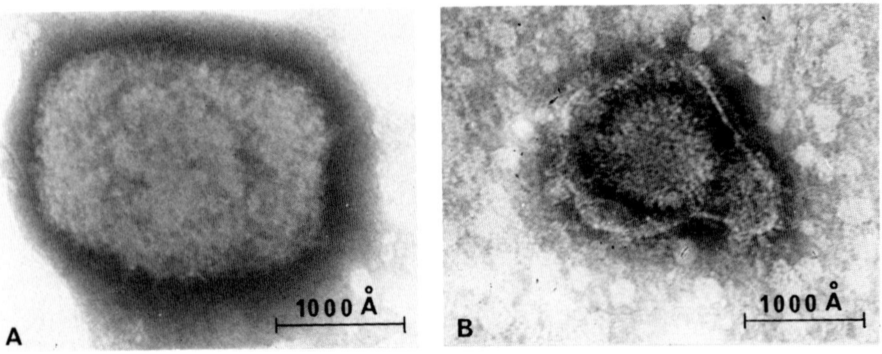

FIG. 8. Particles found in vesicle fluid of patient diagnosed as suffering from (A) variola and (B) varicella.

to attempt culture from specimens taken from crusts late in infection, whereas electron microscopy has proved very successful with such specimens.

Electron microscopy cannot, of course, differentiate between different herpesviruses or different pox viruses (with the exception of orf virus) but this is usually less important than the differentiation of herpes and pox viruses.

Electron microscopy is now a firmly established laboratory method in smallpox diagnosis and is described as such in official publications (Department of Health and Social Security, 1969).

Electron microscopy has also been used in diagnosis of cytomegalovirus (Paradis *et al.*, 1969), herpesvirus encephalitis (Loffler *et al.*, 1970), herpes simplex keratitis (Diderholm *et al.*, 1969), and herpetic iritis (Kaufman *et al.*, 1971).

The relevance of electron microscopy in clinical diagnosis with particular reference to herpesviruses has been discussed in a number of recent articles (e.g., Spradbrow and Francis, 1969; Blank *et al.*, 1970; Long *et al.*, 1970; Bedson, 1971).

V. Morphology and Classification of Herpesviruses

Morphology has become one of the most useful criteria for assigning a virus to the herpes group. Altough it may be dangerous to classify a virus on the basis of only one attribute, it seems reasonable to make at least a presumptive classification of a virus as a member of the group on morphological grounds alone. Thus, whenever a virus has been classified as a herpesvirus on other grounds, its morphology, where known, has always been of the characteristic form. Conversely, no virus showing the characteristic morphology has ever been shown to differ from herpesviruses in other properties characteristic of the group.

On the other hand, because the morphology is so characteristic of the group as a whole, it provides no grounds for subdividing the herpesviruses into subgroups. Any morphological differences between the different viruses are small.

Acknowledgments

I am indebted to Dr. D. G. Rootes, Dr. P. M. Biggs, Dr. K. Hummeler, and Dr. E. A. C. Follett for kindly providing me with the micrographs in Fig. 7. I should like to express my thanks to my colleagues Dr. A. Buchan, Mr. R. W. Honess, and Mrs. C. Sim who read the manuscript and made many helpful comments. I am additionally indebted to Mrs. C. Sim for assistance in checking references. I should like to thank Mrs. J. Davies for typing the manuscript—no mean feat as those familiar with my handwriting will testify. Finally, I should like to express my sincere gratitude and great indebtedness to Professor P. Wildy who first interested me in virus morphology and whose own contributions to the subject so revolutionized our ideas on the structure of viruses.

References

Andrewes, C. H., and Pereira, H. G. (1967). *In* "Viruses of Vertebrates," 2nd ed., p. 278. Ballière, London.

Bedson, H. S. (1971). *Pub. Health* **85**, 171.

Benedetti, E. L., and Emmelot, P. (1965). *J. Cell Biol.* **266**, 299.

Berezesky, I. K., Grimley, P. M., Tyrell, S. A., and Rabson, A. S. (1971). *Exp. Mol. Pathol.* **14**, 337.

Bhatt, P. N., Percy, D. H., Craft, J. L., and Jonas, A. M. (1971). *J. Infec. Dis.* **123**, 178.

Blank, H., Davis, C., and Collins, C. (1970). *Brit. J. Dermatol.* **83**, Suppl., 69.

Breese, S. S., and Dardiri, A. H. (1968). *Virology* **34**, 160.

Brenner, S., and Horne, R. W. (1959). *Biochim. Biophys. Acta* **34**, 103.

Burtscher, H., and Schumacher, A. (1966). *Pathol. Vet.* **3**, 506.

Caspar, D. L. D., and Klug, A. (1962). *Cold Spring Harbor Symp. Quant. Biol.* **27**, 1.

Clark, H. F., Zeigel, R. F., Fabian, F. B., and Karzon, D. T. (1968). *Bacteriol. Proc.* p. 149.

Clarkson, M. J., Thorpe, E., and McCarthy, K. (1967). *Arch. Gesamte Virusforsch.* **22**, 219

Cornwell, H. J. C., Weir, A. R., and Follett, E. A. C. (1967). *Vet. Rec.* **81**, 267.

Crawford, L. V., Crawford, E. M., and Watson, D. H. (1962). *Virology* **18**, 170.

Cruickshank, J. G., Bedson, H. S., and Watson, D. H. (1966). *Lancet* **2**, 527.

Dalton, A. J., and Zeve, V. H. (1967). *Cancer Res.* **27**, 2465.

Daniel, M. D., Meléndez, L. V., King, N. W., Fraser, C. E. O., Barahona, H. H., Hunt, R. D., and Garcia, F. G. (1971). *Proc. Soc. Exp. Biol. Med.* **138**, 835.

Department of Health and Social Security. (1969). "Diagnosis of Smallpox Medical Memorandum." HM Stationery Office, London.

Diderholm, R., Stenram, U., Tegner, K. B., and Willen, R. (1969). *Acta Med. Scand.* **186**, 181.

Elford, W. J., Perdrau, J. R., and Smith, W. (1933). *J. Pathol. Bacteriol.* **36**, 49.
Epstein, M. A. (1962a). *J. Cell. Biol.* **12**, 589.
Epstein, M. A. (1962b). *J. Exp. Med.* **115**, 1.
Epstein, M. A., and Holt, S. J. (1963). *Nature* (*London*) **198**, 509.
Epstein, M. A., Achong, B. G., and Barr, Y. M. (1964). *Lancet* **1**, 702.
Evans, A. S., and Melnick, J. L. (1949). *Proc. Soc. Exp. Biol. Med.* **71**, 283.
French, E. L., Purchase, H. G., and Nazerian, K. (1972). *J. Gen. Virol.* (in press).
Gravell, M., Granoff, A., and Darlington, R. W. (1968). *Virology* **36**, 467.
Hinze, H. C. (1971). *Infec. Immunity* **3**, 350.
Horne, R., and Wildy, P. (1961). *Virology* **15**, 348.
Hsiung, G. D., Fischman, H. R., Fong, C. K., and Green, R. H. (1969). *Proc. Soc. Exp. Biol. Med.* **130**, 80.
Kaufman, H. E., Kanai, A., and Ellison, E. P. (1971). *Amer. J. Ophthamol.* **71**, 465.
Loffler, H., Bienz, E., Schmid, U., and Eigenheer, F. (1970). *Pathol. Microbiol.* **36**, 324.
Long, G. W., Nobel, J., Murphy, F. A., Hermann, U. L., and Lourie, B. (1970). *Appl. Microbiol.* **20**, 497.
Ludwig, H., Biswal, N., Bryans, T., and McCombs, R. M. (1971). *Virology* **45**, 534.
McCarthy, K., Thorpe, E., Laursen, A. C., Heymann, C. S., and Beale, A. J. (1968). *Lancet* **2**, 856.
McCombs, R. M., Brunschwig, J. P., Mirkovic, R., and Benyesh-Melnick, M. (1971). *Virology* **45**, 816.
Macrae, A. D., Field, A. M., McDonald, J. R., Meurisse, E. V., and Porter, A. A. (1969). *Lancet* **2**, 313.
Malherbe, H., and Strickland-Cholmley, M. (1970). *Lancet* **1**, 785.
Markham, R., and Smith, K. M. (1949). *Parasitology* **39**, 330.
Meléndez, L. V., Hunt, R. D., King, N. W., Barahona, H. H., Davies, M. D., Fraser, C. E. O., and Garcia, F. G. (1972). *Nature* (*London*) *New Biol.*, **235**, 182.
Melnick, J. L., Midulla, M., Wimberly, I., Barrera-Oro, J. G., and Levy, B. M. (1964). *J. Immunol.* **92**, 596.
Middelkamp, J. N., Patrizi, G., and Reed, C. A. (1967). *J. Ultrastruct. Res.* **18**, 85.
Miyamoto, K. (1971). *J. Virol.* **8**, 534.
Miyamoto, K., and Morgan, C. (1971). *J. Virol.* **8**, 910.
Monroe, J. H., Shibley, G. P., Schidlovsky, G., Nakai, T., Howatson, A. F., Wivel, N. W., and O'Connor, T. E. (1968). *J. Nat. Cancer Inst.* **40**, 135.
Morgan, C., Ellison, S. A., Rose, H. M., and Moore, D. H. (1954). *J. Exp. Med.* **100**, 195.
Morgan, C., Rose, H. M., Holden, M., and Jones, E. P. (1959). *J. Exp. Med.* **110**, 643.
Morgan, D. G., Epstein, M. A., Achong, B. G., and Meléndez, L. V. (1970). *Nature* (*London*) **228**, 170.
Nagler, F. P. O., and Rake, G. (1948). *J. Bacteriol.* **55**, 45.
Nazerian, K., and Burmester, B. R. (1968). *Cancer Res.* **28**, 2454.
Nazerian, K., Lee, L. F., Witter, R. L., and Burmester, B. R. (1971). *Virology* **43**, 442.
Nesburn, A. B. (1969). *J. Virol.* **3**, 59.
O'Callaghan, D. J., Hyde, J. M., Gentry, G. A., and Randall, C. C. (1968). *J. Virol.* **2**, 793.
Paradis, N., Martineau, B., and Cote, J. R. (1969). *Union Med. Can.* **98**, 1287.
Plummer, G., and Waterson, A. P. (1963). *Virology* **19**, 412.
Prezbindowski, K. S., Sun, F. F., and Crane, F. L. (1968). *Exp. Cell Res.* **50**, 241.
Roizman, B., Spring, S. B., and Schwartz, J. (1969). *Fed. Proc., Fed. Amer. Soc. Exp. Biol.* **28**, 1890.
Ruska, E. (1943). *Science* **37**, 16.
Smith, W., and Mackay, J. M. (1969). *J. Comp. Pathol.* **79**, 421.

Spradbrow, P. B., and Francis, J. (1969). *Vet. Rec.* **84**, 244.
Spring, S. B., Roizman, B., and Schwartz, J. (1968). *J. Virol.* **2**, 384.
Sydiskis, R. J. (1969). *J. Virol.* **4**, 283.
Watrach, A. M., Hanson, L. F., and Watrach, M. A. (1968). *Virology* **35**, 321.
Watson, D. H. (1968). *Symp. Soc. Gen Microbiol.* **18**, 207.
Watson, D. H., and Wildy, P. (1963). *Virology* **21**, 100.
Watson, D. H., Wildy, P., and Russell, W. C. (1964). *Virology* **24**, 523.
Wildy, P., Russell, W. C., and Horne, R. W. (1960). *Virology* **12**, 204.
Wolf, K., and Darlington, R. W. (1971). *J. Virol.* **8**, 525.

Chapter 3

The Physical and Chemical Properties of the Herpesviruses

Glenn A. Gentry and Charles C. Randall

I. Introduction

The earliest physicochemical data on the herpesviruses were obtained in 1910 (although there was no such recognized group then) when Schmiedhoffer (1910) showed that pseudorabies virus would pass through a filter with pores small enough to retain bacteria, a finding confirmed a few years later by Sangiorgi (1914). Not until a decade had passed, however, were similar data obtained for herpes simplex virus (Luger and Lauda, 1921). It was possible by this means to make crude estimates of the size of these viruses. Later, more refined indirect methods (ultracentrifugation, diffusion, etc.) were used to estimate the sizes of the herpesviruses (Kaplan, 1969), but the most accurate measurements have been made with the electron microscope, as described by Watson (see Chapter 2). With the possible exception of the data on filterability, all of the early findings were markedly affected by the purity of the preparation, and virus purification—not always an easy task with herpesviruses—has become so important as to comprise a major part of every study of the chemical properties of the herpesviruses. For that reason, the following sections will include discussions of the methods of preparation and criteria for purity of the herpesviruses.

II. The Herpesvirion—Physical Properties

A. Morphology

Wildy *et al.* (1960) published a key work on the morphology and structure of herpes simplex virus and, in so doing, have provided a set of standards by which all candidate herpesviruses may be judged. Three main parts of the virion have been described on the basis of their appearance in negatively stained preparations in the electron microscope: (1) the core, which contains the genome; (2) the capsid, which surrounds the core and is composed of 162 capsomers, of which each is in turn composed of smaller subunits; and (3) the outer membrane or envelope, which encloses the nucleocapsid. The core is 77.5 nm in diameter; the nucleocapsid, 105 nm; and the complete virion, 180 nm. The morphology of the herpesviruses is discussed in detail by Watson in Chapter 2.

B. Mass of the Herpes Virion

Because of the difficulty in purifying HSV,* much of the work of the previous decade was directed toward solving this problem so that the reliability of analyses could be ensured. As a legacy of this period, there are numerous reports dealing with the density of the virion of HSV. These values were obtained by measurement of the position of the viral band at equilibrium in density gradients, usually of CsCl (but sometimes of potassium tartrate) or,

*For abbreviations of virus names, see Table IX.

more recently, of sucrose, silica gel-polyethylene glycol, or dextran. The findings are summarized in Table I, from which several general findings emerge: (1) Different strains of HSV may have different buoyant densities. (2) The density in CsCl may be different for the same virus, depending on the cell in which it was grown (Spear and Roizman, 1967). (3) The choice of gradient may also affect the observed density. Toplin *et al.* (1971), for example, found that in CsCl the density of the Lucké virus was 0.02 gm/cm^3 higher than in potassium tartrate or sucrose gradients. Klingeborn and Pertoft (1972) found a much larger difference between the density of EAV in silica gel (1.08 gm/cm^3) and in CsCl (1.27 gm/cm^3). The reasons for the higher densities observed with CsCl are not clear, but they could include osmotic effects, as it can be inferred that the herpesvirus envelope is relatively impermeable to CsCl (see Section IV,A).

The reasons for the difference in density of the viral particles grown in different host cells are not clear. Roizman (1969a) has suggested that some of the differences may reflect differences in the composition of the envelope. The variation in density may reflect differences in lipid content of the viral membrane which the virus acquires by budding from the cellular membranes and which may differ in different hosts; the variation in density may also reflect differences in the degree of glycosylation of the viral glycoproteins.

It is of some interest to calculate the density of the virion of HSV by a completely independent method. This may be done using an estimate of the dry mass of the virion obtained by quantitative electron microscopy. This technique is based on the proportionality of the mass of the observed particle to the transmission of visible light by the photographic negative and requires special instrumentation. With small polystyrene spheres of known mass as standards, Lampert *et al.* (1969) determined the dry mass of HSV to be 1.3×10^{-15} gm/virion. If a spherical shape and a diameter of 180 nm (Wildy *et al.*, 1960) are assumed, a value of 0.43 gm/cm^3 is obtained, but it should be emphasized that water is not included. If it is assumed further that the space between the envelope and the capsid (diameter 105 nm; Wildy *et al.*, 1960) is filled with water, then the virion density would be 1.21 gm/cm^3, which is not much different from the values observed in density gradients.

C. *Density of the Individual Components of the Virion*

It has proved difficult to purify any of the three main components of the virions of the herpesviruses, but Lampert *et al.* (1969) have provided, by quantitative electron microscopy, estimates of the dry mass of each. By their method, described in Section II,B, the envelope was 0.6×10^{-15} gm; the empty, naked capsid, 0.5×10^{-15} gm; and the core, 0.2×10^{-15} gm.

In general, one studies the parts of the virion by analyzing particles lacking one or more components. Defective virions can be obtained in a variety of ways. Naked nucleocapsids, some coreless, can be purified from isolated nuclei of infected cells which, during the normal course of viral replication, contain particles lacking the envelope, as shown for PRV by Sydiskis (1970) and for HSV by Spring and Roizman (1968), Stein *et al.* (1970), and Becker *et al.* (1971). However, it is not clear if the particles isolated from the nuclei are indeed devoid of membranes (see Chapter 6). The proportion of incomplete virions can sometimes be enhanced by using a system which produces defective particles. These systems are as follows: Cells are abortively infected with HSV (Spring and Roizman, 1967), in which nucleocapsids are not enveloped; the cells are treated with 5-fluorouracil and infected with PRV, which produce empty virions (Reissig and Kaplan, 1962); HSV-infected cells treated with hydroxyurea, which yield empty capsids (Nii *et al.*, 1968); and EAV-infected cells treated with 5-fluorodeoxyuridine (O'Callaghan *et al.*, 1968). A third alternative is to begin with purified complete virions and to remove each part chemically. Thus far, the outer envelope has been removed by treatment with nonionic detergents, such as Triton X-100 or Nonidet P40, from EAV by Abodeely *et al.* (1970, 1971), PRV by Kaplan and Ben-Porat (1970), and HSV by Olshevsky and Becker (1970) and Roizman and Spear (1971). The different viral components can be separated from each other by virtue of their different densities, as well as by their sizes, by banding in CsCl and sucrose density gradients. Deuterium oxide (heavy water) has also been used in the preparation of sucrose gradients for this purpose (Matis *et al.*, 1971).

The densities of the various subviral particles are shown in Table II. Sydiskis (1969, 1970) has identified the cores by showing that the DNA contained therein had the density in CsCl corresponding to that of PRV-DNA (1.730–1.732 gm/cm^3). The cores were not found unless the lysate of infected cells had first been treated with formaldehyde, which stabilized them as well as the other components, an observation made earlier by Spring and Roizman (1967).

III. The Herpesvirion—Chemical Properties

A. Purification

1. Source of Virus

The purity of preparations of herpesviruses has continued to be a difficult problem, and of the various methods used, each has its own drawbacks. In early studies, brain and other tissues from animals were used as sources of

Type 2	HAASE MAX SCHAT$_2$	1.267	CsCl		Schiek (1967)
PRV[b]		1.278	CsCl	Same value whether stabilized with formaldehyde or not	Kaplan (1969)
		1.28	CsCl		Sydiskis (1969)
EAV[c]		1.18	Sucrose		Darlington and Randall (1963)
		1.18	Potassium tartrate		Darlington and Randall (1963)
		1.08	Silica gel		Klingeborn and Pertoft (1972)
		1.27	CsCl		Klingeborn and Pertoft (1972)
		[illegible]	Silica gel		Pertoft (1970a,b)

more recently, of sucrose, silica gel-polyethylene glycol, or dextran. The findings are summarized in Table I, from which several general findings emerge: (1) Different strains of HSV may have different buoyant densities. (2) The density in CsCl may be different for the same virus, depending on the cell in which it was grown (Spear and Roizman, 1967). (3) The choice of gradient may also affect the observed density. Toplin *et al.* (1971), for example, found that in CsCl the density of the Lucké virus was 0.02 gm/cm³ higher than in potassium tartrate or sucrose gradients. Klingeborn and Pertoft (1972) found a much larger difference between the density of EAV in silica gel (1.08 gm/cm³) and in CsCl (1.27 gm/cm³). The reasons for the higher densities observed with CsCl are not clear, but they could include osmotic effects, as it can be inferred that the herpesvirus envelope is relatively impermeable to CsCl (see Section IV,A).

The reasons for the difference in density of the viral particles grown in different host cells are not clear. Roizman (1969a) has suggested that some of the differences may reflect differences in the composition of the envelope. The variation in density may reflect differences in lipid content of the viral membrane which the virus acquires by budding from the cellular membranes and which may differ in different hosts; the variation in density may also reflect differences in the degree of glycosylation of the viral glycoproteins.

It is of some interest to calculate the density of the virion of HSV by a completely independent method. This may be done using an estimate of the dry mass of the virion obtained by quantitative electron microscopy. This technique is based on the proportionality of the mass of the observed particle to the transmission of visible light by the photographic negative and requires special instrumentation. With small polystyrene spheres of known mass as standards, Lampert *et al.* (1969) determined the dry mass of HSV to be 1.3×10^{-15} gm/virion. If a spherical shape and a diameter of 180 nm (Wildy *et al.*, 1960) are assumed, a value of 0.43 gm/cm³ is obtained, but it should be emphasized that water is not included. If it is assumed further that the space between the envelope and the capsid (diameter 105 nm; Wildy *et al.*, 1960) is filled with water, then the virion density would be 1.21 gm/cm³, which is not much different from the values observed in density gradients.

C. *Density of the Individual Components of the Virion*

It has proved difficult to purify any of the three main components of the virions of the herpesviruses, but Lampert *et al.* (1969) have provided, by quantitative electron microscopy, estimates of the dry mass of each. By their method, described in Section II,B, the envelope was 0.6×10^{-15} gm; the empty, naked capsid, 0.5×10^{-15} gm; and the core, 0.2×10^{-15} gm.

In general, one studies the parts of the virion by analyzing particles lacking one or more components. Defective virions can be obtained in a variety of ways. Naked nucleocapsids, some coreless, can be purified from isolated nuclei of infected cells which, during the normal course of viral replication, contain particles lacking the envelope, as shown for PRV by Sydiskis (1970) and for HSV by Spring and Roizman (1968), Stein *et al.* (1970), and Becker *et al.* (1971). However, it is not clear if the particles isolated from the nuclei are indeed devoid of membranes (see Chapter 6). The proportion of incomplete virions can sometimes be enhanced by using a system which produces defective particles. These systems are as follows: Cells are abortively infected with HSV (Spring and Roizman, 1967), in which nucleocapsids are not enveloped; the cells are treated with 5-fluorouracil and infected with PRV, which produce empty virions (Reissig and Kaplan, 1962); HSV-infected cells treated with hydroxyurea, which yield empty capsids (Nii *et al.*, 1968); and EAV-infected cells treated with 5-fluorodeoxyuridine (O'Callaghan *et al.*, 1968). A third alternative is to begin with purified complete virions and to remove each part chemically. Thus far, the outer envelope has been removed by treatment with nonionic detergents, such as Triton X-100 or Nonidet P40, from EAV by Abodeely *et al.* (1970, 1971), PRV by Kaplan and Ben-Porat (1970), and HSV by Olshevsky and Becker (1970) and Roizman and Spear (1971). The different viral components can be separated from each other by virtue of their different densities, as well as by their sizes, by banding in CsCl and sucrose density gradients. Deuterium oxide (heavy water) has also been used in the preparation of sucrose gradients for this purpose (Matis *et al.*, 1971).

The densities of the various subviral particles are shown in Table II. Sydiskis (1969, 1970) has identified the cores by showing that the DNA contained therein had the density in CsCl corresponding to that of PRV-DNA (1.730–1.732 gm/cm^3). The cores were not found unless the lysate of infected cells had first been treated with formaldehyde, which stabilized them as well as the other components, an observation made earlier by Spring and Roizman (1967).

III. The Herpesvirion—Chemical Properties

A. *Purification*

1. Source of Virus

The purity of preparations of herpesviruses has continued to be a difficult problem, and of the various methods used, each has its own drawbacks. In early studies, brain and other tissues from animals were used as sources of

TABLE I

Density of the Herpesvirion

Virus	Strain	Density (gm/cm^3)	Gradient	Comments	References
			CsCl		Schiek (1967)

TABLE II
DENSITIES[a] OF CORES, CAPSIDS, AND NUCLEOCAPSIDS

Virus	Cores	Capsids	Nucleo-capsids	Complete Virions	References
PRV[b]	1.50–1.53	1.325–1.350		1.280	Sydiskis (1969)
			1.295	1.280	Sydiskis (1970)
HSV[c]			1.305	1.270	Spring and Roizman (1967) and Spring *et al.* (1968)
HSV[b]	1.37–1.45		1.325	1.285	Spring and Roizman (1967) Spring *et al.* (1968)
EAV			1.30	1.270	Klingeborn and Pertoft (1972)

[a] Densities in gm/cm^3; determined in CsCl gradients.
[b] Stabilized with formaldehyde.
[c] Lysates centrifuged without formaldehyde treatment.

crude virus (Holden, 1932). For chemical studies of virus structure, however, it would be difficult to imagine a more unsatisfactory source, and even today the question of contamination with host material continues to be debated.

Although material from infected cell cultures is the most common starting source for preparing herpesviruses, there is one important exception, EAV, which may be prepared from the plasma of infected Syrian hamsters. In this system, concentrations of more than 10^{11} virions/ml of plasma may be reached, and it is a simple matter to prepare large quantities of high-quality virus from it (Darlington and Randall, 1963).

When material from infected cell cultures is used as a starting source, several factors must be taken into consideration. For example, supernatant from infected cultures, containing complete virions but no host cells, offer some advantages (Kaplan and Ben-Porat, 1970; Spear *et al.*, 1970). The main limitation, however, is that in some systems the concentration of virus may be low. This has been especially true for the cell-associated herpesviruses, varicella–zoster virus in particular (Trlifajová *et al.*, 1970; Ludwig *et al.*, 1972b).

Sonicates of infected cells generally contain a mixture of naked and enveloped virions, some with cores and some empty (Olshevsky and Becker, 1970; Becker *et al.*, 1971, Halliburton, 1972). This can be an advantage in providing a source of various types of defective particles. For this purpose, it has usually been more fruitful to begin the operation by separating the infected cells into cytoplasmic and nuclear fractions. The nuclear virus is freed by disruption of the nuclei by brief sonic oscillation or by freezing and thawing. The cytoplasm or extracellular fluid serve as sources for enveloped virions, whereas the nuclei contain a mixture of naked empty and full capsids (Ben-Porat *et al.*, 1970; Olshevsky and Becker, 1970).

2. Procedures

For EAV, plasma is obtained using appropriate anticoagulants,* and cellular elements are removed by sequential differential filtration, ending with a minimum porosity of 450 nm. Virus is sedimented by high-speed centrifugation (24,000 *g* for 30 minutes), and the pellet, usually a pale iridescent green tinged with red, is resuspended in buffer by brief sonic oscillation (90 kcycles, 90 watts, 30–60 seconds). At this point, the preparation consists of complete virions and little else, as determined by electron microscopy (Abodeely *et al.*, 1970). Further purification, however, may be required as described in the section on virion-associated enzymes (Randall *et al.*, 1972).

The methods of purifying virions from cell culture material, whether supernatant fluids or homogenates, either of whole cells, nuclei, or cytoplasm, almost always begin with a low-speed centrifugation (4,000–5,000 *g*) of the virus-containing material in order to eliminate cell debris which may be considerable, especially in case of homogenates of infected cells. This may be followed by high speed (20,000–80,000 *g*) sedimentation of the virus onto a "cushion" of sucrose (60–70%) which is denser than the virus. The virus-containing material may then be centrifuged through a preformed sucrose density gradient (Table III) one or more times, as desired. Equilibrium CsCl density gradients have also been used but have certain limitations which will be mentioned below. Other steps in the purification, such as immune precipitation (Shimono *et al.*, 1969), treatment with nucleases, and chromatography on calcium phosphate columns (Taverne and Wildy, 1959; Wildy *et al.*, 1960; Russell, 1962; Robinson and Watson, 1971) have also been used. More recently, dextran has been used to provide density gradients with reduced osmolarity. This apparently permits better separation of the virus from membranous cell vesicles. Dextran-prepared virus was further purified on discontinuous sucrose (20–50%) or potassium tartrate (10–50%) gradients, (Spear and Roizman, 1972). Silica gel gradients have also been used for purification of herpesviruses (Pertoft, 1970a,b; Klingeborn and Pertoft, 1972). Table III shows that selection of conditions of purification through sucrose gradients has been somewhat empirical.

*If infectivity assays are contemplated, heparin should be avoided, as it will interfere with the assay. Its mode of action will be discussed later in this chapter.

TABLE III
SUCROSE DENSITY GRADIENTS USED TO PURIFY HERPESVIRUSES

Virus	Gradient (%)	Centrifugal force (× *g*)[a]	Time	References
EAV	30–52	32,600	120 minutes	Abodeely *et al.* (1970)
PRV	15–30	10,000	140 minutes	Ben-Porat *et al.* (1970)
HSV	12–52	60,000	40 minutes	Olshevsky and Becker (1970)
	5–40	16,000	90 minutes	Robinson and Watson (1971)
	20–50[b]	81,500	18 hours	Spear and Roizman (1972)
Lucké	10–60	57,300[c]	60 minutes	Toplin *et al.* (1971)
MDV	12–52	81,500	45 minutes	Chen *et al.* (1972)

[a] At midpoint of tube (except c).
[b] A discontinuous gradient, in steps of 50, 40, 30, and 20% sucrose. Virus was initially in the 50% sucrose, and floated to the 40–50% interface during centrifugation.
[c] Maximum centrifugal force, in rate-zonal rotor.

3. LIMITATIONS

Several of the steps commonly used in the purification of other viruses may have an undesirable effect on the herpesviruses. First, fluorocarbon treatment, useful in removing cell debris, may under some circumstances also inactivate PRV (Ivaničová, 1961) and HSV (Norcross *et al.*, 1963) probably by damaging the envelope. In contrast, Toplin *et al.* (1971) reported that IBRV was unaffected by trichlorotrifluoroethane.

Second, various detergents sometimes used to lyse cells and to disperse debris and membranous material may have similar effects. It is worth noting that removal of the herpes envelope has been accomplished with detergents (Kaplan and Ben-Porat, 1970; Olshevsky and Becker, 1970; Abodeely *et al.*, 1971; Becker *et al.*, 1971).

Third, CsCl, used in equilibrium density gradients, may cause herpesvirions and subviral components to be disrupted (Spring and Roizman, 1967) with loss of infectivity (Ben-Porat and Kaplan, 1962; Sydiskis, 1969). The disruption can be prevented by use of formaldhyde as a stabilizing agent (Spring and Roizman, 1967; Sydiskis, 1969), but this has the disadvantage of inactivating the virus and also altering the proteins.

4. CRITERIA OF PURITY

The tool most often used to estimate the purity of herpesvirus preparations is the electron microscope. Its principal limitation is that it will not detect soluble proteins. For this reason, homogenates of labeled, uninfected cells are sometimes mixed with unlabeled, infected cells, and the virus purified. The degree to which the virus may be freed of label is used as an estimate of the effectiveness of the purification. These and other criteria are described further in the section on protein analyses.

B. Composition of the Complete Virion

1. Proof that Herpesviruses Contain DNA

a. Early Studies. In addition to the direct study of rather impure preparations referred to above, another line was developing which ultimately led to the demonstration that herpesviruses contain DNA. This began with the suggestion made by Lipschütz (1921) and by Goodpasture and Teague (1923) that the inclusion bodies observed in virus infections were composed, at least in part, of the elementary bodies of the virus. This view was not readily accepted, and the nature of the inclusions was a subject of much controversy, although Baumgartner (1935) finally showed that HSV inclusions contained infectious virus. The importance of these studies was that if the inclusions contained virus, it might be possible to draw conclusions about the chemical nature of the virus; hence Cowdry (1928) stained inclusions of HSV-infected cells for DNA by the Feulgen reaction, but his results were ambiguous. By the late 1940's, it was suspected that HSV contained DNA, as had been shown for rabbit papilloma (Taylor *et al.*, 1942) and vaccinia (Hoagland *et al.*, 1940) viruses. Lépine and Sautter (1946), for example, unable to obtain a Feulgen-positive stain of HSV inclusions, concluded that no virus was present. Crouse *et al.* (1950), however, later found that the HSV inclusions were indeed Feulgen-positive if the cells were stained early enough and suggested, on this basis, that HSV did contain DNA. Randall and Bracken (1957), in describing the Feulgen-positive inclusion of EAV, implied that this, too, was a DNA virus.

b. HSV and PRV. The first evidence independent of staining that the herpesviruses contain DNA was reported by Kaplan and Ben-Porat (1961), who found that 5-fluorouracil, an inhibitor of DNA synthesis, blocked the formation of infectious PRV. The block was bypassed when thymidine was present in the medium, and on this basis it was suggested that PRV contained DNA. Later, more direct data were published showing that HSV and PRV both contained DNA, of about 73 moles % G + C (Ben-Porat and Kaplan, 1962), close to currently accepted values. Virus labeled with ^{32}P was purified from culture fluids on a CsCl gradient and showed coincident peaks of DNA and infectivity but essentially no RNA. The viral DNA was hydrolyzed, unlabeled carrier nucleotides were added, and the mixture was separated by column chromatography. The base composition was estimated by the ratio of counts between the different nucleotides which had been labeled uniformly. This experiment illustrates the considerable ingenuity required for analyses when the quantity of virus is limiting, a difficulty which has continued to be a hindrance in many studies of herpesviruses.

Also in 1962, three other groups reported that HSV contained DNA. First, Russell (1962) reported that HSV purified by centrifugation, chromatography on calcium sulfate, and treatment with RNase and DNase contained DNA but no significant amount of RNA. Furthermore, Smith and Melnick (1962) described a staining method using DNase and uranyl acetate by which the presence of viral DNA could be shown with the electron microscope. Epstein (1962) made similar findings. A year later, Norcross *et al.* (1963) purified HSV by fluorocarbon treatment and banding on a potassium tartrate density gradient and by direct assay found a DNA content of 10–11% of dry weight.

c. EAV. Further evidence that EAV contained DNA was reported by Gentry *et al.* (1962), in an autoradiographic study of DNA labeling of hepatic parenchymal cell nuclei of infected hamsters. On the basis of the pattern of labeling, which showed grains scattered over the inclusions and not over the marginated host chromatin, and on the basis of preliminary assays of purified EAV (see also Darlington and Randall, 1963), it was suggested that this virus, like PRV and HSV, also contained DNA. In the following year, chemical assays of virus purified directly from plasma of infected hamsters showed that it contained DNA with a G + C content of 56 moles % (Darlington and Randall, 1963).

d. CMV. McAllister *et al.* (1963), using human CMV, confirmed and extended earlier findings of Feulgen-positive inclusions (Cowdry, 1928), by showing that areas within the inclusions were Feulgen positive and that the DNA contained therein was resistant to DNase unless the sections were first treated with pepsin. It was inferred from this that the DNA was located inside protein structures and thus protected from the action of DNase. Goodheart *et al.* (1963) showed that 5-fluorodeoxyuridine blocked the multiplication of CMV and that thymidine reversed the block, providing further evidence that the cytomegaloviruses contain DNA.

e. Molecular Weight. The first molecular weights for herpesvirus DNase were reported by Crawford and Lee (1964) for human CMV, by Kaplan and Ben-Porat (1964) for PRV, and by Russell and Crawford (1964) for HSV, PRV, EAV, and IBRV. These values were based on banding the virus DNA in CsCl density gradients. With the publication of a detailed study of EAV DNA (Soehner *et al.*, 1965), the essential nature of the DNA of the herpesviruses was established; although as new herpesviruses have been found, it has been customary to confirm their DNA content with a variety of by now standard techniques. It is possible that a new period of discovery lies ahead, and if confirmed, the straightforward report of Lando and Ryhiner (1969) of the preparation of infectious HSV DNA may eventually be looked back on as one of the gateposts.

2. Chemical Analyses of the Herpes Virion

Improved methods of purification have permitted analyses of purified virions. These are summarized in Table IV. Because of the variety in the manner of reporting data, it was necessary to convert the values to the same units where possible, using the dry weight as standard in some cases, and the known molecular weight of the DNA as an estimate of the DNA content per virion in others. One of the important limitations to this type of presentation is the tendency for preparations of herpesviruses to consist of mixtures of complete virions and various defective particles, as discussed in Section III, A, 1. The proportion of empty virions would affect the values obtained for the DNA content of the virion, and a preparation consisting largely of naked nucleocapsids would yield low values for lipids. It is likely, as will be pointed out in Section III, C, that the complete virion contains carbohydrate associated with the envelope proteins. The quantity per virion, however, is not known, and no conclusions about it can be drawn from Table IV, as the DNA deoxyribose alone could account for the carbohydrate content of HSV reported by Russell *et al.* (1963).

A discrepancy exists between the dry weight determinations based on particle counts (Russell *et al.*, 1963; Darlington and Randall, 1963) and on quantitative electron microscopy (Lampert *et al.*, 1969), the latter giving somewhat lower values. Because a similar discrepancy exists between DNA content based on particles counts and on molecular weight, it is possible that the particle counts in question were low. Basing the DNA content on the molecular weight depends on the assumption that each virion contains one genome. This appears to be independently justified by genetic studies (Brown *et al.*, 1972) which have produced no evidence to the contrary.

The significance of the spermine and spermidine content of the HSV virion is not clear, although Gibson and Roizman (1971) have pointed out that there is sufficient spermine within the nucleocapsid to neutralize 40% of the negative charge on the DNA. The spermidine appears to be contained only within the envelope, as it is selectively lost when this structure is disrupted.

3. Amino Acid Composition

The amino acid composition of complete EAV has been determined recently by O'Callaghan *et al.* (1972). Virus was prepared as described by Abodeely *et al.* (1970) and purified further by an additional centrifugation

TABLE IV
CHEMICAL COMPOSITION OF HERPESVIRIONS[a]

Virus	Dry weight	Protein	DNA	Lipid	Carbo-hydrate	Spermine	Spermidine
HSV	4.3–5.7	3–4[b]	0.3–0.4[b]	1.0–1.3[b]	0.1[b]		
	1.3[c]		0.14[d], 0.17[e]			0.014[f]	0.029[f]
PRV		2.1[g]	0.12[h]				
EAV	4.5[i]		0.42[i]				
			0.15[j]				

[a] All values expressed in units of 10^{-15} gm/virion.

[b] Calculated from data of Russell *et al.* (1963). The expected value for carbohydrate would be 0.12—0.16, based on that present in the DNA as deoxyribose, assuming an average nucleotide of 322 daltons. The authors used the anthrone reaction (Hewitt, 1958), which would measure deoxyribose. Other values based on the DNA content/virion. Dry weight: total of individual values, excluding carbohydrates.

[c] Dry mass determined by quantitative electron microscopy (Lampert *et al.*, 1969).

[d] By calculation, from data of Norcross *et al.* (1963), indicating a DNA content of 10–11% of dry weight, and the dry mass of 1.3×10^{-15} gm (Lampert *et al.*, 1969).

[e] Based on a molecular weight of 99×10^6 daltons (Kieff *et al.*, 1971), and the assumption that each virion contains one genome.

[f] By calculation, from data of Gibson and Roizman (1971). Values based on the estimate of 0.17×10^{-15} gm of DNA/virion.

[g] By calculation, from data of Ben-Porat and Kaplan (1962).

[h] Based on a molecular weight of 70×10^6 daltons (Kaplan and Ben-Porat, 1964) and the assumption that each virion contains one genome.

[i] Darlington and Randall (1963).

[j] Based on a molecular weight of 92×10^6 daltons (Soehner *et al.*, 1965) and the assumption that each virion contains one genome.

through a potassium tartrate gradient; purity was assessed by polyacrylamide gel electrophoresis and electron microscopy. The total proteins were hydrolyzed with 6 *N* HCl at 110°C and the hydrolysates were analyzed with a Beckman/Spinco automatic amino acid analyzer. In addition, Dreesman *et al.* (1972) have reported the amino acid composition of naked nucleocapsids of HSV-1 and HSV-2. Nucleocapsids were isolated from lysates of infected cells, treated with Nonidet P-40, centrifuged through a discontinuous sucrose gradient and treated further with deoxycholate and Tween 80. Purity was assessed by electron microscopy, by removal of radioactivity from a mixture of unlabeled infected cell lysates and lysates of uninfected cells labeled with [^{3}H]leucine or [^{3}H]thymidine, and by testing the ability of the nucleocapsids to act as immunogens for the production of specific antiviral antibody. The amino acid composition was determined by procedures similar to those of O'Callaghan *et al.* (1972). The results of these two studies are included in Table V.

TABLE V
AMINO ACID COMPOSITION OF INTACT EQUINE ABORTION VIRUS, AND OF HERPES SIMPLEX VIRUS NUCLEOCAPSIDS

Amino acid	EAV[a]	HSV-1[b]	HSV-2[b]
Lysine (moles %)	3.5	6.3	7.6
Histidine (moles%)	2.4	2.8	2.0
Arginine (moles %)	6.8	4.7	3.9
Aspartic acid (moles %)	9.1	8.8	10.1
Threonine (moles %)	8.0	4.8	4.4
Serine (moles %)	7.7	6.1	6.9
Glutamic acid (moles %)	9.7	12.4	13.3
Proline (moles %)	5.6	6.1	6.4
Glycine (moles %)	8.6	10.2	11.3
Alanine (moles %)	10.2	10.4	9.6
Half-cystine (moles %)	0.5	2.0	3.0
Valine (moles %)	8.4	6.6	5.6
Methionine (moles %)	1.7	< 1.0	< 1.0
Isoleucine (moles %)	3.8	5.3	4.4
Leucine (moles %)	9.2	8.6	8.9
Tyrosine (moles %)	2.8	1.1	1.1
Phenylalanine (moles %)	3.5	3.9	4.4
Tryptophan (moles %)	ND[c]	ND	ND

[a]O'Callaghan *et al.* (1972).
[b]Dreesman *et al.* (1972).
[c]Not determined.

While it is clearly difficult to draw conclusions from a comparison of the amino acid composition of intact virions of one herpesvirus with that of nucleocapsids of another, a few points should be mentioned about the data in Table V. First, the total mole percent content of amino acids which tend not to participate in α helix formation (val, ile, ser, cys, thr, gly, pro) (Fasman, 1963) is remarkably similar between EAV (42.6), HSV-1 (41.1), and HSV-2 (42.0). Furthermore, the total mole percent content of nonpolar amino acids (pro, gly, ala, val, met, ile, leu, phe) for intact EAV (51.0) is also very close to that of HSV-1 (51.1) and of HSV-2 (50.6). These similarities may be a reflection of the similar capsid conformation of these viruses, although it is obvious that analysis of the respective capsids would give more reliable information on this point.

An interesting difference is that the HSV nucleocapsids contained more lysine than arginine, while the reverse was true for EAV virions. Although it cannot be determined if this difference would disappear if enveloped HSV were analyzed, labeling studies suggest that HSV core proteins do contain significant amounts of arginine (Olshevsky and Becker, 1970).

Finally, no important differences were noted between the amino acid compositions of HSV-1 and HSV-2 nucleocapsids.

4. Virion-Associated Enzymes

One other area which has been limited by difficultyin purifying the herpesviruses is the study of virion-associated enzymes, or enzyme activities that appear to be an integral part of purified virus. Recently, protein kinase activity has been found associated with EAV (Randall *et al.*, 1972). In this reaction the [γ-^{32}P]phosphate from ATP is apparently transferred to the serine and threonine residues of each of the various EAV proteins. Before maximum activity can be demonstrated, however, removal of a significant proportion of an [α-^{32}P]ATPase, which apparently interferes with kinase activity by cleaving phosphate from ATP to yield adenosine, is required. This may be accomplished by suspending virus in EDTA (0.001 *M* in 0.01 *M* Tris-HCl, pH 7.4) and centrifugation on 20–42% potassium tartrate density gradients. Virions thus purified appear complete as judged by electron microscopy and contain only trace amounts of [α-^{32}P]ATPase activity although [γ-^{32}P]ATPase activity is still associated with viral fractions (H.W. Rogers and C.C. Randall, unpublished observations). The [α-^{32}P]-ATPase appears to be a host-derived contaminant.

The origin of the protein kinase, which has also been reported in HSV (Rubenstein *et al.*, 1972; Silberstein *et al.*, 1972) is not clear, but there is no evidence that it is coded by the virus genome. Since at the present time the kinase appears to be associated with those animal viruses possessing a membranous envelope (Strand and August, 1971), it is possible that a host-coded enzyme is incorporated into the virion at the time of envelopment. An alternative possibility, at least for the herpesviruses, is that the enzyme could be derived from host cell chromatin, which is known to contain kinase activity (Takeda *et al.*, 1971). For the moment, the question of its origin remains unresolved.

C. *Analysis of Proteins*

In no other area of study of the herpesviruses has the problem of purity been so difficult as in the analysis of viral structural proteins. This stems from several biological features of these viruses: (1) They are unstable and tend to lose their envelopes easily; (2) they have a tendency to aggregate; (3) a large proportion of the progeny virus remains intracellular; and (4) cellular debris, in particular membrane fragments, often contaminates preparations of partially purified virus and is difficult to remove. The solution to the problem of purity has depended on improved methods of preparation, discussed in Section III, A, and on special tests for purity.

1. Tests for Purity

The criteria that have been used to prove the purity of a virus preparation are fraught with difficulty, often requiring considerable ingenuity and sometimes generating controversy. It is worthwhile to consider some of them.

1. Electron microscopy is perhaps one of the more widely used criteria of purity, and from it one can draw conclusions about the nature of the virions present, i.e., whether they are enveloped or naked nucleocapsids, or whether or not they contain a core. One limitation is that the proportion of empty, enveloped capsids may appear to be much higher than it really is, because phosphotungstic acid, used to stain the cores, does not readily penetrate the herpesvirus envelope (Watson, 1968). Another limitation is that electron microscopy cannot detect impurities such as soluble or adsorbed host proteins, which are too small to be resolved.

2. Mixed labeling procedures have also been used effectively as criteria of purity. Generally, host cells are labeled with appropriate radioactive amino acids, ^{14}C, for example, and the host proteins thus labeled are mixed with material from cultures labeled during infection with the corresponding ^{3}H-labeled amino acids. It is assumed that in the latter case, the main proteins labeled will be viral, and the success of the purification depends on the degree of selective elimination of ^{14}C-containing material from the preparation. Various forms of this criterion have been used by a number of investigators (Kaplan and Ben-Porat, 1970; Ben-Porat and Kaplan, 1970; Olshevsky and Becker, 1970; Robinson and Watson, 1971; Chen *et al.*, 1972; Spear and Roizman, 1972).

3. Another criterion, employed by Robinson and Watson (1971), was the disappearance with purification of the lines seen in immunodiffusion assays of crude virus with antisera to host cells (rabbit or baby hamster kidney). Although the immunodiffusion precipitin assay is relatively insensitive when compared to other serological procedures, it is obviously useful when sufficient materials are available.

4. The omission of sodium dodecyl sulfate from the gels has also been used by Robinson and Watson (1971). In this case, no stainable bands of protein were seen, whereas they were observed with crude preparations. The implication here is that the only protein present in purified virus was that comprising the virions, which had to be solubilized by the detergent. This criterion would not, however, detect particulate contamination.

There is little doubt that there is something to be gained by using all criteria mentioned above, but criteria (1) and (2), used most frequently, have been sufficient to insure the general uniformity of results achieved by different laboratories with the viruses to be discussed below.

2. Methods of Analysis

The proteins of the herpesviruses have been analyzed by immunological procedures, by separation of the various proteins on acrylamide gels, or by a combination of both. One of the most helpful techniques in the study of viral proteins has been polyacrylamide gel electrophoresis (Maizel, 1966) which has been improved by Dimmock and Watson (1969) and by Laemmli (1970). A detergent, usually sodium dodecyl sulfate (SDS), a polyanion, is generally included to dissociate aggregates of polypeptides; SDS also ensures that the molecules will migrate according to molecular weight, not according to charge. Because the rate of migration through the gel depends largely upon molecular weight (smaller proteins moving faster), it has been possible to estimate the molecular weights of protein within individual peaks by including standard proteins of known molecular weight (Shapiro *et al.*, 1967).

The various bands of proteins may be identified by direct staining, if there is sufficient virus, or by autoradiography of the labeled viral proteins, the latter involving the slicing of the gel lengthwise and placing it on a photographic plate for exposure. Since the gels are very flexible, care must be taken with alignment when comparing the autoradiograph thus produced with the staining profiles. An alternative method of locating the protein bands of labeled virus is also useful. In this method, the gels are cut into slices, each 1–2 mm thick, and the individual slices are assayed for radioactivity. Differentially labeled standard proteins may also be included, providing internal markers. The resolution of this method, however, is often poor compared with autoradiography or staining. It seems clear that further improvements in resolution would be helpful in obtaining the maximum information from gel electrophoretic analyses.

3. Analysis of the Viral Proteins

a. Immunological Analysis. In the first of these studies, Watson and Wildy (1963) found that antisera to uninfected host cells would agglutinate enveloped HSV particles but not naked nucleocapsids, whereas antisera to HSV exclusively agglutinated naked nucleocapsids. The authors concluded that envelopes and capsids do not share common antigens, and that the envelopes are derived at least in part from host material.

In further serological studies, Tokomaru (1965a,b) suggested that HSV-infected cells contained multiple antigens, and Watson *et al.* (1966) showed that HSV-infected cells had as many as ten virus-specified protein antigens. In a more recent report, Miyamoto *et al.* (1971), by comparing early and late

7 S and 19 S antibodies to HSV, have obtained evidence that cores may have one or more antigens not shared by capsids. These studies, taken together, imply that the herpesviruses consist of several different proteins and that each of the different components of the virion probably has its own unique antigens.

b. ANALYSIS BY ACRYLAMIDE GEL ELECTROPHORESIS. An examination of the published patterns of distribution of the viral protein after acrylamide gel electrophoresis reveals a considerable degree of similarity, even between the viruses within the herpes group which have little genetic relatedness. Figure 1 illustrates the electrophoretic profile of the proteins and glycoproteins of PRV, obtained by slicing the gel and ascertaining the amount of radioactivity in the slices. Figure 2 shows the electrophoretic profile of HSV obtained from the absorbance profiles of the proteins stained by Coomassie Brilliant Blue. Despite the differences in technique, it is clear that the profiles of the proteins of HSV and PRV are similar. Weinberg and Becker (1969) have reported that the electrophoretic profiles of EBV and HSV are also similar. Chen *et al.* (1972) have compared the proteins of MDV with those of PRV and HSV and have also found that there were only minor differences between the electrophoretic profiles of the proteins of these three viruses. A summary of the molecular weights of the various structural proteins of several of the herpesviruses is given in Table VI.

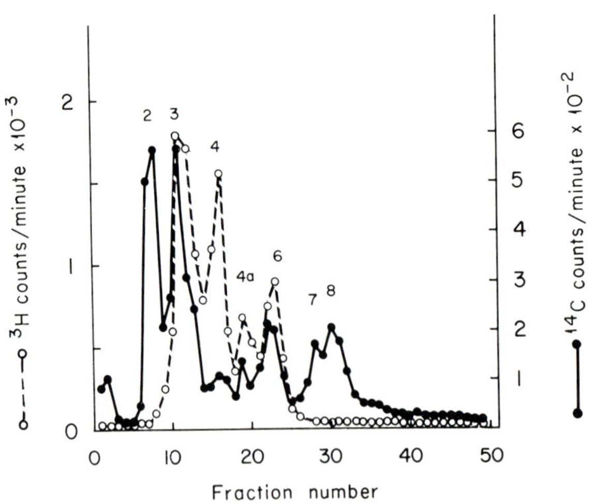

FIG. 1. Electrophoretogram of the proteins of PRV. Infected rabbit kidney cells were labeled simultaneously with [^{3}H]glucosamine and [^{14}C]leucine for 16 hours postinfection, virus was purified, and viral proteins were separated by polyacrylamide gel electrophoresis. [^{14}C] Leucine, solid lines; [^{3}H] glucosamine, dashed lines. (From Kaplan and Ben-Porat, 1970.)

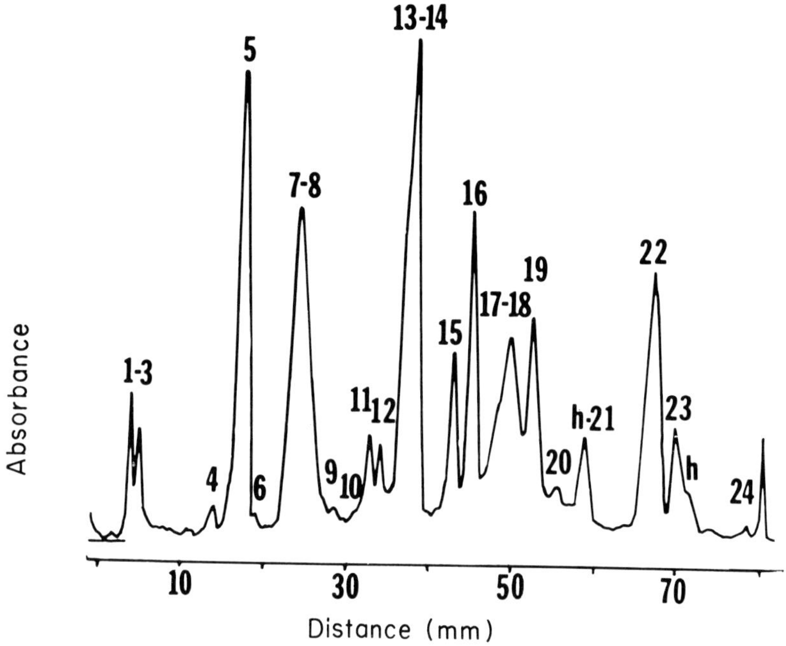

FIG. 2. Electrophoretogram of purified HSV, strain F. Absorbance profile of Coomassie Brilliant Blue-stained proteins. (From Spear and Roizman, 1972).

Most of the information available about the proteins which make up the different viral structures is derived from information obtained after slicing the acrylamide gel and ascertaining the distribution of the labeled viral proteins in the slices. As mentioned above, the main limitation of this technique is its relatively poor resolution. It is possible that some of the proteins seen as a single entity may in reality consist of two or more overlapping peaks. Indeed, this may be inferred from the profiles presented by Spear and Roizman (1972). This can also be deduced from the data of Ben-Porat *et al.* (1970) who showed that at least two polypeptides with different amino acid composition are present in some of the peaks. Furthermore, there may be numerous minor structural proteins, but it is still difficult to identify these with certainty. It is clear, however, that when the proteins of purified preparation of the herpesviruses are examined by staining the gels instead of slicing them many more individual proteins may be resolved. Thus by the staining technique the proteins of EAV were resolved into 20 distinct peaks (Abodeely *et al.*, 1971) and those of herpes simplex into 24 (see Fig. 2 and Spear and Roizman, 1972).

TABLE VI
MOLECULAR WEIGHTS OF THE PROTEINS OF THE HERPESVIRUSES
MOLECULAR WEIGHT[a]/AUTHOR'S DESIGNATION

		HSV		PRV	MDV[b]	EAV
Protein		*c*	*d*	*e,f,g*	*h*	*i*
Capsid	1	110/II	155/VP5	120/2	110/VPI	
	2	34/VIII		30/7		
	3			25/8		
Core	1			100/3		
	2	51/VI		65/4a		
	3	37/VII		45/6		
Envelope	1	101/III	126/VP8–7	100/3	101/VPII	115/1
	2	85/IV	79/86/VP14–12	82/4		95/2, 80/3
	3	58/V	53–59/VP19–17	65/4a	58/VPIV	75/4
	4			45/6		

[a]Molecular weights in units of 10^3 daltons.
[b]Molecular weights based entirely on similarities with data on HSV proteins. Envelope proteins located by labelled glucosamine incorporation. See Olshevsky and Becker (1970).
[c]From Olshevsky and Becker (1970).
[d]From Spear and Roizman (1972).
[e]From Ben Porat *et al.* (1970).
[f]From Ben-Porat and Kaplan (1970).
[g]From Kaplan and Ben-Porat (1970).
[h]From Chen *et al.* (1972).
[i]From Abodeely *et al.* (1971).

i. The capsid. It has been possible to purify naked, empty virions (i.e., capsids) of HSV (Olshevsky and Becker, 1970) and PRV (Ben-Porat and Kaplan 1970; Ben-Porat *et al.* 1970). Such material is obtained from nuclei of infected cells and can be purified by centrifugation in a sucrose density gradient. As observed in the electron microscope, the capsid lacks both envelope and core.

There appears to be one principal capsid protein in the herpesviruses with a molecular weight variously reported from 110×10^3 to 155×10^3 daltons (see Table VI). Spear and Roizman (1972), who reported the higher figure, described some anomalies in the migration of polypeptides larger than 100×10^3 daltons in polyacrylamide gels and based their estimate on the use of myosin (MW 220×10^3 daltons) and β-galactosidase (MW 130×10^3 daltons) as standards. The principal capsid protein comprises about 28% of the proteins of HSV (Olshevsky and Becker, 1970), and appears to be the major antigen of at least HSV and PRV (Shimono *et al.*, 1969; Courtney *et al.*, 1971).

Such a capsid protein has been identified in each herpesvirus thus far studied and has been reported to be the major protein present in mature herpesviruses. Earlier procedures which did not suggest this in EAV (Abodeely *et al.*, 1971) or in HSV (Spear *et al.*, 1970) have since been modified (Spear and Roizman, 1972; H. W. Rogers and C. C. Randall, personal communication) so that there is now general agreement about it.

From the labeling patterns of the viral proteins with different amino acids, it can be deduced that the major capsid protein in HSV contains significant quantities of arginine, leucine (Olshevsky and Becker, 1970; Halliburton, 1972), and tryptophan (Stevens *et al.*, 1969). Similarly, it is clear that PRV also contains significant proportions of these three amino acids (Ben-Porat *et al.*, 1970; Kaplan *et al.*, 1970).

In addition to the major capsid protein, the capsid also contains at least two more proteins of lower molecular weight and may contain others which have not been resolved.

ii. The nucleocapsids. By removal of the envelope from purified virus, the proteins in the nucleocapsid can be identified. This has been done for HSV (Olshevsky and Becker, 1970; Robinson and Watson, 1971), PRV (Kaplan and Ben-Porat 1970), and EAV (Abodeely *et al.*, 1971). The electrophoretic profiles of the nucleocapsids of HSV and PRV seem indistinguishable. The differences observed between the different viruses are less marked than those obtained for the same virus in different laboratories. The number of proteins in the nucleocapsid was estimated at 6 for PRV by Kaplan and Ben-Porat (1970), 4 for HSV by Olshevsky and Becker (1970), and 11 for HSV by Robinson and Watson (1971). The lower numbers may represent an underestimation for the reasons discussed above.

Spear and Roizman (1972) have also treated purified virions with detergent to remove the envelope and have separated the proteins remaining with the nucleocapsids. In these experiments most of the protein peaks, including some nonglycosylated species, were reduced in size with the main exception of the major capsid protein. Furthermore, while some of the glycosylated species were almost completely removed by the detergent, others remained in reduced but substantial amounts. The authors raised the possibility that this was due to the partial removal of some of the proteins of the nucleocapsids, as well as to incomplete removal of the enveloped proteins.

In a more recent series of experiments with HSV, Gibson and Roizman (1972) have compared the polyacrylamide gel profiles of the proteins of nucleocapsids and empty capsids obtained from nuclei of infected cells and nucleocapsids prepared from mature cytoplasmic virus by removal of the envelopes with detergent treatment. As expected, the major capsid protein referred to above was the principal component of the empty capsids as well as of both kinds of nucleocapsids. The empty capsids also contained somewhat smaller amounts of at least two other species (53×10^3 and 33×10^3 daltons). Each of these three is also present in profiles of the nucleocapsids and of complete virions. The profiles of the nuclear-derived nucleocapsids from cells infected with HSV-1 and HSV-2 were identical.

After removal of the envelope of EAV, analysis of the nucleocapsid revealed 16 remaining proteins; all the glycoproteins and lipoproteins had been removed (Abodeely *et al.*, 1971). Although the major capsid protein was missing from the profile, it has since been located migrating more slowly than the envelope proteins (H. W. Rogers and C. C. Randall, personal communication).

iii. Core proteins. The core proteins of the herpesviruses are the most elusive of all, probably because the core is unstable as a unit when the capsid is removed and therefore very difficult to purify. Although the separation of formaldehyde-stabilized cores has been reported (Sydiskis, 1969), information about the proteins contained therein has come from comparisons of profiles of labeled complete virions or nucleocapsids with those of labeled empty capsids purified from nuclei of infected cells. Olshevsky and Becker (1970) tentatively identified two core proteins (see Table VI) in HSV, and Kaplan and Ben-Porat (1970) have also considered that three of the PRV proteins may be associated with the core. An obvious difficulty is that one or more core proteins may have nearly identical molecular weights with either capsid or envelope proteins and for that reason may be difficult to resolve.

iv. Envelope proteins. Several methods have been exploited to obtain information about the envelope proteins. In principle, it should be possible to identify envelope proteins by their absence from naked nucleocapsids purified from nuclei of infected cells (Ben-Porat and Kaplan, 1970; Olshevsky and Becker, 1970). Nucleocapsids isolated from nuclei, however, may in some cases be associated with envelope components (Spring and Roizman, 1968; Ben-Porat *et al.*, 1970). Envelope material can also be removed from complete virions by a detergent such as Nonidet P-40 or Triton X-100 (Kaplan and Ben-Porat, 1970; Olshevsky and Becker, 1970; Abodeely *et al.*, 1971; Spear and Roizman, 1972).

The envelope proteins appear to constitute a significant fraction of the total virion proteins. Indeed, Kaplan and Ben-Porat (1970) have reported that 40% of the PRV proteins are in the envelope, and it may be estimated from the data of Olshevsky and Becker (1970) that a similar situation obtains with HSV. Both HSV and PRV contain significant quantities of lecithins and sphingomyelin (Asher *et al.*, 1969; Ben-Porat and Kaplan, 1971). It may be expected, however, that the lipid component of the virus will vary in composition, depending on the host cell in which it is grown. Ben-Porat and Kaplan (1971) have shown that the envelope of PRV appears to be derived in large measure from the inner nuclear membrane. This is based on the almost identical phospholipid composition of the viral envelope and that of the inner nuclear membrane. The envelope, however, is not derived from preexisting inner nuclear membrane but from areas newly synthesized after infection (Ben-Porat and Kaplan, 1971, 1972). The biogenesis of the viral envelope will be discussed in detail in Chapter 6.

Table VI shows the molecular weights, as well as the number, of proteins found by different laboratories to be associated with the viral envelope. The data obtained from the different viruses are similar with respect to molecular weight. Most laboratories have reported the herpesviruses to be surrounded by an envelope which is composed of between two to four glycoproteins. It is probable, however, that these proteins are not completely resolved. Indeed, Spear and Roizman (1972) have reported that the envelope proteins can be resolved into at least eight polypeptides.

Three of the envelope proteins in EAV are lipoproteins, as indicated by the data of Abodeely *et al.* (1971). All four envelope proteins of this virus are glycosylated, as inferred from the fact that they all stain for carbohydrate. Envelope protein 1 in EAV is glycosylated but does not contain significant amounts of lipid.

From Table VII, it can be seen that the most highly glycosylated envelope protein is not always the most abundant. For example, in HSV-1, the three envelope proteins are present in roughly equal amounts, based on amino acid labeling; however, envelope protein 1 is labeled most heavily with glucosamine. It also appears that the relative abundance of the different envelope proteins differs in different viruses. Thus, in contrast to the nucleocapsids of the different herpesviruses, which may be composed of similar proteins, differences seem to exist in the proteins contained in the viral envelope of different viruses. Keller *et al.* (1970) have reported that the proteins in the envelope of different strains of HSV differ from each other, at least with respect to their degree of glycosylation (Table VIII). It should be mentioned that some differences in the envelope proteins may be host-controlled, although direct evidence supporting this is lacking for the herpesviruses.

There are some other similarities, in addition to molecular weights, between the envelope proteins of different herpesviruses. Envelope protein 1 of PRV thus appears to contain less leucine than the other viral proteins, based on labeling ratios with radioactive arginine and leucine, and tryptophan and leucine (Ben-Porat *et al.*, 1970). A similar situation seems also to exist in HSV envelope protein 1, since this protein appears less prominent when the virus is labeled with leucine than when it is labeled with a mixture of amino acids (Olshevsky and Becker, 1970).

TABLE VII

RELATIVE ABUNDANCE AND DEGREE OF GLYCOSYLATION OF ENVELOPE PROTEINS

Envelope protein	HSV[a]		HSV[b]		PRV[c]		MDV[d]		EAV[e]	
	A.A.[h] (%)	Gluc[h] (%)	A.A.[f]	Gluc[g]	A.A.[f]	Gluc[g]	A.A.[h] (%)	Gluc[g]	A.A.[i]	Gluc[i]
1	30	52	+ + +	+ + +	+ + +	+ + + +	66	+ + +	+ + +	+ + +
2	30	19	+ +	+	+	+ + +			+ +	+ +
3	40	29	+ +	+ +	+	+	34	+ +	+ + +	+ + +
4					+ +	+ +			+	+

[a]From Olshevsky and Becker (1970).
[b]From Spear and Roizman (1972).
[c]From Kaplan and Ben-Porat (1970).
[d]From Chen *et al.* (1972).
[e]From Abodeely *et al.* (1971).
[f]Envelope proteins labeled with amino acids, estimated by inspection of electrophoretic acrylamide gel profiles.
[g]Envelope proteins labeled with glucosamine, estimated as in *f*.
[h]Based on author's figures.
[i]Estimated by inspection of electrophoretic acrylamide gel profiles stained for carbohydrates or proteins.

TABLE VIII
RELATIVE ABUNDANCE OF GLUCOSAMINE LABEL IN ENVELOPE PROTEINS OF DIFFERENT STRAINS OF HSV[a]

Envelope protein		Virus strains				
		HF[b,c]	VR3[d]	F[d]	MP[d]	G[d]
d						+ + +
e	1	+ + + +	+ + + +	+ + + +	+	+ +
fg			+	+	+ +	
ij	2	+ +	+ +	+ +	+ +	+ +
1	3	+ +	+ +	+ +	+ + +	+ +

[a]Estimated by visual inspection of labelling profiles of glycosylated proteins in partially purified virus preparations.
[b]HF, VR3, and F are HSV type 1; MP is a macroplaque mutant of HSV type 1; and G is HSV type 2.
[c]From Olshevsky and Becker (1970).
[d]From Keller *et al.* (1970).

4. CONCLUSIONS

Several conclusions seem possible about the proteins of the herpesviruses.

1. There is a major capsid protein with a molecular weight at least 120×10^3 daltons or larger. This has been identified in each of the herpesviruses thus far studied.

2. The envelope proteins include the bulk of the glucosamine residues, most if not all of the lipids, and comprise approximately 40% of the total virion proteins.

3. There is reasonable agreement in overall findings with respect to the major proteins from one herpesvirus to the next. This may well reflect the identical morphology of the various herpesviruses, as revealed by the electron microscope. For example, it appears that the herpesvirus capsid can be assembled only from a rather limited variety of specialized polypeptides of given molecular weight.

4. Differences in the relative amounts, as well as the relative degree of glycosylation, of the envelope proteins between the different viruses seem to exist. The degree of host modification of these proteins is not clear.

5. There are many questions remaining to be answered. One of the immediate problems is to evaluate the significance of the numerous minor bands observed in the experiments using stained gels.

D. *Analysis of DNA*

1. Location within the Virion

The DNA, or genome, of the herpesvirus is located in the core, or nucleoid, which is the central structure of the virion. Several lines of evidence support this.

First, viral nucleic acid stands out after staining with uranyl acetate and may be visualized by electron microscopy. That the stained material is DNA is shown by its removal from virions incubated with DNase prior to staining. Such procedures have been used to show the location of the DNA within the cores of HSV (Smith and Melnick, 1962; Epstein, 1962), and of Lucké virus (Zambernard and Vatter, 1966). Virions with "empty" cores have also been produced by infecting cells with PRV in the presence of fluorouracil, an inhibitor of DNA synthesis (Reissig and Kaplan, 1962). A similar observation has been made with EAV-infected cells blocked with fluorodeoxyuridine (O'Callaghan *et al.*, 1968).

Second, the volume occupied by the DNA, assumed to be the radiosensitive target volume, is less than the volume of the core (Bonet-Maury, 1948; Powell, 1959; Wildy *et al.*, 1960). This evidence, obviously indirect, depends on the assumption that the radiosensitive target volume can be equated with the genome, a concept which has been questioned by Luria (1955), who described some inconsistencies arising when viruses of different sizes were compared.

Finally, more direct evidence has been obtained by Sydiskis (1969), who isolated PRV cores from formaldehyde-stabilized material from infected cell cultures. The DNA present in the cores had a G + C content typical of PRV DNA.

2. Properties of the DNA of the Herpesviruses

It has gradually emerged that all the various herpesviruses contain DNA that is double-stranded, linear, without unusual components, of variable guanine–cytosine (G + C) content, and of high molecular weight. There is little controversy at present about the first three points. First, part of the currently accepted definitions of a herpesvirus is that it must contain DNA. Second, whenever the viral DNA has been denatured thermally it has shown that the molecule is double-stranded. Third, that it is linear may be inferred from the electron microscopic studies of EAV DNA (Soehner *et al.*, 1965), of HSV DNA (Becker *et al.*, 1968), and from the alkaline sucrose gradient studies of HSV and MDV DNA's (Bachenheimer *et al.*, 1971). Finally, it may be inferred from the report of Erikson and Szybalski (1964) of the density of HSV DNA in Cs_2SO_4 that it is not glycosylated, and from the chromatographic studies included in Table IX, as well as the work of Low *et al.* (1969, 1971) with HSV and PRV, that herpesvirus DNA is not methylated. The remaining two aspects, G + C content and molecular weight, being somewhat more variable in the laboratory, if not in nature, deserve more detailed discussion.

a. Guanine–Cytosine Content of Herpesvirus DNA. The guanine–cytosine (G + C) contents of the DNA's of a number of herpesviruses have been measured and are summarized in Table IX. From these results several things are clear. First and foremost, the use of equilibrium banding in cesium chloride in the analytic ultracentrifuge is a very popular technique for measuring G + C content, and is reasonably reproducible from laboratory to laboratory. There are pitfalls, however, for which one should watch. For example, the final density is almost always measured relative to a known standard. Because of this one ought to choose two standards which give sharp peaks relatively close above and below the unknown DNA. This reduces errors from two sources: first from imprecision in determining the position of the standard, and, second, nonlinearity of the gradient between widely separated peaks. Another pitfall, sadly not well-documented, is that caused by the presence of contaminating species of DNA, usually *Mycoplasma*. This has often been a problem when DNA from infected cells was analysed directly, but it has been shown that in EAV contaminated with *Mycoplasma*, the virus and the *Mycoplasma* band together on potassium tartrate gradients. The virus band then contains both *Mycoplasma* as well as EAV DNA's, which will appear on a preparative CsCl gradient as two peaks of radioactivity (Gentry and Stock, 1969).

Second, when purified virus is hard to obtain as in the case of the cell-associated herpesviruses, one must resort to one of the two following methods: direct analysis with the analytical centrifuge of DNA from infected cells, or the collection of fractions from a preparative CsCl gradient containing DNA from cells labeled with [^{3}H]TdR or ^{32}P during infection. The latter is used when there is not enough virus DNA present to meet even the minimum needs of the analytic method. Ideally, an independent standard of known density labeled with a different isotope should be included. Often, however, the host DNA has been used as the reference. As already mentioned (Gentry and Stock, 1969) *Mycoplasma* DNA can confuse the issue, especially when one cannot use optical density to estimate the relative quantity of DNA in each peak.

Third, thermal denaturation, direct chromatographic analysis, and the $e_{260/280}$ method all require purified viral DNA freed from significant amounts of host DNA, and these procedures ordinarily give values similar to those obtained by the CsCl method.

TABLE IX

G & C CONTENT OF THE DNA'S OF THE HERPESVIRUSES

Virus[a]	G + C (moles %)	Method[b]	References
HSV, type 1	73	Chromat. analysis of [^{32}P] DNA from virus purified by prep. CsCl	Ben-Porat and Kaplan (1962)
	68	Analyt. CsCl, t_m, $e_{260/280}$	Russell and Crawford (1963)
	68	Analyt. CsCl	Russell and Crawford (1964)
	65.1 ± 2.8	Direct chromat. analysis	Lando *et al.* (1965)
	68.3	Analyt. CsCl, DNA from infected cells	Goodheart *et al.* (1968)
	68	Analyt. CsCl, DNA from infected cells	Plummer *et al* (1969b)
	67	Analyt. CsCl, t_m	Kieff *et al.* (1971)
	66.3	Analyt. CsCl	Graham *et al.* (1972)
	65.7	t_m	Graham *et al.* (1972)
	69.9	Direct chromat, analysis	Graham *et al.* (1972)
	66.7	Prep. CsCl, [^{3}H] or [^{14}C] DNA from purified virus	Halliburton (1972)
HSV, type 1 MP var.	68	Analyt, CsCl, DNA from infected cells	Plummer *et al.* (1970)
HSV, type 2	70.4	Analyt. CsCl, DNA from infected cells	Goodheart *et al.* (1968)
	70	Analyt. CsCl, DNA from infected cells	Plummer *et al.* (1969b)
	69	Analyt. CsCl	Kieff *et al.* (1971)
	68	Analyt. CsCl	Ludwig *et al.* (1971)
	68.4	Analyt. CsCl	Graham *et al.* (1972)
	66.0	t_m	Graham *et al.* (1972)
	72.0	Direct chromat. analysis	Graham *et al.* (1972)
	68.9	Prep. CsCl, [^{3}H] or [^{14}C] DNA from purified virus	Halliburton (1972)

EBV	62	Analyt. CsCl, DNA from Burkitt cells	Goodheart (1969)
	61	Prep. CsCl, [^{3}H] DNA from purified virus	Weinberg and Becker (1969)
	59	Prep. CsCl, [^{3}H] DNA from purified virus	Schulte-Holthausen and zur Hausen (1970)
	56–58	Analyt. and prep. CsCl, DNA from purified virus	Wagner *et al.* (1970)
	60	Prep. CsCl, [^{3}H] DNA from purified virus	Becker and Weinberg (1971)
CMV human	58	Analyt. CsCl	Crawford and Lee (1964)
	57	Analyt. CsCl, DNA from infected cells	Plummer *et al.* (1969b)
V-Z	46	Analyt. CsCl	Ludwig *et al.* (1972b)
HV saimiri	70	Analyt. CsCl, DNA from infected cells	Goodheart (1970)
HV tamarinus	67	Analyt. CsCl, DNA from infected cells	Plummer *et al.* (1969b)
Vervet CMV	51	Analyt. CsCl, DNA from infected cells	Plummer *et al.* (1969b)
PRV	73	Chromat. analysis of [^{32}P] DNA from virus purified by prep. CsCl	Ben-Porat and Kaplan (1962)
	74	Analyt. CsCl	Russell and Crawford (1964)
	73	Analyt. CsCl	Kaplan and Ben-Porat (1964)
	71–73	Prep. CsCl, [^{3}H] DNA from purified virus, and from cores	Sydiskis (1969)
	72	Analyt. CsCl, DNA from infected cells	Plummer *et al.* (1969b)
	72	Analyt. CsCl	Ludwig *et al.* (1971)
	72.4	Analyt. CsCl	Graham *et al.* (1972)
	73.5	t_m	Graham *et al.* (1972)
	76.7	Direct chromat. analysis	Graham *et al.* (1972)
	72.9	Prep. CsCl, [^{3}H]- or [^{14}C] DNA from purified virus	Halliburton (1972)

TABLE IX (*continued*)

Virus[a]	G + C (moles %)	Method[b]	References
EAV	56	Direct chromat. analysis	Darlington and Randall (1963)
	55	Analyt. CsCl	Russell and Crawford (1964)
	57	Analyt. CsCl, t_m	Soehner *et al.* (1965)
	57	Analyt. CsCl, DNA from infected cells	Plummer *et al.* (1969b)
	57	Analyt. CsCl, DNA from infected cells	Plummer *et al.* (1969a)
	55	Analyt. CsCl	Ludwig *et al.* (1971)
EHV-2	56	Analyt. CsCl	Russell and Crawford (1964)
	58	Analyt. CsCl, DNA from infected cells	Plummer *et al.* (1969b)
	58	Analyt. CsCl, DNA from infected cells	Plummer *et al.* 1969a)
EHV-3	57	Analyt. CsCl, DNA from infected cells	Plummer *et al.* (1969a)
ECE	66	Analyt. CsCl	Ludwig *et al.* (1971)
Equine CMV	57	Analyt. CsCl, DNA from infected cells	Plummer *et al.* (1969a)
IBRV	71	Analyt. CsCl	Russell and Crawford (1964)
	72	Analyt. CsCl, DNA from infected cells	Plummer *et al.* (1969b)
	71	Analyt. CsCl	Ludwig *et al.* (1971)
	71.4	Analyt. CsCl	Graham *et al.* (1972)
	71.5	t_m	Graham *et al.* (1972)
BMV	64	Analyt. CsCl, DNA from infected cells	Martin *et al.* (1966)
AV	65	Analyt. CsCl, DNA from infected cells	Martin *et al.* (1966)
Dog HV	33	Analyt. CsCl, DNA from infected cells	Plummer *et al.* (1969b)
	65–67	Prep. CsCl, [^{3}H] DNA from purified virus	Aurelian (1969)
	66	Prep. CsCl, [^{3}H] DNA from purified virus	Lust and Carmichael (1971)
Cat HV	46	Analyt. CsCl, DNA from infected cells	Plummer *et al.* (1969b)
Mouse CMV	58, 63	Analyt. CsCl, DNA from infected cells	Plummer *et al.* (1969b)

Rabbit LV	34	Analyt. CsCl, DNA from infected cells	Goodheart (1972)
GPHV	57	Prep. CsCl, [^{3}H] DNA from purified virus	Nayak (1971)
ILT	45	Analyt. CsCl, DNA from infected cells	Plummer *et al.* (1969b)
MDV	56–57	Prep. CsCl, [^{3}H] DNA from sucrose grad. purified virus	Lee *et al.* (1969)
	46	Prep. CsCl, labeled DNA from infected cells	Burg *et al.* (1970)
	46	Analyt. CsCl	Lee *et al.* (1971b)
	46	Analyt. CsCl	Bachenheimer *et al.* (1971)
THV	46–47	Analyt. CsCl	Lee *et al.* (1971a)
Lucké	45–47	Analyt. CsCl	Wagner *et al.* (1970)
	45	t_m	Gravell (1971)
FV4	56	Prep. CsCl, [^{3}H] DNA from purified virus	Gravell (1971)

[a]Complete names for the viruses follow in order of appearance in the table. Additional references are included where needed for clarity. HSV, herpes simplex virus. MP var. is the macroplaque variant of Hoggan and Roizman (1959b). EBV, Epstein-Barr virus. CMV, cytomegalovirus. V-Z, varicella–zoster virus. HV saimiri, monkey lymphoma virus (Melendez *et al.*, 1969). HV tamarinus, marmoset herpes virus (Holmes *et al.*, 1964; Melnick *et al.*, 1964). Vervet CMV, vervet cytomegalovirus (Black *et al.*, (1963). PRV, pseudorabies virus. EAV, EHV-1; equine abortion virus, equine herpesvirus 1. EHV-2, equine herpesvirus 2. EHV-3, equine herpesvirus 3. ECE, equine coital exanthema virus. Equine CMV, equine cytomegalovirus, equine herpesvirus 4. IBRV, infectious bovine rhinotracheitis virus. BMV, bovine mammilitis virus. AV, Allerton virus (related to BMV). Dog HV, canine herpesvirus (Strandberg and Carmichael, 1965; Stewart *et al.*, 1965). Cat HV, feline herpesvirus (Ditchfield and Grinyer, 1965). Mouse CMV, mouse cytomegalovirus; mouse salivary gland virus. GPHV, guinea pig herpesvirus. CLV, cottontail rabbit lymphoma virus (Hinze, 1971). ILT, infectious laryngotracheitis virus (galline). MDV, Marek's disease virus (galline). THV, turkey herpesvirus (related to MDV). Lucké, Lucké virus of frogs. FV4, frog virus 4 (Rafferty, 1965).

[b]Principal references and/or remarks for the methods used: Prep. CsCl, equilibrium banding in a preparative cesium chloride density gradient, with location of virus DNA by radioactivity. Analyt. CsCl, equilibrium banding in an analytical cesium chloride density gradient; with location of virus DNA by absorbance. Unless otherwise indicated, DNA from purified virus was used, so that contamination with other DNA species could be minimized. In order to facilitate comparisons with G + C content obtained by other methods, densities were converted to G + C mole% in those cases in which density alone was reported; the linear relationship described by Schildkraut *et al.* (1962) was used. t_m, determination of G + C from thermal denaturation (melting) temperature; the G + C content is proportional to the melting point provided the other conditions (salt concentration, other solutes, etc.) are held constant (Marmur and Doty, 1959). $e_{260/280}$, pH 3 (Fredericq *et al.*, 1961). Direct chromat. analysis, isolation and quantitation of component bases of purified viral DNA by either UV or radioactivity.

b. GUANINE–CYTOSINE CONTENT AND CLASSIFICATION. It was at first thought that one of the unique characteristics of the herpesviruses was a DNA with relatively high G + C. That this was a natural assumption may be seen from Table IX; the first report of herpesvirus DNA's with less than 55–56 moles% of G + C was made in 1969 (Plummer *et al.*, 1969b). That herpesviruses may have G + C contents significantly lower than that of mammalian cells has been suggested by Goodheart (1972) who reported a G + C of 34 moles % for rabbit lymphoma virus DNA. It is clear that the DNA G + C content is not very helpful in deciding if a candidate virus belongs to the herpes group. On the other hand, the G + C content can be very useful in differentiating between members of the herpes group. For example, it still seems the most reliable way of distinguishing between HSV types 1 and 2. The major problem in using DNA G + C contents in identifying the various herpesviruses occurs with those which have DNA G + C contents near that of host cell DNA. As Kaplan and Ben-Porat (1963) pointed out, it is easy to separate HSV DNA (68–69% G + C) from mammalian DNA (40–45% G + C; Davidson, 1965) in CsCl density gradients. It is not, however, so simple to distinguish MDV DNA (46% G + C) from chicken DNA (43% G + C; Davidson, 1965). The report of Lee *et al.* (1971b), which finally established the G + C content of MDV DNA, shows the lengths to which one must go when the G + C content of the virus DNA is so close to that of the host DNA. Basically, in order to show that host cell DNA has not in some way contaminated the final preparation, it is essential to begin with highly purified virus, and it is very helpful to use some independent methods such as hybridization to show that the virus DNA really is different from host DNA. It appears that similar procedures will be required to settle the controversy over the G + C content of canine herpesvirus (see Table IX), for which there is no published explanation.

c. MOLECULAR WEIGHTS OF HERPESVIRUS DNA. Molecular weights have been determined for the DNA of many of the herpesviruses, and these are summarized in Table X. The most reliable figures are those found by a variety of methods, among which there is no large discrepancy. Of the various herpesviruses, it appears that the genomes of only four (HSV-1, HSV-2, PRV, and EAV) have been measured by more than a single method. One might suspect, however, that most of the herpesviruses should have genome sizes approaching 100×10^6 daltons. Values less than 100×10^6 daltons have been generally reported earlier and as techniques have improved, the values obtained more recently tend toward the higher figure. The single exception is PRV, for which the values 16×10^6 and 22×10^6 daltons were reported recently (Graham *et al.*, 1972). The authors suggest that the molecules may have been sheared during preparation or centrifugation. Another source of fractional values may arise when alkaline sucrose gradients are used. In this case the DNA is denatured, and the effects of nicks in one strand or the other will be seen in the appearance of various fragments. This phenomenon has been observed by Kieff *et al.* (1971) and Roizman and Frenkel (1972), who reported that HSV-1 and HSV-2 DNA's contain single strand breaks which give rise, in alkaline sucrose zone sedimentation, to seven fragments of reproducible size, ranging from 49.5×10^6 (intact single strand) to 10.1×10^6 daltons. The fragments less than 49.5×10^6 daltons can be arranged in three pairs, each totalling 49×10^6 to 50×10^6 daltons, and Roizman and Frenkel (1972) have suggested that the genome may be put together out of specific fragments by the ligase which in some cases fails to join all the pieces.

d. HYBRIDIZATION STUDIES. One of the more recent developments in the study of herpesviruses has been the use of nucleic acid hybridization methods for a variety of purposes. The simplest is to rule out the presence of contaminating DNA's, as in the work of Lee *et al.* (1971b) with MDV. In this case, assumed MDV DNA was tested to see if it would bind labeled RNA from normal and from MDV-infected duck cells. It bound only the latter, and this was used as evidence for the purity of the MDV DNA.

A second purpose is the measurement of genetic relatedness between different herpesviruses. Several reports related to this are summarized in Table XI. At present it appears that hybridization procedures do not show much genetic relatedness between the various pairs thus far tested, except for HSV-1 and HSV-2. These findings are in general agreement with those of Subak-Sharpe *et al.* (1966), who used a form of nearest-neighbor analysis, the doublet frequency, to show that EAV, HSV, and PRV DNA's all were different from each other and were unrelated to vertebrate DNA. Although one cannot draw any conclusion about the amount of genetic relatedness between viral genomes, for example, from comparative doublet frequency patterns, such an analysis nevertheless remains a sensitive and useful method in studying genetic relatedness. The comparison in which hybridization studies have proven most useful is that between HSV types 1 and 2. Bronson *et al.* (1972), using RNA–DNA hybridization, have reported homology between HSV-1 and 2 from 14 to 48%, depending on which member of the pair provided the labeled RNA (see Table XI). Limitations in measuring genetic relatedness by RNA–DNA hybridization are that different parts of the viral genome are transcribed at different times after infection (Huang *et al.*, 1971; Rakusanova *et al.*, 1971; Wagner, 1972). Furthermore, virus-specific RNA can be divided into two populations—one abundant, and one scarce (Roizman and Frenkel, 1972)–which may also affect to some extent the results obtained during hybridization experiments. The use of DNA–

TABLE X

MOLECULAR WEIGHTS OF HERPESVIRUS DNA

Virus[a]	MW[b]	Method[c]	References
HSV, type 1	51	Band width in CsCl	Russell and Crawford (1963)
	54	Sedimentation	Russell and Crawford (1963)
	68	Sedimentation	Russell and Crawford (1964)
	100	Electron Microscopy	Becker *et al.* (1968)
	110	Zone sedimentation in sucrose	Becker *et al.* (1968)
	99	Zone sedimentation in sucrose	Kieff *et al.* (1971)
	95	Renaturation kinetics	Frenkel and Roizman (1971)
	87.7	Sedimentation	Graham *et al.* (1972)
HSV, type 1 MP. var.	95	Zone sedimentation in sucrose	Bachenheimer *et al.* (1971)
HSV, type 2	99	Zone sedimentation in sucrose	Kieff *et al.* (1971)
	87.7	Sedimentation	Graham *et al.* (1972)
EBV	100	Zone sedimentation in sucrose	Weinberg and Becker (1969)
CMV human	32	Band width in CsCl	Crawford and Lee (1964)
PRV	70	Band width in CsCl	Kaplan and Ben-Porat (1964)
	68	Sedimentation	Russell and Crawford (1964)
	16.07	Sedimentation; two components observed	Graham *et al.* (1972)
	22.2		

EAV (EHV-1)	92.2	Sedimentation, band width in CsCl, and electron microscopy	Soehner *et al.* (1965)
EHV-2	84	Sedimentation	Russell and Crawford (1964)
IBRV	54	Sedimentation	Russell and Crawford (1964)
BMV	34	Band width in CsCl	Martin *et al.* (1966)
AV	32	Band width in CsCl	Martin *et al.* (1966)
MDV	120	Zone sedimentation in sucrose	Lee *et al.* (1971b)
	103	Zone sedimentation in sucrose	Bachenheimer *et al.* (1971)

[a] See footnote *a* for Table X.

[b] Molecular weight in units of 10^6 daltons.

[c] Principal references and remarks for the methods used: Band width in CsCl (Thomas and Berns, 1961), this method is based on the ratio of the width to the height of the band of DNA at equilibrium in a CsCl density gradient. It depends heavily on having a homogeneous population of molecules; any significant contamination with broken molecules will cause low values to be obtained. It requires further an empirical correction factor without which the values will be approximately half those found with other methods. Sedimentation (Burgi and Hershey, 1963), the sedimentation constant (s) is calculated from the sedimentation velocity of the boundary in the analytical ultracentrifuge, and from s the molecular weight is calculated. Zone sedimentation in sucrose (Studier, 1965), a small volume (band) of viral DNA is layered onto a sucrose density gradient and its rate of sedimentation measured in the preparative ultracentrifuge; s is determined by comparison with known marker DNA's. From s the molecular weight is calculated. Electron microscopy (von Kleinschmidt and Zahn, 1959), molecular weight is calculated from the length of individual molecules measured by electron microscopy, using the conversion factor $1 \mu m = 1.92 \times 10^6$ daltons (Thomas and MacHattie, 1967). The success of this method depends, in part, on choosing the right molecules for measurement. In practice, one seeks a fairly large number of molecules all with similar lengths, approximating the maximum length seen in the preparation.

DNA hybridization, which is not subject to this criticism, has confirmed a substantial degree of genetic relatedness between HSV-1 and HSV-2 (Kieff *et al.*, 1972; Ludwig *et al.*, 1972a).

TABLE XI
NUCLEIC ACID HYBRIDIZATION AND THE GENETIC RELATEDNESS OF THE HERPESVIRUSES

DNA in excess	Labeled species	Homology (%)	References
HSV-1	HSV-2 RNA[a]	48[b]	Bronson *et al.* (1972)
HSV-2	HSV-1 RNA	14	Bronson *et al.* (1972)
HSV-1	HSV-2 DNA	47–50	Kieff *et al.* (1972)
HSV-1	HSV-2 DNA	69.8	Ludwig *et al.* (1972a)
HSV-2	HSV-1 DNA	40–47	Kieff *et al.* (1972)
HSV-2	HSV-1 DNA	68.3	Ludwig *et al.* (1972a)
HSV-1	IBRV RNA	0	Bronson *et al.* (1972)
HSV-1	PRV RNA	1	Bronson *et al.* (1972)
HSV-2	IBRV RNA	1	Bronson *et al.* (1972)
HSV-2	PRV RNA	2	Bronson *et al.* (1972)
IBRV	PRV RNA	2	Bronson *et al.* (1972)
IBRV	HSV-1 RNA	9	Bronson *et al.* (1972)
IBRV	HSV-2 RNA	4	Bronson *et al.* (1972)
PRV	IBRV RNA	6	Bronson *et al.* (1972)
PRV	HSV-1 RNA	2	Bronson *et al.* (1972)
PRV	HSV-1 DNA	8	Ludwig *et al.* (1972a)
PRV	HSV-2 RNA	6	Bronson *et al.* (1972)
PRV	HSV-2 DNA	8	Ludwig *et al.* (1972a)
ECEV	HSV-1 RNA	0	Ludwig *et al.* (1971)
MDV	HSV-1 RNA	1–2	Bachenheimer *et al.* (1971)
MDV	HSV-2 RNA	1–2	Bachenheimer *et al.* (1971)
EBVC[c]	HSV DNA	6	zur Hausen *et al.* (1970)
MDVT[d]	EBV DNA	0	zur Hausen *et al.* (1970)
CMVC[e]	EBV DNA	0	zur Hausen *et al.* (1970)
Lucké	FV4 DNA	2	Gravell (1971)

[a] RNA was extracted from cells labeled during infection.
[b] Percent homology = (cpm bound, heterologous reaction)/(cpm bound, homologous reaction) × 100.
[c] EBVC is DNA extracted from a Burkitt tumor cell line which contains substantial EBV DNA.
[d] MDVT is DNA extracted from a tumor of Marek's disease.
[e] CMVC is DNA extracted from cells infected with cytomegalovirus.

IV. Resistance of the Herpesviruses to Inactivation

The resistance of viruses to various physical and chemical treatment was a preoccupation of early virologists, and some of their work with HSV was extended by Holden (1932). Much of this work, however, is hard to interpret because of the unavailability of purified virus. To study HSV during that period one usually used brain tissue from infected animals, either as a suspension or in a dried state. Despite the presence of much extraneous materials, it was found (Holden, 1932) that HSV was inactivated by lipid solvents, a test still used to help identify herpesviruses.

A. Stability to Chemicals

The role played by the envelope in the infectivity of the herpes viruses has been the subject of considerable discussion (Darlington and Moss, 1969) and is detailed in Chapter 5. Briefly, the envelope is thought to aid in attachment and penetration of the virus. Indeed it appears that the report of Lando and Ryhiner (1969) of the preparation of infectious DNA of HSV has finally confirmed what has long been assumed, that the ultimate infectivity of HSV lies in the DNA, and that the function of the rest of the virion is to package and deliver the genome. Regarding the envelope, however, several aspects should be mentioned here. First, any chemical agent which removes the envelope dramatically reduces the infectivity of the herpesviruses. Because the envelope contains considerable amounts of lipid, the herpesviruses are especially sensitive to lipid solvents (Darlington and Moss, 1969; Smith, 1959; Kaplan, 1969; Roizman, 1969a). These include ethyl ether (Andrewes and Horstmann, 1949; Kaplan and Vatter, 1959), sodium deoxycholate (Bedson and Gostling, 1958), and chloroform (Roizman and Roane, 1963), but in general any lipid solvent would be expected to inactivate the herpesviruses. While the effects of fluorocarbons appear to be variable, these chemicals in some cases can inactivate herpesviruses by altering the envelopes, as shown for PRV (Ivaničová, 1961) and HSV (Norcross *et al.*, 1963). The herpesviruses are sensitive to several enzymes, which also probably alter the envelope in some way. These include trypsin [as shown for HSV (Gresser and Enders, 1961), for PRV (Kaplan, 1969), for EAV (Bartha *et al.*, 1969; Romváry *et al.*, 1969; Agthe and Schmidt, 1971)] and for HSV, acid and alkaline phosphatases (Amos, 1953), and phospholipase C and pronase (Spring and Roizman, 1968).

The envelope may also play a role in controlling the penetration of agents which disrupt the capsid or inactivate the core. In this respect Vilagines (1969) suggested that the temperature dependency of inactivation of HSV by ethidium bromide reflected the speed of penetration across the viral membrane. The envelope also appears to be impermeable to CsCl, as complete virions are more stable in CsCl density gradients than are naked nucleocapsids (Spring and Roizman, 1968; Roizman, 1969b). Furthermore, phosphotungstic acid, a stain used in electron microscopy, does not penetrate the envelope readily (Watson, 1968). Another implication regarding the permeability of the envelope arises from the work with EAV (Randall *et al.*, 1972). Because all the EAV proteins are phosphorylated in the reaction, some mechanism by which the phosphate is transferred across the envelope may be inferred. That this transfer may be limiting is also supported by the fact that the reaction is stimulated by Nonidet P-40, as well as by dithiothreitol, both capable of disrupting the envelope (Olshevsky and Becker, 1970; Abodeely *et al.*, 1971; Gainer *et al.*, 1971; Spear and Roizman, 1972). It is interesting that the envelope of HSV is also sufficiently impermeable to prevent the loss of spermidine (Gibson and Roizman, 1971).

Chemicals which appear to inactivate the core are ethidium bromide (Vilagines, 1969) and nitrous acid (Ivaniĉová *et al.*, 1963), while 5-bromouracil is a special case. When present in the DNA in small amounts 5-bromouracil behaves as a mutagen and has been used to provide a variety of temperature-sensitive and other mutants of HSV (Brown *et al.*, 1972; Timbury, 1971). When sufficient amounts of 5-bromouracil have been incorporated into the DNA, the virion density increases in density gradients, and much less infectious virus may be obtained, as shown for PRV (Kaplan *et al.*, 1965) and for HSV (Schiek and Schiek, 1969). 7,12-Dimethylbenzanthracene, a carcinogen which inactivates HSV-1 and HSV-2 at different rates (Docherty *et al.*, 1971), may also act on the viral genome.

Other chemicals, including urea, detergents (Kaplan, 1969; Roizman, 1969a), and CsCl (Spring and Roizman, 1968), probably act by disaggregating the total virus structure. A recent addition to the list is dithiothreitol, a reducing agent which appears to disrupt the entire PRV virion (Gainer *et al.*, 1971).

B. Stability to Heat

The effect of temperature on the herpesviruses has received considerable attention. HSV is relatively thermosensitive under ordinary conditions (Kaplan, 1969), with a half-life at 37°C of 1.5 hours (Scott *et al.*, 1961) to 3 hours (Farnham and Newton, 1959). It is possible, however, to stabilize HSV against heat inactivation by a variety of agents, including 1 *M* Na_2SO_4 or Na_2HPO_4 (Wallis and Melnick, 1965), and, in general, it is difficult to draw valid comparisons between viruses heated under different conditions (Roizman, 1969a). Thermal inactivation of HSV appears to follow first-order kinetics (Scott *et al.*, 1961; Farnham and Newton, 1959), but a second component in the inactivation curve has been described by Kaplan (1957), Hoggan and Roizman (1959a), and Plummer and Lewis (1965). Kaplan (1969) suggested that the second component indicated that some of the virus had clumped, or that more than one step was needed to heat-inactivate a single infectious virion.

A related area is that of temperature-sensitive HSV mutants, which will not grow at raised temperatures of incubation but which are otherwise as heat-resistant as the wild type (Brown *et al.*, 1972; Timbury, 1971; Schaffer *et al.*, 1970, 1971). It is thought that in some of these mutants certain virus-specific nonstructural proteins may not function at the elevated temperature, but this is still not clear.

C. Stability to Irradiation

The herpesviruses are inactivated exponentially by X, γ, or ultraviolet (UV) irradiation (Powell, 1959; Scott *et al.*, 1961; Kaplan, 1962; Pfefferkorn *et al.*, 1965; Sullivan *et al.*, 1971). With X rays, 14,000 R lowered the titer of HSV by 90% (Powell, 1959), and a similar reduction was described for PRV with a dose of 200,000 R of γ rays (Kaplan and Ben-Porat, 1966). With UV, a 90% reduction in titer of PRV was achieved with a dose of 440 ergs/mm^2 (Kaplan, 1962). Further studies of the complete inactivation with ultraviolet light have been completed by Dilovski (1969) for PRV and by Smith *et al.* (1971) for HSV types 1 and 2. In the latter work it was found that HSV type 2 was inactivated more rapidly. Wallis and Melnick (1964) have demonstrated the photosensitization of HSV by neutral red, toluidine blue, and proflavine, and Schneweis (1969) has more recently described the increased UV inactivation of HSV which contains 5-bromo- or 5-iodouracil in its DNA. Pfefferkorn *et al.* (1965, 1966) have described the photoreactivation of UV-inactivated PRV.

It has been shown by Zavadova and Zavada (1968) for PRV, and by Bockstahler and Lytle (1970) for HSV that the UV-inactivation curves of these two herpesviruses have two components. Whether the slowly inactivated component is related to repair or not remains to be demonstrated, although the work of Rabson *et al.* (1969) suggests that if repair is involved, it is by a host-coded mechanism. This may be inferred from this study because HSV partially inactivated with UV grew much more poorly in cell cultures from patients with xeroderma pigmentosum (XP), a genetic disease in which the patient lacks the DNA repair mechanism. Nonirradiated HSV grew well in the XP cells, as did UV-irradiated HSV in control cells. Ross *et al.* (1971) have also implicated the repair process, or possibly recombination, in a study of small plaque production by UV-inactivated HSV.

Another related area is the demonstration that some functions of the herpesviruses are more sensitive to UV inactivation than others. Tokumaru

(1969) has reported that partially inactivated HSV retains the ability to cause tissue lesions in guinea pigs and rabbits, but no longer causes fatal tonic convulsions or giant cells in these host. Miyamoto and Morgan (1971) have reported that UV irradiation of HSV prevents the release of its DNA, but that if the dose is increased, fusion also is prevented. It is at best difficult to relate these two works to the direct effect of UV on the DNA itself. Other studies of considerable interest describe the induction of genetic changes in mammalian cells by UV-irradiated HSV. One of the basic papers in this area is that of Waubke *et al.* (1968), who showed that the capacity of HSV to induce chromosomal aberrations was only one-fourth as sensitive to UV as was infectivity. Making use of the relatively higher sensitivity of infectivity, Munyon *et al.* (1971) transferred the genetic information for thymidine kinase, still "intact" despite the overall loss of infectivity, from UV-inactivated HSV to mammalian host cells that lack thymidine kinase. Along similar but slightly less specific lines, Duff and Rapp (1971a,b) have reported that UV-inactivated HSV type 2 could transform hamster cells *in vivo*.

D. *Inhibitors of Adsorption*

Another agent, not strictly inactivating but whose action seems to be primarily physical is heparin, which blocks adsorption of the virus to the host cell, as originally reported for HSV by Vaheri and Cantell (1963). The mechanism is not clear, but may be related to the high negative charge that this molecule carries, because Tytell and Neuman (1963) have shown that the effect of heparin can be reversed by the addition of the polycation protamine sulfate. In addition to heparin other sulfated polyanions, including those in agar, may also block adsorption of the herpesviruses. This phenomenon has been summarized by Roizman (1969a) and studied further by Hochberg and Becker (1968); the latter found that heparin could also remove adsorbed HSV from host cells. This phenomenon was also studied by Germanov and Sokolov (1969) and Sokolov and Germanov (1969), who have selected HSV mutants resistant to the sulfated agar polysaccharides. More recently, Falke and Kahl (1971) have reported that compound 48/80 (a mixture of oligomers of 4-methoxyphenethyl-*N*-methylamine), as well as heparin, both could block penetration of host cells by HSV. There are, however, some differences in the action of these two compounds; 48/80 liberates histamine and heparin does not, and while the effect of heparin on HSV penetration can be reversed that of 48/80 cannot. To have a complete understanding of the action of polyanions in this system requires a knowledge of the nature of herpesvirus adsorption. Little, however, is known about the electrical aspects of this beyond the fact that these viruses and their host cells carry net negative charges (Weiss and Horoszewics, 1971; Matis and Zuffa, 1969) and that electrolytes, in particular magnesium and calcium, are required (Farnham and Newton, 1959). In any case, the sulfated agar polysaccharides and heparin have from time to time interfered with experiments in a manner most puzzling to the virologist who was not aware of them.

E. Practical Aspects

Both Kaplan (1969) and Roizman (1969a) have commented on the difficulty of storing HSV. When suspended in medium containing serum, it is stable for several months at −70° C, and for several weeks at +4° C. Oddly, however, at −20° C, HSV loses titer rapidly, dropping as much as 1 log in 2 weeks (Stoker and Ross, 1958; Schneweis, 1961). The suspending medium also affects the low temperature storage of herpesviruses. Meurisse (1969), for example, reported that varicella–zoster virus stored in frozen cell cultures was stable for several years at −65° C or −184° C. For long-term storage the best method is probably lyophilization. Popescu *et al.* (1969) have shown that lyophilized PRV is stable for 3–4 years, and Calnek *et al.* (1970) have shown that cell-free MDV can be lyophilized if stabilized with ethylene diamine tetraacetate (EDTA). On the other hand, Kottaridis *et al.* (1969) reported that MDV was inactivated by lyophilization, although it survived well at −60° C in blood from infected chickens. Human CMV also is somewhat stable in blood, persisting for 28 days in whole banked blood and for 3 months in freshly frozen plasma (Armstrong *et al.*, 1971). As a rule while MDV is stable enough in the dust of poultry houses (Jurajda and Klimes, 1970), cell-free MDV has not been very stable in the laboratory, and several technical improvements have been suggested in its handling. Mikami and Bankowski (1970), citing the report by Wallis and Melnick (1968) that dimethylsulfoxide stabilized HSV, used this compound together with fetal calf serum to help preserve MDV during its preparation. Cook and Spears (1970) have used water as an effective suspending agent for cell-free MDV—a time-honored procedure for HSV (Munk and Ackermann, 1953). Furthermore, the growing interest in the epidemiology of HSV, especially type 2, has generated at least two recent papers (Rodin *et al.*, 1971; Nahmias *et al.*, 1971) describing media for the transport of HSV at ambient temperatures. These media should considerably improve the handling of clinical specimens. One should, however, test new procedures carefully, especially when dealing with clinical material. A case in point is the experience of Doherty *et al.* (1967), who found that IBRV was inactivated by calcium alginate wool swabs especially intended for clinical use.

Effective procedures for destroying the infectivity of herpesviruses may be based in part on the sensitivity of the envelope to various solvents, as well as to agents which inactivate proteins. Sery and Furgiuele (1961), Blackwell and Chen (1970), and Oxford *et al.* (1971) have described the effects of a variety of agents on HSV as well as other viruses.

V. Conclusion

The importance of reliable physicochemical data to the proper classification of the herpesviruses should be obvious. While the certification of a candidate virus as a member of the herpes group is now usually based first of all on morphology (Wildy *et al.*, 1960), the intragroup classification depends heavily on physicochemical properties. Perhaps the best example of this dependence is seen in the difference between HSV types 1 and 2. Nahmias and Dowdle (1968) have summarized the differences between these two types, which include greater sensitivity of type 2 to UV irradiation (Duff and Rapp, 1971b; Smith *et al.* 1971) and thermal inactivation (Schneweis, 1962; Figueroa and Rawls, 1969), to temperature of incubation (Ratcliffe, 1971), and to 7, 12-dimethylbenzanthracene (Docherty *et al.*, 1971). Although Roizman *et al.* (1970) proposed that there exists a spectrum of types between HSV 1 and 2, the 2% difference in G + C content of the DNA has remained quite constant, and no intermediates have been found by this criterion. Most recently this has been confirmed by Halliburton (1972) for a variety of fresh isolates of both type 1 and type 2. Halliburton (1972) further reported differences in the basic proteins seem in the extracts of cells infected with HSV types 1 and 2. These should complement the studies of genetic relatedness summarized in Section III and lead to a better understanding of the physicochemical differences between HSV types 1 and 2 at an unprecedented level of detail.

Acknowledgments

Several persons have provided indispensable assistance. In particular we thank Susan Conerly, Susan Brown, Cathi Hesselbein, Kathy Ellis, and Jeanette Mize who have assisted with the typing and collecting of references. We also are grateful to the staff of the Rowland Medical Library of the University of Mississippi Medical Center for many extra favors above and beyond the call of duty. We especially thank Dr. Dennis O'Callaghan of the Department of Microbiology for the generous use of his private library and for his thorough editorial comments, and Dr. Clyde Goodheart for some valuable suggestions. Glenn A. Gentry is a Research Development Career Awardee of the National Institute of Allergy and Infectious Diseases (5-K3-AI-7021).

References

Abodeely, R. A., Lawson, L. A., and Randall, C. C. (1970). *J. Virol.* **5**, 513–523.

Abodeely, R. A., Palmer, E., Lawson, L. A., and Randall, C. C. (1971). *Virology* **44**, 146–152.

Agthe, V., and Schmidt, R. (1971). *Acta Virol.* (*Prague*), *Engl. Ed.* **15**, 421–424.

Amos, H. (1953). *J. Exp. Med.* **98**, 365–372.

Andrewes, C. H., and Horstmann, D. M. (1949). *J. Gen. Microbiol.* **3**, 290–297.

Armstrong, D., Ely, M., and Steger, L. (1971). *Infec. Immunity* **3**, 159–163.

Asher, Y., Heller, M., and Becker, Y. (1969). *J. Gen. Virol.* **4**, 65–76.

Aurelian, L. (1969). *J. Virol.* **4**, 197–202.

Bachenheimer, S. L., Kieff, E. D., Lee, L. F., and Roizman, B. (1971). *In* "Oncogenesis and Herpesviruses" Int. Agency Res. Cancer, Lyon (P. M. Biggs *et al.*, eds.), pp. 74–81. Elsevier, Amsterdam.

Bartha, A., Belak, S., and Benyeda, J. (1969). *Acta Vet.* (*Budapest*) **19**, 97–99.

Baumgartner, G. (1935). *Schweiz. Med. Wochenschr.* **16**, 759–760.

Becker, Y., and Weinberg, A. (1971). *Isr. J. Med. Sci.* **7**, 561–567.

Becker, Y., Dym, H., and Sarov, I. (1968). *Virology* **36**, 184–192.

Becker, Y., Levitt-Hadar, J., Dym, H., and Olshevsky, U., (1971). *Isr. J. Med. Sci.* **7**, 656–662.

Bedson, S. P., and Gostling, J. V. T. (1958). *Brit. J. Exp. Pathol.* **39**, 502–509.

Ben-Porat, T., and Kaplan, A. S. (1962). *Virology* **16**, 261–266.

Ben-Porat, T., and Kaplan, A. S. (1970) *Virology* **41**, 265–273.

Ben-Porat, T., and Kaplan, A. S. (1971). *Virology*, **45**, 252–264.

Ben-Porat, T., and Kaplan, A. S. (1972). *Nature* (*London*) **235**, 165–166.

Ben-Porat, T., Shimono, H., and Kaplan, A. S. (1970). *Virology* **41**, 256–264.

Black, P. H., Hartley, J. W., and Rowe, W. P. (1963). *Proc. Soc. Exp. Biol. Med.* **112**, 601–605.

Blackwell, J. H., and Chen, J. H. S. (1970). *J. Ass. Offic. Anal. Chem.* **53**, 1229–1236.

Bockstahler, L. E., and Lytle, C. D. (1970). *Biochem. Biophys. Res. Commun.* **41**, 194–189.

Bonet-Maury, P. (1948). *In* "Les Ultravirus des Maladies Animales" (C. Levaditi, P. Lepine, and J. Verge, eds.), p. 165. Maloine, Paris.

Bronson, D. L., Graham, B. J., Ludwig, H., Benyesh-Melnick, M., and Biswal, N. (1972). *Biochim. Biophys. Acta* **259**, 24–34.

Brown, S. M., Ritchie, D. A., and Subak-Sharpe, J. H. (1972). *Proc. Int. Congr. Virol., 2nd, 1971* p. 287.

Burg, R., Morris, C. A. Adler, S. A., and Maag, T. A. (1970). *Bacteriol. Proc.* 170.

Burgi, E., and Hershey, A. D. (1963). *Biophys. J.* **3**, 309–321.

Calnek, B. W., Hitchner, S. B., and Aldinger, H. K. (1970). *Appl. Microbiol.* **20**, 723–726.

Chen, J. H., Lee, L. F., Nazerian, K., and Burmester, B. R. (1972). *Virology* **47**, 434–443.

Cook, M. K., and Spears, J. F. (1970). *J. Virol.* **5**, 258–261.

Courtney, R. J., McCombs, R. M., and Benyesh-Melnick, M. (1971). *Virology* **43**, 356–365.

Cowdry, E. V. (1928). *Science* **68**, 40–41.

Crawford, L. V., and Lee, A. J. (1964). *Virology* **23**, 105–107.

Crouse, H. V. Coriell, L. L., Blank, H., and Scott, T. F. McN. (1950). *J. Immunol.* **65**, 119–128.

Darlington, R. W., and Moss, L. H., III. (1969). *Progr. Med. Virol.* **11**, 16–45.

Darlington, R. W., and Randall, C. C. (1963). *Virology* **19**, 322–327.

Davidson, J. N. (1965). "The Biochemistry of the Nucleic Acids," 5th ed., p. 62. Wiley, New York.

Dilovski, M. (1969). *Zentralbl. Veterinaermed, Reihe B* **16**, 346–352.

Dimmock, N. J., and Watson, D. H. (1969). *J. Gen. Virol.* **5**, 499–509.

Ditchfield, J., and Grinyer, I. (1965). *Virology* **26**, 504–506.

Docherty, J. J., Goldberg, R. J., and Rapp, F. (1971). *Proc. Soc. Exp. Biol. Med.* **136**, 328–333.

Doherty, P. C., Simmons, G. C., and Payne, E. (1967). *Aust. Vet. J.* **43**, 257–260.

Dreesman, G. R., Suriano, J. R., Swartz, S. K., and McCombs, R. M. (1972). *Virology* **50**, 528–534.

Duff, R., and Rapp, F. (1971a). *Nature (London) New Biol.* **233**, 48–50.
Duff, R. and Rapp. F. (1971b). *J. Virol.* **8**, 469–477.
Epstein, M. A. (1962). *J. Exp. Med.* **115**, 1–11.
Erikson, R. L., and Szybalski, W. (1964). *Virology* **22**, 111–124.
Falke, D. (1963). *Zentralbl. Bakteriol., Parasitenk., Infektionskr. Hyg., Abt. 1: Orig.* **191**, 247–252.
Falke, D., and Kahl, G. F. (1971). *J. Gen. Virol.* **10**, 273–277.
Farnham, A. E., and Newton, A. A. (1959). *Virology* **7**, 449–461.
Fasman, G. D. (1963). *In* "Methods in Enzymology" (S. P. Colowick and N. O. Kaplan, eds.), Vol. 6, p. 928. Academic Press, New York.
Figueroa, M. E., and Rawls, W. E. (1969). *J. Gen. Virol.* **4**, 259–267.
Fredericq, E., Oth, A., and Fontaine, F. (1961). *J. Mol. Biol.* **3**, 11–17.
Frenkel, N., and Roizman, B. (1971). *J. Virol.* **8**, 591–593.
Frenkel, N., and Roizman, B. (1972) *Proc. Nat. Acad. Sci. U.S.* **69**, 2654–2658.
Gainer, J. H., Long, J., Jr., Hill, P., and Capps, W. I. (1971). *Virology* **45**, 91–100.
Gentry, G. A., and Stock, D. A. (1969). *Int. Symp. Mycoplasma Dis. Man* 1968 pp. 173–177 and 337–338.
Gentry, G. A., Walker, B. M., and Randall, C. C. (1962). *Virology* **16**, 460–465.
Germanov, A. B., and Sokolov, M. I. (1969). *Arch. Gesamte Virusforsch.* **28**, 77–84.
Gibson, W., and Roizman, B. (1971). *Proc. Nat. Acad. Sci. U.S.* **68**, 2818–2821.
Gibson, W., and Roizman, B. (1972). *J. Virol.* **10**, 1044–1052.
Goodheart, C. R. (1969). *Bacteriol. Proc.* 153.
Goodheart, C. R. (1970). *J. Amer. Med. Ass.* **211**, 91–96.
Goodheart, C. R. (1972). *Proc. Int. Congr. Virol. 2nd. 1971*, p. 75.
Goodheart, C. R., Filbert, J. E., and McAllister, R. M. (1963). *Virology* **21**, 530–532.
Goodheart, C. R., Plummer, G., and Waner, J. L. (1968). *Virology* **35**, 473–475.
Goodpasture, E. W., and Teague, O. (1923). *J. Med. Res.* **44**, 139–184.
Graham, B. J., Ludwig, H., Bronson, D. L., Benyesh-Melnick, M., and Biswal, N. (1972). *Biochim. Biophys. Acta* **259**, 13–23.
Gravell, M. (1971). *Virology* **43**, 730–733.
Gresser, I., and Enders, J. F. (1961). *Virology* **13**, 420–426.
Halliburton, I. W. (1972). *In* "Oncogenesis and Herpesviruses" Int. Agency Res. Cancer, Lyon. (P. M. Biggs *et al.*, eds.), pp. 432–438.
Hewitt, B. R. (1958). *Nature (London)* **182**, 246–247.
Hinze, H. C. (1971). *Infec. Immunity* **3**, 350–354.
Hoagland, C. L., Lavin, G. I., Smadel, J. E., and Rivers, T. M. (1940). *J. Exp. Med.* **72**, 139–147.
Hochberg, E., and Becker, Y. (1968). *J. Gen. Virol.* **2**, 231–241.
Hoggan, M. D., and Roizman, B. (1959a). *Virology* **8**, 508–524.
Hoggan, M. D., and Roizman, B. (1959b). *Amer. J. Hyg.* **70**, 208–219.
Holden, M. (1932). *J. Infec. Dis.* **50**, 218–236.
Holmes, A. W., Caldwell, R. G., Dedmon, R. E., and Deinhardt, F. (1964). *J. Immunol.* **92**, 602–610.
Huang, H. L., Szabocsik, J. M., Randall, C. C., and Gentry, G. A. (1971). *Virology* **45**, 381–389.
Ivaničová, S. (1961). *Acta Virol. (Prague), Engl. Ed.* **5**, 328.
Ivaničová, S., Škoda, R., Mayer, V., and Sokol, F. (1963). *Acta Virol. (Prague), Engl. Ed.* **7**, 7–15.
Jurajda, V., and Klimes, B. (1970). *Avian Dis.* **14**, 188–190.
Kaplan, A. S. (1957). *Virology* **4**, 435–457.
Kaplan, A. S. (1962). *Virology* **16**, 305–313.
Kaplan, A. S. (1969). *Virol. Monogr.* **5**, 1–115.

Kaplan, A. S., and Ben-Porat, T. (1961). *Virology* **13**, 78–92.
Kaplan, A. S., and Ben-Porat, T. (1963). *Virology* **19**, 205–214.
Kaplan, A. S., and Ben-Porat, T. (1964). *Virology* **23**, 90–95.
Kaplan, A. S., and Ben-Porat, T. (1966). *J. Mol. Biol.* **19**, 320–322.
Kaplan, A. S., and Ben-Porat, T. (1970). *Proc. Nat. Acad. Sci. U.S.* **66**, 799–806.
Kaplan, A. S., and Vatter, A. E. (1959). *Virology* **7**, 394–407.
Kaplan, A. S., Ben-Porat, T., and Kamiya, T. (1965). *Ann. N.Y. Acad. Sci.* **130**, 226–239.
Kaplan, A. S., Shimono, H., and Ben-Porat, T. (1970). *Virology* **40**, 90–101.
Keller, J. M., Spear, P. G., and Roizman, B. (1970). *Proc. Nat. Acad. Sci. U.S.* **65**, 865–871.
Kieff, E. D., Bachenheimer, S. L., and Roizman, B. (1971). *J. Virol.* **8**, 125–132.
Kieff, E., Hoyer, B., Bachenheimer, S. L. and Roizman, B. (1972). *J. Virol.* **9**, 738–745.
Klingeborn, B., and Pertoft, H. (1972). *Virology* **48**, 618–623.
Kohlhage, H. (1964). *Arch. Gesamte Virusforsch.* **14**, 358–365.
Kottaridis, S. D., Luginbuhl, R. E., and Fredrickson, T. N. (1969). *Amer. J. Vet. Res.* **30**, 1851–1855.
Laemmli, U. K. (1970). *Nature (London)* **227**, 680–684.
Lampert, F., Bahr, G. F., and Rabson, A. S. (1969). *Science* **166**, 1163–1165.
Lando, D., and Ryhiner, M. L. (1969). *C. R. Acad. Sci.* **269**, 527–530.
Lando, D., deRudder, J., and Privat de Garilhe, M. (1965). *Bull. Soc. Chim. Biol.* **67**, 1033–1042.
Lee, L. F., Roizman, B., Spear, P. G., Kieff, E. D., Burmester, B. R., and Nazerian, K. (1969). *Proc. Nat. Acad. Sci. U.S.* **64**, 952–956.
Lee, L. F., Armstrong, R. L., and Nazerian, K. (1971a), *Bacteriol. Proc.* p. 170.
Lee, L. F., Kieff, E. D., Bachenheimer, S. L., Roizman, B., Spear, P. G., Burmester, B. R., and Nazerian, K. (1971b). *J. Virol.* **7**, 289–294.
Lépine, P., and Sautter, V. (1946). *Ann. Inst. Pasteur, Paris* **72**, 174–183.
Lipschütz, B. (1921). *Zentralbl. Bakteriol., Parasitenk. Infektranskr. Abt. I: Orig.* **87**, 303.
Low, M., Hay, J., and Keir, H. M. (1969). *J. Mol. Biol.* **46**, 205–207.
Low, M., Mechie, M. I., and Hay, J. (1971). *Biochem. J.* **124**, 63P.
Ludwig, H. O., Biswal, N., and Benyesh-Melníck, M. (1972a). *Virology* **49**, 95–101.
Ludwig, H., Biswal, N., Bryan, J. T., and McCombs, R. M. (1971). *Virology* **45**, 534–537.
Ludwig, H., Haines, H. G., Biswal, N., and Benyesh-Melnick, M. (1972b). *J. Gen. Virol.* **14**, 111–114.
Luger, A., and Lauda, E. (1921). *Z. Gesamte Exp. Med.* **24**, 289–292.
Luria, S. E. (1955). *In* "Radiation Biology" (A. Hollaender, ed.), Vol. 2, pp. 333–364. McGraw-Hill, New York.
Lust, G., and Carmichael, L. E. (1971). *J. Inferr. Dis.* **124**, 572–580.
McAllister, R. M., Straw, R. M., Filbert, J. E., and Goodheart, C. R. (1963). *Virology* **19**, 521–531.
Maizel, J. V., Jr. (1966). *Science* **151**, 988–990.
Marmur, J., and Doty, P. (1959). *Nature (London)* **183**, 1427–1429.
Martin, W. B., Hay, D., Crawford, L. V., Le Boúvier, G. L., and Crawford, E. M. (1966). *J. Gen. Microbiol.* **45**, 325–332.
Matis, J., and Zuffa, A. (1969). *Acta Virol. (Prague), Engl. Ed.* **13**, 371–378.
Matis, J., Leššo, J., and Čiampor, F. (1971). *Acta Virol. (Prague), Engl. Ed.* **15**, 521.
Melendez, L. V., Daniel, M. D., Garcia, F. G., Fraser, C. E. O., Hunt, R. D., and King, N. W. (1969). *Lab. Anim. Care* **19**, 372–377.
Melnick, J. L., Midulla, M., Wimberly, I., Barrera-Ora, J. G., and Levy, B. M. (1964). *J. Immunol.* **92**, 596–601.
Meurisse, E. V. (1969). *J. Med. Microbiol.* **2**, 317–325.
Mikami, T., and Bankowski, R. A. (1970). *J. Nat. Cancer Inst.* **45**, 319–333.

Miyamoto, K., and Morgan, C. (1971). *J. Virol.* **8**, 910–918.
Miyamoto, K., Morgan, C., Hsu, K. C., and Hampar, B. (1971). *J. Nat. Cancer Inst.* **46**, 629–646.
Munk, K., and Ackermann, W. W. (1953). *J. Immunol.* **71**, 426–430.
Munyon, W., Kraiselburd, E., Davis, D., and Mann, J. (1971). *J. Virol.* **7**, 813–820.
Nahmias, A., Wickliffe, E., Pipkin, J., Leibovitz, A., and Hutton, R. (1971). *Appl. Microbiol.* **22**, 451–454.
Nahmias, A. J., and Dowdle, W. R. (1968). *Progr. Med. Virol.* **10**, 110–159.
Nayak, D. P. (1971). *J. Virol.* **8**, 579–588.
Nii, S., Rosenkranz, H. S., Morgan, C., and Rose, H. M. (1968). *J. Virol.* **2**, 1163–1171.
Norcross, C., McCrea, J. F., and Angerer, S. (1963). *Virology* **21**, 522–525.
O'Callaghan, D. J., Hyde, J. M., Gentry, G. A., and Randall, C. C. (1968). *J. Virol.* **2**, 793–804.
O'Callaghan, D. J., Rogers, H. W., and Randall, C. C. (1972). *Virology* **47**, 842–844.
Olshevsky, U. and Becker, Y. (1970). *Virology* **40**, 948–960.
Oxford, J. S., Potter, C. W., McLaren, G., and Hardy, W. (1971). *Appl. Microbiol.* **21**, 606–610.
Pertoft, H. (1970a). *Virology* **41**, 368–372.
Pertoft, H. (1970b). *Anal. Biochem.* **38**, 506–516.
Pfefferkorn, E. R., Rutstein, G., and Burge, B. W. (1965). *Virology* **27**, 457–459.
Pfefferkorn, E. R., Burge, B. W., and Coady, H. M. (1966). *J. Bacteriol.* **92**, 856–861.
Plummer, G., and Lewis, B. (1965). *J. Bacteriol.* **89**, 671–674.
Plummer, G., Bowling, C. P., and Goodheart, C. R. (1969a). *J. Virol.* **4**, 738–746.
Plummer, G., Goodheart, C. R., Henson, D., and Bowling, C. P. (1969b). *Virology* **39**, 134–137.
Plummer, G., Waner, J. L., Phuangsab, A., and Goodheart, C. R. (1970). *J. Virol.* **5**, 51–59.
Popescu, A., Aderca, I., and Bem, S. (1969). *Lucr. Inst. Cercet. Vet. Bioprep. Pasteur* **6**, 455–466.
Powell, W. F. (1959). *Virology* **9**, 1–19.
Rabson, A. S., Tyrrell, S. A., and Legallais, F. Y. (1969). *Proc. Soc. Exp. Biol. Med.* **132**, 802–806.
Rafferty, K. A., Jr. (1965). *Ann. N. Y. Acad. Sci.* **126**, 3–21.
Rakusanova, T., Ben-Porat, T., Himeno, M., and Kaplan, A. S. (1971). *Virology* **46**, 877–889.
Randall, C. C., and Bracken, E. C. (1957). *Amer. J. Pathol.* **33**, 709–727.
Randall, C. C., Rogers, H. W., Downer, D. N., and Gentry, G. A. (1972). *J. Virol.* **9**, 216–222.
Ratcliffe, H. (1971). *J. Gen. Virol.* **13**, 181–183.
Reissig, M., and Kaplan, A. S. (1962). *Virology* **16**, 1–8.
Robinson, D. J., and Watson, D. H. (1971). *J. Gen. Virol.* **10**, 163–171.
Rodin, P., Hare, M. J., Barwell, C. F., and Withers, M. J. (1971). *Brit. J. Vener. Dis.* **47**, 198–199.
Roizman, B. (1969a). *Curr. Top. Microbiol. Immunol.* **49**, 1–79.
Roizman, B. (1969b). *In* "The Biochemistry of Viruses" (B. B. Levy, ed.), pp. 415–482. Dekker, New York.
Roizman, B., and Aurelian, L. (1965). *J. Mol. Biol.* **11**, 528–538.
Roizman, B., and Frenkel, N. (1972). *In* "Molecular Basis for Viral Neoplasia," Proc. 25th annual symp., M. D. Anderson Hospital and Tumor Inst. in press.
Roizman, B., and Roane, P. R., Jr. (1961). *Virology* **15**, 75–79.
Roizman, B., and Roane, P. R., Jr. (1963). *Virology* **19**, 198–204.
Roizman, B., and Spear, P. G. (1971). *In* "Nucleic Acid-Protein Interactions—Nucleic Acid Synthesis in Viral Infection" (D. W. Ribbons, J. F. Woessner, and J. Schultz, eds.), pp. 435–460. North-Holland Publ., Amsterdam.
Roizman, B., Keller, J. M., Spear, P. G., Terni, M., Nahmias, A., and Dowdle, W. (1970). *Nature* (*London*) **227**, 1253–1254.
Romváry, J., Toth, B., and Vizy, L. (1969). *Acta Vet.* (*Budapest*) **19**, 311–317.

Ross, L. J. N., Wildy, P. D., and Cameron, K. R. (1971). *Virology* **45**, 808–812.
Rubenstein, A. S., Gravell, M., and Darlington, R. W. (1972). *Abstr. Annu. Meet. Amer. Soc. Microbiol.* p. 199.
Russell, W. C. (1962). *Virology* **16**, 355–357.
Russell, W. C., and Crawford, L. V. (1963). *Virology* **21**, 353–361.
Russell, W. C., and Crawford, L. V. (1964). *Virology* **22**, 288–292.
Russell, W. C., Watson, D. H., and Wildy, P. (1963). *Biochem. J.* **87**, 26P–27P.
Sangiorgi, G. (1914). *Pathologica* **6**, 201–204.
Schaffer, P. A., Vonka, V., Lewis, R., and Benyesh-Melnick, M. (1970). *Virology* **42**, 1144–1146.
Schaffer, P. A., Courtney, R. J., McCombs, R. M., and Benyesh-Melnick, M. (1971). *Virology* **46**, 356–368.
Schiek, W. (1967). *Z. Immuitaetsforsch., Allerg. Klin. Immunol.* **132**, 207–217.
Schiek, W., and Schiek, E. (1969). *Arch. Gesamte Virusforsch.* **28**, 229–238.
Schiek, W., and Schneweis, K. E. (1968). *Arch. Gesamte Virusforsch.* **23**, 280–283.
Schildkraut, C. L., Marmur, J., and Doty, P. (1962). *J. Mol. Biol.* **5**, 109–118.
Schmiedhoffer, J. (1910). *Z. Infektionskr. Haustiere* **8**, 383–405.
Schneweis, K. E. (1961). *Z. Hyg. Infektionskr.* **147**, 319–326.
Schneweis, K. E. (1962). *Z. Immunitaetsforsch. Allerg. Klin. Immunol.* **124**, 24–48.
Schneweis, K. E. (1969). *Arch. Gesamte Virusforsch.* **28**, 203–211.
Schulte-Holthausen, H., and zur Hausen, H. (1970). *Virology* **40**, 776–779.
Scott, T. F. McN., McLeod, D. L., and Tokumaru, T. (1961). *J. Immunol.* **86**, 1–12.
Sery, T. W., and Furgiuele, F. P. (1961). *Amer. J. Ophthalmol.* **51**, 42–57.
Shapiro, A. L., Vineula, E., and Maizel, J. V., Jr. (1967). *Biochem. Biophys. Res. Common.* **28**, 815–820.
Shimono, H., Ben-Porat, T., and Kaplan, A. S. (1969). *Virology* **37**, 49–55.
Silberstein, H., McAuslan, B. R., and August, J. T. (1972). *Fed. Proc., Fed. Amer. Soc. Exp. Biol.* **31**, 407.
Smith, J. W., Rodriguez, J. E., and McKee, A. P. (1971). *Appl. Microbiol.* **21**, 350–357.
Smith, K. O., and Melnick, J. L. (1962). *Virology* **17**, 480–490.
Smith, M. G. (1959). *Progr. Med. Virol.* **2**, 171–202.
Soehner, R. L., Gentry, G. A., and Randall, C. C. (1965). *Virology* **26**, 394–405.
Sokolov, M. I., and Germanov, A. B. (1969). *Acta Virol. (Prague), Engl. Ed.* **13**, 119–123.
Spear, P. G., and Roizman, B. (1967). *Nature (London)* **214**, 713–714.
Spear, P. G., and Roizman, B. (1972). *J. Virol.* **9**, 143–159.
Spear, P. G., Keller, J. M., and Roizman, B. (1970). *J. Virol.* **5**, 123–131.
Spring, S. B., and Roizman, B. (1967). *J. Virol.* **1**, 294–301.
Spring, S. B., and Roizman, B. (1968). *J. Virol.* **2**, 979–985.
Spring, S. B., Roizman, B., and Schwartz, J. (1968). *J. Virol.* **2**, 384–392.
Stein, S., Todd, P., and Mahoney, J. (1970). *Can. J. Microbiol.* **16**, 953–957.
Stevens, J. G., Kado-Boll, G. J., and Haven, C. B. (1969). *J. Virol.* **3**, 490–497.
Stewart, S. E., David-Ferreira, J., Lovelace, E., Landon, J., and Stock, N. (1965). *Science* **148**, 1341–1343.
Stoker, M. G. P., and Ross, R. W. (1958). *J. Gen. Microbiol.* **19**, 250–267.
Strand, M., and August, J. T. (1971). *Nature (London), New Biol.* **233**, 137–140.
Strandberg, J. D., and Carmichael, L. E. (1965). *J. Bacteriol.* **90**, 1790–1792.
Studier, F. W. (1965). *J. Mol. Biol.* **11**, 373–390.
Subak-Sharpe, J. H., Bürk, R. R., Crawford, L. V., Morrison, J. M., Hay, J., and Keir, H. M. (1966). *Cold Spring Harbor Symp. Quant. Biol.* **31**, 737–748.
Sullivan, R., Fassolitis, A. C., Larkin, E. P., Read, R. B., Jr., and Peeler, J. T. (1971). *Appl. Microbiol.* **22**, 61–65.
Sydiskis, R. J. (1969). *J. Virol.* **4**, 283–291.

Sydiskis, R. J. (1970). *J. Virol.* **6**, 280–285.
Takeda, M., Yamamura, H., and Ohga, Y. (1971). *Biochem. Biophys. Res. Commun.* **42**, 103–110.
Taverne, J., and Wildy, P. (1959). *Nature (London)* **184**, 1655–1656.
Taylor, A. R., Beard, D., Sharp, D. G., and Beard, J. W. (1942). *J. Infec. Dis.* **71**, 110–114.
Thomas, C. A., Jr., and Berns, K. I. (1961). *J. Mol. Biol.* **3**, 277–288.
Thomas, C. A., Jr., and MacHattie, L. D. (1967). *Annu. Rev. Biochem.* **36**, 485.
Timbury, M. (1971). *J. Gen. Virol.* **13**, 373–376.
Tokumaru, T. (1965a). *J. Immunol.* **95**, 181–188.
Tokumaru, T. (1965b). *J. Immunol.* **95**, 189–195.
Tokumaru, T. (1969). *Proc. Soc. Exp. Biol. Med.* **131**, 1099–1106.
Toplin, I., Mizell, M., Sottong, P., and Monroe, J. (1971). *Appl. Microbiol.* **21**, 132–139.
Trlifajová, J., Šourek, J., and Ryba, M. (1970). *Acta Virol. (Prague), Engl. Ed.* **14**, 25–34.
Tytell, A. A., and Neuman, R. E. (1963). *Proc. Soc. Exp. Biol. Med.* **113**, 343–346.
Vaheri, A., and Cantell, K. (1963). *Virology* **21**, 661–662.
Vilagines, R. (1969). *C. R. Acad. Sci., Ser. D.* **269**, 400–402.
von Kleinschmidt, A., and Zahn, R. K. (1959). *Z. Naturforsch. B* **14**, 776–779.
Wagner, E. K. (1972). *Virology* **47**, 502–506.
Wagner, E. K., Roizman, B., Savage, T., Spear, P. G., Mizell, M., Durr, F. E., and Sypowicz, D. (1970). *Virology* **42**, 257–261.
Wallis, C., and Melnick, J. L. (1964). *Virology* **23**, 520–527.
Wallis, C., and Melnick, J. L. (1965). *J. Bacteriol.* **90**, 1632–1637.
Wallis, C., and Melnick, J. L. (1968). *J. Virol.* **2**, 953–954.
Watson, D. H. (1968). *Symp. Soc. Gen. Microbiol.* **18**, 207–228.
Watson, D. H., and Wildy, P. (1963). *Virology* **21**, 100–111.
Watson, D. H., Shedden, W. I. H., Tetsuka, T., Elliot, A., Wildy, P., Bourgaux-Ramoisy, D., and Gold, E. (1966). *Immunology* **11**, 399–408.
Waubke, R., zur Hausen, H., and Henle, W. (1968). *J. Virol.* **2**, 1047–1054.
Weinberg, A., and Becker, Y. (1969). *Virology* **39**, 312–321.
Weiss, L., and Horoszewicz, J. S. (1971). *Int. J. Cancer* **7**, 149–159.
Wildy, P., Russell, W. C., and Horne, R. W. (1960). *Virology* **12**, 204–222.
Zambernard, J., and Vatter, A. E. (1966). *Virology* **28**, 318–324.
Zavadova, Z., and Zavada, J. (1968). *Acta Virol. (Prague), Engl. Ed.* **12**, 507–514.
zur Hausen, H., Schulte-Holthausen, H., Klein, G., Henle, W., Henle, G., Clifford, P., and Santesson, L. (1970). *Nature (London)* **228**, 1056–1058.

Chapter 4
Replication—Biological Aspects

Robert W. Darlington and Allan Granoff

I. Introduction

In this chapter the most thoroughly studied herpesviruses (principally herpes simplex and pseudorabies viruses) will be used as models to delineate the biological aspects of the growth of this group of ubiquitous viruses. Because of a lack of information about many of the subgroups, they will not be discussed in this chapter. A certain amount of information regarding the biological activities of these herpesviruses may be found in the chapters dealing with specific virus subgroups.

It should be kept in mind that herpesviruses exhibit variation in their biologic behavior not only within the large heterogenous group but also within subgroups. Thus, a member of a subgroup (e.g., herpes simplex, type 1) might exhibit differences in behaviour from other members of the subgroup (e.g., herpes simplex, type 2) (Figueroa and Rawls, 1969; Lowry *et al.*, 1971; Radcliffe, 1971).

II. Host Range

A. In Vivo

1. Herpes Simplex Virus

Herpes simplex virus (HSV), as far as is known, causes natural disease only in man. However, a wide variety of animals can be infected with HSV experimentally. Gruter (1920) and Lowenstein (1919) demonstrated that inoculation of rabbit corneas with the contents of vesicles results in a severe keratitis which is transmissible to other rabbits. Soon after this report, Doerr (1920) and Doerr and Vochting (1920) pointed out that central nervous system (CNS) signs sometimes result from experimental keratitis in rabbits. Infection of the CNS results also from subdural or intracerebral injection of HSV-containing vesicle fluid into rabbits (Blanc, 1921). Intravenous injection of HSV may also produce an encephalitis but usually requires a potentiating agent such as histamine (Good and Campbell, 1945). The usual result of intravenous injections is infection of the viscera with necrotic lesions in the liver and other organs (Cooke *et al.*, 1942). Dermal inoculation of rabbits may result in crops of vesicles in 5–7 days. If tar is applied to the skin prior to inoculation, vesicles appear sooner (3–4 days) and are zoster-like. Virus can be found in the corresponding spinal ganglia (Teague and Goodpasture, 1923). Rabbits may also be infected by intranasal instillation of HSV, the virus apparently spreading via the trigeminal nerves. Findings which may provide a model for disseminated disease in the human newborn are those of Biegeliesen *et al.* (1957) and Middlekamp *et al.* (1967), who demonstrated that herpes simplex virus given intravenously to a pregnant rabbit could cross the placenta and infect the fetus.

Mice are also extremely susceptible to experimental infection with HSV. Andervont (1929) found that inoculation of mice with HSV by the intracranial route was the most effective way of initiating infection but that infection was also possible by corneal, intracutaneous, intraperitoneal, and intravenous routes. Lennette and Koprowski (1944) reported that mice over 14 days old are considerably less susceptible to intraperitoneal, intracranial, or subcutaneous infection by HSV than are younger animals, a finding that has been substantiated by several workers and is quite generally accepted. However, it should be kept in mind that susceptibility depends not only on the age of the animal, but also on its genetic constitution and most importantly on the strain of virus used. It is imperative that this age-related susceptibility be tested in designing experiments because the factors enumerated above result in great variation.

In addition to its infectivity for rabbits and mice, HSV will also infect many other species of mammals. It has been transmitted to rats by the intracorneal (Teissier *et al.*, 1922) and intracerebral (Wenner, 1944) routes. Hamsters (Zarafonetis *et al.*, 1944), guinea pigs (Urbain and Schaefer, 1929), and cotton rats (Florman and Trader, 1947) have also been experimentally infected.

It is obvious from the preceding that there are many species having greater or lesser susceptibility to experimental infection with HSV and that infection can be accomplished by a number of routes. One of the most striking aspects of HSV infections is the predilection of the virus for neural tissue regardless of the route of infection. The pattern of spread of HSV to the CNS has been well documented by Johnson (1964) and Wildy (1967).

Herpes simplex virus is quite pathogenic for the embryonated egg (Anderson, 1940) infecting the chorioallantois and also causing cutaneous, pharyngeal, amniotic, and peritoneal infections of the embryo following injection into the allantoic fluid.

2. Pseudorabies Virus

Several other herpesviruses have wide experimental host ranges similar to HSV. Probably the best known of these is pseudorabies virus (PRV). This virus naturally infects pigs, cattle, sheep and probably other species. Experimentally, PRV infects rabbits (Hurst, 1934) via intradermal, intramuscular, subcutaneous, or intracerebral routes; inoculation by these routes results eventually in CNS infections via either hematogenous or neural spread, or both. Intravenous infection results in foci of viral multiplication in various organs. Mice (King, 1940) and Syrian hamster (R. W. Darlington, unpublished observations) are also highly susceptible to infection by various routes. Monkeys (*Macaca mulatta*) can be infected with PRV virus by inoculation into peripheral or central nervous system tissue (Hurst, 1936). In the chick embryo, PRV multiplies in the tissues of the central nervous system, as well as in the chorioallantoic membrane (Albrecht *et al.*, 1963).

3. B Virus

One of the most interesting viruses with respect to host range is herpesvirus simiae or "B" virus of monkeys. This virus causes lesions in monkeys much like the "fever blisters" resulting from HSV infection of man. However, when man is accidentally infected by a monkey bite (Sabin and Wright, 1934) or by working with infected monkey tissue cultures (Davidson and Hummeler, 1960), a central nervous system infection of high mortality ensues. This virus also infects rabbits (Sabin, 1934) and guinea pigs (Chappell, 1960). The host range is probably much wider than has been indicated here, but the extreme lethality of the virus for man has understandably limited experimental work.

4. Equine Abortion Virus

Another herpesvirus with a relatively wide experimental host range is equine abortion virus (EAV, equine herpes 1) which will infect Syrian hamsters (Anderson and Goodpasture, 1942). When injected intraperitoneally, the virus causes a rapidly fatal hepatitis with the liver parenchymal cells showing characteristic inclusions. Mice can be infected by both the intraperitoneal and intramuscular routes (R. W. Darlington, unpublished observations). Chick embryos can also be infected with this virus (Randall, 1955a). In animal, as well as cell culture systems, this virus requires adaptation before it will readily infect new systems.

5. Infectious Bovine Rhinotracheitis Virus

Another herpesvirus which is similar to those discussed above in that a considerable number of apparently intact virus particles are released from infected cells is infectious bovine rhinotracheitis virus (IBR). This virus has a much narrower experimental host range, however. Cattle are the natural hosts and only goats have been infected experimentally (McKercher, 1959). Rabbits inoculated intradermally or intratesticularly (Armstrong *et al.*, 1961) developed localized lesions but inclusions were not seen and attempts at serial passage were unsuccessful.

The viruses which have been discussed have the broadest experimental host ranges of any of the herpesviruses that have been studied in any detail.

From this it should not be concluded that they are unique in this respect. The fact is that many of the more recently isolated herpesviruses have not been studied thoroughly with regard to range of animals susceptible to infection. Newer isolates are often not examined in animals at all, investigators relying completely on cell culture systems.

6. Varicella–Zoster and Cytomegaloviruses

In contrast to the viruses discussed above, which have wide experimental host ranges, varicella–zoster virus and the cytomegaloviruses are limited to the one species they normally infect. There has been one report (Rivers, 1926) that varicella–zoster vesicle fluid when inoculated into monkey testes induces focal collections of cells with intranuclear inclusions.

B. *In Vitro*

The host range of herpesvirus infectivity for cell cultures frequently parallels the *in vivo* host range; those viruses which infect the widest variety of animals in the laboratory also will infect a large number of cultured cells from various species.

A list of some of the cells which will support the growth of various herpesviruses is given in Table I. This list is not meant to be exhaustive either with respect to cells or to viruses. One should be cautious in making the assumption that if a particular cell type is not listed, the virus will not grow in it. It simply may not have been tested, or, if tested, not reported. Examination of Table I makes it obvious that there is a gradation within the herpesvirus group with respect to host range. This range is widest for HSV and PRV. It extends through varicella–zoster (V–Z) which will grow only in a limited number of cells derived from the species which the virus naturally infects. One of the more puzzling aspects of the growth of V–Z is that, with one exception, no workers have been able to achieve passage of cell-free virus from infected cell cultures. In contrast, cell-free virus from vesicle fluid readily infects susceptible cells. In addition, virus from vesicle fluid will remain viable for long periods when stored at −65°C, while frozen cell–virus complexes lose infectivity rapidly (Weller *et al.*, 1958). The exception noted above is the report of Caunt (1963) who recovered cell-free V–Z virus by sonication of infected human thyroid cell cultures. The various cytomegaloviruses are somewhat similar to V–Z virus, spreading initially from cell to cell and only late in infection releasing infectious virus into the culture fluid (McAllister *et al.*, 1963). The appearance of cell-associated virus may precede released virus by 2–5 days (Vonka and Benyesh-Melnick, 1966).

TABLE I
GROWTH OF HERPESVIRUSES IN CELL CULTURE[a]

Virus	Cells	Reference
Herpes simplex	Chick embryo	Stulberg and Schapira (1953)
	Rabbit kidney	Barski *et al.* (1955) Sosa-Martinez *et al.* (1955) Kaplan (1957)
	Marmoset kidney	Schur and Holmes (1965)
	Hamster kidney	Watson and Wildy (1963)
	Chinese hamster	Hampar and Ellison (1963)
	Feline kidney	Crandell (1959)
	Swine kidney	Hancock *et al.* (1959)
	HeLa	Scherer and Syverton (1954), Stoker (1959)
	KB	Hinze and Walker (1961)
	HEp-2	Kaplan (1957)
	Human amnion	Ousterhout and Tamm (1959)
	Rat lung, rabbit lung	Szántó (1960)
	Human fibroblasts	Enders (1953)
	Mouse fibroblasts	Scherer (1953)
	Rous sarcoma	Nankervis *et al.* (1959)
	Tortoise kidney	Fauconnier (1963)
Pseudorabies	Mouse fibroblasts	Scherer (1953)
	HeLa	Scherer and Syverton (1954)
	Rabbit kidney	Kaplan and Vatter (1959)
	Swine kidney	Singh (1962), McFerran and Dow (1962)
	Lamb kidney	Ceccarelli and Del Mazza (1958)
	Dog kidney	Aurelian and Roizman (1964)
	Monkey kidney	von Kerékjártó and Rhode (1957)
	Chick embryo	Albrecht *et al.* (1963), Béládi and Ivánovics (1954), Csery-Pechany *et al.* (1951)
EAV (equine herpes 1)	Horse	Randall (1955b)
	Fetal cat	Randall (1954)
	HeLa	Randall (1957)
	Horse kidney	Shimizu *et al.* (1957)
	Mouse fibroblasts (L)	Randall and Lawson (1962)
	Hamster kidney (BHK)	Darlington and James (1966)
IBR	Bovine embryonic kidney	Madin *et al.* (1956)
	HeLa	Cabasso *et al.* (1957)
	Human amnion	Cheatham and Crandell (1957)
	Porcine kidney	Schwarz *et al.* (1957)
	Monkey kidney	Rouhandeh (1963)

TABLE I (*Continued*)

Virus	Cells	Reference
Infectious laryngotracheitis (avian)	Chick embryo	Atherton and Anderson (1957)
	HeLa	Webster (1959)
Marek's disease (avian)	Chick kidney	Churchill and Biggs (1967)
	Duck embryo fibroblasts	Salomon *et al.* (1968)
Varicella–zoster	Primary human cells	Weller *et al.* (1958)
	Monkey kidney	Slotnick and Rosanoff (1963)
	Human embryonic lung (diploid)	Rapp and Benyesh-Melnick (1963)
	Human thyroid	Caunt (1963)
	HeLa	Svedmyr (1965)
Cytomegalovirus (human)	Primary human cells	Weller *et al.* (1957)
	Human embryonic lung (diploid)	Hanshaw (1966)

[a]Expanded from Kaplan (1969).

The growth in cell culture of those herpesviruses which have been implicated as oncogenic agents is of interest both from the standpoint of providing model systems for oncogenesis in general and the study of human oncogenic agents specifically.

Marek's disease virus (MDV) causes lymphoproliferative disease in its natural host, the chicken. There is essentially no infectious virus in the transformed cells, the feather follicle epithelium providing the main source of infectious virus (Calnek *et al.*, 1970a,b). The virus was first isolated in chick kidney (Churchill and Biggs, 1967) and duck embryo fibroblast cells (Salomon *et al.*, 1968). The virus has now been shown to replicate in a variety of cells from avian species but not in cells from other species, and it, like varicella–zoster, remains largely cell associated (Nazarian, 1972).

The oncogenic monkey herpesviruses, herpesvirus saimiri (HVS) and herpesvirus ateles (HVA) have a somewhat broader host range in cell culture. Herpesvirus saimiri multiplies best in cells derived from owl, squirrel, or marmoset monkeys. It also replicates to a lesser degree in human embryonic skin, muscle, and lung cells and in fetal dog lung cells (Melendez *et al.*, 1972). Herpesvirus ateles has a similar cell culture host range (Melendez *et al.*, 1972). These viruses, in contrast to MDV, are released from the cell in an infectious form and have a considerably less restricted host range, multiplying in a variety of cells from different species, ranging from human to hamster and including goats, rabbits, and dogs.

Examples of viruses having the most restricted range are the Epstein-Barr virus (EBV) of humans and the herpesvirus seen in the Lucké tumor of frogs. Epstein-Barr virus, although observed in cell suspension culture lines from certain African, American, and New Guinea lymphomas (Epstein *et al.*, 1964b; O'Conor and Rabson, 1965; Pope *et al.*, 1968), has not been grown in any other cell lines but there are unconfirmed reports of its passage in monkeys (Epstein *et al.*, 1964b) and hamsters (Stewart *et al.*, 1965). The virus seen in the Lucké tumor has not been propagated in cell cultures or animal systems. A herpesvirus which can be propagated in tissue culture was isolated from a tumor-bearing frog (Rafferty, 1965; Gravell *et al.*, 1968), but this subsequently proved to be a different herpesvirus from that seen in the tumor (Gravell, 1971).

III. Environmental Factors Affecting Virus Growth

There is a limited amount of information on the physical and chemical factors influencing the growth of the herpesviruses, and in many instances the significance of these reports is somewhat vague, the reports appearing as isolated observations.

A. Physical Factors

1. Temperature

The optimum temperature for herpesvirus growth is a resultant of two factors: the rate of virus production and the rate of thermal inactivation of the virus. Thus, a temperature at which there is minimal inactivation of virus infectivity and where the most virus is produced should be optimum. As can be seen from the following reports, this optimum for those herpesviruses which have been studied is between 35° and 37°C.

Studies in cell culture have demonstrated a marked effect of temperature on the yield of virus and on the growth curve of HSV. Thompson and Coates (1942) reported that with chick embryo fragment cultures maximum virus concentrations were found at 35°C and that no infectious virus could be detected in cultures grown at 40°C. In HeLa cells, 35°C incubation produced the highest titers of HSV and incubation at 27.7°C or below for 3 days produced little or no infectious virus (Wheeler, 1958). Farnham and Newton (1959) found that the length of the latent period of HSV in HeLa cells at 30°C was increased by 3–4 hours as compared to 37°C. The maximum cell-associated and released-virus yield was at 31°–33°C while little virus was found at 40°C. The lower yields at the higher temperature correlated with virus inactivation at the elevated temperature. The half-life of HSV infectivity was calculated to be 13, 3, and 0.4 hours at 30°, 37°, and 44°C, respectively. Similar findings have been reported by Hoggan and Roizman (1959a). Recent research has indicated that there are qualitative differences in temperature requirements for types 1 and 2 HSV (Radcliffe, 1971). Type 1 strains produced cytopathogenic effect in Vero cells at temperatures from 35°–40.3°C whereas the infectivity of type 2 strains was reduced 100-fold at 40.3°C but was not affected at the lowest temperature.

Mice held at 37°C (rectal temperature = 40°C) were more resistant to HSV infection than were mice held at 24°C (rectal temperature = 37°C). In the mice held at the higher temperature, there was apparently more inactivation of the infecting dose as considerably less virus could be isolated from the brains of these animals as compared to those held at the lower temperature (Schmidt and Rasmussen, 1960).

As one might expect, the herpesviruses which infect poikilotherms have quite different temperature requirements from those which infect homeotherms. A herpesvirus isolated from leopard frogs (Rafferty, 1965; Gravell *et al.*, 1968) multiplies at 25°C, while another herpesvirus associated with the frog renal tumor (see Chapter 19) is detected in tumor cells *in vivo* or *in vitro* only at temperatures from 4°–10°C and not at 20°–25°C as reviewed by Granoff (1972).

A herpesvirus isolated from an iguana (Clark and Karzon, 1972) will replicate at 36°C but not as well as at 30°C. At 36°C, however, little or no infectious virus is found in the cell culture fluid, while at 30°C, there is abundant released infectious virus. This may reflect inactivation at the higher temperature as the half-life of this virus at 37°C is 13 hours, and at 23° and 4°C there is no appreciable inactivation for 48 hours. The common catfish virus, a herpesvirus of ictalurid fish, also has a temperature optimum of between 25° and 35°C. Growth curves at these temperatures (Wolf and Darlington, 1971) are essentially the same as those for HSV at 35° and 37°C. At temperatures of 10° to 25°C the slope of the exponential rise is unchanged but the eclipse period is lengthened and the final titer reached is reduced as the temperature is lowered.

2. Preirradiation

The synthetic processes of herpesviruses that have been examined are much more resistant to ultraviolet and X-irradiation than are host cells. Rabbit kidney cells irradiated with as much as 40,000 R of X-irradiation continued to produce HSV although the yield was about 30% less than unirradiated cells (Kaplan, 1957). When the cells received 10,000 R, and were infected within 3 days after irradiation, their capacity to produce virus was unimpaired although synthetic processes were effectively stopped in uninfected cells. Similar results have been reported for HSV grown in X-irradiated L cells (Powell, 1959).

The growth of PRV in embryo rabbit kidney cells is also greatly resistant to UV irradiation. Essentially no reduction in the capacity of the cells to form infective centers was observed after a dose of 660 ergs/mm^2. At this dose the ability of this same cell population to form colonies was reduced by 99% (Kaplan, 1962). These results indicate that the reproductive capacity of cells is much more sensitive to irradiation than is their capacity to produce virus, and therefore the host cell components affected by irradiation are not required for virus synthesis.

B. Chemical Factors

1. pH

It has been shown that infection of HeLa cells by HSV causes the production of lactic acid and a concomitant fall in pH of the medium (Fisher and Fisher, 1959). This lowered pH has been shown to be a factor in the inactivation of the virus and thus one of the limiting factors in virus yield (Farnham and Newton, 1959). Maximum yields of HSV from HeLa cells were obtained when the pH of the medium was maintained between 7.0 and 7.5. Decreases in yield were attributed to the lability of the virus at pH values above and below the optimum and not to interference with virus synthesis. Roizman (1965a) has suggested that different strains of HSV have different pH optima and that these optima are genetically determined by the virus genome and not the cell. However, there is little experimental evidence supporting this suggestion.

2. Nutritional Factors

It has been shown that glucose is required for the synthesis of herpesvirus by HeLa cells (Lewis and Scott, 1962) and that glutamine, in the absence of serum, is also required. The amount of glutamine in serum is apparently sufficient to provide the concentration essential for growth. In addition, the absence of these two substances does not affect adsorption or penetration; hence, the effect is on virus synthesis.

Of the amino acids, arginine is a requirement for herpesvirus synthesis (Tankersley, 1964), and growth is inhibited by the lack of any one of ten other amino acids. If arginine is omitted from the culture medium, neither cytopathogenic effect nor virus replication is observed in human cells. The omission of lysine, however, results in increased yields of virus, indicating that this amino acid has an inhibitory effect.

IV. Virus Growth Cycle

The interaction of viruses with cells is conventionally divided into a number of phases. The first is *adsorption* or the *attachment* of the viral particle to the cell. The second phase is *penetration* or the entry of the virus into the cell. Once the particle gains entry, it is uncoated and this uncoating marks the beginning of the *eclipse* phase during which infectious virus cannot be detected within the infected cells. The appearance of the first intracellular infectious viral particle marks the end of the eclipse period and the beginning of the *latent period* which ends with the release of the first infectious particle into the surrounding medium. The last phase of the growth cycle is the *period of exponential growth* (or exponential virus increase) during which most of virus is produced. The end of this period represents the end of the virus growth curve. It should be noted that the classical growth cycle as described above was originally developed from work with bacteriophage and that events in animal virus replication, particularly for a complex virus such as herpesvirus, are not as clear-cut. This is particularly true for the eclipse and latent periods which are very difficult to delineate in the virus–animal cell systems with which we are dealing. However, for the purposes of this discussion these conventions will be used, keeping their limitation in mind.

The events in the virus growth curve have been well delineated for most of those members of the herpesvirus group that have short growth cycles; that is, 16–20 hours from infection to the end of the exponential growth phase. These include herpes simplex, pseudorabies, equine abortion, IBR, B virus, etc. Examples of representative growth curves are shown in Fig. 1. Growth curves for varicella–zoster and the various cytomegaloviruses are not accurate, mainly because low virus concentrations prohibit initial infection of all the cells in a culture. Thus, rather than obtaining a one-step growth curve, one is generally looking at a series of successive infections.

A. Adsorption

Adsorption of herpes simplex virus, as is the case with other viruses, requires electrolytes in the medium. Farnham and Newton (1959) found that calcium and magnesium particularly were required for the attachment of herpes simplex virus to HeLa cells.

The relative concentration of virus and cells also influences the rate of adsorption. Farnham (1958) found that the smaller the volume a given amount of virus was contained in, the greater the number of plaques obtained.

Different herpesviruses have different rates of adsorption to cells (Fig. 2).

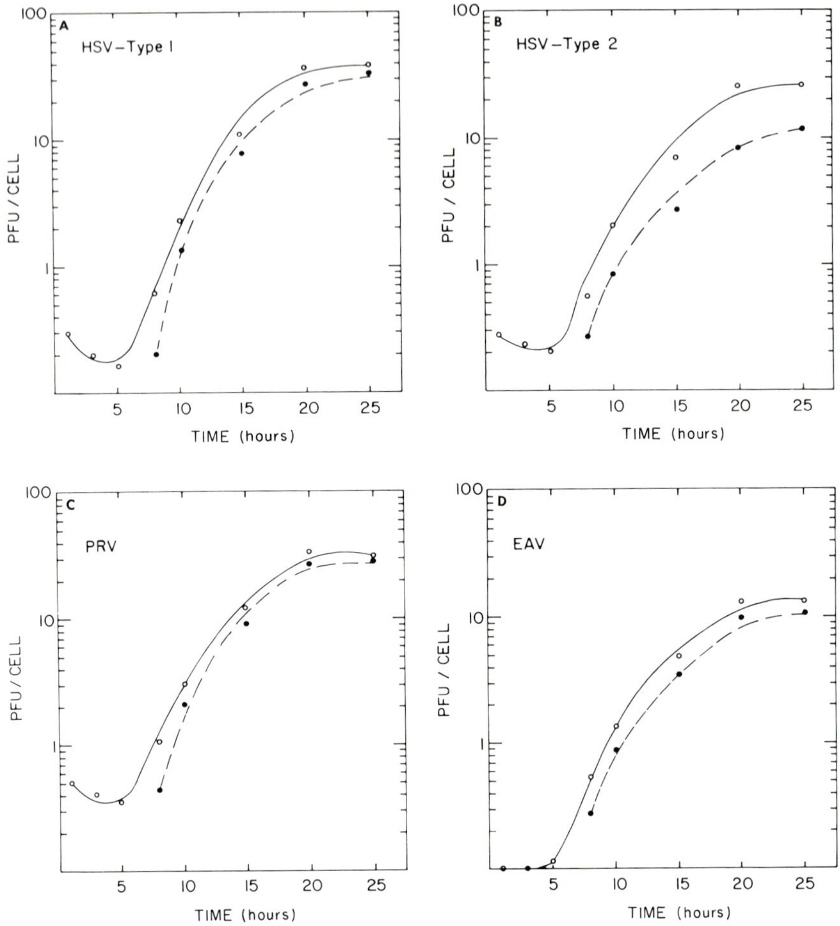

FIG. 1. Representative growth curves for herpesviruses. (A) Type 1 HSV (H_4 strain) in BHK 21 cell monolayers. (B) Type 2 HSV in BHK 21 cell monolayers. (C) PRV in BHK 21 cell monolayers. (D) EAV in L cell suspension cultures. Solid line represents cell associated virus. Dashed line represents released virus. The multiplicity of infection was approximately 5 PFU/cell in all cases.

When comparable amounts of H4 HSV and EAV were used to infect BHK 21 cells under identical conditions, 90% or more of the H4 HSV had attached by 1 hour while only 62% of the EAV had attached. Identical virus strains may also have different rates of adsorption depending on the cells used. Herpes simplex virus (HFEM strain) adsorbs rapidly to HeLa cells (Watkins, 1960) while this strain adsorbs chick embryo cells much more slowly (Waterson, 1958). The same is true for PRV which adsorbs to rabbit kidney cells

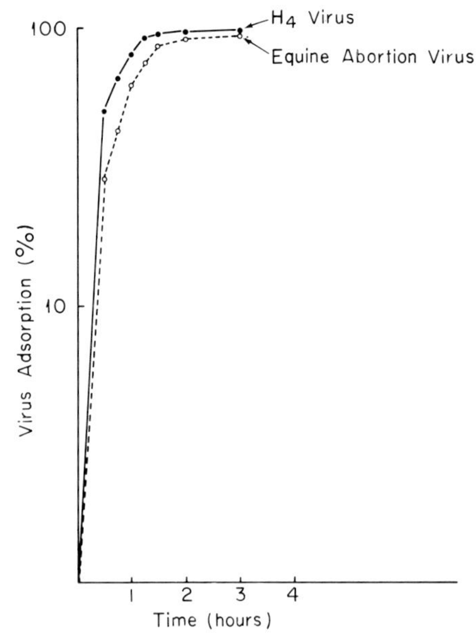

FIG. 2. Adsorption curves for HSV (H_1 strain) and EAV in BHK 21 cells.

more rapidly (Kaplan and Vatter, 1959) than it does to chick embryo cells (Béládi, 1962). Electron microscopy also revealed that herpesviruses attach rapidly (90% attached by 45 minutes after infection) to cells (Holmes and Watson, 1963). Enveloped particles adsorbed more readily than unenveloped and fewer particles attached at 0°C than at higher temperatures.

B. Penetration

Penetration of virus particles into cells after adsorption may be followed by direct visualization with electron microscopy or by the use of antiserum or low pH to determine when the virus becomes inaccessible to inactivation. Both of these methods have been used to examine the penetration of herpesviruses into cells. Information gained by electron microscopy is covered in another chapter in this volume (Chapter 3). The information to be gained by electron microscopy is limited by the small sample size. More quantitative information has been obtained by taking advantage of the fact that while adsorbed particles are sensitive to inactivation by antibody or low pH, viruses which have penetrated are insensitive to such inactivation.

Farnham and Newton (1959) added anti-herpesvirus serum to HeLa cell cultures at selected times after infection with HSV. At 37°C practically all of the virus inoculum was insensitive to the action of antiserum by 3 hours.

At 30° C, about 70% of the virus was neutralized, and, at 4° C, over 80% was still neutralizable by antiserum. These experiments again demonstrate the temperature dependence of the adsorption process. Huang and Wagner (1964) using resistance to acid (pH 3) as a criterion for penetration of HSV found that at 37° C over 90% of attached virus had penetrated the cell by 10 minutes, while at 25° C, 20 minutes were required for 90% penetration. At 4° C less than 1% of the virus had penetrated by 1 hour. The above findings were based on the use of acid to inactivate virus which had not penetrated the cell. Under the same conditions, antisera could not neutralize 15% of the virus at 4° C indicating that virus attached to the cell membrane is more resistant to neutralization by antibody than is free virus. Thus, resistance to acid pH is a better indication of virus penetration than is resistance to inactivation by antisera.

C. Eclipse Period

By definition, the eclipse period is that time span during which no infectious virus can be detected within the infected cell. During this period, however, many synthetic activities are taking place. Virus-specific enzymes appear, and viral DNA and structural protein begin to be synthesized until they reach a critical level so that virus assembly may begin. The length of the eclipse period is dependent on both the virus strain and on the cell strain and may also be dependent on the multiplicity of infection (Kaplan, 1957).

The major problem in determining the length of the eclipse period in cell–virus systems is the confusion introduced by the failure to remove all of the residual virus inoculum. This may be overcome, at least in part, by extensive washing of the infected cells (Kaplan, 1957) or by mild treatment of the infected cells with ultraviolet light, followed by washing (Yoshino *et al.*, 1960). Cell suspensions, because of the ease of removal of residual virus by washing, are probably the best system to most accurately measure the length of the eclipse period. When the growth curves of EAV were done (Darlington and James, 1966) in monolayer and suspension L cells, even after extensive washing it was not possible to reduce the residual virus in monolayer cultures much below 10^4 plaque-forming units (PFU), while in suspension cultures (Fig. 1D) the residual virus was not detectable.

Evidence that the cell may have an influence on the length of the eclipse period was provided by Kaplan (1957). The eclipse period for HSV in rabbit kidney was 4 hours, and in chorioallantoic membrane it was 10–12 hours. Conversely, the eclipse period for EAV in L (suspension and monolayer), HeLa, and BHK cells was roughly the same (Darlington and James, 1966). Roizman (1963), using two strains of HSV which could be easily distinguished by their plaque morphology (micro- and macroplaque strains), found that if cells were first infected by one strain, subsequent infection by the other resulted in appreciably shortened eclipse periods. This would appear to indicate that enzymes or viral structural components synthesized by the first virus can also be utilized by the second, resulting in a shorter time needed to begin virus assembly.

D. Latent Period

Determination of the latent period in viral infections is complicated by the fact that it is difficult to obtain synchronized infection. This may be due to cells being infected at different times, although this problem may be overcome to some extent by using high multiplicities of infection. Allowing attachment at 4°C and raising the temperature to 36°C of all the cultures at once also provides some degree of synchrony.

Monolayer or suspension mass cultures have been utilized to obtain an approximation of the latent period of herpesviruses by simple inspection of the growth curves for cell-associated and released virus (Fig. 1 and Table II). The latent period is the time between the rise above background for cell-associated virus subtracted from the time of such an increase for released virus. Figure 1 shows that HSV, types 1 and 2, as well as PRV, have essentially the same latent periods in BHK21 cells, infected in each case under identical conditions. In other cells and under different conditions, the length of the latent period may vary. The latent period appears to be about 2–3 hours for EAV (Darlington and James, 1966) in both monolayer and suspension cultures of L cells. A more accurate estimate of the latent period may be made by following the rate of intracellular development and extracellular accumulation of virus particles and determining the average release time by the equation derived by Rubin *et al.* (1955): $1/k = (t_2 - t_1)/r(\ln C_2 - \ln C_1)$ where $1/k$ is the average release time; r is the constant ratio of extracellular virus to intracellular virus at any time during the exponential rise; and $\ln C_1$, $\ln C_2$ are the natural logarithms of the concentrations of extracellular virus at times t_1 and t_2. Kaplan (1957) using this formula found the release time for the H4 strain of HSV to be 2.3–3.5 hours in rabbit kidney cells and Powell (1959) found the release time for the HRE strain of HSV in L cells to be 30–40 minutes. Some reservations are required, however, about the validity of such quantitation in the face of the uncontrollable variables such as lack of synchronization of infection and/or of cells. At any rate, by whatever method used for its estimation, the latent period for herpesviruses having a short growth cycle and which are readily released from cells appears to be about 1–3 hours. The latent period determined from monolayer or suspension mass cultures is a minimal estimation, since the infective process may not be synchronized and all the cells in the culture are not releasing virus

TABLE II
MULTIPLICATION OF HERPES SIMPLEX, PSEUDORABIES, AND EQUINE ABORTION VIRUSES[a]

		Exponential				
Virus (strain)	Cells	Eclipse (hours)	Latent (hours)	Increase (hours)	Virus yield (PFU/cell)	References
Herpes simplex (H_4)	Rabbit kidney monolayers	5	8	10	300	Kaplan (1957)
Herpes simplex (HFEM)	HeLa monolayers	12	16	15		Stoker and Ross (1958)
Herpes simplex (H_4)	Rabbit kidney suspension	4	5–7	7	100–300	Kaplan (1957)
Herpes simplex (HRE)	L suspension	5	8.5	4–5		Powell (1959)
Pseudorabies	Rabbit kidney suspension	3	5	5	1000	Kaplan and Vatter (1959)
Pseudorabies	Rabbit kidney monolayers		5	5	820	Kaplan and Vatter (1959)
Pseudorabies	Monkey kidney monolayers		12	12		von Kerékjártó and Rhode (1957)
Equine abortion (Ky.D)	L monolayers		8	9		Darlington and James (1966)
Equine abortion (Ky.D)	L suspension	6	8	4–5		Darlington and James (1966)
Equine abortion (Ky.D)	BHK monolayer		6	4–5		Darlington and James (1966)

[a]Expanded from Kaplan (1969).

at the same time. If individual infected cells are cultured in a drop of medium, the latent period for each cell may be determined. HeLa cells infected with HSV and cultured individually (Wildy *et al.*, 1959) had latent periods of between 16 and 26 hours. Pseudorabies virus in individual rabbit kidney cells had latent periods from 6–10 hours (Reissig and Kaplan, 1960). Even the shortest of these latent periods is longer than the latent periods determined for these viruses in mass culture systems. A similar phenomenon was reported for poliovirus in individual monkey kidney cells (Lwoff *et al.*, 1955). It was suggested that this was due to selection of those cells (termed late releasers) in the early phase of the infective process which were still able to attach to the glass surface. This could not be true, however, for the experiments with PRV (Reissig and Kaplan, 1960), because the individual cells were infected after attachment to the glass. It seems likely therefore that the longer latent periods in single cells are due to the different experimental conditions which are probably unfavorable.

E. Exponential Virus Increase

As can be seen from the growth curves (Fig. 1A–D), after the end of the latent period, virus replication occurs exponentially for a variable period of time. The time periods for some herpesviruses are given in Table II. Variables which influence virus growth are the virus strain, the type of cell, and the type of culture (monolayer, suspension, or single cell). One would assume that the reason for the exponential synthesis of virus is the exponential synthesis of a rate-limiting substance, and since DNA is the only macromolecule known to be replicating exponentially in this system, it should be the limiting factor. It has been shown, however, that DNA synthesis is not the limiting factor (Kaplan, 1962; Kaplan and Ben-Porat, 1966). Thus, increasing rates of an essential precursor or increasing levels of activity of an essential enzyme are probably responsible for the observed kinetics.

The ultimate yield of virus produced by infected cells also varies depending on the type of cell, the type of culture, the thermostability of the virus, and the temperature of incubation. This yield has been reported as 1000 PFU/cell for suspension-grown rabbit kidney cells infected with PRV (Kaplan and Vatter, 1959). These same cells grown as monolayers yielded about 820 PFU/cell, and when grown individually (Reissig and Kaplan, 1960), the yield varied from 63 to 500 PFU/cell. Herpes simplex virus has shown the same variation; Wildy *et al.* (1959) found that HeLa monolayers yielded about 300 PFU/cell while individual HeLa cells produced only about 8 PFU/cell.

There is a considerable variation, not only in virus yield, but in the number of physical virus particles required to produce one infectious unit in different systems. The virus strain used seems to be the major determinant, although the cell system and other factors probably also play a role. Under ideal conditions, the best particle to infectivity ratio for HSV is about 10 (Watson *et al.*, 1963). The value for PRV in BHK cells is similar (L. H. Moss and R. W. Darlington, unpublished observations). There is a tendency for the herpesviruses to be released from cells as aggregates of virus particles. These virus aggregates are not easily disaggregated, as dilution or treatment with nucleases does not increase the titer, and the relationship between virus concentration and the number of plaques is not affected by dilution (Kaplan, 1957). Titers of aggregated virus can be increased by procedures which disaggregate the clumps of viruse such as freezing and thawing or sonic oscillation (Kaplan, 1957; Smith, 1963).

F. *Analysis of the Infective Process by Other Methods*

Studies with bacteriophage have provided useful tools for probing the intracellular events which occur during the latent period of virus development. The two approaches to this problem have been (a) the Luria–Laterjet type of experiment (Luria and Laterjet, 1947) where the virus–cell complexes are irradiated with ultraviolet light or X-rays at various times after infection and (b) photoreactivation in which ultraviolet light irradiated virus in infected cells is reactivated by visible light (Dulbecco, 1950).

The Luria–Laterjet type experiments employing X-rays and ultraviolet light (Powell, 1959) have been used to analyze HSV–cell complexes, and similar experiments, utilizing ultraviolet light alone, were employed to analyze PRV–cell complexes (Kaplan, 1962). In both instances the capacity of the host cells to support virus growth was found to be much more resistant to irradiation than was survival of free virus. This finding is qualitatively the same as that for the T-even bacteriophages and their hosts. A family of survival curves of decreasing slopes (single hit type) was observed when the virus–cell complexes were irradiated at various times after infection. This suggests that multiplicity reactivation is the basis for the progressive stabilization of the complexes to irradiation damage since the increased resistance with time is dependent on DNA synthesis.

Ultraviolet light (UV) irradiation causes the formation of thymine dimers from adjacent thymine bases on a DNA chain (Setlow and Setlow, 1962), and this damage can be repaired by an enzyme activated by visible light (Rupert, 1962a,b). Lethal damage to the bacteriophage genome caused by UV irradiation can be reversed in virus infected cells but not in free virus by exposure to light of a longer wavelength (Dulbecco, 1955).

Photoreactivation by irradiation with visible light in the range of 300 to 420 nm has been demonstrated for herpes simplex and pseudorabies virus-infected cell complexes inactivated by irradiation with UV light at 260 nm (Pfefferkorn *et al.*, 1965, 1966). As with bacteriophage T2, photoreactivation occurred only in infected cells and not with free virus. Little photoreactivation occurred within the first 20 minutes after adsorption but after 20 minutes photoreactivation increased rapidly and reached a maximum at about 100 minutes after adsorption. This would suggest that it requires a minimum of 20 minutes for the virus particle to be uncoated.

G. *The Relationship of the Herpesvirus Envelope to Infectivity*

The question of whether the herpesvirus envelope is necessary for the infectivity of the virus is an essential one and has not been answered satisfactorily. Much of the evidence bearing on this question has been obtained by electron microscopy and is covered in Chapter 2. Here we will briefly consider some other experiments pertinent to the question.

It has been reported (Spring and Roizman, 1968) that at 8 hours after infection with HSV 67% of the infectivity is associated with the nucleus. The particles responsible for this infectivity banded in cesium chloride at a density corresponding to unenveloped nucleocapsids while the cytoplasmic infective particles banded at a density corresponding to enveloped virus. The infectivity of the nuclear fraction could be abolished by treatment with either pronase or phospholipase C, and the authors suggested that infectious nuclear virus was either partially enveloped or had on its surface a lipid or lipoprotein constituent which was essential for infectivity.

Ben-Porat and Kaplan (1970) found that the only DNA-containing particles which could be isolated from the nucleus were those associated with at least some envelope material. This suggests that the multitude of unenveloped DNA-containing particles seen by electron microscopy in the infected cell nucleus are unstable and, unless stabilized by at least a partial envelope, lose their DNA and therefore their infectivity upon release from the nucleus.

It is obvious from the above that the question of the necessity of the herpesvirus envelope for infectivity is not completely established. It is equally clear that the preponderance of infectivity is associated with enveloped or at least partially enveloped particles. This is not unexpected when one considers that the envelope is not simply an unaltered bit of nuclear or other cellular membrane wrapped around the virus. Recent work (Kaplan and Ben-Porat, 1970; Ben-Porat and Kaplan, 1972; Spear and Roizman, 1972) indicates that the envelope is newly synthesized and that the glycoproteins, at least, are specified by the viral genome. Therefore, the envelope is virus specific and not cell specific and as such probably has a specific function in attachment or some other step as well as serving as a protective coat for the nucleocapsid.

V. Cytopathogenic Effect and Quantitation of Virus Growth

A. General Cytopathology

Interactions between viruses and cells which result in cellular alterations are termed cytopathogenic effect (CPE). These include morphological and physiological changes which may or may not result in visible changes in the affected cells. The two types of cytopathology most commonly seen in herpesviruses-infected cells are (1) rounding and degeneration often preceded by macrocytosis or ballooning of the infected cell, and (2) formation of syncytia or polykaryocytes which are large multinucleated cells. These two types of cellular degeneration were first described by Lauda and Rezek (1926). They have since been described in virus-infected cells from human patients (Blank *et al.*, 1951; Womack and Randall, 1953) and in HSV-infected cell cultures (Scherer, 1953; Stulberg and Schapira, 1953; Enders, 1953; Scherer and Syverton, 1954; Kaplan and Vatter, 1959; Scott and McLeod, 1959; Hoggan and Roizman, 1959b).

The first type of cellular degeneration starts with cytoplasmic granulation followed by conversion of the cells into a rounded refractile state. These rounded cells increase with time until there are piled up masses of cells in discrete foci, and eventually the infected cells lyse.

It is not necessary that infectious virus be formed for the development of the cytopathological changes. When virus maturation is inhibited in PRV-infected rabbit kidney monolayers by 5-fluorouracil or mitomycin C, the characteristic cytopathic changes still occur (Reissig and Kaplan, 1962). This suggests that the events leading to cytologic changes are independent of virus maturation events.

The kind of effect (rounding or syncytia formation) seen in herpesvirus-infected cell cultures is dependent on the genetic constitution of the infecting virus. Variants of HSV which produce one or the other effect have been isolated by a number of workers (Scott and McLeod, 1959; Nii and Kamahora, 1961; Hoggan and Roizman, 1959b; Munk and Donner, 1963; Wheeler, 1964; Kohlhage and Schieferstein, 1965). Similar variants of pseudorabies virus also exist (Tokumaru, 1957). Phenotypic expression of the cytopathic changes may be influenced by the external environment even though the variants breed true.

The type of cell infected also seems to affect the cytopathology of the virus–cell complex (Munk and Donner, 1963; Kohlhage and Schieferstein, 1965). Thus, although the basic cytopathology is determined by the virus genome, its phenotypic expression is subject to modification by the host cell.

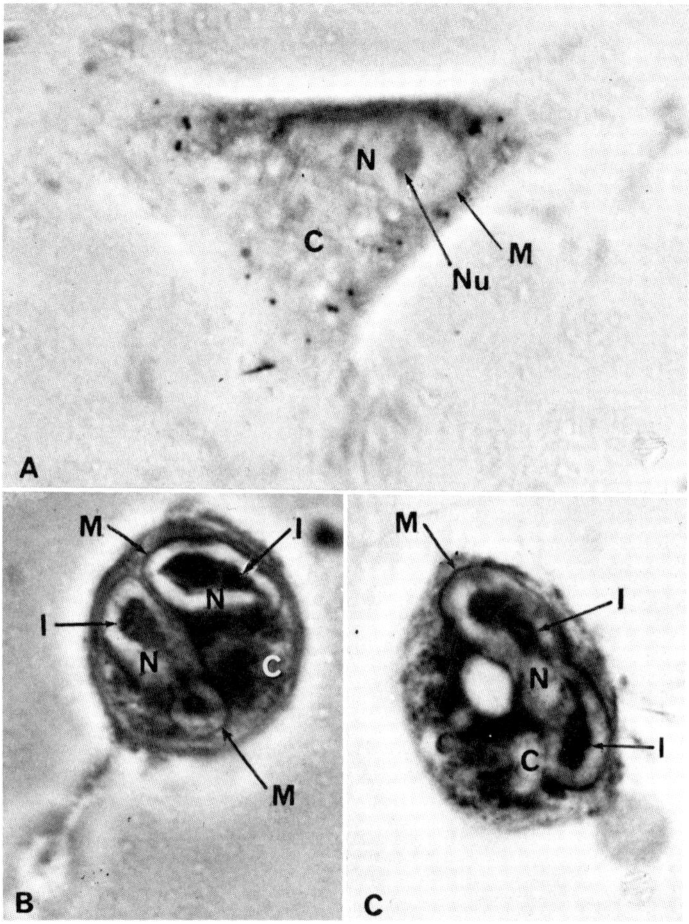

FIG. 3. Nuclear division in rabbit kidney (RK) cells infected with PRV. C, cytoplasm; N, nucleus; Nu, nucleolus; I, intranuclear inclusion; M, nuclear membrane. (A) A single living RK cell photographed before virus inoculation. The cell has only one nucleus. (B) The same cell shown in (A) fixed and stained with the crystal violet–citric acid solution 10 hours after inoculation. The cell is now binucleated and both nuclei have intranuclear inclusions. (C) Another cell, fixed and stained 10 hours after virus inoculation, which shows an elongated nucleus markedly constricted and containing an intranuclear inclusion. The magnification is approximately × 1000. All the cells, which were attached to the bottom of petri plates, were photographed with a phase microscope, using a Leitz 50× water-immersion objective. (From Reissig and Kaplan, 1960).

B. Inclusion Formation

Formation of intranuclear inclusions (Cowdry, 1934) is the characteristic cellular lesion resulting from infection with members of the herpesvirus group. The fully formed inclusion (Cowdry, type A) is eosinophilic and surrounded by marginated chromatin (Fig. 3). The marginated chromatin is often clearly separated from the eosinophilic inclusion in cells fixed by formaldehyde. This effect, however, is probably an artifact of fixation because it is not seen in cells fixed with osmium (Reissig and Melnick, 1955). The inclusions are seen as a result of infection with any of the herpesviruses with the possible exception of the EB virus. Nuclear alterations are present in lymphoblast cells carrying EB virus, but they do not appear to be typical Cowdry type inclusions (Rabson *et al.*, 1966). Cells infected with members of the cytomegalovirus group contain typical intranuclear inclusions but the cells are enlarged and the cytoplasm may contain small basophilic granules (Smith, 1959). Varicella–zoster virus also produces cellular hypertrophy in addition to the inclusions (Weller *et al.*, 1958).

C. Polykaryocyte Formation

One of the most striking types of cytopathogenic effect from certain virus infections is polykaryocytosis (Fig. 4) which is the formation of multinucle-

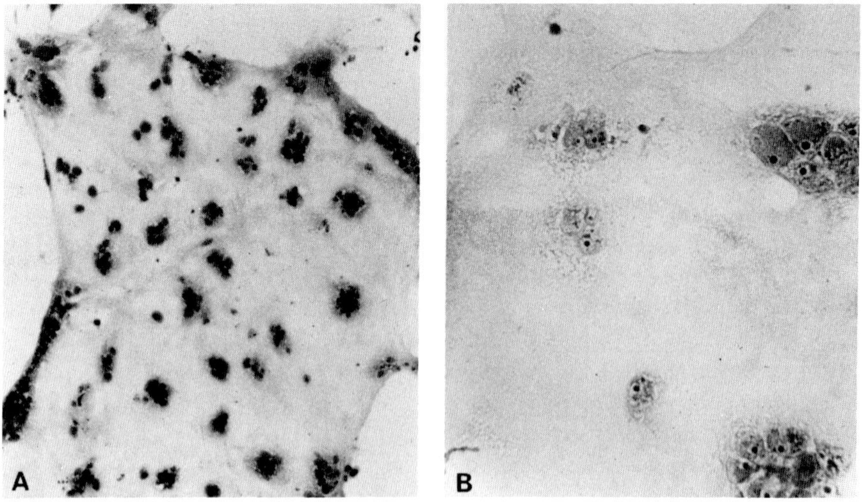

FIG. 4. Polykaryocyte resulting from infection of brown bullhead cells with the common catfish herpesvirus. (A) Low power showing focal collections of nuclei in the cell cytoplasm. (B) Higher power showing individual nuclei.

ated cells variously termed polykaryocytes, syncytia, or giant cells. Polykaryocytosis is induced by several groups of viruses and is particularly prevalent as a result of herpesvirus infections.

There is a question as to whether polykaryocytosis arises as a result of repeated amitotic nuclear division of the same cell or by fusion of several cells. Most evidence indicates that cell fusion is the more important mechanism in the case of virus-induced polykaryocytosis, although amitotic division may be occasionally responsible. This section will be concerned with that evidence relating to herpesvirus polykaryocytosis. However, the reader should be aware that there is a considerable body of evidence relating to polykaryocytosis by other viruses (Poste, 1970).

1. Mechanism of Polykaryocyte Formation

Direct evidence that polykaryocytes can arise by fusion has been provided by time-lapse cinematography of HSV-infected cells (Barski and Robineaux, 1959; Bungay and Watkins, 1964) and of herpes B virus-infected cells (Falke and Richter, 1961a,b).

Another method of determining if fusion or amitosis is responsible for the formation of polykaryocytes is by counting nuclei. If viral polykaryocytes are formed by successive amitotic nuclear division of the same cell rather than by cell fusion, it would be expected that the number of nuclei in cultures containing polykaryocytes would be significantly increased. Ross and Orlans (1958) and Stoker (1959) have made such counts in cell cultures containing polykaryocytes induced by HSV and have found no increase in the number of nuclei.

Virus infection of single isolated cells *in vitro* should lead to polykaryocyte formation if amitotic nuclear division is responsible for the formation of polykaryocytes. Wildy *et al.* (1959) infected single HeLa cells with HSV and found that of 40 cells so infected, only 2 divided and no polykaryocytes were formed. In contrast, the same virus strain growing in confluent HeLa cell monolayers (Stoker, 1959) produced polykaryocytes in 9–12 hours.

The preponderance of the evidence then points to cell fusion as the primary mechanism for polykaryocyte formation, and as Roizman (1962a) has pointed out, it is difficult to understand how polykaryocytes containing several hundred nuclei could be produced by repeated amitosis as the parent nucleus could not provide even one chromosome to each of the nuclei in the polykaryocyte. However, it is clear that even though cell fusion is the primary method of polykaryocyte formation, amitotic nuclear division may be responsible for small polykaryocytes in cell cultures infected with herpesvirus. These have been reported for HSV (Scott *et al.*, 1961), pseudorabies (Kaplan and Ben-Porat, 1959), herpes zoster (Weller *et al.*, 1958), and herpesvirus B (Falke, 1961). In all of these cultures containing the small polykaryocytes ascribed to amitosis there were larger polykaryocytes arising presumably from cell fusion.

2. Requirements for Cell Fusion

It has been suggested (Roizman, 1962a,b) that virus-induced polykaryocytes are formed only by fusion of cells which differ in some respect, that is, infected and uninfected cells or cells at different stages of infection. This was based on the finding that cells infected with high multiplicities of HSV rarely fused, while in cells infected at low multiplicities polykaryocytosis was the predominant CPE. This opinion implies that when all the cells in a culture are infected simultaneously polykaryocytosis cannot occur. This view has also been proposed by others (Stoker, 1959; Bungay and Watkins, 1964).

Despite the views cited above, there is a considerable body of evidence to show that fusion occurs even when all the cells are infected. Siminoff (1964) using a PFU/cell ratio of 5 showed that over 71% of the cells at 12 hours after infection were polykaryocytes in an HSV–HeLa cell system. Similar results were obtained by Nii and Kamahora (1963) and Tokamaru (1968). In fact, it has been reported that when high multiplicities of PRV are used in rabbit kidney cells ($\geqq$ 5 PFU/cell) polykaryocytes appear sooner than when lower multiplicities are used (Kaplan and Vatter, 1959).

It seems inescapable that polykaryocyte formation by herpesvirus-infected cells is the result, in most cases, of fusion of single cells. In some instances polykaryocytes may be formed from single cells by amitotic nuclear division. From the evidence presented, it is clear that herpesvirus-induced cell fusion does not require that infected cells fuse only with uninfected cells. Fusion can occur between infected cells and even between polykaryocytes (Poste, 1970).

3. Factors Influencing Polykaryocyte Formation

a. The Cell. Formation of polykaryocytes by the herpesviruses is greatly dependent on the host cell. It has been shown that the P strain of HSV produces large polykaryocytes in HeLa cells but not in diploid human lung cells even though the virus grows to higher titers in the lung cells (Albanese *et al.*, 1966). Similarly, Roizman's (1962b) macroplaque strain of HSV produced twenty times as many polykaryocytes in HEp2 cells as in ME cells, and the GCA-3 strain of HSV (Waddell and Sigel, 1966) produced polykaryocytes in rabbit kidney but not in KB cells. Tokumaru (1968) found that the cytopathogenic effect of H strain of HSV varied widely depending on its host cells, producing extensive polykaryocytes in rabbit kidney cultures, small polykaryocytes and cell rounding in BHK cells, and only cell rounding in human embryonic kidney, human amnion, and mouse MCN cells. Similarly, T virus, a monkey herpesvirus, produced markedly different amounts of cell fusion in different host cells (Daniel and Melendez, 1968).

The above reports and similar work with other viruses appear to indicate that malignant cells and cells from established cell lines have a higher fusion capacity than primary and secondary diploid cells. An exception to this appears to be the mouse L cell which is refractory to polykaryocyte formation by not only herpesvirus but by other viruses as well (Poste, 1970).

b. The Virus. Formation of polykaryocytes is ultimately dependent upon the genetic constitution of the virus even though it may be influenced to some degree by the host cell. Herpesvirus populations appear to contain variants which differ in their effect on cells. Gray *et al.* (1958) isolated HSV from a case of stomatitis which produced cell rounding, cell proliferation, and polykaryocytosis in HeLa cells. From this parent strain, Scott *et al.* (1961) isolated two variants, one of which produced polykaryocytes and the other of which produced cell proliferation. Several groups of workers have reported isolation of strains of HSV producing one or the other of these effects, so it appears that most HSV isolates are mixtures of viruses that vary with respect to CPE and probably to other characteristics as well. This subject is discussed more fully in Section VI. It is imperative, then, to use plaque isolations in order to reduce chances of working with virus stocks containing a mixture of viruses differing in biologic or other properties.

c. The Environment. Environmental factors are probably responsible for minor variations in the formation of polykaryocytes reported by different laboratories using the same cell–virus system. Such factors as serum concentration and type, presence or absence of glutamine, or even the type of culture (roller versus stationary) have all been reported to influence polykaryocyte formation (Poste, 1970).

4. Virus Multiplication and Cell Fusion

Polykaryocyte formation may be of two types: early (usually within 3 hours after infection) or late, which occurs a number of hours or days after infection and usually coincides with the period of maximum virus multiplication. Early fusion usually requires massive virus inocula and in certain cases may be effected with UV (Okada and Tadakoro, 1962) or propiolactone-inactivated virus (Neff and Enders, 1968). The phenomenon of early fusion by inactivated virus is particularly characteristic of the paramyxoviruses, especially Sendai virus (Hosaka and Koshi, 1968). In contrast, HSV completely loses its ability to fuse cells when it is inactivated by UV irradiation (Cocuzza and Russo, 1966).

Productive infections are not always required for polykaryocyte formation by the herpesviruses. The macroplaque (MP) strain of HSV (Aurelian and Roizman, 1964) does not form infectious virus in dog kidney (DK) cells although small amounts of viral DNA and antigen are produced. By 24 hours after infection, a few polykaryocytes are formed in DK cells infected with high multiplicities of MP-HSV. Similarly, infectious bovine rhinotracheitis virus (IBR) which grows at 37°C but not at 42°C in bovine kidney cells, produces polykaryocytes at both temperatures although at the higher temperature no evidence of viral DNA synthesis was detected (Stevens, 1966). Viral protein synthesis was detected at both temperatures. These experiments indicate that synthesis of complete virus particles is not required for polykaryocyte formation by the herpesviruses.

5. Inhibitors and Polykaryocytosis

a. DNA Inhibition. Inhibition of viral DNA synthesis by mitomycin C in HSV-infected HeLa cells (Munk and Sauer, 1964) had no effect on cell fusion and polykaryocyte formation. Ben-Porat *et al.* (1961) found that noninfectious "coreless" PRV particles, produced by infection of rabbit kidney cells in the presence of mitomycin C, when absorbed to fresh cells were able to induce cell fusion.

Inhibition of DNA synthesis by the halogenated pyrimidines does not affect polykaryocyte formation although the production of infectious virus may be completely suppressed. This has been demonstrated in HSV-cell culture systems with 5-iododeoxyuridine (IUdR) (Tokumaru, 1968) and 5-bromodeoxyuridine (BUdR) (Siminoff, 1964). Equine abortion virus synthesis was inhibited by 5-fluorodeoxyuridine (FUdR), but polykaryocyte production was not affected (O'Callaghan *et al.*, 1968). In contrast to the above, Bungay and Watkins (1964) reported that IUdR, if added to the culture within 6 hours after infection, inhibited both polykaryocytosis and virus production in HSV-infected HeLa cells. Similarly, Falke (1965) found that IUdR and FUdR inhibited polykaryocytosis if added within 2 hours of infection of rabbit kidney cells with HSV. Production of infectious virus in this system was sensitive to the action of the inhibitors up to 4 hours after infection.

Use of other inhibitors of DNA synthesis have also resulted in conflicting reports of their effect on polykaryocytosis. Preincubation of rabbit kidney cells with 5-fluorouracil did not inhibit polykaryocyte formation by PRV (Kaplan, 1962; Reissig and Kaplan, 1962). Daunomycin, on the other hand, prevented polykaryocyte formation by the MP strain of HSV in KB cells when given up to 9 hours after infection (DiMarco *et al.*, 1968).

b. RNA Inhibition. Inhibition of DNA-dependent RNA synthesis by actinomycin C (Falke and Peterknecht, 1968) or by proflavine (Falke, 1965) prevented polykaryocyte formation by HSV in rabbit kidney cells. These inhibitors were only effective if added within 2 hours after infection. As one would expect, these inhibitors had no effect on polykaryocytosis by RNA viruses (Poste, 1970).

c. Protein Inhibition. Falke (1965) also found that polykaryocyte formation by HSV in rabbit kidney cells was inhibited by the protein inhibitory agents cycloheximide and *p*-fluorophenylalanine if they were given within 2 or 3 hours after infection.

d. Conclusions. The results of the studies of polykaryocyte inhibition by various metabolic inhibitors, even though conflicting in many instances, suggest that for the herpesviruses, synthesis of virus-specified messenger and early protein is required for cell fusion and therefore for polykaryocyte formation. This is certainly not true for all polykaryocyte formation, however, particularly for early fusion by the paramyxovirus group and for fusion by chemical and physical agents such as silicon or glass (Poste, 1970).

D. Herpesvirus-Induced Chromosome Aberrations

It is quite clear that chromosome anomalies are associated with or cause various human diseases. It is also clear that mammalian viruses, of which the herpesviruses are prominent examples, induce chromosomal and mitotic irregularities and are mutagenic agents. What is not so clear is the relationship, if any, of these virus-induced chromosomal anomalies to mammalian disease.

1. Types of Anomalies

The most frequently encountered aberrations in virus-infected cells are chromatid breaks (for review, see Stich and Yohn, 1970). These may be breaks in one or both arms of the chromosome and lead to the formation of acentric fragments which are not connected to the remaining chromosome. The acentric fragment may be detached, dislocated, or may remain in its original position. At anaphase, only chromosome pieces with centromeres move toward the spindle poles, the acentric fragments being left behind. Chromosome fragmentation is the term used when chromatid breaks are present in all or most chromosomes of a metaphase plate.

Several different viruses have been implicated in the production of another anomaly known as chromosome pulverization. In this anomaly the entire chromosome complement appears broken up into pieces about the size of chromatid granules seen in interphase nuclei.

Chromatid exchanges are common in cells with chromatid breaks because of the tendency of the broken chromatid ends to fuse with other broken chromatid ends. A great variety of configurations can arise, depending on the locations of breaks and the chromatids involved in the joining process.

One of the causes of the formation of abnormal chromosome numbers and of multinucleated cells are anomalies of the mitotic apparatus, that is, of the microtubules composing the spindle figure and the centrosome. In addition to breaks, there are a number of other chromosome aberrations such as erosions, ruffled chromosomes, haziness, stickiness, etc., which appear to be the result of coiling anomalies of the chromatid and are referred to as coiling deficiencies. Some of these aberrations resemble those induced by treatment with colchicine (Cooper *et al.*, 1968) and have been termed colchicine-like mitosis or C. mitosis.

2. Virus-Induced Chromosome Anomalies in Cultured Cells

Chromosome anomalies of the types discussed above have been attributed to infection with members of several virus groups, some of which contain DNA and some RNA. Induction of detectable chromosome damage is dependent upon viral dose, type of host cell, and the presence of defective virus in the inoculum, and obviously, these factors are not defined for all virus–cell systems. Many viruses, particularly the DNA viruses, which replicate in the nucleus, inhibit DNA synthesis and cell division. Thus, damage to chromosomes or to the mitotic apparatus, which can be observed only at metaphase or anaphase, would be obscured in the absence of cell division. The herpesviruses fit the above description quite well, and yet there have been several reports of chromosome aberrations as a result of infection with these viruses (Table III).

From the table it is obvious that the chromosomes of a variety of cells are damaged by herpesviruses and that a full spectrum of chromosomal aberrations are induced. These aberrations are produced in both aneuploid (Hampar and Ellison, 1961, 1963) and diploid Chinese hamster cells (Stich *et al.*, 1964) and in both primary and continuous cell cultures.

Many investigators have attempted to identify lesions on specific chromosomes as a result of infection with a particular virus. Stich *et al.* (1964) asserted that there was a nonrandom distribution of chromosome breakage in Chinese hamster cells infected with HSV. They found a higher incidence of breaks in particular regions of chromosomes 1 and X. This report was based solely on morphological observations, however, and attempts to localize virus DNA in terms of a site on a particular chromosome or chromosomes representing a site of viral integration have not been successful (Moorhead, 1970). An interesting observation is that of Kohn *et al.* (1967) who

TABLE III

INDUCTION OF CHROMOSOME ABERRATIONS IN CULTURED CELLS BY HERPESVIRUSES[a]

Virus	Host cell	Chromosome aberrations[b]	References
Herpes simplex	Chinese hamster	B	Hampar and Ellison (1961, 1963)
Herpes simplex	Chinese hamster	B,C	Mazzone and Yerganian (1963)
Herpes simplex	Chinese hamster	B,F,P,C	Stich *et al.* (1964)
Herpes simplex	Human lung	B,F,P,C	Stich *et al.* (1964)
Herpes simplex	Mastomys	B,F,P	Huang (1967)
Herpes simplex	Monkey kidney		Boiron *et al.* (1966)
Herpes simplex	BHK 21	B,F,C	Waubke *et al.* (1968)
Herpes zoster	Human lung	B,F,C,M	Benyesh-Melnick *et al.* (1964)
EB virus	Burkitt lymphoma		Kohn *et al.* (1967)
EB virus	Human leukocytes		Henle *et al.* (1967)

[a]Adapted from Stich and Yohn (1970).

[b]B, chromatid breaks; F, fragmentation; P, pulverization; C, coiling deficiencies; M, C-mitosis.

found that C group chromosomes (probably number 10) of 20–30% of the cells of the Burkitt lymphoma have a constriction of the long arm. Henle *et al.* (1967) have reported that normal human leukocytes, transformed with cell-free extracts of Burkitt lymphoma cells carrying the EB virus, also have the C group constriction after but not before transformation.

The precise mechanism by which virus infection produces chromosome damage is not known. However, there are some findings which bear on this problem. It is clear that infectious virus is required, since UV-irradiated HSV or HSV grown in the presence of IUdR does not produce chromosome abnormalities in diploid Chinese hamster cells (Rapp and Hsu, 1965). Heat and antibody-inactivated HSV is also ineffective in producing these aberrations (Tanzer *et al.*, 1964). Radioautography (Rapp and Hsu, 1965; Waubke *et al.*, 1968) has not demonstrated any connection between cell chromosomes and virus nucleic acid synthesis in cells infected with HSV, leading these authors to conclude that the chromosome damage is a result of the presence of an early enzyme under control of the viral genome and not a result of interaction of viral DNA with the cell chromosome.

3. CONCLUSION

It is clear from the preceding discussion that herpesviruses may induce extensive chromosome damage in human and other animal cells. Additionally, the herpesviruses are only one of a large number of virus groups capable of causing this damage (see Stich and Yohn, 1970). There is, as yet, no real information bearing on the role of viruses in somatic cell mutagenesis and therefore in the causation of congenital defects or cancer. Because of the ubiquity of viruses and their mutagenic potential it is possible that they are responsible for a significant proportion of mutations and genetic variation in germ and somatic cell populations.

E. Cytotoxicity

Herpes simplex virus, under certain conditions, has been shown to have cytotoxic effects, both *in vivo* and *in vitro*, which are separable from productive infection. Tokumaru (1963) found that heat-inactivated virus had a pyrogenic effect in guinea pigs. This effect could be partially neutralized by antiserum. Results reported by Vantsis and Wildy (1962) indicate that cell killing and infective center formation by HSV are due to separate populations of particles. Smith (1963) found that HSV has a marked cytotoxic effect on human embryonic fibroblast cells even when infectious virus synthesis is completely suppressed by IUdR although some viral products are produced. These results clearly indicate that HSV exerts a cytotoxic effect which is not connected with viral replication. This effect is viral as it can be eliminated or suppressed with antiviral serum. It is unclear as to what component(s) of the virion is responsible for this effect.

F. Plaque Formation

Plaque formation by viruses in general results from the infection of a single cell when progeny virus from this cell is prevented by some means from infecting cells other than those immediately adjacent to the initially infected one. The size of the plaques varies according to the strain of the virus, the type of cell, and also to some extent the metabolic state of the cell. Herpes simplex virus (H4 strain) PRV and EAV have very similar patterns of plaque development (Darlington and Moss, 1968) in BHK cells (Fig. 5). Plaques first appear at about 2 days and reach maximum size in 4–5 days. However, PRV plaques are considerably larger than those formed by HSV or EAV. The size of HSV plaques varies considerably depending on the cells used for assay. In rabbit kidney cells (Kaplan, 1957) and chick embryo fibroblasts (DeMaeyer and Schonne, 1964), the maximum size is 1–2 mm, while in HeLa cells, somewhat smaller plaques are formed (Farnham, 1958), and in human amnion cells, larger plaques are formed (Ousterhout and Tamm, 1959). It is clear also that plaque size is a phenotypic expression of the virus genotype as illustrated by the large and small plaque variants of HSV (Roizman and Aurelian, 1965).

In order to limit the spread of virus to those cells immediately adjacent to the initially infected cell, it is necessary to either inactivate released virus or restrict its diffusion. This can be accomplished in a variety of ways. Anti-

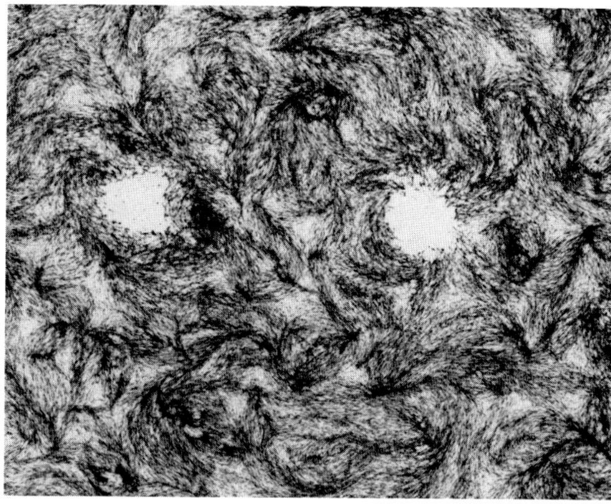

FIG. 5. HSV (H_4 strain) plaques in BHK 21 cells.

serum has been used to inactivate herpes B virus released from monkey kidney cell cultures thus restricting spread of the virus to cell-to-cell transmission (Black and Melnick, 1955). The more usual method of restricting virus is by overlaying the infected cell sheet with a substance such as agar, starch gel, or methylcellulose. This overlay prevents the spread of virus to distant cells but does not interfere with infection of adjacent cells. The efficiency of plaque formation by the herpesviruses under agar is rather low because of the presence in agar of a sulfated polysaccharide which inhibits virus growth (Takemoto and Fabisch, 1964). Other polyanions such as sodium dextran sulfate and heparin can also inhibit growth by preventing virus attachment (Vaheri and Cantell, 1963; Nahmias *et al.*, 1964). This problem can be overcome by adding a polycation such as protamine sulfate to the agar (Tytell and Newman, 1963) or more easily by using a purified agar preparation such as Agarose (Sea-Kem Corp., Los Angeles, Calif.) (Wolf and Darlington, 1971). Visualization of the plaques can be accomplished by incorporating neutral red into the overlay but here one has to be cognizant of the fact that neutral red through photodynamic action (Green and Opton, 1959) can reduce plaque counts and destroy certain host cells. This can be avoided by keeping cultures containing neutral red in the dark or by adding a second overlay containing neutral red near the end of the incubation period.

Quantitation of herpes zoster and the cytomegaloviruses in tissue culture is more difficult for a variety of reasons than is quantitation of those herpesviruses that are readily released from cells. These viruses remain largely cell associated, and herpes zoster, at least, requires the use of infected cells

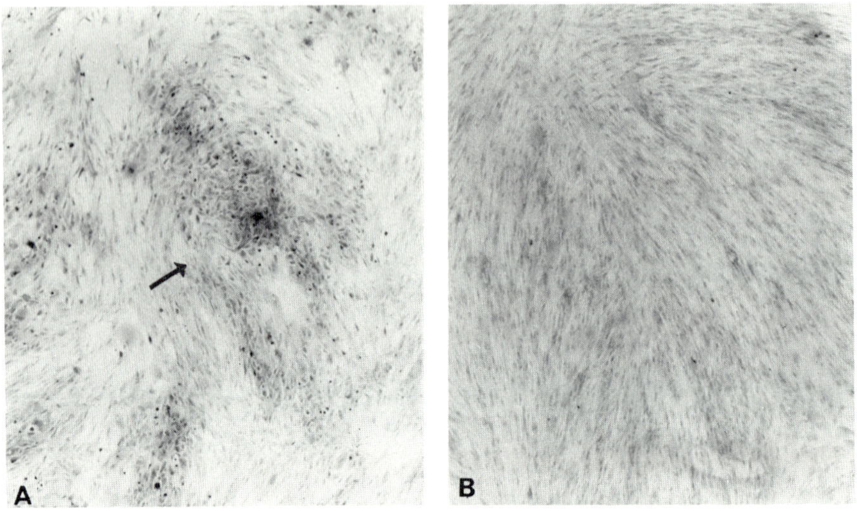

FIG. 6. Varicella–zoster virus infection of WI-38 cells. (A) Infected, (B) control.

as inoculum. The longer growth cycle of these viruses also presents problems in maintaining cells.

Varicella–zoster virus produces a focal lesion (Fig. 6) which spreads radially from the point of initial infection. As transmission of this virus is apparently from cell to cell, it might be expected that a plaque assay would be possible without the use of an overlay. This does not appear to be true, however, as Rapp and Benyesh-Melnick (1963) found it necessary to add agar or methylcellulose overlays in order to obtain plaques. Titration of the cytomegaloviruses is usually accomplished by end-point dilution methods, although Rapp *et al.* (1963) have reported an immunofluorescent focus assay method.

VI. Variation and Genetics

As discussed earlier in this chapter, there are many differences among members of the herpesvirus group—not only between the various subgroups, but also within a particular strain. Until recently, mutants of herpesviruses were usually obtained by passage of the virus through animals or tissue culture; these act as a selection pressure for the emergence of new strains. With this method, virus populations were found to be mixed and to contain viruses differing in a number of properties, including virulence, cytopathology, ability to alter cell membranes, antigenicity, host range, altered physical and chemical properties, ability to induce thymidine kinase, altered plaque type, drug resistance when passaged in the presence of certain drugs (e.g. IUdR or BUdR), and intracellular development as studied by electron microscopy (see review by Kaplan, 1969; Schwartz and Roizman, 1969). Mutants of herpesvirus can be obtained or can emerge with relative ease, thus attesting to the high degree of mutability of this virus group. The fact that mutants can be obtained by simply plating a virus stock and isolating plaques indicates the high frequency of mutants in the virus population (Rapp, 1963). Similar results have been obtained with the limiting dilution method (Kohlhage and Siegert, 1962). The apparent readiness with which the herpesviruses mutate may partially explain why they are the most ubiquitous of all viruses, with hosts ranging from fish to man.

A. Naturally Occurring Mutants

Naturally occurring mutants of a number of animal viruses have been of practical value where attenuated strains have been used for live vaccines. However, with herpesvirus, they have been used mainly to learn more about the biology of this group of viruses, particularly in relation to virus reproduction and effects on cells and hosts (reviewed by Kaplan, 1969; Roizman, 1969). For example, conditional lethal mutants of herpesvirus which can multiply in one host (HEp-2 cells) cannot multiply in another (dog kidney cells). Although infectious progeny is not produced, virus-specific products such as viral antigen and DNA are made and cytopathology occurs. Presumably, some protein(s) needed for infectious virus production is not synthesized or is synthesized but is not functional (Aurelian and Roizman, 1964, 1965, Roizman and Aurelian, 1965; Roizman, 1965b).

Differences in surface properties of herpesviruses may account for the changes in "social behavior" of cells infected with the virus. It has been suggested that virus-specific products modify host cell membranes which subsequently envelope the nucleocapsid. The amount of altered membrane exceeds that required for envelopment of virus, and the virus product bound to this membrane has been considered responsible for the altered "social behavior" of the infected cells (Roizman, 1962a; Roane and Roizman, 1964; Ejercito *et al.*, 1968). An alternate hypothesis is that modification of the cell surface, specifically of the glycoproteins, is produced by lysosomal enzymes released onto the cell surface (Poste, 1970). The subject is dealt with fully in Chapter 6. Since membranes have been assigned considerable importance in the regulation of cellular functions including alterations leading to malignancy, the herpesvirus group may be useful in studying membrane alterations leading to uncontrolled growth. This is an especially good possibility because a number of herpesviruses have proven oncogenic in animals and others are suspect in man (Biggs *et al.*, 1972).

An outstanding example of the practical use of a naturally occurring mutant is found in Marek's disease, a lymphoproliferative malignancy of chickens caused by a herpesvirus [Marek's disease virus (MDV)]. Spontaneous mutants of this virus or an antigenically related turkey herpesvirus have been used to control the disease (see Chapter 17 for details). Numerous mutants of MDV differing in plaque type, antigenicity, and virulence have been isolated (Mikami and Bankowski, 1971; Purchase *et al.*, 1971) illustrating further the mutability of herpesvirus.

B. Chemically Induced Mutants

Chemically induced temperature-sensitive (ts) conditioned lethal mutants of herpes simplex virus types 1 and 2 (HSV-1, HSV-2) have been obtained by growing the virus in the presence of BUdR or nitrosoguanidine or by exposing it to ultraviolet light (Subak-Sharpe, 1969; Brown *et al.*, 1973; Schaffer *et al.*, 1970, 1973; Timbury, 1971). The permissive temperature of type 1 has been 34°–35°C, and the nonpermissive temperature, 39°–40°C (Schaffer *et al.*, 1970, 1973); with type 2, 31° and 38°C have been used (Timbury, 1971). A large number of HSV-1 mutants have been tested for complementation and recombination. In one study (Schaffer *et al.*, 1973), 22 ts mutants fell into 15 nonoverlapping complementation groups, and recombination frequencies of up to 50% were obtained (Schaffer *et al.*, 1972). Based on these results, a partial, additive linkage map has been constructed. Members of four complementation groups did not synthesize viral DNA at nonpermissive temperature, and at 39°C the infectivity of several mutants was inactivated more rapidly than wild-type infectivity, suggesting that the mutants possess altered temperature-sensitive structural proteins. In another study (Brown *et al.*, 1973), nine HSV-1 ts mutants fell into eight complementation groups, and with a three-factor cross, a linear genetic map was constructed that locates nine cistrons spanning about 25 recombination units.

An interesting result has been obtained with several DNA+ ts mutants. These mutants failed to induce thymidine kinase at permissive temperature (Aron *et al.*, 1972), confirming previous observations that virus-induced thymidine kinase activity is not necessary for replication (Kit and Dubbs, 1963; Dubbs and Kit, 1964; Kit *et al.*, 1967). Preliminary characterization of another of the HSV-1 ts mutants suggests a defect in glycoprotein synthesis (Schaffer *et al.*, 1971). Although complementation between HSV-2 mutants has been reported (Timbury, 1971), it has been more difficult to demonstrate, and the degree of complementation has varied considerably from experiment to experiment with the same mutant crosses. The mutants tested appear to belong to ten complementation groups.

Preliminary results indicate that both complementation and recombination occur between HSV-1 and HSV-2 ts mutants (Timbury and Subak-Sharpe, 1973; Schaffer *et al.*, 1973).

Thus far the results with ts mutants of herpes simplex virus account for only a fraction (about 10%) of the total number of cistrons of the virus genome. Although the large genome of herpesvirus (100×10^6 MW) makes identification of each viral function a difficult task, conditional lethal mutants should provide information on a number of important viral gene functions.

References

Albanese, M., Bynoe, M. L., and Tyrrell, D. A. J. (1966). *Arch. Gesamte Virusforsch.* **18**, 356.

Albrecht, P., Blaškovič, J., Jakubik, J., and Leššo, J. (1963). *Acta Virol. (Prague), Engl. Ed.* **7**, 289.

Anderson, K. (1940). *Amer. J. Pathol.* **16**, 137.

Anderson, K., and Goodpasture, E. W. (1942). *Amer. J. Pathol.* **18**, 555.

Andervont, H. B. (1929). *J. Infec. Dis.* **45**, 366.

Armstrong, J. A., Pereira, H. G., and Andrewes, C. H. (1961). *Virology* **14**, 276.

Aron, G. M., Courtney, R. J., Schaffer, P. A., and Benyesh-Melnick, M. (1972). *Abstr. Annual Meeting. Amer. Soc. Microbiol.* p. 203.

Atherton, J. G., and Anderson, W. (1957). *Aust. J. Exp. Biol. Med. Sci.* **35**, 335.

Aurelian, L., and Roizman, B. (1964). *Virology* **22**, 452.

Aurelian, L., and Roizman, B. (1965). *J. Mol. Biol.* **11**, 539.

Barski, G., and Robineaux, R. (1959). *Proc. Soc. Exp. Biol. Med.* **101**, 632.

Barski, G., Lamy, M., and Lépine, P. (1955). *Ann. Inst. Pasteur, Paris* **89**, 415.

Béládi, I. (1962). *Acta Vet. (Budapest)* **12**, 417.

Béládi, I., and Ivánovics, G. (1954). *Acta Microbiol.* **11**, 151.

Ben-Porat, T., and Kaplan, A. S. (1970). *Virology* **41**, 265.

Ben-Porat, T., and Kaplan, A. S. (1972). *Nature (London)* **235**, 165.

Ben-Porat, T., Reissig, M., and Kaplan, A. S. (1961). *Nature (London)* **190**, 33.

Benyesh-Melnick, M., Stich, H. F., Rapp, F., and Hsu, T. S. (1964). *Proc. Soc. Exp. Biol. Med.* **117**, 546.

Biegeliesen, J. Z., Riley, L. H., Jr., and Scott, L. V. (1957). *Virology* **4**, 182.

Biggs, P. M., de-Thé G., and Payne, L. N., eds. (1972), "Oncogenesis and Herpesviruses." Int. Agency Res. Cancer, Lyon.

Black, F. L., and Melnick, J. L. (1955). *J. Immunol.* **74**, 236.

Blanc, G. (1921). *Acad. Sci.* **172**, 725.

Blank, H., Burgoon, C. F., Baldridge, G. D., McCarthy, P. L., and Urbach, F. (1951). *J. Amer. Med. Ass.* **146**, 1410.

Boiron, M., Tanzer, J., Thomas, M., and Hampe, A. (1966). *Nature (London)* **209**, 737.

Brown, S. M., Ritchie, D. A., and Subak-Sharpe, J. H. (1973). *J. Gen. Virol.* **18**, 273.

Bungay, C., and Watkins, J. F. (1964). *Brit. J. Exp. Pathol.* **45**, 48.

Cabasso, V. J., Brown, R. G., and Cox, H. R. (1957). *Proc. Soc. Exp. Biol. Med.* **95**, 471.

Calnek, B. W., Ubertini, T., and Adldinger, H. K. (1970a). *J. Nat. Cancer Inst.* **45**, 341.

Calnek, B. W., Adldinger, H. K., and Kahn, D. E. (1970b). *Avian Dis* **14**, 219.

Caunt, E. A. (1963). *Lancet* **2**, 982.

Ceccarelli, A., and Del Mazza, I. (1958). *Zooprofilassi* **13**, 159.

Chappell, W. A. (1960). *Ann. N.Y. Acad. Sci.* **85**, 931.
Cheatham, W. J., and Crandell, R. A. (1957). *Proc. Soc. Exp. Biol. Med.* **96**, 536.
Churchill, A. E., and Biggs, P. M. (1967). *Nature (London)* **215**, 528.
Clark, H. F., and Karzon, D. T. (1972). *Infec. Immunity* **5**, 559.
Cocuzza, G., and Russo, G. (1966). *Boll. Ist. Sieroter, Milan.* **45**, 228.
Cooke, B. T., Hurst, E. W., and Swan, C. (1942). *Aust. J. Exp. Biol. Med. Sci.* **20**, 129.
Cooper, J. E. K., Yohn, D. S., and Stich, H. F. (1968). *Exp. Cell Res.* **53**, 225.
Cowdry, E. V. (1934). *Arch, Pathol.* **18**, 527.
Crandell, R. A. (1959). *Proc. Soc. Exp. Biol. Med.* **102**, 508.
Csery-Pechany, E., Béládí, I., and Ivánovics, G. (1951). *Acta Physiol.* **2**, 229.
Daniel, M. D., and Melendez, L. V. (1968). *Arch. Gesamte Virusforsch* **25**, 8.
Darlington, R. W., and James, C. (1966). *J. Bacteriol.* **92**, 250.
Darlington, R. W., and Moss, L. H., III. (1968). *J. Virol.* **2**, 48.
Davidson, W. L., and Hummeler, K. (1960). *Ann. N.Y. Acad. Sci.* **85**, 970.
DeMaeyer, E., and Schonne, E. (1964). *Virology* **24** 13.
DiMarco, A., Terni, M., Silvestrini, R., Scarpinato, E., Biagioli, E., and Antonelli, A. (1968). *G. Microbiol.* **16**, 25.
Doerr, R. (1920). *Klin. Monatsbl. Augenheilk.* **65**, 104.
Doerr, R., and Vochting, K. (1920). *Rev. Gen. Ophthalmol.*, (*Paris*) **34**, 409.
Dubbs, D. R., and Kit, S. (1964). *Virology* **22**, 493.
Dulbecco, R. (1950). *J. Bacteriol.* **59**, 329.
Dulbecco, R. (1955). *In* "Radiation Biology" (A. Hollaender, ed.), Vol. 2, pp. 455–486. McGraw-Hill, New York.
Ejercito, P. A., Kreff, E. D., and Roizman, B. (1968). *J. Gen. Virol.* **2**, 357.
Enders, J. F. (1953). *Proc. Soc. Exp. Biol. Med.* **82**, 100.
Epstein, M. A., Achong, B. G., and Barr, Y. M. (1964a). *Lancet* **1**, 702.
Epstein, M. A., Woodall, J. P., and Thomson, A. D. (1964b). *Lancet* **2**, 288.
Falke, D. (1961). *Virology* **14**, 492.
Falke, D. (1965). *Arch. Gesamte Virusforsch.* **15**, 387.
Falke, D., and Peterknecht, W. (1968). *Arch. Gesamte Virusforsch.* **24**, 267
Falke, D., and Richter, I. E. (1961a). *Arch. Gesamte Virusforsch.* **11**, 73.
Falke, D., and Richter, I. E. (1961b). *Arch. Gesamte Virusforsch.* **11**, 86.
Farnham, A. E. (1958). *Virology* **6**, 317.
Farnham, A. E., and Newton, A. A. (1959). *Virology* **7**, 449.
Fauconnier, B. (1963). *Ann. Inst. Pasteur, Paris* **105**, 439.
Figueroa, M. E., and Rawls, W. E. (1969). *J. Gen. Virol.* **4**, 259.
Fisher, T. N., and Fisher, E. (1959). *Proc. Soc. Exp. Biol. Med.* **100**, 780.
Florman, A., and Trader, F. W. (1947). *J. Immunol.* **55**, 263.
Good, R. A., and Campbell, B. (1945). *Proc. Soc. Exp. Biol. Med.* **59**, 305.
Granoff, A. (1972). *In* "Oncogenesis and Herpesviruses" (P. M. Biggs *et al.*, eds.), p. 171. Int. Agency Res. Cancer, Lyon.
Gravell, M. (1971). *Virology* **43**, 730.
Gravell, M., Granoff, A., and Darlington, R. W. (1968). *Virology* **36**, 467.
Gray, A., Tokumaru, T., and Scott, T. F. McN. (1958). *Arch. Gesamte Virusforsch.* **8**, 59.
Green, R. W., and Opton, E. M. (1959). *Proc. Soc. Exp. Biol. Med.* **102**, 519.
Grüter, W. (1920). *Ber. Deut. Ophthalmol. Ges.* **42**, 162.
Hampar, B., and Ellison, S. A. (1961). *Nature (London)* **192**, 145.
Hampar, B., and Ellison, S. A. (1963). *Proc. Nat. Acad. Sci. U.S.* **49**, 474.
Hancock, B., Bohl, E. H., and Birkeland, J. M. (1959). *Amer. J. Vet. Res.* **20**, 127.
Hanshaw, J. B. (1966). *Pediat. Clin. N. Amer.* **13**, 279.

Henle, W., Diehl, V., Kohn, G., zur Hausen, H., and Henle, G. (1967). *Science* **157**, 1064.
Hinze, H. C., and Walker, D. L. (1961). *J. Bacteriol.* **82**, 498.
Hoggan, M. D., and Roizman, B. (1959a). *Virology* **8**, 508.
Hoggan, M. D., and Roizman, B. (1959b). *Amer. J. Hyg.* **70**, 208.
Holmes, I. H., and Watson, D. H. (1963). *Virology* **21**, 112.
Hosaka, Y., and Koshi, Y. (1968). *Virology* **34**, 419.
Huang, A. S., and Wagner, R. R. (1964). *Proc. Soc. Exp. Biol. Med.* **116**, 863.
Huang, C. C. (1967). *Chromosoma* **23**, 162.
Hurst, E. W. (1934). *J. Exp. Med.* **59**, 729.
Hurst. E. W. (1936). *J. Exp. Med.* **63**, 449.
Johnson, R. T. (1964). *J. Exp. Med.* **119**, 343.
Kaplan, A. S. (1957). *Virology* **4**, 435.
Kaplan, A. S. (1962). *Virology* **16**, 305.
Kaplan, A. S. (1969). "Virology Monographs." Springer-Verlag, Berlin and New York.
Kaplan, A. S., and Ben-Porat, T. (1959). *Virology* **8**, 352.
Kaplan, A. S., and Ben-Porat, T. (1966). *Proc. Int. Congr. Microbiol., 9th, 1966* pp. 463–482.
Kaplan, A. S., and Ben-Porat, T. (1970). *Proc. Natl. Acad. Sci. U.S.* **66**, 799.
Kaplan, A. S., and Vatter, A. E. (1959). *Virology* **7**, 394.
King, L. S. (1940). *J. Exp. Med.* **72**, 573.
Kit, S., and Dubbs, D. R. (1963). *Biochem. Biophys. Res. Commun.* **13**, 500.
Kit, S., Dubbs, D. R., and Anken, M. (1967). *J. Virol.* **1**, 238.
Kohlhage, H., and Schieferstein, G. (1965). *Arch. Gesamte Virusforsch.* **14**, 358.
Kohlhage, H., and Siegert, R. (1962). *Arch. Gesamte Virusforsch.* **12**, 273.
Kohn, G., Mellman, W. J., Moorhead, P. S., Loftus, J., and Henle, G. (1967). *J. Nat. Cancer Inst.* **38**, 209.
Lauda, E., and Rezek, P. (1926). *Virchows. Arch, Pathol. Anat. Physiol.* **262**, 827.
Lennette, E. H., and Koprowski, H. (1944). *J. Immunol.* **49**, 175.
Lewis, V. J., Jr., and Scott, L. V. (1962). *J. Bacteriol.* **83**, 475.
Lowenstein, A. (1919). *Muenchen. Med. Wochenschr.* **66**, 769.
Lowry, S. P., Melnick, J. L., and Rawls, W. E. (1971). *J. Gen. Virol.* **10**, 1.
Luria, S. E., and Laterjet, R. (1947). *J. Bacteriol.* **53**, 149.
Lwoff, A., Dulbecco, R., Vogt, M., and Lwoff, M. (1955). *Virology* **1**, 128.
Madin, S. H., York, C. J., and McKercher, D. G. (1956). *Science* **124**, 721.
Mazzone, H. M., and Yerganian, G. (1963). *Exp. Cell. Res.* **30**, 591.
McAllister, R. M., Straw, R. M., Filbert, J. E., and Goodheart, C. R. (1963). *Virology* **19**, 521.
McFerran, J. B., and Dow, C. (1962). *Brit. Vet. J.* **118**, 386.
McKercher, D. G. (1959). *Advan. Vet. Sci.* **5**, 299.
Melendez, L. V., Hunt, R. D., Daniel, M. D., Fraser, C. E. O., Barahona, H. H., Garcia, F. G., and King. N. W. (1972). *In* "Oncogenesis and Herpesviruses" (P. M. Biggs *et al.*, eds.), pp. 451–461. Int. Agency Res. Cancer, Lyon.
Middlekamp, J. N., Reed, U. A., and Patrizi, G. (1967). *Proc. Soc. Exp. Biol. Med.* **125**, 757.
Mikami, T., and Bankowski, R. A. (1971). *Amer. J. Vet. Res.* **32**, 303.
Moorhead, P. S. (1970). *Univ. Tex. M. D. Anderson Hosp. Tumor Inst. 23rd Annu. Symp. Funda. Cancer Res.* pp. 281–306.
Munk, K., and Donner, D. (1963), *Arch. Gesamte Virusforsch.* **13**, 529.
Munk, K., and Sauer, G. (1964). *Virology* **22**, 153.
Nahmias, A. J., Kibrick, S., and Bernfield, P. (1964). *Proc. Soc. Exp. Biol. Med.* **115**, 993.
Nankervis, G. A., Gray, T. A., and Morgan, H. R. (1959), *J. Nat. Cancer Inst.* **22**, 283.
Nazarian, K. (1972). *In* "Oncogenesis and Herpesviruses" (P. M. Biggs *et al.*, eds.), pp. 59–73. Int. Agency Res. Cancer, Lyon.

Neff, J. M., and Enders, J. F. (1968). *Proc. Soc. Exp. Biol. Med.* **127**, 260.
Nii, S., and Kamahora, J. (1961). *Biken's J.* **4**, 255.
Nii, S., and Kamahora, J. (1963). *Biken's J.* **6**, 33.
O'Callaghan, D. J., Hyde, J. M., Gentry, G. A., and Randall, C. C. (1968). *J. Virol.* **2**, 793.
O'Conor, G. T., and Rabson, A. S. (1965). *J. Nat. Cancer Inst.* **35**, 899.
Okada, Y., and Tadakoro, J. (1962). *Exp. Cell Res.* **26**, 108.
Ousterhout, S., and Tamm, I. (1959). *J. Immunol.* **83**, 442.
Pfefferkorn, E. R., Rutstein, C., and Burge, B. W. (1965). *Virology* **27**, 457.
Pfefferkorn, E. R., Burge, B. W., and Coady, H. M. (1966). *J. Bacteriol.* **92**, 856.
Pope, J. H., Achong, B. G., and Epstein, M. A. (1968). *Int. J. Cancer* **3**, 171.
Poste, G. (1970). *Advan. Virus Res.* **16**, 303.
Powell, W. F. (1959). *Virology* **9**, 1.
Purchase, H. G., Burmester, B. R., and Cunningham, C. H. (1971). *Infec. Immunity* **3**, 295.
Rabson, A. S., O'Conor, G. T., Baron, S., Whang, J. J., and Legallais, F. Y. (1966). *Int. J. Cancer* **1**, 89.
Radcliffe, H. (1971). *J. Gen. Virol.* **13**, 181.
Rafferty, K. A., Jr. (1965). *Ann. N.Y. Acad. Sci.* **126**, 3.
Randall, C. C. (1954). *Fed. Proc., Fed. Amer. Soc. Exp. Biol.* **13**, 1445.
Randall, C. C. (1955a). *Proc. Soc. Exp. Biol. Med.* **90**, 176.
Randall, C. C. (1955b). *Amer. J. Pathol.* **31**, 1165.
Randall, C. C. (1957). *Proc. Soc. Exp. Biol. Med.* **95**, 508.
Randall, C. C., and Lawson, L. A. (1962). *Proc. Soc. Exp. Biol. Med.* **110**, 487.
Rapp, F. (1963). *J. Bacteriol.* **86**, 985.
Rapp, F., and Benyesh-Melnick, M. (1963). *Science* **141**, 433.
Rapp, F., and Hsu, T. C. (1965). *Virology* **25**, 401.
Rapp, F., Rasmussen, L. E., and Benyesh-Melnick, M. (1963). *J. Immunol.* **91**, 709.
Reissig, M., and Kaplan, A. S. (1960). *Virology* **11**, 1.
Reissig, M., and Kaplan, A. S. (1962). *Virology* **16**, 1.
Reissig, M., and Melnick, J. L. (1955). *J. Exp. Med.* **101**, 341.
Rivers, T. M. (1926). *J. Exp. Med.* **43**, 275.
Roane, P. R., Jr., and Roizman, B. (1964). *Virology* **22**, 1.
Roizman, B. (1962a). *Cold Spring Harbor Symp. Quant. Biol.* **24**, 327.
Roizman, B. (1962b). *Proc. Nat. Acad. Sci. U.S.* **48**, 228.
Roizman, B. (1963). *Proc. Nat. Acad. Sci. U.S.* **49**, 165.
Roizman, B. (1965a). *Proc. Soc. Exp. Biol. Med.* **119**, 1021.
Roizman, B. (1965b). *Virology* **27**, 113.
Roizman, B. (1969). *Curr. Top. Microbiol. Immunol.* **49**, 1.
Roizman, B., and Aurelian, L. (1965). *J. Mol. Biol.* **11**, 528.
Ross, R. W., and Orlans, E. (1958). *J. Pathol. Bacteriol.* **76**, 393.
Rouhandeh, H. (1963). *(London) Nature* **200**, 386.
Rubin, H., Baluda, M., and Hotchin, J. E. (1955). *J. Exp. Med.* **101**, 205.
Rupert, C. S. (1962a). *J. Gen. Physiol.* **45**, 707.
Rupert, C. S. (1962b). *J. Gen. Physiol.* **45**, 725.
Sabin, A. B. (1934). *Brit. J. Exp. Pathol.* **15**, 321.
Sabin, A. B., and Wright, A. M. (1934). *J. Exp. Med.* **59**, 115.
Salomon, J. J., Witter, R. L., Nazarian, K., and Burmester, B. R. (1968). *Proc. Soc. Exp. Biol. Med.* **127**, 173.
Schaffer, P. A., Vonka, V., Lewis, R. T., and Benyesh-Melnick, M. (1970). *Virology* **42**, 1144.
Schaffer, P. A., Courtney, R. J., McCombs, R. M., and Benyesh-Melnick, M. (1971). *Virology* **46**, 356.

Schaffer, P. A., Lewis, R. T., and Benyesh-Melnick, M. (1972). *Annu. Meet. Amer. Soc. Microbiol.* p. 203.
Schaffer, P. A., Aron, G. M., Biswal, N., and Benyesh-Melnick, M. (1973). *Virology* **52**, 57.
Scherer, W. F. (1953). *Amer. J. Pathol.* **29**, 113.
Scherer, W. F., and Syverton, J. T. (1954). *Amer. J. Pathol.* **30**, 1057.
Schmidt, J. R., and Rasmussen, A. F. Jr. (1960). *J. Infec. Dis.* **107**, 356.
Schur, V. A., and Holmes, A. W. (1965). *Proc. Soc. Exp. Biol. Med.* **119**, 950.
Schwartz, J., and Roizman, B. (1969). *J. Virol.* **4**, 879.
Schwarz. A. J. F., York, C. J., Zirbel, L. W., and Estela, L. A. (1957). *Proc. Soc. Exp. Biol. Med.* **96**, 453.
Scott, T. F. McN., and McLeod, D. L. (1959). *Ann. N.Y. Acad. Sci.* **81**, 118.
Scott, T. F. McN., McLeod, D. L., and Tokumaru, T. (1961). *J. Immunol.* **86**, 1.
Setlow, R. B., and Setlow, J. K. (1962). *Proc. Nat. Acad. Sci. U.S.* **48**, 1250.
Shimizu, T., Ishizaki, R., Kone, Y., Ishii, S., and Matsumoto, M. (1957). *Jap. J. Exp. Med.* **27**, 175.
Siminoff, P. (1964). *Virology* **24**, 1.
Singh, K. V. (1962). *Cornell Vet.* **52**, 237.
Slotnick, V. B., and Rosanoff, E. I. (1963). *Virology* **19**, 589.
Smith, K. O. (1963). *J. Immunol.* **91**, 582.
Smith, M. C. (1959). *Progr. Med. Virol.* **2**, 171.
Sosa-Martinez, J., Gutierrez-Villegas, L., and Sosa, R. M. (1955). *J. Bacteriol.* **70**, 391.
Spear, P. G., and Roizman, B. (1972). *J. Virol.* **9**, 143.
Spring, S. B., and Roizman, B. (1968). *J. Virol.* **2**, 979.
Stevens, J. G. (1966). *Virology* **29**, 570.
Stewart S. E., London, J., Lovelace, E., and Parker, G. (1965). *Wistar Inst. Symp. Monogr.* **4**, 93.
Stich, H. F., and Yohn, D. S. (1970). *Progr. Med. Virol.* **12**, 78.
Stich, H. F., Hsu, T. C., and Rapp, F. (1964). *Virology* **22**, 439.
Stoker, M. G. P. (1959). *Symp. Soc. Gen. Microbiol.* **9**, 142.
Stoker, M. G. P., and Ross, R. W. (1958). *J. Gen. Microbiol.* **19**, 250.
Stulberg, C. S., and Schapira, R. (1953). *J. Immunol.* **70**, 51.
Subak-Sharpe, J. H. (1969). *Proc. Int. Congr. Virol., 1st, 1968* p. 252.
Svedmyr, A. (1965). *Arch. Gesamte Virusforsch.* **17**, 495.
Szántó, J. (1960). *Acta Virol. (Prague), Engl. Ed.* **4**, 380.
Takemoto, K. K., and Fabisch, P. (1964). *Proc. Soc. Exp. Biol. Med.* **116**, 140.
Tankersley, R. W., Jr. (1964). *J. Bacteriol.* **87**, 609.
Tanzer, J., Stoitchkov, Y., Boiron, M., and Bernard, J. (1964). *Ann. Inst. Pasteur, Paris* **107**, 366.
Teague, O., and Goodpasture, E. W. (1923). *J. Amer. Med. Ass.* **81**, 377.
Teissier, P., Gastriel, P., and Reilly, J. (1922). *C. R. Soc. Biol.* **86**, 75.
Thompson, R. L., and Coates, M. S. (1942). *J. Infec. Dis.* **71**, 83.
Timbury, M. C. (1971). *J. Gen. Virol.* **13**, 373.
Timbury, M. C., and Subak-Sharpe, J. H. (1973). *J. Gen. Virol.* **18**, 347.
Tokumaru, T. (1957). *Proc. Soc. Exp. Biol. Med.* **96**, 55.
Tokumaru, T. (1963). *Fed. Proc., Fed. Amer. Soc. Exp. Biol.* **22**, 616.
Tokumaru, T. (1968). *Arch. Gesamte Virusforsch.* **24**, 104.
Tytell, A. A., and Newman, R. E. (1963). *Proc. Soc. Exp. Biol. Med.* **113**, 343.
Urbain, A., and Schaefer, W. (1929). *Ann. Inst. Pasteur, Paris* **43**, 369.
Vaheri, A., and Cantell, K. (1963). *Virology* **21**, 661.
Vantsis, J. T., and Wildy, P. (1962). *Virology* **17**, 225.
Vonka, V., and Benyesh-Melnick, M. (1966). *J. Bacteriol.* **91**, 213.
von Kerékjártó, B., and Rhode, B. (1957). *Z. Naturforsch. B* **12**, 292.

Waddell, G. H., and Sigel, M. M. (1966). *Arch. Gesemte Virusforsch.* **19**, 130.
Waterson, A. P. C. (1958). *Arch. Gesemte Virusforsch.* **8**, 592.
Watkins, J. F. (1960). *J. Gen. Microbiol.* **22**, 57.
Watson, D. H., and Wildy, P. (1963). *Virology* **21**, 100.
Watson, D. H., Russell, W. C., and Wildy, P. (1963). *Virology* **19**, 250.
Waubke, R., zur Hausen, H., and Henle, W. (1968). *J. Virol.* **2**, 1047.
Webster, R. G. (1959). *N.Z. Vet. J.* **7**, 67.
Weller, T. H., McCauley, J. E., Craig, J. M., and Wirth, P. (1957). *Proc. Soc. Exp. Biol. Med.* **94**, 4.
Weller, T. H., Witton, H. M., and Bell, E. J. (1958). *J. Exp. Med.* **108**, 843.
Wenner, H. A. (1944). *Amer. J. Dis. Child.* **67**, 247.
Wheeler, C. E. (1958). *J. Immunol.* **81**, 98.
Wheeler, C. E. (1964). *J. Immunol.* **93**, 749.
Wildy, P. (1967). *J. Hyg.* **65**, 173.
Wildy, P., Stoker, M. G. P., and Ross, R. W. (1959). *J. Gen. Microbiol.* **20**, 105.
Wolf, K., and Darlington, R. W. (1971). *J. Virol.* **8**, 525.
Womack, C. R., and Randall, C. C. (1953). *Amer. J. Med.* **15**, 633.
Yoshino, K., Tanaguchi, H., and Tanaguchi, S. (1960). *Virology* **19**, 97.
Zarafonetis, C. J. D., Smadel, J. E., Adams, J. W., and Haymarker, W. (1944). *Amer. J. Pathol.* **20**, 429.

Chapter 5
Replication of the Viruses—Morphological Aspects

D. H. Watson

I. Introduction

A survey of the literature since 1954 shows that there are at least 200 papers in which replication of herpesviruses has been studied with the electron microscope. In this chapter the various stages of the growth cycle will be described with reference to some of these papers; in general, reference will not be made to studies with individual members of the group where these only confirm conclusions drawn from work on herpes simplex virus.

Morgan and Rose (1959) have stated that "electron microscopy by itself dissociated from allied or complementary techniques can raise new questions, but it cannot provide the answers." The scope of this chapter creates such a dissociation even where it does not exist in the original work. This may, however, be appropriate since a large number of electron microscopic studies have been completely divorced from even the most elementary biological data. In many cases, it is not even known whether single cycle growth is occuring in the system studied. Admittedly, this defect has now been remedied for herpes simplex virus, but technical difficulties in assay of some of the more recently discovered herpesviruses or in growing these in high titer stocks have meant that many studies on these viruses have been made under multicycle conditions.

It should also be noted that infections of cultured cells with herpes simplex virus are notoriously asynchronous. Thus, even when conditions of single-step infection have apparently been attained, it is often not possible to detect synthesis of virus-specific proteins or virus DNA before a rise in the number of virus particles (Russell *et al.*, 1964).

To these biological difficulties must be added the sampling problems encountered in thin sectioning, which mean that only very small volumes of a small number of cells may have been examined in any particular study.

It is important to bear these problems in mind because the temptation is to arrange what may be an arbitrary selection of micrographs into what appears to be a logical sequence of development of virus growth. It is then all too easy to make dynamic interpretations of such static images, and the literature abounds with micrographs purporting to show "particles being engulfed by pinocytotic vesicles," "release of DNA from infecting particles," "envelopment of newly synthesized particles," etc.

II. Attachment and Penetration

Electron microscopic studies on attachment and penetration have usually used infection with up to 1000 physical particles per cell in order to provide a reasonable number of particles in the thin sections. It is quite possible that only a very few particles undergo the specific processes leading to infection and that the rest are treated nonspecifically by the cells. It is important to remember this major difficulty in considering all conclusions derived from electron microscopic studies of attachment and penetration.

A. Attachment

Gostling and Bedson (1956) and Farnham and Newton (1959) had shown that if herpes simplex virus was adsorbed in the cold, virus multiplication only occurred on warming the cells. Farnham and Newton (1959) further showed that virus adsorbed in the cold only became insensitive to antibody after warming and therefore concluded that while virus could attach to cells in the cold, penetration required elevation of the temperature. Holmes and Watson (1963) used these observations in their morphological studies of the early stages of herpes infection; the processes of attachment and penetration were separated by adsorbing the virus at 4° C and then allowing penetration to occur by warming to 37° C.

Both naked and enveloped particles were seen on the outer surface of BHK 21 cells treated with herpes simplex virus at 4° C (Fig. 1). Less than 20% of the particles were inside the cell and most of these were in vesicles near the cell membrane and hence may not have been entirely enclosed within the cell. Particle counts on extracts of cells which were disrupted after attachment showed that there was a higher proportion of enveloped particles attached to the cells than had been present in the inoculum. It was concluded that enveloped particles were about twice as likely to be adsorbed as naked particles. Similar conclusions were drawn by Siegert and Falke (1966).

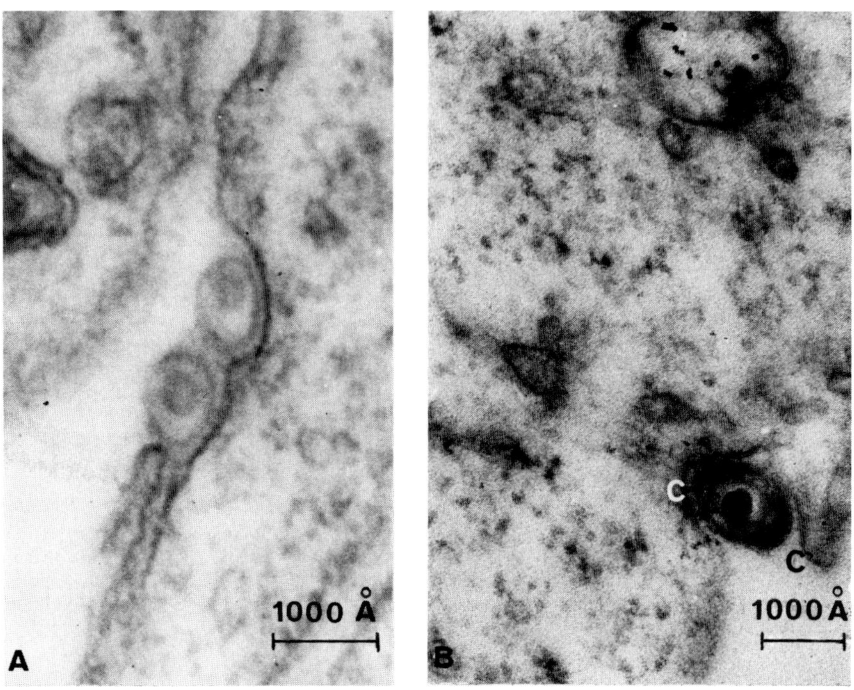

FIG. 1. Thin sections of BHK 21 cells after 45 minutes exposure to herpes simplex virus showing (A) naked and (B) enveloped particles in cell surface (C, cell membrane).

B. Penetration

Holmes and Watson (1963) observed the process of penetration by warming BHK 21 cells to which herpes simplex virus had been adsorbed in the cold. Thin sections showed both enveloped and naked particles in cytoplasmic vesicles (Fig. 2). These seemed to be pinocytotic vesicles, and when these were marked by including colloidal thorium dioxide in the growth medium, virus particles and thorium dioxide were present in the same vesicles (Fig. 2B). They accordingly concluded, as did Epstein *et al.* (1964) and Siegert and Falke (1966), that virus entered the cells by pinocytosis or "viropexis" as had been described for adenovirus and vaccinia virus by Dales (1962). Nucleocapsids were occasionally found free in the cytoplasm, possibly as a result of release of particles from the vesicles. It is difficult to detect release of DNA from the particles by thin-sectioning techniques

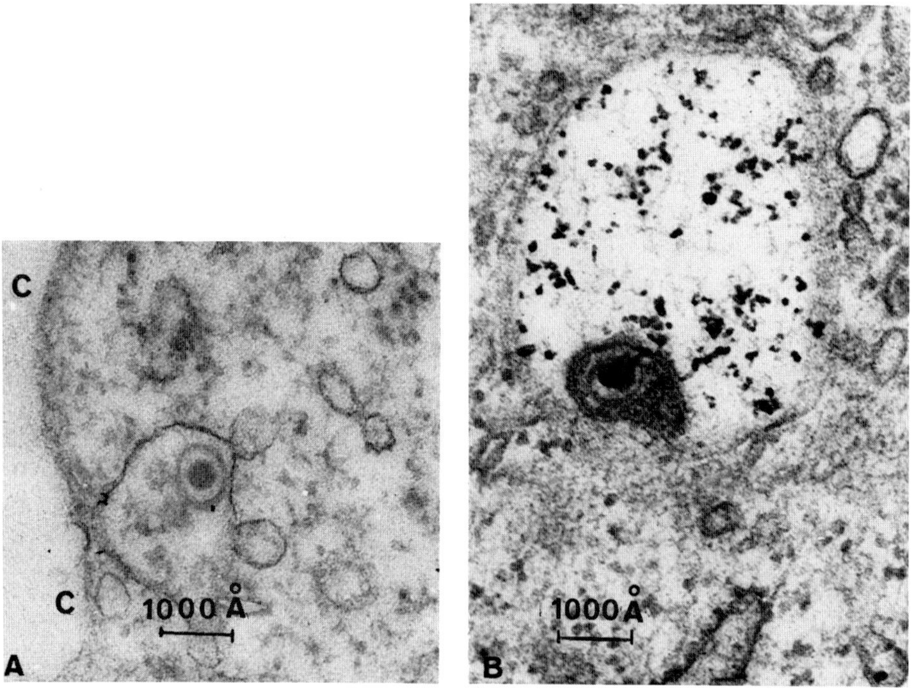

FIG. 2. Thin sections of BHK 21 cells infected with herpes simplex virus at 4°C and then incubated at 37°C for 30 minutes showing (A) naked and (B) enveloped particles in pinocytotic vesicles. The cell in (B) was incubated in medium containing colloidal thorium dioxide so that pinocytotic vesicles are "marked" with small dense grains (C, cell membrane).

alone. However, Hummeler *et al.* (1969) were able to follow this stage in penetration by using autoradiographic techniques in association with electron microscopy. They infected BHK 21 cells with virus labeled with [^{3}H]-thymidine and located parental virus DNA by autoradiography after thin sectioning. They found silver grains in the cytoplasm associated with free naked particles which frequently showed morphological evidence of digestion to leave an isolated dense core. They also observed cytoplasmic silver grains in the absence of any morphological evidence of the virus itself and at later times after infection found silver grains in the nucleus.

Morgan *et al.* (1968) have challenged the view that virus enters the cell by pinocytosis or viropexis. Although they found particles in vesicles, they also observed enveloped virus particles apparently fusing with the plasma membrane (Fig. 3). They also found naked particles lying free in the cytoplasm and concluded that these were produced by release from enveloped particles which had earlier fused with the plasma membrane. They stress that they found few particles in the midst of fusion and speculated that it might be a rare event or might occur very rapidly.

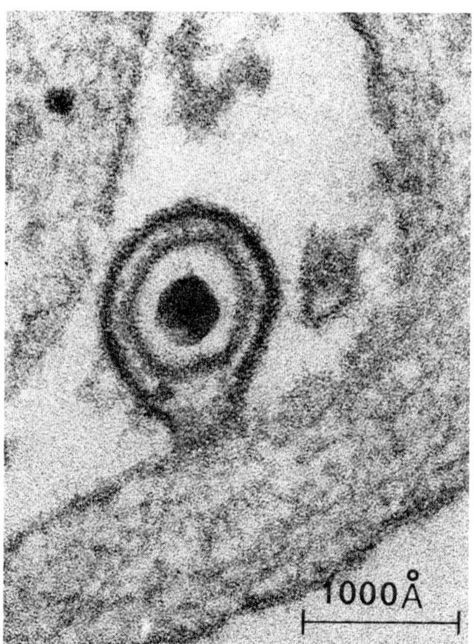

FIG. 3. Enveloped particles of herpes simplex virus on surface of HeLa cell showing apparent fusion of the virus envelope and the cell membrane. (Reproduced by kind permission of Dr. C. Morgan and the American Society for Microbiology).

This work has recently been extended by Miyamoto and Morgan (1971) who have claimed that there are two types of enveloped particles (Fig. 4). One, the "dense capsid" form, shows more electron-dense material between capsid and core than the other, "light capsid," form. The dense forms are described as unstable because they are apparently disintegrated near the cell membrane, and indeed about half of them are stated to be partially disintegrated before entry into the cell. The light capsid forms are apparently more stable and shortly after infection form a higher proportion of the particles found. Only this form is found inside the cell. Later, predominantly empty or coreless capsids are found. The authors speculate that the DNA released from the dense forms codes for a virus-specific enzyme which renders the light capsids permeable and allows them to release "infectious DNA." They thus envisage that both particles have a role in the infectious process. This conclusion would, of course, have far-reaching implications for the kinetics of infection with herpesviruses. If such a mechanism were operative at high multiplicity, it would presumably also be necessary for infection at low multiplicity, and this would demand that herpes infection (at any rate, infection of HeLa cells with this strain of virus) should show two hit kinetics. The authors, however, do consider the possibility that the dense particles play no part in the infection process and that the light particles contain a DNA/RNA polymerase although there is so far no evidence for such an enzyme in herpesvirus particles. They do not, however, consider the possibility that only the dense particles play any part in the infective process with the conversion of the light particles to coreless forms by nonspecific digestion.

Dales and Silverberg (1969) have opposed the view that infection occurs by fusion of the virus envelope with the cell membrane. Like Miyamoto and Morgan (1971), they found particles with broken envelopes in the inoculum, and they suggested that the apparent fusion was caused by apposition of such broken particles to the cell membrane. Hummeler *et al.* (1969) found some evidence of fusion but found that most of their particles of H strain herpes simplex virus entered BHK 21 cells by pinocytosis. They therefore argued on quantitative grounds that this was more likely to be the mode of infection, although such quantitative arguments may not be valid. Morgan *et al.* (1968) have pointed out that pinocytosis is nonspecific and acts on any particulate matter in the growth medium, and, therefore, they argue that it is not surprising to find some virus particles in pinocytotic vesicles. However, Miyamoto and Morgan (1971) claimed that particles in vesicles formed a very small proportion of those found in the cell; this seems in contradiction to the results of Holmes and Watson (1963) and Hummeler *et al.* (1969), and it is possible that the difference may be due to the fact that these authors

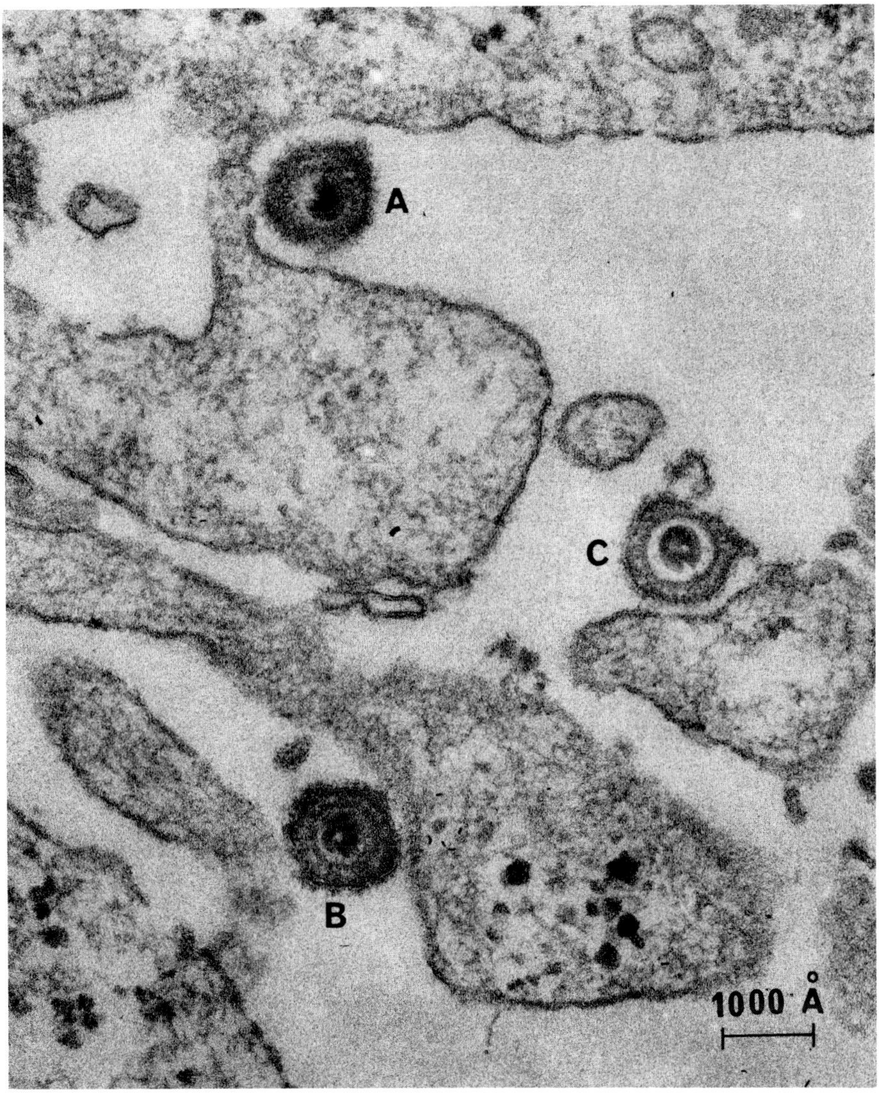

FIG. 4. Enveloped particles of herpes simplex virus on surface of HeLa cell. Particles A and B are dense capsids, and C, light capsid forms. (Reproduced by kind permission of Dr. C. Morgan and the American Society for Microbiology.)

used BHK 21 cells rather than HeLa cells which were used by Morgan *et al.* (1968) and Miyamoto and Morgan (1971). BHK 21 cells grow more rapidly than HeLa cells and may therefore be more active in pinocytosis. One might then predict that infection of BHK 21 cells might be less efficient than infection of less metabolically active cells (because a higher proportion of particles would be pinocytosed before they could fuse with the membrane), whereas in general this appears not to be the case: Studies in this laboratory show that higher plaque numbers are obtained by assay of herpes simplex in BHK 21 cells than in HeLa, HEp 2, or RK 13 cells. This prediction would only hold if virus particles in pinocytotic vesicles were potentially infective, and it appears that at least some of them must be, since infective virus particles, insensitive to antibody (Farnham and Newton, 1959) or low pH (Huang and Wagner, 1964), can be recovered by disruption of infected cells. Plainly, enveloped particles in pinocytotic vesicles could still release their capsids into the cytoplasm by fusion with the vesicle membrane, in which case there would be no real conflict between the two views on penetration. However, both Dales and Silverberg (1969) and Hummeler *et al.* (1969) presented evidence for digestion of particles within vesicles.

Hummeler *et al.* (1969), Morgan *et al.* (1968), and Miyamoto and Morgan (1971) make little reference to uptake of naked particles in their experiments. Their inocula must have contained naked particles because they, like Holmes and Watson (1963), prepared their inocula by disruption of infected cells by ultrasonic vibration. At first sight, it would appear that such particles could only enter the cell by pinocytosis. However, Morgan *et al.* (1969) have claimed that adenovirus particles can pass into the cytoplasm by direct penetration of the cell membrane rather than from pinocytotic vesicles. A similar process with herpesvirus could account for some of the cytoplasmic naked particles observed by Morgan *et al.* (1968).

Abodeely *et al.* (1970) have described entry of both enveloped and naked particles of equine abortion virus by pinocytosis. Zee and Talens (1971), on the other hand, favor the fusion process for infection of bovine kidney cells with infectious bovine rhinotracheitis. McCracken and Clarke (1971) also observed fusion of partially digested, enveloped pseudorabies particles with the cell membrane; enveloped particles were only occasionally seen in pinocytotic vesicles.

A final conclusion on the process of penetration is plainly impossible by electron microscopy alone for the reasons outlined in this section. Furthermore, biochemical studies on the process suffer from many of the difficulties which beset electron microscopic studies. A final solution would demand the isolation of a class of particles with uniform properties with a high efficiency of infection.

III. Growth of the Virus

This section describes the various stages observed in electron microscopic studies of the growth of herpesviruses. No attempt will be made to describe the growth cycles for individual herpesviruses because, although differences have been observed, it is by no means certain that these are significant. Indeed, there are greater differences between the various studies on herpes simplex virus than between different herpesviruses; this may not be surprising in view of the differences described by Schwartz and Roizman (1969a) in the electron microscopic appearance of cells infected with freshly isolated and laboratory strains of herpes simplex virus. What follows then is a composite picture of the morphological aspects of the growth of herpesviruses that will be illustrated with reference to individual studies. These references are not intended to be comprehensive but rather to illustrate the frequency with which individual structures have been observed. Results with different herpesviruses are also cited, again without any claim of being comprehensive but in order to give some idea of the number of different virus systems showing a particular structure.

A. Early Stages

The early stages of the growth cycle are defined as those before newly formed particles are seen in the nucleus. [It should be noted that particle counts of infected cell extracts during the growth cycle (Watson *et al.*, 1964) show that the number of particles begins to increase at a point when there are still apparently appreciable numbers of residual inoculum particles. It, therefore, follows that it is not possible to be certain that the intranuclear particles seen in thin sections are newly formed. However, the work of Hummeler *et al.* (1969), in which cells were infected with labeled virus, gave no evidence for complete particles from the inoculum passing to the nucleus, and it therefore seems reasonable to assume that intranuclear naked particles in thin sections represent progeny virus.]

A number of different structures have been observed in the nuclei of infected cells, and most of these structures are described in the published literature by a number of workers in this field. It is, of course, difficult to distinguish structures with a role to play in virus replication from those structures merely representing break-down products of cellular organelles. Thus, large aggregates are observed near the nuclear membranes early in infection. These aggregates seem to correspond to the marginated chromatin observed by light microscopy of infected cells after Feulgen staining. This correspondence has been confirmed by Schwartz and Roizman (quoted in

Roizman, 1969) who showed that these aggregates contained DNA by autoradiography of cells labeled with [^{3}H]thymidine before infection.

The nucleoli gradually disappear after infection with herpes simplex virus, and some of the intranuclear bodies found early in infection seem to have the characteristic granular structure of nucleoli (Fig. 5) (Watson *et al.*, 1964) and are similar to bodies seen in the nuclei of cells treated with inhibitors (Bernhard, 1966). However, Miyamoto *et al.* (1971) using immunoferritin tagging have found virus-specific antigen in structures which they describe as disaggregated nucleoli, although no antigen was found in the nucleolar matrix.

Fine-grained dense aggregates were observed early in the nuclei of BHK 21 cells infected with herpes simplex virus by Watson *et al.* (1964). These aggregates differed in staining characteristics and granularity from aggregates of interchromatin granules or nucleolar fragments (Fig. 5), and they seem to be characteristic of the virus-infected cells. Naked particles are often found near these granules later in infection. In some places, individual grains 100 Å in diameter are seen at the edge of these granules (Fig. 5). Similar aggregates were described by Schwartz and Roizman (1969a) in cells infected with herpes simplex virus, by Tournier *et al.* (1957) in cells infected with varicella virus, by Felluga (1963) in cells infected with pseudorabies virus, and by Pinkerton *et al.* (1964) in cells infected with human cytomegalovirus.

The aggregates observed by Stackpole (1969) in nuclei of cells from the Lucké adenocarcinoma seem to have a structure similar to the aggregates described in the preceding paragraph, although Stackpole quotes the diameter of the individual granules as 200–400 Å. He showed by autoradiographic methods that thymidine was incorporated into these aggregates. Nii *et al.* (1968a) and Miyamoto *et al.* (1971) used ferritin tagging to show that in cells infected with herpes simplex similar aggregates contained virus antigen. Hampar *et al.* (1971) also observed these structures in Burkitt tumor lymphoblasts containing EB virus and showed that they contained virus antigen reacting with human heterophil-positive infectious mononucleosis sera.

These aggregates may correspond to the A granules described in cytochemical studies of herpes-infected HeLa cells by Love and Wildy (1963) and shown by them to contain both DNA and nonhistone protein.

The role of these aggregates is, of course, uncertain, but because they seem to contain virus antigen and DNA and because virus particles are often found near them, they seem likely to be related to formation of new virus particles.

Of more doubtful significance are the less densely packed aggregates of granules, about 200 Å in diameter, described by Morgan *et al.* (1959), by

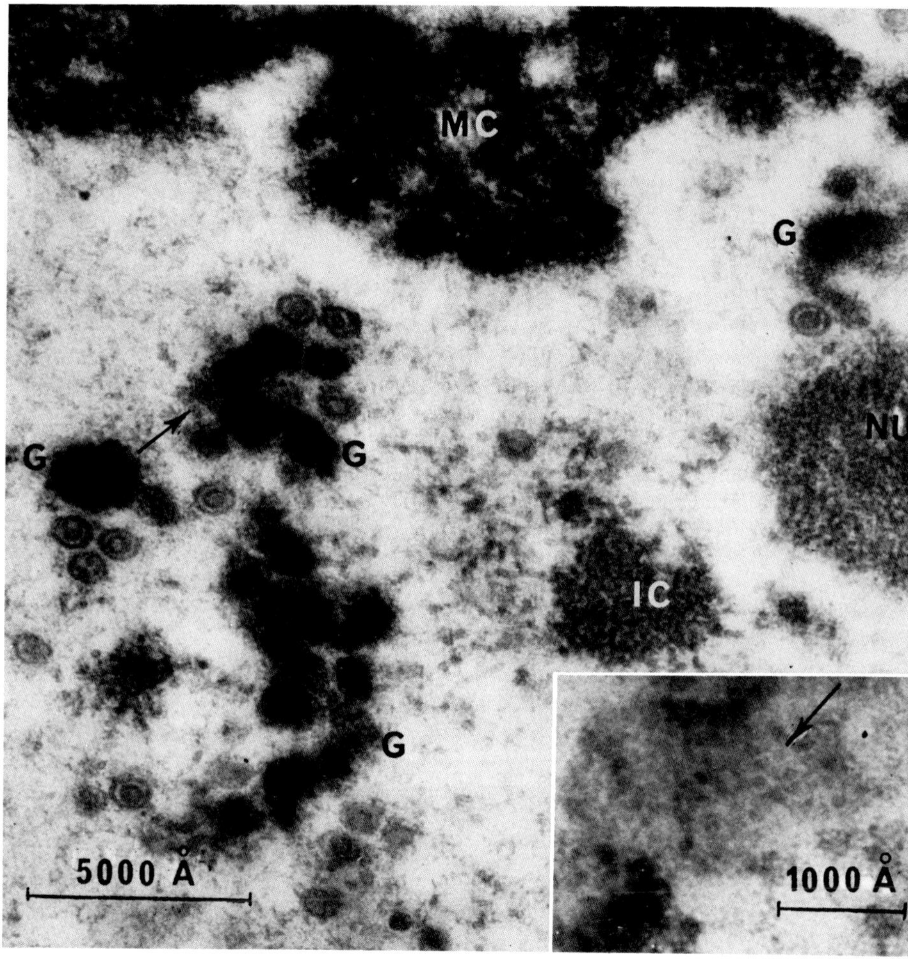

FIG. 5. Section of BHK 21 cell infected with herpes simplex virus showing intranuclear fine-grained aggregates (G). The aggregates differ in grain and in staining characteristics from an aggregate of interchromatin granules, 200 Å in diameter (IC), from a nucleolar fragment (NU), and from the marginated chromatin (MC). The arrow indicates 100 Å granules at the edge of one of the aggregates. The inset shows a higher magnification view of similar granules at the edge of another fine-grained aggregate.

Schwartz and Roizman (1969a), and by Nii (1971) in cells infected with herpes simplex virus. These granules generally appeared hollow. Similar structures were observed in cells infected with Marek's disease virus (Epstein *et al.*, 1968). Nii (1971) has suggested these granules may be virus cores, as has Roizman (1969) who has related them to the 250 Å bodies he found in CsCl gradients of formaldehyde treated lysates from infected cells (see Chapter 2). However, the role of this type of aggregate must be regarded as much less certain than that of the dense, fine-grained aggregates described in the preceding paragraphs. Although they have been described by a number of workers, a puzzling feature is the variability in the frequency of their occurrence. Morgan *et al.* (1959) found large numbers of granules in HeLa cells infected with the JM strain of herpes simplex virus but the same group makes no mention of them in studies of HeLa or FL cells infected with Miyama strain (Nii *et al.*, 1968a,b) or of BHK 21 cells infected with the 1-MAL strain (Miyamoto *et al.*, 1971). They were observed frequently by Schwartz and Roizman (1969a) in HEp 2 cells infected with either of two freshly isolated strains (F, an oral isolate, and G, a genital isolate) or with either of two laboratory strains (mP and MP). The structures described by them look very similar to those labeled interchromatin granules described by Watson *et al.* (1964) (see Fig. 5). These are also present in uninfected cells (Bernhard and Granboulan, 1963) although they are seen more frequently in infected cells. However, the "clearing" of the nucleus by margination of the chromatin which occurs after herpes infection may perhaps allow them to be detected more readily after infection. These structures must therefore be regarded as being of doubtful significance until autoradiography or immunoferritin techniques allow them to be related to synthesis of virus DNA or protein.

All the structures so far described in this section are intranuclear, although Fujiwara and Kaplan (1967) showed that virus structural proteins were first formed in the cytoplasm. Correspondingly, using ferritin tagging, Miyamoto *et al.* (1971) showed the presence of virus antigens in both the cytoplasm and nucleus during early stages of infection of BHK 21 cells with herpes simplex virus. These workers made use of the differing specificities of early (7-day) and later (7-week) rabbit anti-herpes simplex virus sera and used IgG and IgM fractions to give them four reagents which had differing immunological specificities. In this way, they showed that while the early antigens in the nucleus reacted with both early and late antisera, the early antigens in the cytoplasm reacted only with the early sera. This would certainly show that some of the intranuclear antigen differs from the cytoplasmic antigen, but this must not necessarily be taken as evidence that this particular antigen is synthesized in the nucleus. There may well have been some antigenic modification of cytoplasmic antigens transferred to the nucleus. Miyamoto *et al.* (1971) observed ferritin-tagged material in the nuclear pores and interpreted this to be transfer of cytoplasmic antigen to the nucleus. Such a transfer would agree with the evidence of Spear and Roizman (1968) that herpesvirus proteins are made in the cytoplasm and transferred to the nucleus.

B. Formation of Naked Particles

Particle counts on extracts of cells infected with herpes simplex virus show an increase in the number of naked particles 1–2 hours before increased numbers of enveloped particles are found (Watson *et al.*, 1964). Thin sections of the infected cells at this stage of the cycle show naked particles usually scattered singly throughout the nucleus (Fig. 6). Autoradiography of thin sections of cells infected with labeled virus shows that progeny particles are not usually found in the vicinity of parental DNA (Hummeler *et al.*, 1969).

The cores may either be dense or hollow and less dense (Fig. 6) (Watson *et al.*, 1964; Nii *et al.*, 1968b; Nii, 1971). Usually both types of core are represented in the early particles (Watson *et al.*, 1964; Nii, 1971), although Nii *et al.* (1968b) found only hollow cores in particles observed early in infection. The differences may well be explained by the results of Nii (1971), who noted that even when cells were infected at high multiplicity, sections of adjacent nuclei often showed particles of different core morphology. However, even where both forms were found simultaneously, the proportion of dense cores rose later in the cycle (Watson *et al.*, 1964). McCracken and Clarke (1971) working with pseudorabies virus and Strandberg and Aurelian (1969) with canine herpesvirus also noted higher proportions of dense core forms later in infection.

Nii *et al.* (1968c) found only particles with hollow cores in cells infected with herpes simplex virus in the presence of 50 m*M* hydroxyurea; this chemical completely inhibited production of infective virus. They accordingly suggested that the hollow core particles do not contain DNA without necessarily implying that they were a precursor to dense core forms containing DNA. Miyamoto *et al.* (1971) showed the presence of virus antigen in hollow cores using immunoferritin tagging but were unable to determine the reactivity of dense cores with ferritin-labeled antibody, possibly because the dense core capsids are less permeable to the conjugate.

Heine *et al.* (1971) studied particles of herpesvirus saimiri in infected WI 38, African green monkey kidney, and owl monkey kidney cells. A higher proportion of hollow core particles was found in WI 38 cells than in the other two cells, and the infectivity yield was correspondingly lower, which may be in accord with the idea that the hollow core particles contain no DNA. On the other hand, Stackpole (1969) showed with autoradiographic methods that hollow cores of Lucké virus in tumor explants incorporated thymidine, and with pulse chase experiments he showed that these particles were later converted to the dense core form.

The significance of hollow and dense cores has, therefore, not been established rigorously. The difference could, of course, be artifactual, and

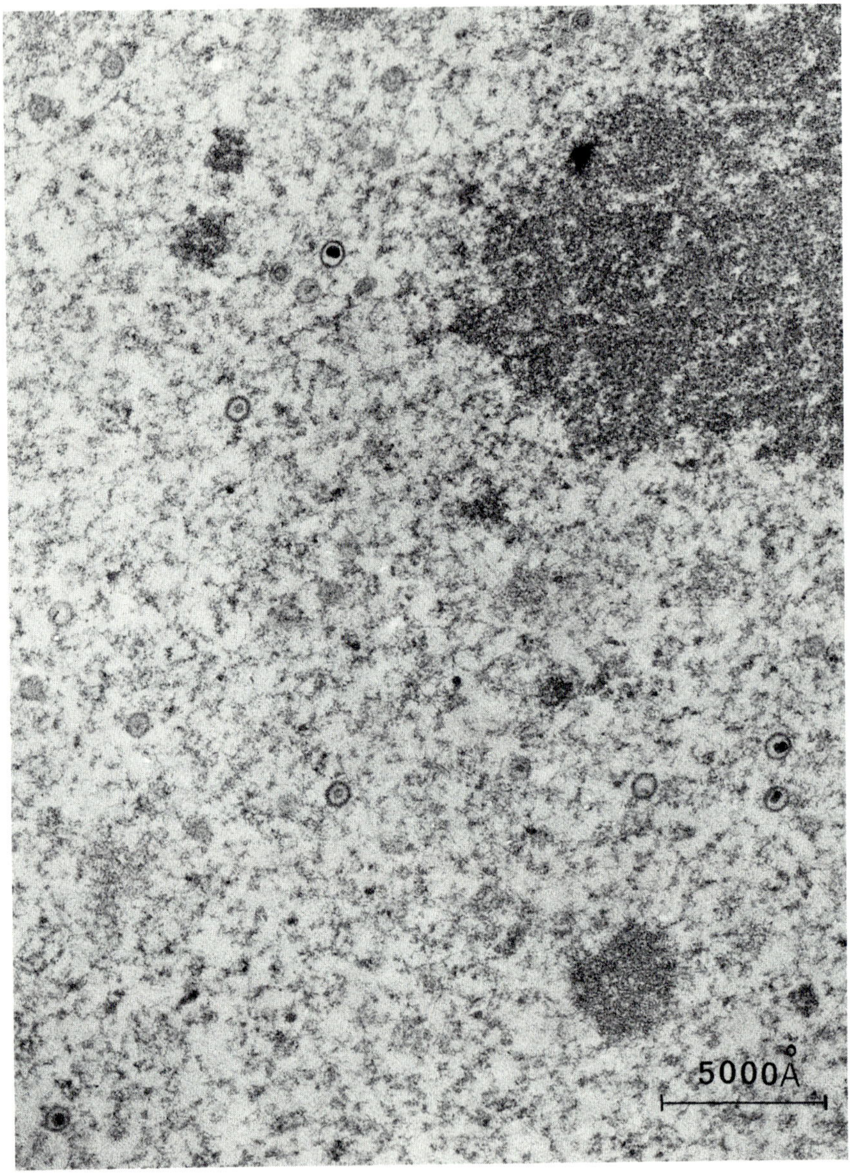

FIG. 6. Scattered naked particles of herpes simplex virus in nucleus of infected HeLa cell. Both hollow and dense cores are present. (Reproduced by kind permission of Dr. C. Morgan and the American Society for Microbiology.)

Kellenberger *et al.* (1967) and Granboulan *et al.* (1971) have drawn attention to the difficulties involved in the fixation and staining of intracellular bacteriophage particles, which may or may not contain DNA. All enveloped particles have dense cores, but this may be related to their location in the cytoplasm because most of the cytoplasmic naked particles also have a dense core.

The granular cores found in some herpesvirus particles have been described in Chapter 2. They will not be described in detail here, but Miyamoto (1971) has proposed that they are a precursor of the dense core particle.

Apparently empty or coreless capsids are also observed in infected cells, and examples of these capsids are seen in at least some micrographs in all the published studies. It is again difficult to be sure of their significance. Watson *et al.* (1964) showed by serial sectioning that a capsid may appear coreless in one section but possess a core in the next section (see Fig. 11). However, higher proportions of coreless particles have been observed in certain cases. Thus, Stackpole (1969) published micrographs of areas in Lucké tumour cells where nearly all the virus particles are empty. O'Callaghan *et al.* (1968) also observed large numbers of empty capsids in cells infected with equine abortion virus in the presence of 5-fluorodeoxyuridine (FUdR). Plainly, the empty particles observed here must be considered to be real. However, the assembly of empty particles either in the presence or absence of metabolic inhibitors does not mean that this process is a necessary step in the assembly of infective virus particles.

As indicated earlier, particles observed early in the cycle are usually found scattered throughout the nucleus. Later in infection, groups of particles are found near the fine-grained aggregates referred to in Section III, A (Fig. 5). Aggregates surrounded by a number of particles (Fig. 7) have also been observed in cells infected with herpes simplex virus (Watson *et al.*, 1964), pseudorabies virus (Felluga, 1963), and cytomegalovirus (Pinkerton *et al.*, 1964).

Still later, when greater numbers of particles are present, the formation of large aggregates of particles ("crystals," Fig. 8) has been observed by a number of workers (Morgan *et al.*, 1959; Melnick *et al.*, 1968; Schwartz and Roizman, 1969; Miyamoto, 1971; Nii, 1971). Schwartz and Roizman (1969a) found crystals more frequently in cells infected with a freshly isolated oral strain of herpes simplex than in cells infected with either of two laboratory strains or with a freshly isolated genital strain. However, even strain differences may not account for all the variations: Stoker *et al.* (1959) found no crystals in HeLa cells infected with herpes simplex HFEM strain, whereas D. H. Watson and P. Wildy (unpublished observations) later observed crystals in the same virus–cell system. It seems likely that crystal formation is a quantitative effect; there are wide differences in the numbers of particles

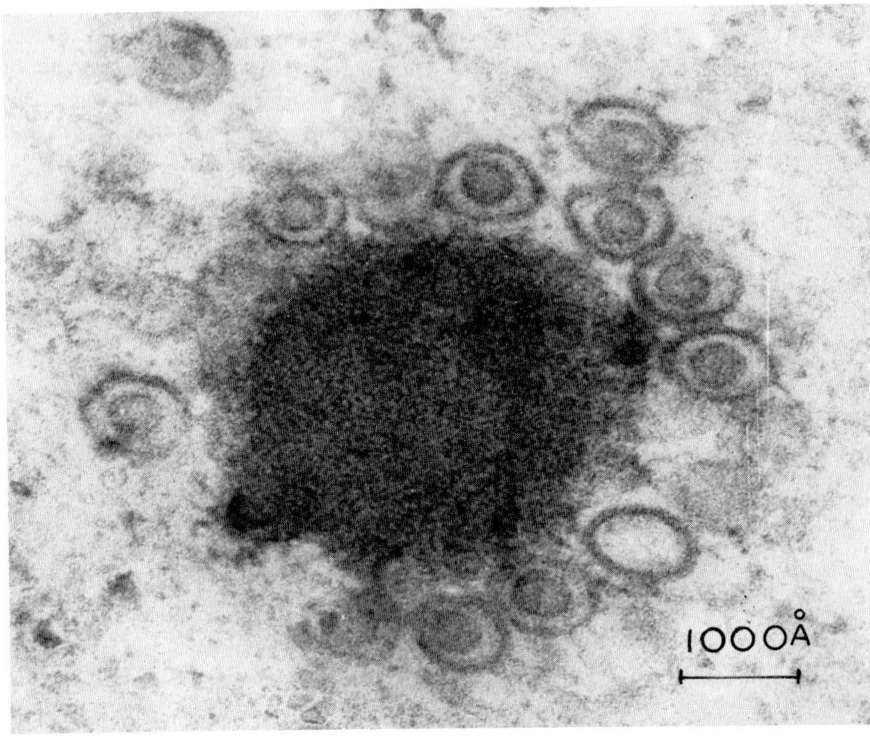

FIG. 7. Naked particles of herpes simplex virus surrounding fine-grained dense aggregate in nucleus of infected BHK 21 cell.

produced in different cells by different strains at different passage levels, and it is possible that crystals are formed of necessity whenever large numbers of particles are manufactured. Similar conclusions have recently been reached by Nii and Ono (1971).

The intranuclear particles are frequently observed in association with tubules or filaments. They were observed in cells infected with avian laryngotracheitis virus (Watrach, 1962), in cells of mice infected with herpes simplex type 2 (Murphy *et al.*, 1967), and in cells of the chorioallantoic membrane also infected with a type 2 strain of herpes simplex virus (Couch and Nahmias, 1969). Schwartz and Roizman (1969a) also observed these intranuclear particles in cells infected with a type 2 strain and have concluded that they are more typical of type 2 than of type 1 infections. The filaments described by these workers all have the form of microtubules with densely stained membranes arranged in pairs. The filaments described by

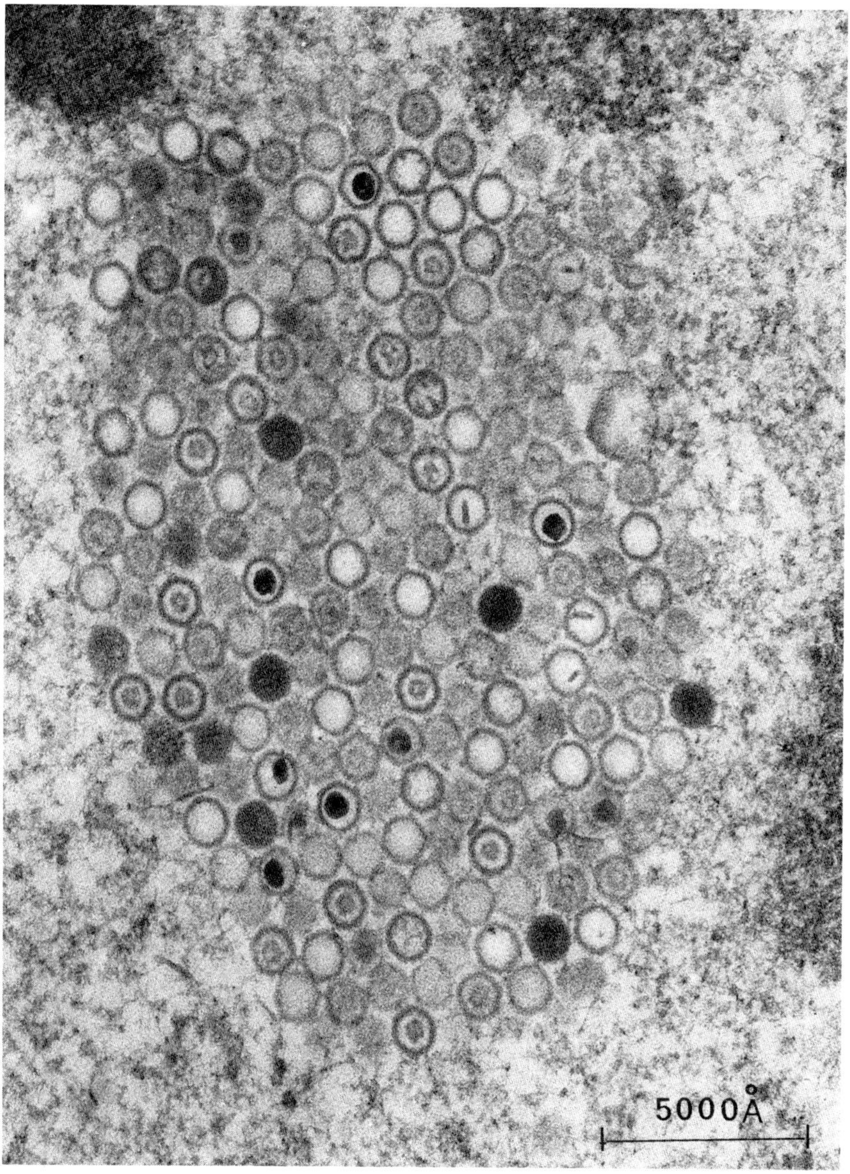

FIG. 8. "Crystal" of naked particles of herpes simplex virus in nucleus of infected HeLa cell. Cores are of either dense or hollow form. (Reproduced by kind permission of Dr. C. Morgan and the American Society for Microbiology.)

Abraham and Tegtmeyer (1970) in cells infected with feline herpesviruses have a different appearance—tightly packed bundles of single membranes. Finally, Stackpole and Mizell (1968) have described two kinds of tubules in frog tumor cells containing Lucké virus: these are 350 and 600 Å in diameter, respectively. They believe that the smaller tubules are related to core material, and they propose that the larger ones are formed by layering capsid material onto the smaller ones, although at the moment, there is no firm evidence for these ideas.

Miyamoto *et al.* (1971) have suggested that the capsid surface of herpes simplex virus possesses at least two separate antigenic specificities. Using immunoferritin techniques, they showed that both early IgM and late IgG antibodies reacted with virus capsids in infected cells. The conjugated late IgG still reacted with the capsids after pretreatment with unconjugated early IgM showing that the two reagents react with different sites.

C. Envelopment of Naked Particles

1. Mechanism of Envelopment

Particle counts on extracts of cells during growth show that the number of enveloped particles usually rises following the rise in the number of naked particles, and, correspondingly, the proportion of enveloped particles increases (Watson *et al.*, 1964). Even using the same strain of virus there seem to be differences in the proportion of enveloped particles observed. Thus, preparations of HFEM strain of herpes simplex virus grown in HeLa cells contain a higher proportion of enveloped particles than preparations of the same strain grown in BHK 21 cells (Watson and Wildy, 1963). It is, therefore, likely that the mechanism, or at any rate the efficiency, of envelopment differs from cell to cell, and this difference may well account for some of the apparently conflicting views on virus envelopment.

The problem of dynamic interpretation of static images (see Section I) becomes particularly acute in studies of virus envelopment. Morgan *et al.* (1954) noted enveloped particles of herpes simplex virus in the cytoplasm of infected chorioallantoic membranes of chick embryos while the particles in the nucleus were naked. They accordingly suggested that the envelope was acquired in the cytoplasm. Reissig and Melnick (1955) studied the growth of herpes B virus in monkey kidney cells and also noted enveloped particles in the cytoplasm, but they did observe occasional enveloped particles in the nucleus as Stoker *et al.* (1959) did in HeLa cells infected with herpes simplex virus. Two further studies of HeLa cells infected with herpes simplex virus by Morgan *et al.* (1959) and Falke *et al.* (1959) both described reduplication of the nuclear membrane which was extensively invaginated. They postulated that this process was related to virus envelopment which they thought took place either within the nucleus or at its periphery. Falke *et al.* (1959) demonstrated envelopment by the inner nuclear membrane, and the observation of Morgan *et al.* (1959) of enveloped particles between the inner and outer nuclear membrane would seem to be consistent with this view. Nii *et al.* (1968b) extended observations on the reduplication of nuclear membranes. They showed that reduplicated nuclear membranes often extended into the nucleus near groups of naked particles (Fig. 9A). Sometimes, the reduplicated membranes seemed to have fused to give thicker lamellae and capsids could be seen enclosed by them (Fig. 9b). Watson *et al.* (1964), studying BHK 21 cells infected with herpes simplex virus, noted vesicular structures in the cytoplasm which apparently derived from the nuclear membrane (Fig. 10). Sometimes, these contained naked particles apparently partly enveloped (Fig. 11). Correspondingly, Nii *et al.* (1968b) reported proliferation of reduplicated nuclear membranes into the cytoplasm of infected HeLa cells and showed budding of naked particles into cytoplasmic vacuoles (Fig. 12). Thus, in both BHK 21 cells and HeLa cells, envelopment may occur in the cytoplasm but although intranuclear enveloped particles were often found in HeLa cells, they were never found in BHK 21 cells, and Watson *et al.* (1964) only noted one enveloped particle between the inner and outer nuclear membranes. This quantitative difference may account for the higher proportion of enveloped particles in virus grown in HeLa cells. However, Darlington and Moss (1968) also used BHK 21 cells in their studies of the growth of herpes simplex, pseudorabies, and equine abortion viruses. They found large numbers of enveloped particles within vacuoles at the edge of the nucleus, although these vacuoles were often continuous with the perinuclear cisternae. Cytoplasmic envelopment was also observed occasionally, and in one case particles were seen apparently acquiring an envelope by budding from the cytoplasm into the outer nuclear membrane.

Similar observations on envelopment have been made for cytomegalovirus (McGavran and Smith, 1965) and varicella–zoster virus (Tournier *et al.*, 1957), infectious bovine rhinotracheitis virus (Armstrong *et al.*, 1961), turkey herpesvirus (Nazerian *et al.*, 1971), and herpesvirus saimiri (Heine *et al.*, 1971), although once again there are variations in the number of intranuclear enveloped particles reported. Thus, they were observed quite frequently by McGavran and Smith (1965) and not at all by Armstrong *et al.* (1961).

McGavran and Smith (1965), Darlington and Moss (1968), and Schwartz and Roizman (1969a) have all noted that the nuclear membrane is frequently thickened at the point of contact with a naked particle, suggesting that the membrane is modified before it envelopes the capsid. It is likely that this

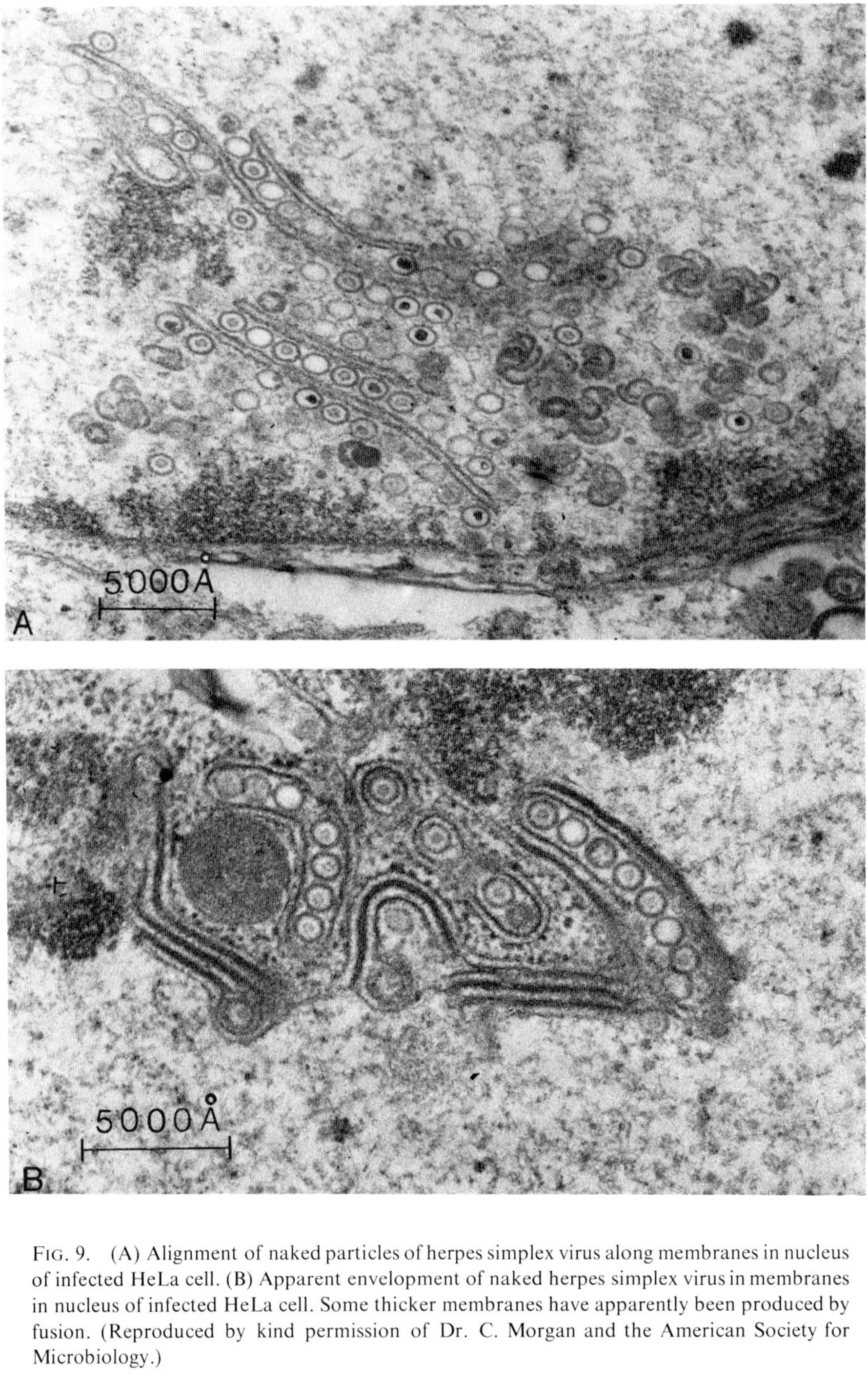

FIG. 9. (A) Alignment of naked particles of herpes simplex virus along membranes in nucleus of infected HeLa cell. (B) Apparent envelopment of naked herpes simplex virus in membranes in nucleus of infected HeLa cell. Some thicker membranes have apparently been produced by fusion. (Reproduced by kind permission of Dr. C. Morgan and the American Society for Microbiology.)

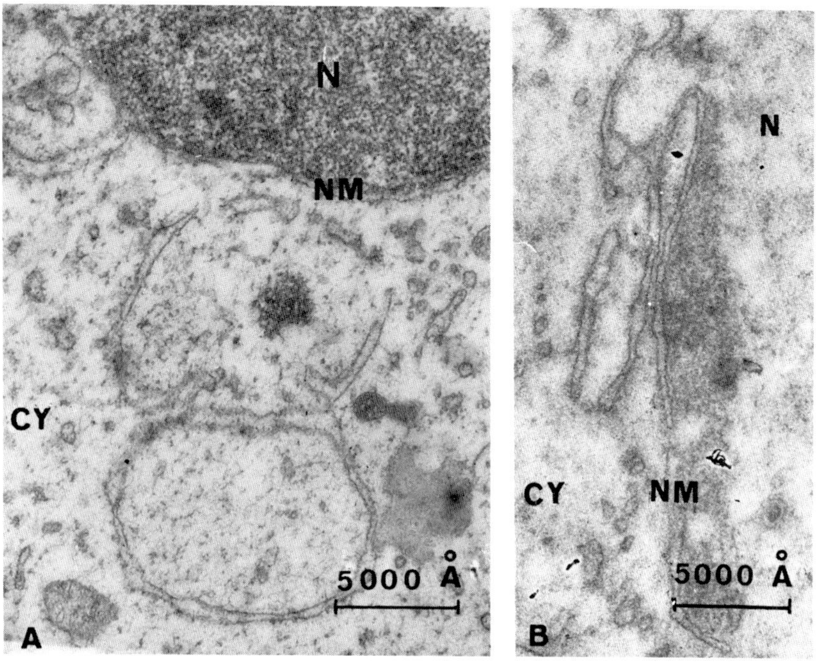

FIG. 10. (A) Membranous structures in cytoplasm of BHK 21 cell infected with herpes simplex virus, (B) suggests that these originate from the nuclear membrane. (CY, cytoplasm; N, nucleus; NM, nuclear membrane.)

thickening is related to the virus-specific antigen detected with immunoferritin tagging by Miyamoto *et al.* (1971) on the inner side of the nuclear membrane enclosing capsides. This material had a different antigenic specificity from the outer surface of enveloped particles, since it reacted only with early IgG and late IgM antibodies, whereas the early IgM and late IgG antibodies reacted with the envelope surface.

Schwartz and Roizman (1969a) have noted that the capsid is always maintained at a fixed distance from the enveloping nuclear membrane and deduce that this is due to the presence of an inner envelope. Felluga (1963) has described an elaborate series of intermediates in envelopment of pseudorabies virus in pig kidney cells. The naked particles (A forms) are described as being enveloped by nuclear membrane to give B particles which later acquire additional layers at cytoplasmic membranes to give C and D particles.

As has already been noted by Darlington and Moss (1969), in their review

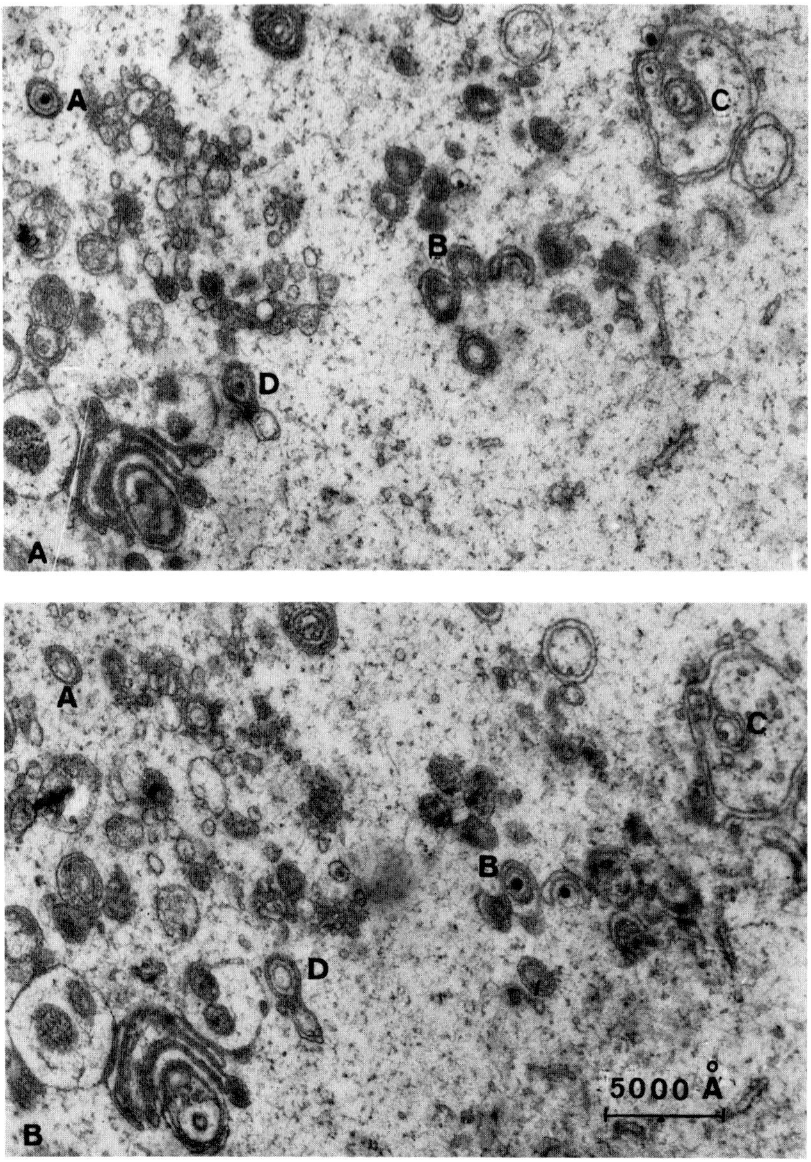

FIG. 11. Two consecutive serial sections of part of the cytoplasm of BHK 21 cell infected with herpes simplex virus. Corresponding particles in the two sections marked A, B, C, D. (Note that A and D are coreless in (B) but not in (A), while B is coreless in (A) but not in (B). At C, envelopment of naked particles is apparently occurring in vacuolar structures similar to those in Fig. 10.

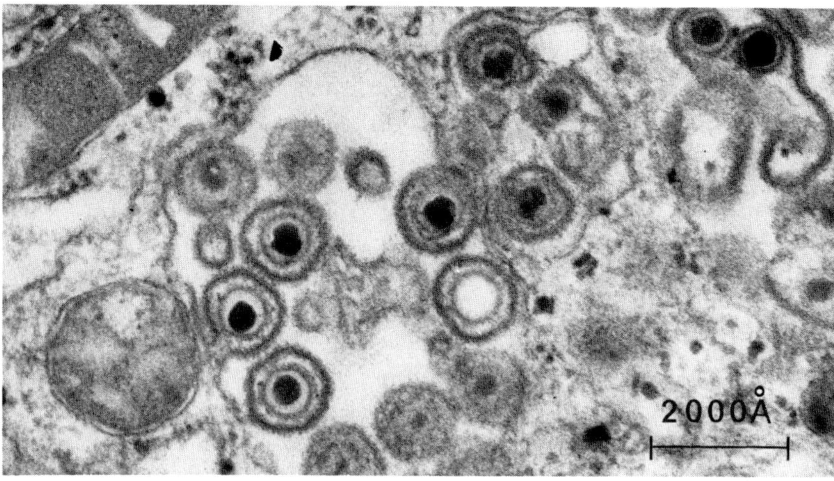

FIG. 12. Part of the cytoplasm of HeLa cell infected with herpes simplex, showing enveloped particles in vacuole; a naked particle is apparently acquiring an envelope by budding into the vacuole. (Reproduced by kind permission of Dr. C. Morgan and the American Society for Microbiology.)

on the envelope of herpesviruses, virtually all workers have noted naked particles in the cytoplasm. This is not surprising in view of the apparent dissolution of the nuclear membrane (Fig. 10). However, Roizman (1971) has observed naked particles in the cytoplasm of infected cells where the nucleus appears to be intact. He has related this observation to the work of Stackpole (1969) who has suggested that after Lucké virus is enveloped by the inner nuclear membrane, the virus becomes unenveloped by the outer nuclear membrane and then enveloped once again by membranes of the Golgi network. Darlington and Moss (1969), however, also account for cytoplasmic naked particles on the basis of breaks in the nuclear membrane and suggest that envelopment occurs wherever a particle comes into contact with a cell membrane, be it nuclear or cytoplasmic. A logical extension of this view would be the envelopment of naked particles at the cell membrane as described by Epstein (1962) and Simonoff and Menefee (1966), although Nii *et al.* (1968b) have questioned this interpretation and suggested that some of the particles observed by Epstein (1962) may, in fact, represent entering particles being uncoated.

2. Significance of the Envelope

The overall picture of envelopment in Section III,C,1 is of an almost random process which is underlined by the occurrence of envelopes containing two or even more nucleocapsids. Pirie (1957) first questioned the relevance of the envelope for the infectivity of the virus. Smith (1964) separated naked and enveloped particles on cesium chloride density gradients and found infectivity only in fractions containing enveloped particles. However, Ben-Porat and Kaplan (1962), Watson *et al.* (1964), and Spring and Roizman (1968) have all drawn attention to the poor recoveries of infectivity when herpes simplex virus is centrifuged through cesium chloride density gradients, and Smith's (1964) results may, therefore, only indicate preferential loss of infectivity of naked particles under these conditions. Watson *et al.* (1964) found that the infective titers of herpes simplex preparations were often significantly greater than the number of enveloped particles in the preparations and concluded that naked particles might be infective. Stein *et al.* (1970) separated naked and enveloped particles by centrifuging in sucrose density gradients. They found most of the infectivity was associated with fractions containing only enveloped particles, but considered that the low infectivities associated with naked particles were significant and not due to contamination with enveloped particles. Abodeely *et al.* (1970) used detergent to strip the envelopes from equine abortion virus particles in order to produce particles which appeared naked in the electron microscope. The detergent treatment destroyed over 99.99% of the infectivity of the preparation but they considered the residual infectivity of the de-enveloped particles was greater than could be accounted for by contaminating enveloped particles, since they saw no enveloped particles in a total of 27,000 particles counted.

Spring and Roizman (1968) approached the problem by using cell fractionation techniques. They showed that 75% of the infectivity present in HEp 2 cells 8 hours after infection with herpes simplex virus was associated with the nuclei. Nuclei may, of course, contain enveloped particles (Section III,C, 1), but Spring and Roizman (1968) showed that the infective nuclear particles were unstable on sedimentation in cesium chloride density gradients, whereas the infective cytoplasmic particles were not. However, because the infectivity of the nuclear particles was sensitive to phospholipase, Roizman (1969) believes that the nuclear infectivity is associated with naked particles possessing an inner but not an outer envelope.

Darlington and Moss (1969) also used cell fractionation to study this problem in BHK 21 cells infected with pseudorabies. The virus from the nuclear fraction was largely naked [presumably the enveloped particles observed in vesicles near the surface of the nucleus in this system by Darlington and Moss (1968) must have been removed with the cytoplasmic fraction]. The residual infectivity of these nuclear preparations was less than the number of enveloped particles, but Darlington and Moss (1969) argued that if enveloped particles accounted for all the infectivity, the enveloped particle to infectivity ratio would have been between 7 and 15, whereas the particle to infectivity ratio for preparations containing mostly enveloped particles was five to ten times higher than this figure. They concluded that both naked and enveloped particles are infective although not necessarily with equal efficiencies. Plainly, they cannot rule out the possibility that their infective naked particles have an inner envelope, since Roizman (1969) has postulated that this structure is permeable to phosphotungstate and therefore not detected in negatively stained preparations. Roizman's (1969) views are particularly important in emphasizing that there may be more than two classes of particle and that the division into enveloped and naked viruses on morphological grounds alone may be an oversimplification.

Defects in envelopment have been held responsible for absence of infective virus in infected cells. Thus, Spring *et al.* (1968) found naked but no enveloped particles in the abortive infection of dog kidney cells with their DK^- mutant. It is possibly significant, however, that all the naked particles in their micrograph have a hollow core. Cook and Stevens (1968) observed that the envelopes of varicella–zoster virus growing in human amnion cells were often incomplete, resulting in loss of the central dense cores, and they have related this to the lack of cell-free infectious virus in this system.

Finally, we may note that although Watson and Wildy (1963) were unable to detect agglutination of enveloped particles with antiserum to herpes-specific antigens (Watson *et al.*, 1966) it has been possible to show such agglutination using better antisera (R. W. Honess and K. L. Powell, personal communication). This is in accord with the observation of the virus-specific antigen on the outer surface of the envelope using immunoferritin tagging (Miyamoto *et al.*, 1971).

D. *Release*

Morgan *et al.* (1959) proposed that virus was released by a process of "reverse phagocytosis," whereby vacuoles containing enveloped particles released their contents at the cell surface. Epstein (1962), in addition, suggested that envelopment and release might occasionally occur simultaneously by budding of naked particles through the cell membrane. Epstein (1962) has contrasted this type of release by budding with the release of adenovirus by cell lysis. However, it seems likely that release by disruption can occur with herpesviruses also, at least in some cells. Thus, the supernatant growth medium of BHK 21 cells infected with herpes simplex virus contains largely naked particles (Watson *et al.*, 1964), whereas most of the particles released from infected HEp 2 cells are enveloped (Watson and Wildy, 1963). Jasty and Chang (1972) suggested that naked particles of infectious bovine rhinotracheitis virus could be released following sequestration in folded nuclear membrane.

Darlington and Moss (1969), noting the suggestions of Robertson (1959) and Palay and Karlin (1959) that the cisternae of the endoplasmic reticulum open through the plasma membrane, have suggested that such channels could act as a means of egress for particles after envelopment at the inner nuclear membrane. They observed particles in the cisternae leading toward to the cell exterior, but Porter (1961) has, in fact, opposed the view that the cisternae do open through the cell membrane.

Schwartz and Roizman (1969b) have, however, observed an elaborate network of branched tubules 650 Å in diameter in HEp 2 cells infected with herpes simplex virus. These were sometimes continuous with the outer nuclear membrane and opened through the cell membrane. The branched network was specific for infected cells and was never observed in uninfected cells. They did not occur in dog kidney cells abortively infected with the DK^- mutant. Enveloped particles were frequently present in these channels, and Schwartz and Roizman (1969b) have questioned whether enveloped particles are ever present in closed cytoplasmic vacuoles. They point out that the channels allow the virus to be released through the cytoplasm but at the same time to be separated from it. Since they have shown that infected cells can uncoat superinfecting virus particles for at least 6 hours after the first infection, they therefore suggest that the particles being released through the channels are protected from uncoating enzymes.

Similar release channels have been observed by Strandberg and Aurelian (1969) in cells infected with canine herpesvirus and by Jasty and Chang (1972) in cells infected with infectious bovine rhinotracheitis.

There can be no doubt of the reality of the channels observed by these workers, nor that they open to the cell exterior. What is remarkable is that they should be so numerous and yet not noted by so many workers. Perhaps, once again, there are variations between cells with respect to this property. It is perhaps noteworthy that infected HEp 2 cells not only release a high proportion of enveloped particles into the supernatant medium but also do so with great efficiency.

Another clue to the apparent variations between workers on this point is given by Schwartz and Roizman (1969b) themselves. They found very few of the channels when HEp 2 cells were infected with type 2 herpes simplex virus, and correspondingly claimed that the cytoplasm contained large numbers of partially disaggregated naked particles. It appears, therefore, that the infecting virus itself has some influence in this process.

IV. Conclusion

The overall picture of development of herpesviruses as seen by electron microscopy is not very different now from that given in the pioneering studies of Morgan *et al.* (1954, 1959). A wider range of viruses has been studied, details have been filled in, but the wide variations observed by different workers has often confused rather than clarified our view of the situation. Since it now appears that the enveloped herpesvirus particle may contain up to 24 proteins or glycoproteins (Spear and Roizman, 1972) as well as lipid and DNA, it is inevitable that its assembly must be an extremely complex process. The morphological differentiation of developmental forms can only be crude in relation to such a complex structure. Advances in our knowledge may come, however, by further application of immunoferritin tagging procedures, particularly if these are used in combination with sera specific for individual components of the virus (Watson and Wildy, 1969).

Acknowledgments

I am indebted to Dr. Councilman Morgan and the American Society for Microbiology for permission to reproduce Figs. 3, 4, 6, 8, and 9 from publications in the *Journal of Virology*. I thank my colleagues Dr. A. Buchan, Mr. R. W. Honess, and Mrs. C. Sim for reading the manuscript and making helpful suggestions. Once again, I should like to acknowledge the labors of my long-suffering typist, Mrs. J. M. Davies.

References

Abodeely, R. A., Lawson, L. A., and Randall, C. C. (1970). *J. Virol.* **5**, 513.
Abraham, A., and Tegtmeyer, P. (1970). *J. Virol.* **5**, 617.
Armstrong, J. A. Pereira, H. G., and Ardrewes, C. H. (1961). *Virology* **14**, 276.
Ben-Porat, T., and Kaplan, A. S. (1962). *Virology* **16**, 261.
Bernhard, W. (1966). *Nat. Cancer Inst., Monogr.* **23**, 13.
Bernhard, W., and Granboulan, N. (1963). *Exp. Cell Res., Suppl.* **9**, 19.
Cook, M. L., and Stevens, J. G. (1968). *J. Virol.* **2**, 1458.
Couch, E. F., and Nahmias, A. J. (1969). *J. Virol.* **3**, 228.
Dales, S. (1962). *J. Cell Biol.* **13**, 303.
Dales, S., and Silverberg, H. (1969). *Virology* **37**, 475.
Darlington, R. W., and Moss, L. H. (1968). *J. Virol.* **2**, 48.
Darlington, R. W., and Moss, L. H. (1969). *Progr. Med. Virol.* **11**, 16.
Epstein, M. A. (1962). *J. Cell Biol.* **12**, 589.
Epstein, M. A., Hummeler, K., and Berkaloff, A. (1964). *J. Exp. Med.* **119**, 291.
Epstein, M. A., Churchill, A. E., and Biggs, P. M. (1968). *J. Nat. Cancer* **41**, 805.
Falke, D., Siegert, R., and Vogell, W. (1959). *Arch. Gesamte Virusforsch.* **9**, 484.
Farnham, A. E., and Newton, A. A. (1959). *Virology* **7**, 449.
Felluga, B. (1963). *Ann. Sclavo* **5**, 412.
Fujiwara, S., and Kaplan, A. S. (1967). *Virology* **32**, 60.
Gostling, J. V. T., and Bedson, S. P. (1956). *Brit. J. Exp. Pathol.* **37**, 434.
Granboulan, P., Séchaud, J., and Kellenberger, E., (1971). *Virology* **46**, 407.
Hampar, B., Hsu, K. C., Martos, L. M., and Walker, J. L. (1971). *Proc. Nat. Acad. Sci. U.S.* **68**, 1407.
Heine, U., Ablash, D. V., and Armstrong, G. R. (1971). *Cancer Res.* **31**, 1019.

Holmes, I. M., and Watson, D. H. (1963). *Virology* **21**, 112.
Huang, A. S., and Wagner, R. R. (1964). *Proc. Soc. Exp. Biol. Med.* **116**, 863.
Hummeler, K., Tomassin, N., and Zajac, B. (1969), *J. Virol.* **4**, 67.
Jasty, V., and Chang, P. W. (1972). *J. Ultrastruct. Res.* **38**, 433.
Kellenberger, E., Eiserling, F. A., and de la Tour, E. B. (1967). *J. Ultrastruct. Res.* **21**, 335.
Love, R., and Wildy, P. (1963). *J. Cell Biol.* **17**, 237.
McCracken, R. M., and Clarke, J. K. (1971). *Arch. Gesamte Virusforsch.* **34**, 189.
McGavran, M. H., and Smith, M. G. (1965). *Exp. Mol. Pathol.* **4**, 1.
Melnick, J. L., Rabin, C. R., and Jenson, A. B. (1968). *J. Virol.* **2**, 78.
Miyamoto, K. (1971). *J. Virol.* **8**, 534.
Miyamoto, K., and Morgan, C. (1971). *J. Virol.* **8**, 910.
Miyamoto, K., Morgan, C., Hsu, K. C., and Hampar, B. (1971). *J. Nat. Cancer Inst.* **46**, 629.
Morgan, C., and Rose, H. M. (1959). *Symp. Soc. Gen. Microbiol.* **9**, 256.
Morgan, C., Ellison, S. A., Rose, H. M., and Moore, D. H. (1954). *J. Exp. Med.* **100**, 195.
Morgan, C., Rose, H. M., Holden, M., and Jones, E. P. (1959). *J. Exp. Med.* **110**, 643.
Morgan, C., Rose, H. M., and Mednis, B. (1968). *J. Virol.* **2**, 507.
Morgan, C., Rosenkranz, H. S., and Mednis, B. (1969). *J. Virol.* **4**, 777.
Murphy, F. A., Harrison, A. H., and Whitfield, S. G. (1967). *Arch. Gesamte Virusforsch.* **21**, 463.
Nazerian, K., Lee, L. F., Witter, R. L., and Burmester, B. R. (1971). *Virology* **43**, 442.
Nii, S. (1971). *Biken J.* **14**, 177.
Nii, S., and Ono, N. (1971). *Biken J.* **14**, 57.
Nii, S., Morgan, C., Rose, H. M., and Hsu, K. C. (1968*a*). *J. Virol.* **2**, 1172.
Nii, S., Morgan, C., and Rose, H. M. (1968*b*). *J. Virol.* **2**, 517.
Nii, S., Rosenkranz, H. S., Morgan, C., and Rose, H. M. (1968*c*). *J. Virol.* **2**, 1163.
O'Callaghan, D. J., Hyde, J. M., Gentry, G. A., and Randall, C. C. (1968). *J. Virol.* **2**, 793.
Palay, S. L., and Karlin, L. J. (1959). *J. Biophys. Biochem. Cytol.* **5**, 373.
Pinkerton, H., Sun, C. N., Henson, D., and Neff, J. (1964). *Virology* **24**, 498.
Pirie, N. W. (1957). *Nature of Viruses, Ciba Found. Symp., 1956* p. 56.
Porter, K. R. (1961). *In* "The Cell' (J. Brachet and A. E. Mirsky, eds.), Vol. 2 p. 62. Academic Press, New York.
Reissig, M., and Melnick, J. L. (1955). *J. Exp. Med.* **101**, 341.
Robertson, J. D. (1959). *Progr. Biophys. Biophys. Chem.* **10**, 343.
Roizman, B. (1969). *Curr. Top. Microbiol. Immunol.* **49**, 1.
Roizman, B. (1971). *Proc. Int. Symp. Appl. Med. Virol. 3rd.*, p. 37.
Russell, W. C., Gold, E., Keir, H. M., Omura, H., Watson, D. H., and Wildy, P. (1964). *Virology* **22**, 103.
Schwartz, J., and Roizman, B. (1969*a*). *J. Virol.* **4**, 879.
Schwartz, J., and Roizman, B. (1969*b*). *Virology* **38**, 42.
Siegert, R. S., and Falke, D. (1966). *Arch. Gesamte Virusforsch.* **19**, 230.
Siminoff, P., and Menefee, M. G. (1966). *Exp. Cell Res.* **44**, 241.
Smith, K. O. (1964). *Proc. Soc. Exp. Biol. Med.* **115**, 814.
Spear, P. G., and Roizman, B. (1968). *Virology* **36**, 545.
Spear, P. G., and Roizman, B. (1972). *J. Virol.* **9**, 143.
Spring, S. B., and Roizman, B. (1968), *J. Virol.* **2**, 979.
Spring, S. B., and Roizman, B., and Schwartz, J. (1968), *J. Virol.* **2**, 384.
Stackpole, C. W. (1969). *J. Virol.* **4**, 75.
Stackpole, C. W., and Mizell, M. (1968). *Virology* **36**, 63.
Stein, S., Todd, P., and Mahoney, J. (1970). *Can. J. Microbiol.* **16**, 953.
Stoker, M. G. P., Smith, K. M., and Ross, R. W. (1959). *J. Gen. Microbiol.* **19**, 244.
Strandberg, J. D., and Aurelian, L. (1969). *J. Virol.* **4**, 480.

Tournier, P., Cathala, F., and Bernhard, W. (1957). *Presse Med.* **65**, 1229.
Watrach, A. M., (1962). *Virology* **18**, 324.
Watson, D. H., and Wildy, P. (1963). *Virology* **21**, 100.
Watson, D. H., and Wildy, P. (1969). *J. Gen. Virol.* **4**, 163.
Watson, D. H., Wildy, P., and Russell, W. C. (1964). *Virology* **24**, 523.
Watson, D. H., Shedden, W. I. H., Elliot, A., Tetsuka, T., Wildy, P., Bourgaux-Ramoisy, D., and Gold, E. (1966). *Immunology* **11**, 399.
Zee, Y. C., and Talens, L. (1971). *J. Gen. Virol.* **11**, 59.

Chapter 6
Replication—Biochemical Aspects

Tamar Ben-Porat and Albert S. Kaplan

I. Introduction

Information about the metabolism of virus-infected cells is fundamental to an understanding of the mechanisms controlling virus synthesis and assembly. This information may aid in understanding some of the causes that underlie cellular pathology and may reveal the basis for the oncogenic potential of viruses; it may also provide a rational approach to the chemotherapy of virus infection.

Studies on host–virus interactions at the molecular level were initiated by the pioneer experiments of Cohen (1949), Hershey (1956), and others. This approach has provided a wealth of information about many of the biochemical details of the infective process in bacteriophage-infected bacteria. Among other things, one of the chief reasons for the spectacular success in the biochemical analysis of infected bacteria is the highly quantitative nature of phage experiments. The earlier experiments on the biochemistry of animal virus infections made use of virus-infected animals, and the results of these experiments are difficult to interpret. However, since the development of cell culture techniques and the plaque assay method for the study of animal viruses, the interactions of viruses and their host cells have been analyzed in homogeneous populations of infected cells, and advances in understanding the infective process have consequently ensued.

This chapter will deal mainly with those aspects of the molecular biology of herpesvirus-infected cells which provide information about the mechanisms of control by means of which the infecting virus usurps the metabolic machinery of the host cells, as observed during a virulent interaction between the virus and its host cell. The limited amount of information available concerning possible differences in metabolic processes between herpesvirus-transformed cells and normal cells is summarized in some of the other chapters of this book.

II. Effect of Infection on Macromolecular Synthesis

Initially, the effect of infection with herpesviruses on cellular macromolecular synthesis was investigated using relatively insensitive colorimetric methods. The results of such experiments indicated that after infection there may or may not be an increase in the amount of DNA per cell, but that there is no change in the amount of RNA or protein.

Changes in the rate of synthesis of macromolecules in virus-infected cells are more readily detected by following the incorporation of radioactive isotopes. However, the amount of radioactive precursor incorporated will not necessarily reflect the rate of macromolecular synthesis, because the amount incorporated will also be influenced by the size of the acid-soluble intracellular pool of the precursor, a parameter which may differ in infected and uninfected cells. Unfortunately, in many cases the data available dealing with the incorporation of precursors into macromolecules do not include analyses of the intracellular pools, so that the exact quantitative effect of infection on macromolecular synthesis of the cells cannot be estimated from the results of these experiments. However, it is possible to conclude from these experiments that after infection of cells with the herpesviruses there is a redirection of the metabolic processes from the elaboration of cell-specific to that of virus-specific products. The overall effect of infection on the rate of synthesis of macromolecules will be influenced by three factors.

1. The physiological state of the cells at the time of infection determines the rate of synthesis of cellular macromolecules. Cells infected in logarithmic phase have a high background of synthesis of cellular components and a high level of activity of enzymes; nondividing cells in stationary phase, on the other hand, have a low background of cellular synthesis. Since infection inhibits the synthesis of cell-specific molecules, the effect of infection on the overall rate of macromolecular synthesis in the cells will vary, especially during the early stages of infection, with the physiological state of the cells.

2. The permissiveness of the cells to a given herpesvirus, i.e., the degree to which viral products accumulate in these cells, will also affect the rate of macromolecular synthesis, especially at later stages of infection, during which most viral products are synthesized.

3. The multiplicity of infection of the cells will affect the rate of the inhibition of RNA synthesis (Aurelian and Roizman, 1965), as well as the rate of disaggregation of host-specific polysomes (Sydiskis and Roizman, 1967). It will also affect the rate of accumulation of viral products (Kaplan, 1959). Thus, the rate of macromolecular synthesis in the infected cells will depend upon the multiplicity of infection.

The effect of infection of cells with various members of the herpesvirus group is qualitatively the same. In all cases that have been studied, there has been observed an inhibition of the rate of synthesis of host macromolecules with a more or less abundant accumulation of virus-specific components. In no case has there been a clear-cut demonstration that infection of cells with members of the herpesviruses, which may be oncogenic, induces an increase in the rate of synthesis of cellular components as demonstrated for other viruses which are known to cause cellular transformation.

III. RNA Synthesis

Infection of cells with the herpesviruses leads to a gradual decrease in the rate of incorporation of uridine and other precursors into RNA (Kaplan and Ben-Porat, 1960; Aurelian and Roizman, 1965; Hay *et al.*, 1966; Flanagan, 1967). The decrease in the rate of incorporation of uridine reflects a decrease in the rate of RNA synthesis in these cells, since no difference exists between infected and mock-infected cells in the phosphorylation of externally supplied [^{3}H]uridine nor in the size of the pool of endogenously formed uridine derivatives (Rakusanova *et al.*, 1972). The rates of RNA synthesis in the cells at different times after infection reflect a composite of the decreasing rate of synthesis of cell-specific RNA molecules and of the increasing rate of synthesis of virus-specific RNA molecules.

The analysis of the type of RNA molecules synthesized by infected cells is probably one of the more promising means of uncovering the role played by the cellular and viral genomes in the control of infection. This type of analysis of herpesvirus-infected cells is only in an incipient stage. Neither the virus-specific nor the cell-specific RNA molecules synthesized in the infected cells nor the functions for which they code have been analyzed and characterized sufficiently to shed light on these controlling processes.

A. Cellular RNA Synthesis

The decrease in the rate of RNA synthesis in cells after infection indicates that the synthesis of cell-specific RNA molecules is inhibited, at least partially. Mammalian cells contain at least three types of RNA polymerase systems, each being involved in the synthesis of different types of RNA molecules; virus infection may exert a differential inhibitory effect on the different polymerases. Experiments designed to answer this question suffer, however, from the fact that in uninfected cells the different RNA molecules are processed rapidly after their synthesis, and that infection with the herpesviruses may affect not only the rate of their synthesis but also the rate of their processing. Despite this experimental difficulty, it is possible to conclude from the information available (summarized below) that infection probably does not exert a significant differential inhibitory effect on the synthesis of different types of cellular RNA molecules.

1. Ribosomal RNA (rRNA)

Hay *et al.* (1966) were the first to report that incorporation of uridine into precursor rRNA during a 30-minute pulse was decreased to undetectable levels by 7.5 hours after herpes simplex virus (HSV) infection. During the first few hours after infection, the synthesis of precursor rRNA (as measured by the size of the peak of 45 S precursor rRNA present in the cells after a 30-minute pulse), as well as the mature rRNA (as measured by the accumulation of this RNA in the infected cells during a longer pulse), seemed to be inhibited approximately to the same extent. However, the experiments in which the synthesis of 45 S RNA, and those in which the synthesis of mature rRNA were measured, are not directly comparable because the multiplicity of infection may not have been the same.

Wagner and Roizman (1969a) showed that after infection of cells with HSV, the inhibition of the appearance of newly synthesized mature rRNA was more rapid than was the synthesis of other types of RNA molecules. At 4 hours postinfection, the amount of radioactivity in 45 S RNA present in infected cells labeled for 60 minutes with either uridine or methionine was approximately one-third that present in uninfected cells labeled under the same conditions; the synthesis of mature rRNA was, however, inhibited by more than 90%. The authors concluded that infection of cells with HSV not only inhibits the synthesis of precursor rRNA but also affects the orderly processing of this RNA. Essentially the same results were also obtained in pseudorabies virus (PRV)-infected rabbit kidney (RK) cells (Rakusanova and Kaplan, 1970).

Since precursor rRNA is normally cleaved and since this cleavage may be either retarded or activated by infection, it is possible to determine the extent of inhibition of the synthesis of 45 S RNA, *only* if one compares the amount of radioactivity accumulating in the peak of 45 S RNA from infected and uninfected cells during a very short pulse with labeled precursors. Such an experiment has not been reported. However, if one assumes that precursor rRNA is methylated to the same extent in infected and in uninfected cells, the rate of inhibition of methylation of RNA in the infected cells may be used as a criterion for the rate of synthesis of precursor rRNA. Short-time labeling experiments revealed that the rate of methylation of RNA in the infected cells decreases only slightly more rapidly than does the rate of RNA synthesis, and that the synthesis of precursor rRNA seems thus to be inhibited at approximately the same rate as the overall synthesis of RNA in the cells (A. S. Kaplan, unpublished results). Similar conclusions have been reached by Hay and Low (1970).

2. C-RNA (RNA that Anneals to Cellular DNA)

Hay *et al.* (1966) and Flanagan (1967) reported that while the synthesis of the RNA that anneals to cellular DNA is much reduced after infection of cells with HSV, some C-RNA is still synthesized, even at relatively late stages of infection. Whether this RNA was synthesized by a residual number of uninfected cells in the cultures or whether the infected cells synthesized cell-specific RNA at a reduced rate was, however, not established.

When the rate of RNA synthesis is decreased by approximately 65% in PRV-infected cells (as measured by the amount of uridine incorporated into RNA during a 90-minute pulse), the amount of labeled C-RNA accumulating in the cells is reduced by only 30%. Table I shows that this is so, since whereas after its synthesis in uninfected cells a large proportion of C-RNA turns over rapidly, C-RNA in infected cells turns over to a limited extent only if at all. The rate of synthesis of C-RNA is inhibited by infection approximately to the same degree as is the overall rate of RNA synthesis (Table I). After a short pulse (7 minutes), the amount of labeled C-RNA synthesized by the cells is decreased by infection to the same extent as the amount of total RNA, and the percentage of labeled RNA that anneals to cellular DNA is approximately the same in infected and uninfected cells (1.18 and 0.93%, respectively). After a longer labeling period, however, only 0.25% of the total label in uninfected cells but 1.02% of that in infected cells annealed to DNA, indicating that C-RNA turns over in uninfected cells but not in the infected cells.

Hybridization competition experiments showed that the C-RNA that accumulates in the infected cells differs from that present normally in uninfected cells. At least part of this RNA is synthesized as relatively large molecules which are then cleaved and adenylated; a large proportion of this RNA is found in the cytoplasmic fractions of the infected cells (Rakusanova *et al.*, 1972). However, the actual identity of the C-RNA that accumulates in the infected cells is uncertain at present. This RNA could represent an accumulation within the infected cells of RNA molecules that normally turn over very rapidly in uninfected cells, or it could be the transcript of part of the cell genome not normally transcribed in the uninfected cells.

3. Cellular Messenger RNA (mRNA)

The synthesis of cellular mRNA seems to be inhibited at a more rapid rate after infection of cells with PRV than is the overall synthesis of RNA.

TABLE I
HYBRIDIZATION OF RNA FROM INFECTED AND UNINFECTED RK CELLS LABELED WITH [^{3}H]URIDINE FOR VARIOUS PERIODS OF TIME[a]

Cells	Time of labeling (minutes)	Input (counts /minute)	Hybridized to cellular DNA filter	
			Counts /minute	% input
Infected	7	3,050	36	1.18
	15	6,250	76	1.21
	60	22,600	259	1.13
	90	34,400	376	1.10
	210	69,300	706	1.02
Uninfected	7	10,200	93	0.93
	15	22,600	155	0.68
	60	85,300	335	0.39
	90	110,000	410	0.35
	210	272,000	670	0.25

[a]RK cells were infected or mock-infected. At 7, 15, 60, etc., minutes prior to harvesting, [^{3}H]uridine (100 μCi/ml) was added to different cultures, which were then incubated with the label for the indicated periods of time. All the cultures were harvested at 5.5 hours postinfection, RNA was extracted, and an aliquot was hybridized to cellular DNA (20 μg) fixed to filters. (From Rakusanova *et al.*, 1972.)

This can be deduced from the fact that at early stages of infection (when about 80% as much polysome-associated cellular mRNA is present in the infected as in the uninfected cells) little of the cellular RNA that is synthesized by the cells becomes associated with polysomes (Rakusanova *et al.*, 1972). If one assumes that newly synthesized mRNA can compete successfully with existing polysomal mRNA for association with ribosomes, one is led to conclude that functional cellular mRNA synthesis is inhibited more rapidly in the infected cells than is the overall rate of synthesis of cellular RNA molecules. However, the formation of functional cellular mRNA probably requires an orderly cleavage of precursor molecules, and this cleavage may be adversely affected by infection. Thus, the relatively rapid inhibition of the formation of functional cellular mRNA may not be at the level of transcription but rather at the level of its processing.

4. 4 S RNA

The effect of infection on the rate of synthesis of cell-specific tRNA in the cells has not been measured, although it has been shown that there is a decrease in the level of this RNA in the infected cells (Bell *et al.*, 1971). Ribonucleic acid that anneals to cellular DNA and has a sedimentation value of 4 S is synthesized by infected cells (Hay *et al.*, 1966; Rakusanova *et al.*, 1972). At least part of this RNA is, however, derived from larger molecules and probably represents C-RNA which normally turns over in uninfected cells, but which in infected cells is converted into molecules of relatively low molecular weight (Rakusanova *et al.*, 1972).

In conclusion, evidence currently available shows that infection of cells with the herpesviruses leads to a gradual decrease in the rate of synthesis of cellular RNA, the rate of inhibition being approximately the same for all types of RNA molecules. The inhibition of cell-specific RNA is not complete and even at late stages of infection, the infected cells synthesize cellular RNA. In addition to the virus-induced inhibition of cellular RNA synthesis, infection also inhibits the proper processing of the transcribed RNA molecules.

B. Viral RNA Synthesis

1. mRNA

Viral mRNA is by definition RNA transcribed from viral DNA which has the potential of associating with polysomes and of being translated into a specific protein. A rigorous analysis of the RNA transcribed from the viral genome has not as yet been accomplished, and it is not known whether only informational RNA, i.e., RNA that can be translated into specific proteins, is transcribed. For the sake of simplicity, this will be assumed to be the case, although the possibility that some viral RNA molecules function as regulating units has not been excluded.

The earliest reports on the synthesis of virus-specific RNA in HSV-infected cells were published by Subak-Sharpe and Hay (1965) and by Hay *et al.* (1966), who described the synthesis in the infected cells of RNA that anneals to viral DNA and that has sedimentation values of 20 S and 4 S. Flanagan (1967) showed that in KB cells infected with HSV, viral RNA can be detected at relatively early stages of infection (3 hours). The rate of viral RNA synthesis increases up to 7 hours postinfection and decreases thereafter. The virus-specific RNA showed considerable spread in size, the bulk of the molecules having sedimentation values of 12 S to 32 S. Essentially the same results with respect to time of synthesis and sedimentation values of the bulk of virus-specific RNA molecules were obtained subsequently by Wagner and Roizman (1969a) for HSV-infected KB cells and by Rakusanova *et al.* (1972) for PRV-infected RK cells. However, the size distribution, as well as the time of appearance of viral RNA, will vary for different herpesviruses. For example, the RNA specified by equine abortion virus (EAV) differs from that of HSV with respect to its time of appearance in the infected cells and to its size (Huang *et al.*, 1971; Szabocsik *et al.*, 1972).

The RNA transcribed from the viral genome may be divided into three broad classes, which, to conform to the terminology used for similar classes of RNA molecules synthesized in bacteriophage-infected cells, have been called immediate–early, early, and late RNA. Immediate–early RNA is defined as those RNA molecules which are transcribed in the infected cells without protein synthesis. Early RNA consists of RNA molecules transcribed before the onset of viral DNA synthesis. Late RNA are those molecules of RNA not transcribed unless protein and DNA synthesis occurs in the infected cells.

The genomes of herpesviruses are relatively large (see Chapter 3), and most of the genetic information they contain is unique (Frenkel and Roizman, 1971). Thus, the herpesviruses, in principle, can code for many functions. The division of viral RNA into three classes represents, therefore, an oversimplification, and this subdivision is useful only as a first step in the characterization of the viral RNA molecules. Further characterization of this RNA and the temporal control of its transcription will have to await more refined techniques of RNA analysis, as well as an increase in the amount of information about viral functions.

The synthesis of immediate–early RNA has been detected in PRV-infected RK cells treated with cycloheximide (Rakusanova *et al.*, 1971). Under these conditions, viral RNA molecules (predominantly 26 S) accumulate in the infected cells. Only 25% of the sequences normally transcribed in the infected cells prior to the onset of DNA synthesis (the sequences of the early RNA) are transcribed in cycloheximide-treated infected cells; these are the immediate—early RNA molecules.

An analysis of the virus-specific RNA synthesized in EAV-infected cells (Huang *et al.*, 1971) revealed that approximately 50% of the viral RNA sequences transcribed at late stages of infection are not transcribed at earlier stages, and thus represent so-called late RNA. Similar results have also been reported for HSV-infected cells by Wagner (1972) who demonstrated that only part of the RNA sequences normally synthesized by infected cells were transcribed in cells in which viral DNA synthesis had been inhibited.

Roizman and co-workers (personal communications) have found recently that the entire viral genome of HSV is transcribed in cycloheximide-treated, infected cells, i.e., in the absence of virus-specific protein and DNA synthesis. The method used to detect viral RNA in these experiments was, in contrast to the RNA competition experiments described above, probably sufficiently sensitive to detect relatively infrequent sequences of RNA. While the system used in these experiments permits the synthesis of at least some viral proteins in the presence of cycloheximide (Sydiskis and Roizman, 1967) (viral DNA synthesis is also probably not completely inhibited), it is possible that the control of the transcription of RNA discussed above might be exerted at the level of the *rate* of transcription of different classes of viral RNA. The entire viral genome might thus be available for transcription at any time during the infective process, but certain sequences might be more rapidly transcribed under a given set of conditions.

At least part of the viral mRNA molecules are produced by cleavage of large precursor molecules which are synthesized in the nucleus (Wagner and Roizman, 1969a,b; Roizman *et al.*, 1970). The nucleus of infected cells contains virus-specific RNA with a sedimentation constant larger than that of the virus-specific RNA associated with polysomes, part of these molecules representing the transcript of approximately 10% of the viral genome. Cytoplasmic viral mRNA competes to approximately 80% in DNA–RNA hybridization tests with the larger virus-specific RNA extracted from the nuclei of infected cells.

Cytoplasmic viral RNA contains covalently linked sequences of polyadenylic acid (poly A) (Rakusanova *et al.*, 1972; Bachenheimer and Roizman, 1972). The sequences of Poly A are added to the viral RNA after its synthesis (A. S. Kaplan and T. Ben-Porat, unpublished results; B. Roizman, personal communication), as are the poly A sequences found in cellular mRNA.

In conclusion, the different parts of the viral genome are sequentially transcribed in the infected cells. Currently available information concerning the patterns of synthesis and of processing of viral RNA indicates that the processes are probably the same as those occurring during the formation of cellular mRNA. The RNA is transcribed in the nucleus as relatively large molecules which are subsequently cleaved, adenylated, and transferred to the cytoplasm.

2. Transfer RNA (tRNA)

The ability of the herpesviruses to code for tRNA was first investigated by Subak-Sharpe and his co-workers, who reasoned that because of the large difference in the content of guanine and cytosine and in the CpG doublet frequency between HSV DNA and host cell DNA, the synthesis of viral proteins would require a change in the translation machinery of the cells, and that control could occur at the level of tRNA. These considerations were reinforced by the fact that some viruses are known to specify the synthesis of tRNA molecules.

The earlier experiments (Subak-Sharpe and Hay, 1965; Subak-Sharpe *et al.*, 1966) suffered from problems of experimental design and inadequate technology. On the basis of these experiments, it was concluded that HSV codes for tRNA, in particular, for arginyl tRNA. However, using more stringent criteria, Morris *et al.* (1970) were unable to detect the presence in the infected cells either of arginyl or seryl virus-specific tRNA, a finding later confirmed by Bell *et al.* (1971).

The proteins synthesized by the PRV-infected cells are relatively higher in arginine and are lower in lysine content than are the proteins synthesized by the uninfected cells, a difference which is to be expected on the basis of the overall base composition of the two types of genomes (Kaplan *et al.*, 1970). The difference in the amino acid composition of the proteins synthesized by infected and uninfected cells could require a change after infection in the relative amounts of different tRNA molecules. However, despite the relatively high content of arginine in viral proteins, there is a significant decrease in the cells after infection in the amount of tRNA that can be charged with arginine (Bell *et al.*, 1971). It has not been established, however, whether the ratio of tRNA molecules specific for one amino acid to tRNA molecules specific for another amino acid differ in infected and uninfected cells as do the ratios of one amino acid to another in the proteins synthesized by these cells.

IV. DNA Synthesis

The early experiments showed that between 6 and 9 hours after infection of HeLa cells with HSV, before any increase in infectious virus can be observed, there is an increase in the amount of DNA per cell; by 72 hours postinfection, the infected cells possess nearly twice the normal amount of DNA (Newton and Stoker, 1958; Newton *et al.*, 1962). An increase in the amount of DNA per cell is also observed when RK cells in the stationary phase are infected with PRV. However, monolayer cultures of RK cells infected in the logarithmic phase show no change in their content of DNA, as measured by the diphenylamine reaction (Kaplan and Ben-Porat, 1960). The effect of infection on the synthesis of DNA is thus dependent upon the physiological state of the cells at the time of infection. This is best demonstrated in incorporation experiments with labeled thymidine. Monolayer cultures of uninfected RK cells in the stationary phase incorporate little or no thymidine. As early as 2 hours after infection an increase in the amount of [2-^{14}C]thymidine incorporated into DNA is detected, and by the end of the infective process, the cells will have incorporated 10–20 times more labeled thymidine than uninfected cells during a similar time period. The amount of [2-^{14}C]thymidine incorporated into the DNA of infected and uninfected cells in the logarithmic phase is, on the other hand, approximately the same when the labeled compound is added at the time of infection and incorporation is allowed to proceed throughout the infective process (Kaplan and Ben Porat, 1963). A difference in the rates of DNA synthesis between the infected and uninfected cells can be detected only by "pulse-labeling" experiments. Using this procedure, it was found that there is a virus-induced early suppression, followed by an increase, in the rate of incorporation of thymidine into infected cells (Kaplan and Ben-Porat, 1960; Newton *et al.*, 1962).

A. Synthesis of Cellular DNA in the Infected Cells

Infection of susceptible cells with the herpesviruses generally leads to a decrease in the rate of synthesis of cellular DNA. Although some of the herpesviruses, such as EBV and Marek's disease virus (MDV) (Gerber and Hoyer, 1971; Lee, 1972), confer upon leukocytes the ability to multiply and consequently to synthesize cellular DNA, the synthesis of cellular DNA is inhibited in those EBV-infected cells in which early viral antigens are synthesized (Gergely *et al.*, 1971a,b; Nonoyama and Pagano, 1972).

The type of DNA synthesized by infected cells may be identified in most cases because cellular and viral DNA may differ in base composition, a property that permits their separation by centrifugation in a density gradient of cesium chloride or by chromatography on methylated albumin columns. The following example illustrates the methodology utilized to determine the relative amounts of cellular and viral DNA synthesized at different stages of the infective process in PRV-infected cells. The DNA synthesized by the infected cells at various times after infection was labeled; viral DNA was separated from cellular DNA by isopycnic centrifugation in cesium chloride; and the amount of radioactive label associated with each kind of DNA was determined. Since only the DNA synthesized during the labeling period is radioactive, the relative amounts of viral and cellular DNA synthesized during the labeling period will be proportional to the amount of label incorporated into each and can thus be ascertained. Using this technique, it was found that cells infected in the stationary phase synthesize only viral DNA (Ben-Porat and Kaplan, 1963). There is a gradual decrease in the rate of incorporation of thymidine into cellular DNA after infection of cells in the logarithmic phase and by 7–8 hours after infection, the cells infected with PRV no longer synthesize cellular DNA; concurrently, there is an increase in the incorporation of thymidine into viral DNA (Fig. 1) (Kaplan and Ben-Porat, 1963).

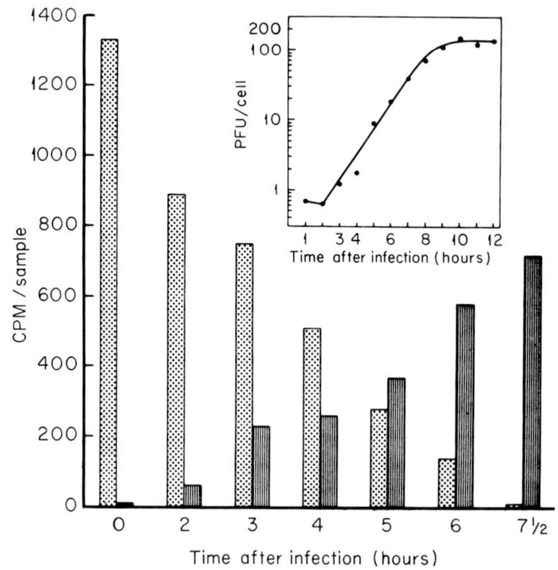

FIG. 1. The decrease in the rate of incorporation of [2-^{14}C]thymidine into cellular DNA and the increase in the rate of its incorporation into viral DNA with time after infection. At various times after infection the cells were incubated for 60 minutes with [2-^{14}C]thymidine. The cells were harvested, DNA extracted, and cellular DNA separated from viral DNA in CsCl gradients. Stippled bars: radioactivity associated with cellular DNA; lined bars; radioactivity associated with viral DNA. (From Kaplan and Ben-Porat, 1963.)

Similar experiments have been carried out in cells infected with HSV (Roizman and Roane, 1964; Russell *et al.*, 1964). After infection, a new type of DNA, with a buoyant density corresponding to that of viral DNA, makes its appearance in the virus-infected cells. As in the case of PRV-infected cells, the rate of synthesis of cellular DNA decreases, and the rate of viral DNA synthesis increases as infection proceeds. Essentially the same results have also been obtained with equine abortion virus (EAV)-infected cells by O'Callaghan *et al.* (1968a) who used methylated albumin chromatographic columns to separate cellular from viral DNA.

B. Synthesis of Viral DNA in the Infected Cells

Since cells in the stationary phase synthesize viral DNA only (see above), it is possible to follow the site of formation of this DNA by autoradiography. Studies of this type have revealed that viral DNA is synthesized within the nucleus, specifically within the intranuclear inclusion (Munk and Sauer, 1963).

It has been clear for some time that most of the herpesviruses which have been studied can replicate and synthesize DNA in cells at different stages of the cell cycle. This was deduced from the fact that infection can be detected at relatively early stages of infection in practically every cell present in an infected nonsynchronized culture. Using synchronously growing cells, Cohen *et al.* (1971a) have provided more rigorous evidence that HSV DNA replication is indeed independent of the growth cycle of the cells. However, the DNA of EAV can replicate only in cells in S phase, i.e., in cells in which cellular DNA is being synthesized (Lawrence, 1971). It seems, therefore, that the synthesis of EAV DNA is dependent upon some cellular function, and it is likely that this virus, unlike some other members of the herpes group of viruses, cannot code for at least one function essential for the replication of its DNA.

The onset of viral DNA synthesis in infected cells varies with different strains of herpesviruses; it is probably also dependent upon the type of cell infected, as well as upon the multiplicity of infection. Viral DNA replicates semiconservatively, and, in principle, replicates in a geometric fashion, i.e., after replication, the two strands of the viral DNA molecule can each serve as a template for the formation of a complementary strand (Kaplan and Ben-Porat, 1964). Indeed the rate of viral DNA synthesis increases (see Fig. 1) as infection proceeds, and this increasing rate may be interpreted as being a reflection of the exponential mode of synthesis of viral DNA within the cell, in which the number of DNA molecules available for replication determines the rate of DNA synthesis. However, this is not the case, as shown by the fact that the infected cells acquire the ability to synthesize viral DNA at increasing rates, even when the accumulation of viral DNA molecules in these cells is inhibited (Kaplan, 1962). Furthermore, only part of the newly synthesized molecules of DNA accumulating in the infected cells participates in the replication process. Even though not integrated into virions, at least part of these molecules do not replicate because rapidly after their synthesis these molecules are converted into a form in which they are insensitive to the action of DNase. This DNase-insensitive DNA is presumably not available as a template for replication (Kaplan, 1964). Relatively few DNA molecules are in the process of being replicated at any given time, and the process of duplication of a DNA molecule is relatively rapid (Kaplan and Ben-Porat, 1966). Immediately after its synthesis, viral DNA seems to consist of nicked strands which are later ligated. However, not all of these nicks are repaired, and they appear in the DNA of mature virions at sites that may be specific (Kieff *et al.*, 1971).

Protein synthesis is necessary to maintain a constant rate of DNA synthesis in infected, as well as in uninfected, cells. The dependence of DNA synthesis upon concomitant protein synthesis in the infected cells is especially marked during the early stages of infection, and may reflect, at least in part, an early requirement of protein synthesis for the formation of some of the early enzymes involved in DNA synthesis that are induced by infection (see Section IX of this chapter). However, viral DNA synthesis is reduced in the infected cells, even when the inhibitors of protein synthesis are added after all the enzymes involved in DNA synthesis have appeared in the cells (Roizman and Roane, 1964; Kaplan and Ben-Porat, 1966), and addition of puromycin to the infected cells at that time results in a rapid drop in the rate of DNA synthesis to about 40% of that of untreated, infected cells; thereafter, the rate of DNA synthesis remains constant (Kaplan and Ben-Porat, 1966). Thus, DNA synthesis in infected, as well as in uninfected, cells is dependent upon concomitant synthesis of protein; however, this dependence decreases as the infective process continues. This is illustrated in Fig. 2 which shows the degree of sensitivity of DNA synthesis of cells to the addition of cycloheximide at different times after infection. (Exactly the same results are obtained with puromycin.) Of special interest is the inverse relationship between the sensitivity of DNA synthesis in infected cells and the activity of enzymes involved in the synthesis of DNA that are induced by infection. The puromycin-sensitive agent is not, however, one of the known enzymes involved in the synthesis of

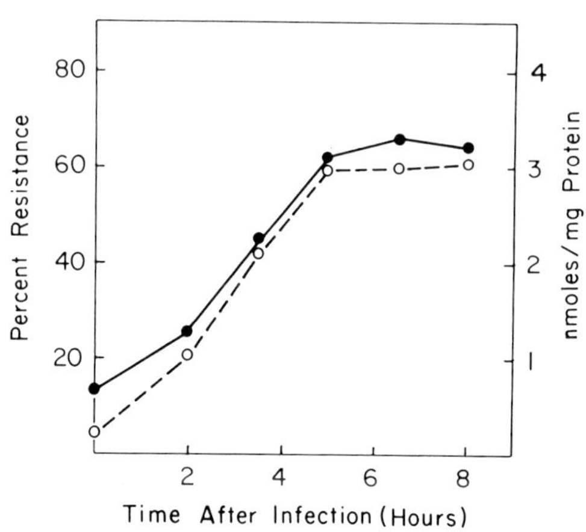

FIG. 2. Effect of cycloheximide on DNA synthesis and induction of early enzymes in infected cells. At various times after infection cycloheximide was added to the cells, and their ability to incorporate thymidine into DNA during the next 60 minutes was compared to that of infected cells to which no cycloheximide was added (closed circles). The ability of extracts of cells at various times after infection to catalyze the incorporation of thymidine into DNA *in vitro* was also measured (open circles). (A. S. Kaplan, unpublished results.)

DNA. The level of activity of these enzymes remains constant in the infected cells after the addition of puromycin (Kaplan and Ben-Porat, 1966). Thus, while protein synthesis is required for the maintenance of the normal rate of DNA synthesis in the infected cells, the synthesis of DNA in these cells is affected to a lesser extent by puromycin than it is in uninfected cells. It is interesting that the residual cellular DNA synthesis that occurs in the infected cells is also less affected by puromycin than it is in uninfected cells. Furthermore, the proteins which permit this synthesis are not used stochiometrically, as DNA synthesis proceeds, but rather seem to function catalytically (A. S. Kaplan, unpublished results). The proteins essential to the maintenance of a maximal rate of DNA synthesis in infected cells thus consist of two types: One type is rapidly lost, as are the proteins performing a similar function in uninfected cells. The loss of these proteins reduces the rate of synthesis of DNA in the infected cells to about 40% of that of untreated, infected cells. A second type consists of molecules which are stable and which allow the synthesis both of cellular and of viral DNA in the infected cells. These proteins appear in the infected cells in parallel with the early enzymes induced by infection (see Fig. 2). One is led to conclude that a protein, which acts catalytically, is necessary for DNA synthesis both in infected and in uninfected cells. This protein is unstable in uninfected cells but is stable, in part, in the infected cells; it is not one of the known enzymes involved in DNA synthesis.

V. Protein Synthesis

A. Rate of Protein Synthesis in Herpesvirus-Infected Cells

Infection of cells with most members of the herpesvirus group which have been studied results in the inhibition of cell-specific protein synthesis and in the induction of virus-specific protein synthesis.

In analyzing the changes in the rate of protein synthesis after infection of cells, one generally determines the rate of incorporation of labeled amino acids into protein. Figure 3 shows the incorporation of three different amino acids into the proteins of RK cells infected with PRV. Under the conditions used [multiplicity, 20 plaque forming units (PFU)/cell], the rate of incorporation of leucine into the proteins does not change during the first 5 hours postinfection. The relatively stable rate of leucine incorporation during the early stages of infection is due to a smooth switch over from the synthesis of cell-specific proteins to the synthesis of virus-specific proteins in this system. When lower multiplicities of infection are used, no change in leucine incorporation is observed up to 8 hours post-

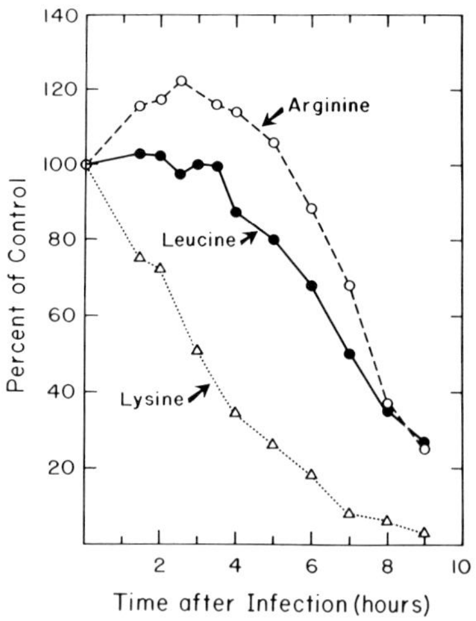

FIG. 3. Incorporation of essential amino acids into proteins at various times after infection. RK cells were infected (adsorbed multiplicity, 20 PFU/cell). At various times postinfection the cells were washed with medium containing one-tenth the usual amount of amino acids and incubated further in the same medium containing either [^{3}H]arginine, [^{3}H]leucine, or [^{3}H]lysine. One hour later the cells were harvested and the amounts of labeled amino acids incorporated into protein was determined. (From Kaplan *et al.*, 1970.)

infection (Hamada and Kaplan, 1965), indicating that the inhibition of cellular protein synthesis induced by the virus is multiplicity-dependent. Figure 3 shows also that the rate of lysine incorporation decreases rapidly after infection, while the rate of arginine incorporation increases during the early stages of infection. The changes in the rates of incorporation of these amino acids after infection are not due to changes in the intracellular pools but reflect a decrease in the rate of synthesis of cellular proteins and a concomitant increase in the synthesis of viral proteins in the cells (Kaplan *et al.*, 1970; Ben-Porat *et al.*, 1971; Saxton and Stevens, 1972). The cellular proteins are relatively richer in lysine and poorer in arginine than are the virus-specific proteins.

In HEp-2 cells infected with HSV, there is a decrease during the early stages of infection in the rate of incorporation of amino acids into proteins, a decrease which reflects the early inhibition in this system of the synthesis of cell-specific proteins. This early decrease is followed by a recovery in the rate of amino acid incorporation that is due to the increasing rate of synthesis of viral proteins (Roizman *et al.*, 1965; Sydiskis and Roizman, 1966). Thus, the effect of infection of cells with the herpesviruses on the overall rate of protein synthesis varies with the different virus–cell systems.

The infecting virus, the multiplicity of infection, and the type of cells infected and their physiological state will all affect the rate of inhibition of the synthesis of cell-specific proteins, as well as the rate of accumulation of virus-specific proteins, and will thereby determine the overall rate of protein synthesis in the infected cells.

B. Synthesis of Cell-Specific Proteins

The type of protein (cell-specific or virus-specific) synthesized by infected cells may be identified by several criteria. These criteria have been used to demonstrate the inhibition of synthesis of cell-specific proteins in cells infected with the herpesviruses.

a. Immune Precipitation. By this method cellular and viral proteins isotopically labeled are precipitated by specific γ-globulins, and the amount of radioactivity associated with the precipitate represents a measure of the amount of antigen synthesized. Experiments of this type (Hamada and Kaplan, 1965) showed that whereas the amount of leucine incorporated into proteins did not change during the first 7–8 hours after infection, the amount of labeled protein synthesized by the infected cells that reacted with γ-globulins specific for cellular proteins decreased; concurrently, the rate of synthesis of proteins that reacted with virus-specific γ-globulins increased. These results were the first demonstration that cell-specific protein synthesis was inhibited in cells infected with a herpesvirus.

b. Differences in Size of Viral and Cellular Polysomes and Disappearance of Cellular mRNA from Polysomes Present in Infected Cells. Sydiskis and Roizman (1966, 1967) showed that the polysomes which are normally present in HEp-2 cells and which have an average sedimentation value of about 170 S are disaggregated after infection (the rate of disaggregation is multiplicity dependent) and are replaced by polysomes which have an average sedimentation value of 220 S to 270 S. Sydiskis and Roizman (1967) concluded that the larger polysomes are probably virus-specific and that infection causes the disaggregation of cellular polysomes with the consequent inhibition of cell-specific protein synthesis.

The polysomes involved in the synthesis of PRV-specific proteins are larger than those involved in the synthesis of host proteins, as demonstrated by the analysis of the types of mRNA molecules associated with polysomes of different sizes present in the infected cells synthesizing both virus-specific and cell-specific proteins. Thus, at 2 hours postinfection, 65% of the viral polysomal mRNA but only 32% of the cellular polysomal mRNA are found in association with polysomes having a sedimentation value greater than 230 S. By 5 hours postinfection, virtually no cellular mRNA remains polysome-associated, indicating a cessation of the synthesis of cellular proteins (Ben-Porat *et al.*, 1971).

c. THE RATIO OF VARIOUS AMINO ACIDS TO EACH OTHER IN VIRAL AND IN CELLULAR PROTEIN. Figure 4 shows the profile of the nascent peptides associated with polysomes isolated from cells at various times after infection with PRV. The nascent peptides present in uninfected cells (Fig. 4A) have a much higher ratio of lysine to leucine than those present in infected cells (Fig. 4C). Of special interest is Fig. 4B, which illustrates the distribution of polysomes present in cells at relatively early stages of infection, when the individual infected cell in the culture is engaged in the synthesis both of virus- and cell-specific proteins (Kaplan *et al.*, 1970). Two types of polysomes are present in these cells: (1) relatively large polysomes (virus-specific) with nascent peptides comparatively poor in lysine and (2) smaller (cell-specific) polysomes with nascent peptides comparatively rich in lysine.

This experiment clearly illustrates the difference in average amino acid content between the proteins specified by the cellular and viral genomes, differences which probably reflect the difference in base composition between the two types of DNA. The dissimilarity in the average amino acid content of the viral and cellular proteins provides a useful tool for monitoring the types of proteins synthesized by the infected cells under various experimental conditions.

d. ELECTROPHORETIC PROFILES OF VIRAL AND CELLULAR PROTEINS. The electrophoretic profiles in sodium dodecyl sulfate (SDS) polyacrylamide gels of the proteins synthesized by HSV-infected cells (Spear and Roizman, 1968), or by PRV-infected cells (Shimono *et al.*, 1969; Kaplan *et al.*, 1970) differ greatly from those synthesized by uninfected cells (Fig. 5). At early stages of the infective process (2.5 hours), the electrophoretic profile of the proteins is intermediate between that of the proteins synthesized by uninfected cells and that of the proteins synthesized by cells at later stages of infection; this reflects the continued synthesis of cellular proteins during the early stages of infection. The differences in electrophoretic patterns between the proteins synthesized by uninfected cells and those synthesized by cells at later stages of infection are of sufficient magnitude to indicate that the synthesis or cell-specific proteins has been greatly reduced by infection.

C. *Synthesis of Viral Proteins*

The early studies on the synthesis of viral proteins in infected cells were performed by following the appearance of complement-fixing antigens which react specifically with antiserum prepared against the virus (Gold *et al.*, 1963; Russell *et al.*, 1964). The appearance in the cells of viral antigens

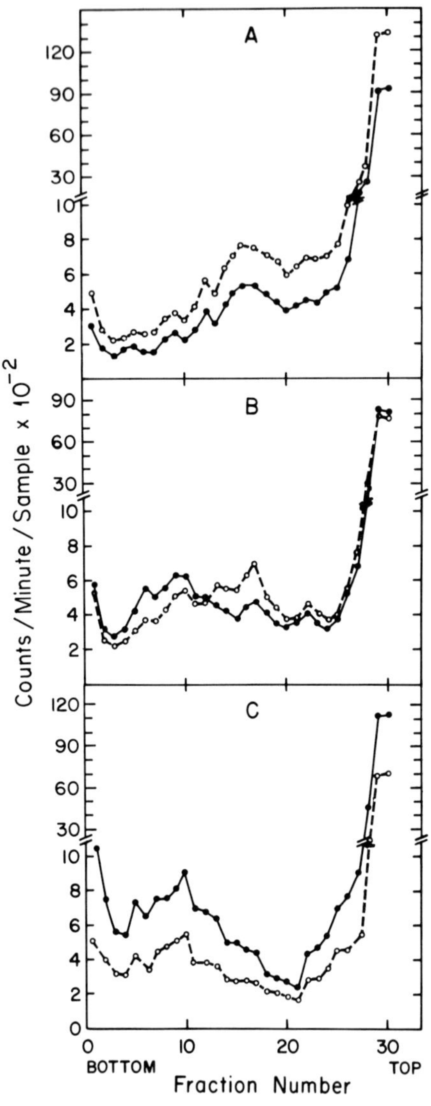

FIG. 4. Ratio of lysine to leucine in the nascent polypeptide chains associated with the polysomes obtained after infection. At various times after infection, the cells were incubated for 2 minutes in medium containing [^{3}H]lysine and [^{14}C]leucine. The cultures were harvested, the polysomes centrifuged in sucrose gradient, and the distribution of radioactivity in the gradient was determined. Open circles, [^{3}H]lysine; filled circles, [^{3}H]leucine. (A) Uninfected cells; (B) 2.5 hours postinfection; (C) 5 hours postinfection. (From Ben-Porat *et al.*, 1971.)

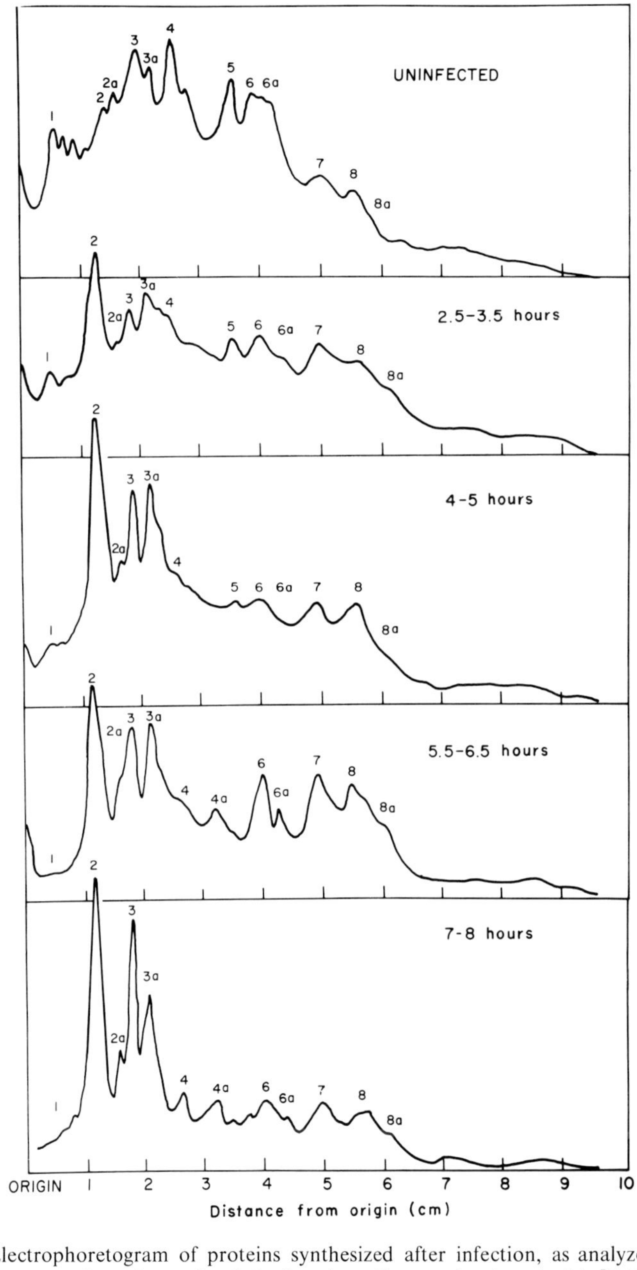

FIG. 5. Electrophoretogram of proteins synthesized after infection, as analyzed by autoradiography. At various times after infection the cells were incubated with [^{14}C]leucine for 1 hour. The cells were harvested, and the proteins extracted and electrophoresed in SDS–polyacrylamide gels. (From Kaplan *et al.*, 1970.)

has also been detected by gel immunodiffusion, polyacrylamide gel immunoelectrophoresis, and by indirect immunoprecipitation tests (Tokumaru, 1965; Watson *et al.*, 1966; Hamada and Kaplan, 1965). These studies revealed that infected cells synthesize virus-specific antigens of varying sizes, that these antigens are synthesized by the infected cells well before the formation of infectious virus begins, and that while some of these antigens become associated in time with mature viral particles, a large proportion remains in soluble form.

The herpesviruses have relatively large genomes and should, in principle, be able to code for about 100 polypeptides. The analysis of the proteins coded by such complex viruses is subject to many pitfalls. The use of SDS–polyacrylamide gels to separate the various viral proteins provides an initially useful tool to identify and characterize the major proteins. This method suffers from relatively low resolution, so that minor protein peaks are difficult to analyze. Furthermore, minor proteins that coelectrophorese with other viral proteins may not be detected.

Analysis by SDS–polyacrylamide gel electrophoresis indicates that the profile of the proteins synthesized during a period when the infected cells are producing viral proteins only is complex. Several major bands and numerous minor bands may be observed (Spear and Roizman, 1968; Kaplan *et al.*, 1970). This is illustrated in Fig. 5, which shows the electrophoretic profile of these proteins as analyzed by autoradiography.

Most of the major peaks have been identified and are, to a large degree, composed of structural viral components which become part of the viral core, capsid, or envelope. (See Chapter 3; also Section V,D below.) The minor proteins have not been identified, but many are probably structural proteins, since purified virions yield minor protein peaks with similar electrophoretic mobilities (Spear and Roizman, 1972).

Electrophoresis in SDS–polyacrylamide gels separates proteins on the basis of molecular weight. The proteins migrating to different peaks in the gel differ, however, not only with respect to their molecular weight but also with respect to their amino acid composition, indicating that each of the peaks consists, to a large degree, of only one or, at the most, a few major proteins. When the cells are labeled with various essential amino acids, different peaks appear, indicating that the total number of proteins in the gels is greater than indicated by labeling the proteins with just one amino acid (Kaplan *et al.*, 1970). Thus, it is clear that the infected cells synthesize a relatively large number of viral proteins in sufficient amounts to give distinct peaks in polyacrylamide gels, as well as to contribute to a characteristic amino acid composition of these protein peaks. Many other proteins, including enzymes, are probably synthesized as well in the infected cells, but they cannot be detected by these methods.

D. Nonstructural Viral Proteins

As mentioned above, the early studies dealing with the viral antigens synthesized by the infected cells revealed the presence of proteins that reacted with virus-specific γ-globulins but did not become part of the viral particles. Whether these were structural viral proteins that were synthesized in excess of the amount required for the formation of viral particles, or whether the antiserum prepared against mature virus also reacted with nonstructural virus-induced proteins was not clear.

That at least part of these are nonstructural viral proteins was demonstrated by the finding that during the early stages of PRV infection, proteins are formed which react with serum prepared against extracts of cells at early stages of infection. These proteins differ antigenically from the proteins found associated with the viral particles and are not precursors of structural viral proteins. They are, thus, true nonstructural viral proteins (Hamada and Kaplan, 1965).

The synthesis of nonstructural viral proteins may also be detected by comparing the electrophoretic profiles of isotopically labeled proteins synthesized by the infected cells (when they synthesize viral proteins only) with those present in the mature virons (Fig. 6). Several proteins from the infected cells migrate to positions in polyacrylamide gels which do not coincide with the positions of structural viral proteins. Two of these protein peaks disappear after a chase, however, and may represent either unstable nonstructural proteins which turn over rapidly or proteins which are precursors of other structural or nonstructural proteins (A. S. Kaplan, unpublished results). At least two stable major nonstructural proteins are synthesized by the infected cells (Fig. 6), which have molecular weights of approximately 90,000 daltons (3a proteins) and 25,000 daltons (8a proteins). (The estimation of the molecular weight of the 3a protein obtained by SDS–gel electrophoresis may be inaccurate since it is a glycoprotein.) There may be several other minor nonstructural proteins which are not resolved by this method. Furthermore, it is impossible to identify proteins by their position in the gel only, because different proteins with the same molecular weight will migrate as one peak. To overcome this difficulty and to determine whether a given peak of protein synthesized by infected cells consists of structural proteins, nonstructural proteins, or both, a method which compares the relative amino acid content of the peaks of proteins derived from infected cells with those derived from purified virus was used. These studies revealed that the ratio of one essential amino acid to another in the proteins in one peak obtained from purified virions was different from that in the proteins migrating to the same position present in the extracts from infected cells (A. S. Kaplan, unpublished results). Thus, at least one peak of proteins synthesized

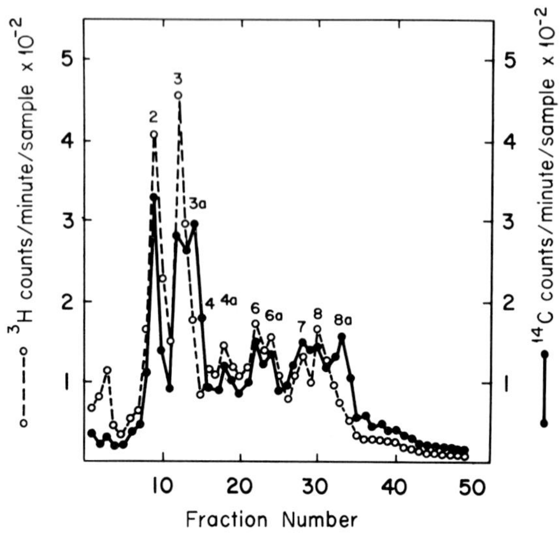

FIG. 6. Electrophoretogram of virion proteins and of proteins synthesized by infected RK cells. Infected cells were incubated with [^{14}C]leucine (closed circles) between 4 and 8 hours after infection, followed by a 1-hour chase with an excess of cold amino acids. Mature virions were purified from infected cultures which had been incubated throughout the infective process with [^{3}H]leucine (open circles). The cells were harvested, mixed with purified virions, and the proteins electrophoresed on SDS–polyacrylamide gels. (A. S. Kaplan, unpublished results.)

by the infected cells represents a mixture of structural and nonstructural proteins. As mentioned above, separation of proteins by SDS–polyacrylamide gel electrophoresis will, of course, only detect proteins which are present in sufficient amounts to contribute appreciably to the amino acid composition of the proteins in the peak. Many of the proteins coded for by the viral genome are probably enzymes involved in the synthesis of the viral components; one would not expect these proteins to accumulate in large amounts in the infected cells, and they would, therefore, not be detectable by gel electrophoresis.

The three nonstructural proteins which have been detected after infection are synthesized in relatively large amounts, but their functions are unknown. Protein 3a is the major glycoprotein synthesized by the infected cells. Stevens *et al.* (1969) described the synthesis in PRV-infected cells of an acid-soluble nonstructural viral protein which becomes attached to cellular chromatin and has postulated that such a protein may play a role in the virus-induced inhibition of cellular DNA synthesis.

In conclusion, it is clear that infected cells synthesize relatively large amounts of nonstructural viral proteins. However, except for their catalytic function, no definite evidence has yet been obtained concerning the role of nonstructural viral proteins in the infective process. The formation of virus-induced enzymes is discussed in Section IX of this chapter.

E. Site of Synthesis and of Accumulation of Viral Proteins

Numerous reports have appeared that are concerned with the site of accumulation of viral antigens in the infected cells; most of these reports deal with the appearance in the cells of antigens reacting with hyperimmune or convalescent sera conjugated to fluorescein or to ferritin. Investigators using these methods have reported variously that viral antigens appear first in the nucleus or in the cytoplasm or in the nuclear and cytoplasmic membranes, in areas surrounding the nuclear membrane, in small or large granules, or a combination of any one of these. These studies are difficult to interpret because different sera react to a different extent both with structural and with nonstructrual proteins, the identity of the proteins reacting in each case being unknown. Antisera against specific structural or nonstructural viral proteins have not yet been produced because these proteins have not been purified. Studies using tagged antisera to localize the site of accumulation of viral proteins suffer also from the fact that viral proteins probably undergo changes in antigenicity, as well as changes in their localization within the cells, during the process of assembly and maturation of the virion. The localization of the viral antigens in the cells (using the same sera) will thus vary somewhat, depending on which stage of the infective process the cells are examined.

Although the experiments using tagged antisera did not reveal the identity of the viral antigens observed in the cytoplasm and the nuclei of the infected cells, they clearly indicated that viral antigens accumulate in both areas. The site of *synthesis* rather than of accumulation of the viral antigen cannot, however, be established by these cytological methods, and these methods failed to determine whether viral capsid proteins are synthesized in the nucleus or whether they are synthesized in the cytoplasm (as are most cellular proteins) and migrate thereafter to the nucleus.

That at least some virus-specific proteins are probably synthesized on cytoplasmic polysomes was suggested by the experiments of Sydiskis and Roizman (1966) who showed that infection of HEp-2 cells with HSV caused an initial breakdown of the polysomes present in the cells at the time of infection, followed by the reformation of larger polysomes which, as seemed likely, were virus-specific, an assumption later proven to be correct. The cytoplasmic site of synthesis of most viral proteins was also indicated by the fact that essentially no difference was found between infected and uninfected cells in the distribution of radioactive proteins between the nuclear and cytoplasmic fractions after a short pulse with radioactive amino acids (Fujiwara and Kaplan, 1967). Furthermore, a flow of proteins, which had been synthesized during a short pulse with labeled amino acids, from the cytoplasm to the nucleus also was detected in infected but not in uninfected cells (Olshevsky *et al.*, 1967; Fujiwara and Kaplan, 1967). The proteins migrating to the nucleus become associated with viral particles and become reactive with antisera prepared against mature virus (Fujiwara and Kaplan, 1967). Furthermore, a large portion of the proteins that are synthesized in the cytoplasm of infected cells and that subsequently migrate to the nucleus have electrophoretic mobility rates in polyacrylamide gels similar to those of the proteins found in mature virions (Spear and Roizman, 1968; Shimono and Kaplan, 1968). These data indicate that most of the structural viral proteins are synthesized in the cytoplasm and thereafter migrate to the nucleus where the capsids are assembled.

The transfer of the structural viral proteins to the nucleus is a relatively slow process both in HSV- and in PRV-infected cells. In the latter case, a flow of radioactive proteins to the nucleus can be detected up to about one hour after a pulse with radioactive amino acids (Fujiwara and Kaplan, 1967). In HSV-infected cells a flow continues for approximately 2 hours and then stops (Olshevsky *et al.*, 1967). A maximum of 50% of the major structural proteins synthesized by the infected cells are, at any given time, found associated with nuclear fractions (Spear and Roizman, 1968; Ben-Porat *et al.*, 1969). This is probably due to the concurrent migration of viral proteins to the nucleus and of completed nucleocapsids from the nucleus to the cytoplasm, since only 20% of the major structural viral proteins synthesized by the cells during a pulse do not eventually become part of the viral particles (Ben-Porat *et al.*, 1969).

The mechanism responsible for the migration of virus-specific proteins from their site of synthesis in the cytoplasm to the nucleus of the infected cell is not known at the present time. The simplest and most appealing explanation for this migration is that it is due to diffusion. Thus, if assembly of structural viral proteins into particles within the nucleus acts as a diffusion sink, a concentration gradient would be established which would lead to an accumulation of these structural proteins in the nucleus. Since assembly of the viral proteins occurs only in the nucleus, the existence either of a nuclear condensing factor or of a cytoplasmic inhibitor of assembly must be postulated.

Structural viral proteins migrate to the nucleus and are assembled into empty capsids, even when little viral DNA accumulates (Ben-Porat *et al.*, 1969). Furthermore, despite the accumulation of viral DNA in arginine-deprived cells, structural proteins do not migrate to the nucleus (Becker *et al.*, 1967; Mark and Kaplan, 1971). Thus, viral DNA is not the factor responsible for the migration of structural viral proteins from the cytoplasm to the nucleus of the infected cells. The factor(s) responsible for this migration are at present not clearly understood. This question is discussed further in Section V,F which deals with the role of arginine in the infective process.

Many of the viral proteins are glycoproteins which become associated with membranes in the infected cells. Spear and Roizman (1970) have shown that the virus-specified glycopeptides present in the smooth membranes are most likely glycosylated *in situ*. This was concluded on the basis of the following evidence: (1) Little glucosamine label was found associated with nascent peptides on polysomes. (2) Puromycin inhibited the incorporation of amino acids into proteins but only partially affected the incorporation of glucosamine into acid-precipitable macromolecules. (3) After a pulse of 1 hour with labeled amino acids and labeled glucosamine, nonglycosylated proteins were present on the membranes. After a chase, however, these proteins disappeared and there was an increase in the amount of the glycosylated proteins present in the membranes.

Thus, most viral proteins are synthesized on cytoplasmic polysomes. The structural viral capsid proteins then migrate to the nucleus where they are assembled into particles. The glycosylation of the viral membrane glycoproteins occurs most likely after the peptides have attached to the membranes. The possibility that some viral proteins are synthesized in the nucleus of the infected cells has not been excluded.

F. The Special Role of Arginine in Herpesvirus Replication

The need for arginine in the replication of herpesviruses was first reported by Tankersley (1964) and confirmed by Roizman *et al.* (1965) and Sharon (1966). Several papers have since appeared dealing with an analysis at the molecular level of the events occurring in arginine-deprived infected cells. The first of these was by Becker *et al.* (1967) who reported that viral DNA synthesis occurred in HSV-infected cells deprived of arginine and that protein synthesis was inhibited by about 50%, but that neither complete nor incomplete viral particles were formed. Essentially the same findings were later reported for PRV-infected, arginine-starved cells (Mark and Kaplan, 1971). Roizman *et al.* (1967) showed by immunofluorescence that at least some viral proteins are synthesized in the arginine-deprived cells, a finding later confirmed by Courtney *et al.* (1970) who used the same methods.

Spring *et al.* (1969) showed that in arginine-deprived HEp-2 cells infected with HSV, the synthesis of proteins of high molecular weight is preferentially inhibited. They interpreted these results to mean that the probability that a given protein will be completed depends on the number of arginine residues in the proteins and that given an equal frequency of arginine in two peptides, the one with the lower molecular weight will have a higher probability of being completed. The special role of arginine in the infective process would thus be the result of the relatively large molecular weight of the viral proteins and their high content of arginine. Although at first glance this explanation seemed plausible, it is not supported by the experimental evidence reported by other laboratories.

Olshevsky and Becker (1970) showed that structural viral proteins are synthesized in infected, arginine-deprived cells and that these proteins become integrated into viral particles, once arginine is supplied to the cells. Whereas capsid proteins and envelope proteins synthesized during arginine deprivation became part of viral particles that are assembled, once arginine was supplied, little, if any, core proteins synthesized during the period of arginine starvation could be detected in these particles. Thus, either these proteins are not synthesized (or are not functional) in arginine-starved cells or core proteins do not form a pool from which proteins can later be chased into particles. These results could, however, also reflect the fact that the core proteins are relatively poor in leucine, since as a result of its design this experiment would not have detected leucine-poor proteins.

Courtney *et al.* (1971) and Mark and Kaplan (1971) analyzed the proteins synthesized in arginine-deprived, infected cells by SDS–polyacrylamide gel electrophoresis and reported that the major viral proteins are synthesized in the cytoplasm of these cells, although at a reduced rate. However, these proteins do not migrate to the nucleus and do not assemble into particles as they do normally but will migrate to the nucleus, once arginine is supplied to the cells (Courtney *et al.*, 1971).

The lack of migration of structural viral proteins in arginine-deprived cells may indicate that a protein which is more affected by arginine deprivation than other proteins plays a role in this phenomenon. Such a protein could act as a condensing factor which would effectively reduce the concentration of the pool of unassembled structural proteins in the nucleus, thus favoring a continued diffusion of these proteins into the nucleus. If this were the case, the condensing protein, in contrast to the structural viral proteins, would have to be synthesized in the nucleus (since otherwise assembly would occur in the cytoplasm). This protein would represent only a small fraction of the virus-specific proteins synthesized by infected cells, since its lack of synthesis cannot be detected in arginine-deprived cells by methods which should show the absence of a major protein.

Viral membrane glycoproteins also are synthesized in arginine-deprived cells but are not integrated into the nuclear membrane as they are in normally infected cells (Mark and Kaplan, 1972). The usual increase in the rate of incorporation of choline into the phospholipids of the nuclear membrane, as well as the flow of phospholipids from the cytoplasmic membranes to the nuclear membranes, also does not occur, indicating that the virus-induced synthesis of nuclear membrane does not take place in arginine-deprived cells (Mark and Kaplan, 1972). The lack of nuclear membrane synthesis in arginine-deprived cells is probably responsible for the absence of viral glycoproteins in this membrane.

Present evidence thus indicates that most of the viral proteins are synthesized in arginine-deprived cells but that they do not assemble into particles in the nuclei of the infected cells. The lack of migration of viral proteins to the nucleus may result from the fact that a protein, the synthesis of which is more affected by arginine deprivation than that of other proteins, plays a central role in the assembly of viral particles. It is also possible, however, that the lack of assembly of viral particles in the nucleus is directly related to the lack of characteristic virus-induced alterations of the nuclear membrane, since the nuclear membrane has been shown to play a role in the assembly of adenovirus (Winters and Russell, 1971).

Although the special role of arginine in the replication of the herpesviruses is not clearly understood at present, its elucidation may provide valuable insight into the processes controlling viral maturation.

VI. Membrane Alterations

Most of the information relating to the changes induced by infection in the membranes of the host cells has been acquired from electron microscopic studies and is discussed in detail elsewhere in this book. The features common to cells infected with most of the members of the herpesvirus group which has emerged from these studies and which are relevant to the present discussion are as follows: (1) The nuclear membrane becomes convoluted. (2) The herpesviruses acquire their envelope by budding from cellular membranes, and although there appears to be some variation observed in different virus–cell systems with respect to the particular membranes which serve as the source of the viral envelope, most of the herpesviruses studied thus far appear to bud from the inner nuclear membrane. (3) Most of the cellular membranes become "altered" and acquire virus-specific antigens.

A. Phospholipid Metabolism in the Infected Cells

The synthesis of lipids and their association with the envelope of the herpesviruses was first studied by Asher *et al.* (1969), who found that infection of BSC_1 cells with HSV did not change the rate of incorporation of $[^3H]$choline into lipids and that both in infected and in uninfected cells choline was incorporated mainly into lecithin. The effect of infection with

PRV on the phospholipid metabolism of RK cells was subsequently investigated (Ben-Porat and Kaplan, 1971, 1972) with the following findings: In this system, there is an increase after infection of about 20% in the incorporation of ^{32}P, [^{3}H] choline, and [^{3}H]*myo*-inositol into phospholipids. While the increase of incorporation of label into the membranes of the cytoplasmic fraction is significant, it is especially marked in the membranes of the nuclear fractions of the infected cells. (In these experiments the phospholipids associated with nuclear fractions, from which all membranes but the inner nuclear membrane had been removed, were compared with those associated with preparations of other cellular fractions, as well as of purified virus. Since phospholipids are found in association only with membranes in infected and in uninfected cells, no attempt was made to isolate the membranes in each fraction. Isolation of the membranes was deemed unnecessary and detrimental since it may lead to errors as a result of poor recovery.)

Infection changed also the relative degree of incorporation of labeled precursor into different phospholipids. Two to three times more label derived from ^{32}P and [^{3}H]choline appeared in sphingomyelin in infected than in unfected cells. Table II shows that the inner nuclear membrane of RK cells is relatively rich in sphingomyelin compared to other cellular membranes. The increase after infection in the relative amount of label incorporated into sphingomyelin probably reflects the large amount of *de novo* synthesis of the inner nuclear membrane as discussed below.

B. The Biogenesis of the Viral Envelope

Although most herpesvirus strains that have been studied acquire their envelopes from the inner nuclear membrane, it has become increasingly clear that different members of the herpes group of viruses may acquire their outer envelope by budding from different cellular membranes. The degree of genetic relatedness between the different members of the group is small (see Chapter 3), and basic differences in the mechanisms regulating the growth processes of these viruses may exist. Thus, at least one member of the herpes group of viruses, herpesvirus saimiri, acquires its envelope by a mechanism that does not involve budding from cellular membranes. The envelope of this virus is laid down around the nucleocapsid within the nucleus (Heine *et al.*, 1971). All other herpesviruses analyzed to the present time, however, acquire their envelope by budding from cellular membranes.

The proteins normally associated with the cellular membranes from which the virus buds are not present in the areas of the membrane from which the viruses acquire their envelope because purified preparations of enveloped virions contain little, if any, of the proteins present in the cells at the time of infection (Ben-Porat and Kaplan, 1970; Spear and Roizman, 1972). How-

TABLE II
DISTRIBUTION OF RADIOACTIVITY AMONG THE PHOSPHOLIPIDS OF VARIOUS FRACTIONS FROM CELLS CULTIVATED IN ^{32}P AND IN VIRUS PRODUCED BY THESE CELLS[a,b]

Fraction	Lysolecithin	Sphingo-myelin	Phosphatidyl-serine	Phosphatidyl-choline + Phosphatidyl-inositol	Phosphatidyl-ethanolamine
Cytoplasmic	2.3[c]	11.0	2.7	61.0	23.0
Outer nuclear	4.2	8.6	3.2	62.3	21.7
Inner nuclear	3.5	20.8	3.7	50.5	21.5
Virus	3.3	21.0	3.5	51.2	21.0

[a]RK cells were seeded and cultivated in medium containing ^{32}P (2 μCi/ml). Part of the culture was infected and part was mock-infected. Incubation was continued in the ^{32}P medium. Virus was harvested from the infected cultures and purified; the various cellular fractions were isolated from the mock-infected cultures. The lipids were extracted and the phospholipids were separated by thin-layer chromatography.
[b]From Ben-Porat and Kaplan, 1971.
[c]Percent of total radioactivity.

ever, this is not the case for the phospholipids of the viral membrane, most of which preexist in the cells at the time of infection (Asher *et al.*, 1969; Ben-Porat and Kaplan, 1971). The viral envelope is derived, therefore, from one of the following: (1) areas of the cellular membranes from which the cellular proteins have been displaced, (2) areas of the membranes which at the time of infection contained little or no proteins, or (3) areas of the membranes that are synthesized *de novo* after infection from newly formed virus-specific proteins and glycoproteins and from phospholipids preexisting in the cells.

The biogenesis of the viral envelope was studied in detail in PRV-infected RK cells (Ben-Porat and Kaplan, 1971, 1972). In this system, most of the virions acquire their envelope by budding from the inner nuclear membrane. This has been observed by electron microscopy and is shown also by the characteristic phospholipid composition of the viral envelope which mimics that of the inner nuclear membrane (Table II).

The viral envelope is not derived from a random area of the nuclear membrane to which viral specific proteins have become attached. This was first indicated by the fact that the areas of the nuclear membrane which the nucleocapsid acquires are metabolically more active than the remainder of the nuclear membrane after infection (Ben-Porat and Kaplan, 1971). Thus, either the virions bud from areas on the membrane that have been synthesized *de novo* after infection, using mostly phospholipids preexisting in the cells, or they bud from areas of the membrane which have experienced an increased rate of turnover.

The convolution of the nuclear membrane observed by electron microscopy in herpesvirus-infected cells suggests that infection may stimulate the synthesis of new nuclear membrane. Evidence that extensive new nuclear membrane is indeed assembled in PRV-infected cells comes from experiments which show that phospholipids present in cytoplasmic membranes at the time of infection become part of the inner nuclear membrane. By 7 hours after infection there is a twofold increase in the amount of phospholipids associated with the nuclear membrane, representing a twofold increase of this membrane (Ben-Porat and Kaplan, 1972).

Thus, in PRV-infected cells, at least, the sections of the nuclear membrane destined to become viral envelopes are synthesized *de novo*, but the phospholipids that become associated with the nuclear membrane are derived, for the most part, from other cellular membranes. The proteins used to build the nascent nuclear membrane are virus-specific exclusively, since the synthesis of cell-specific proteins is inhibited in these cells. The budding of nucleocapsids, is probably restricted solely to the newly synthesized areas of the nuclear membrane, thereby ensuring the presence of only virus-specific proteins in the viral envelope.

The envelope of herpesvirus saimiri is also clearly not derived from preexisting membranes (Heine *et al.*, 1971). On the other hand, other strains of herpesvirus that acquire their envelope by budding from cellular membranes may use "modified" cellular membranes in which the cellular proteins have been displaced by viral proteins. However, evidence that this occurs has as yet not been adduced.

C. *Integration of Viral Proteins into the Plasma Membrane of Infected Cells*

Cells infected with the herpesviruses acquire virus-specific antigens on their surface; the presence of these antigens can be demonstrated by a variety of methods (Roane and Roizman, 1964; Watkins, 1964; Nii *et al.*, 1968c; Pearson *et al.*, 1970; Chen and Purchase, 1970; Lowry *et al.*, 1971). The antigens appearing on the surface of cells infected both with HSV and with the Epstein-Barr virus (EBV) seem to be identical to the antigens present in the mature virions that react with neutralizing antibody (Roizman and Spring, 1967; Pearson *et al.*, 1970). Alterations in the properties of the plasma membranes after infection of the cells by HSV are also indicated by the fact that these cells become susceptible to agglutination by concanavalin A (Tevethia *et al.*, 1972).

In an attempt to identify and characterize the virus-induced proteins that appear in the plasma membrane of infected cells, Roizman and co-workers (Roizman, 1970; Spear *et al.*, 1970; Keller *et al.*, 1970; Heine *et al.*, 1972) have performed a series of experiments which have led them to conclude that these proteins are, in most cases, identical to the proteins that become part of the envelope of mature virions. Their findings may be summarized as follows: The glycoproteins synthesized by HEp-2 cells infected with the F or Vr-3 strains of HSV and present in cell fractions enriched for smooth membranes or in purified preparations of plasma membrane are identical to the glycoproteins in preparations of partially purified virus with respect to electrophoretic mobility. Viral glycoproteins are also present in the smooth membrane fractions from cells infected with the G strain (a genital strain) and the MP strain (a strain producing macroplaques and extensive syncytia). However, the ratio of one of these glycoproteins to another in the cellular membranes is different from the ratio of the glycoproteins associated with the virions. Thus in some cases, all (and in other cases, only part) of the structural viral glycoproteins become associated with smooth membrane fractions. Similar results have been obtained with cells infected with PRV (a virus that gives rise to extensive syncytia); glycosylated proteins similar to the glycoproteins of the viral envelope have been found associated with cellular fractions containing smooth membranes (J. R. Griffin and A. S. Kaplan, unpublished results).

Although these results seem to indicate that most of the viral envelope proteins become associated with the plasma membrane, experiments of this type suffer from two shortcomings: (1) The envelope proteins of the herpesviruses may attach unspecifically to the plasma membrane, as demonstrated by Cohen *et al.* (1971b) for the envelope proteins of vesicular stomatitis virus. Roizman and Spear (1971) have shown that the viral proteins are tightly bound to the cellular membranes; however, this does not eliminate the possibility of unspecific attachment. (2) In all these experiments, the membranes were isolated as fragments. It is possible that during the unavoidable treatment of the infected cells during the course of isolation of membranes, mature viral particles present in the cytoplasm of these cells may be disrupted. Segments of the nuclear membrane (the source of the viral envelope in these systems) which is known to become convoluted and to invaginate into the cytoplasm, also may be fragmented. The segments of the nuclear membrane, as well as the envelopes derived from disrupted virions, may behave during the isolation procedure in a manner similar to that of the fragments of the plasma membranes, and the fraction containing the plasma membranes, although relatively uncontaminated by other cellular membranes, may be contaminated with viral envelope material. Thus, while it is likely that viral envelope proteins are integrated into the plasma membranes of the infected cells, currently available evidence is not clear-cut. Proof that this is the case would be the demonstration of the presence of these proteins in plasma membranes isolated as intact ghosts, and the elimination of possible unspecific adsorption of viral membrane proteins to cellular membranes.

The reason for the virus-induced modification of the plasma membrane in the virus replication is unknown. Electron microscopic data indicate that the virus does not acquire its envelope by budding from this membrane. The integration of virus-specified glycoproteins into the plasma membrane may be of negative survival value to the virus, since it increases the ability of the immune host to combat infection. The change in the plasma membrane, however, occurs in most cells infected with the herpesviruses which have been studied, and mutants which do not bring about these changes have not yet been isolated. There are two possible explanations for the presence of viral proteins in the plasma membrane of the infected cells: (1) These proteins may prevent the interaction of the plasma membranes with virus and the possible consequent inactivation of newly synthesized virus. (2) Viral membrane proteins may become integrated into any membrane in the process of assembly in the infected cells. Plasma membranes normally experience a rapid rate of turnover (Siekevitz, 1972); infection may not inhibit this turnover, and the viral proteins (the only proteins synthesized by the infected cells) consequently may become part of this membrane. Thus, the integration of viral proteins into those cellular membranes, which are not the source of the viral envelope, could simply reflect basic mechanisms of membrane assembly.

In conclusion, the identity of the proteins integrated into the plasma membranes and their functions are not clearly defined at present. However, available data indicate that virus-specific antigens are integrated into the plasma membranes.

D. Alteration of "Cytoplasmic" Membranes

All the cellular membranes of HEp-2 cells infected with the F strain of HSV acquire the same virus-specific glycoprotein (Spear *et al.*, 1970). This is not so for PRV-infected RK cells. In the latter case, the structural viral glycoproteins, i.e., the glycoproteins associated with the envelope of the mature virions, can be found in fractions containing the inner nuclear membrane and the smooth membranes. However, the PRV-infected RK cells also synthesize a virus-specific nonstructural glycoprotein which is made in relatively large amounts. This glycoprotein comprises approximately 10% of the total proteins synthesized by the infected cells and is found associated with membranes of relatively high density only, probably those of the rough endoplasmic reticulum. A large proportion of the glycoproteins is excreted by the infected cells but the function of these membrane proteins is unknown at the present time (Ben-Porat and Kaplan, 1970; T. Ben-Porat, unpublished results).

E. The Social Behavior of the Infected Cells

The herpesviruses cause the infected cells to clump or to fuse; there is a gradation among various strains of the degree to which these changes occur after they infect susceptible cells. Indeed, it seems that infection of the cells with these viruses may increase the "stickiness" of the cell surface (Watkins, 1964). The tendency of infected cells to interact with each other has been termed by Roizman, "social behavior." This terminology will be used because much of the work done to date on this subject has been performed by Roizman and his co-workers.

The relationship of virus multiplication to cell fusion has been reviewed by Poste (1970). Briefly, fusion is not observed when cells are infected with ultraviolet light-irradiated HSV (Roizman, 1965; Coccuzo and Russo, 1966). Cell fusion occurs in the absence of DNA synthesis (Falke, 1967; Falke *et al.*, 1969; Munk and Sauer, 1964; Ben-Porat *et al.*, 1961; Reissig and Kaplan, 1962). However, RNA and protein synthesis are required, at least during the early stages of infection (Falke and Peterknecht, 1968). Cell fusion does not occur when infected cells are deprived of arginine, even though under these conditions most of the virus-specific proteins are synthesized but do not become assembled into particles. Fusion occurs, however, during abortive infection with a host range mutant of HSV unable to grow in canine kidney cells (Aurelian and Roizman, 1965), and a noninfectious particle causing fusion has been reported by Tokumaru (1968). Thus, most of the evidence indicates that, in general, fusion of the infected cells is directly or indirectly mediated by a product specified by the viral genome.

Poste (1970) postulates that infection of cells with fusion-producing viruses causes a decrease in the thickness of the cell membrane, a reduction that results from the virus-induced release of lysosomal enzymes (Poste, 1971a,b; Greenham and Poste, 1971). Indeed, lysosomal stabilizing agents, such as hydrocortisone, inhibit virus-induced cell fusion (Greenham and Poste, 1971; Tokumaru, 1968) without affecting normal replication of the virions. Furthermore, inhibition of lysosomal protease activity induces in the infected cells a reduction in virus-induced cell fusion. Fine *et al.* (1970), however, reported that cells infected with a strain of HSV, which produces extensive cell fusion, retained their lysosomal integrity, whereas cells infected with another strain, which does not produce cell fusion, released a considerable amount of lysosomal enzymes. This finding is at odds with the views held by Poste.

A different hypothesis for the basis of cell fusion has also been advanced by Roizman and co-workers who believe that the insertion of virus-specific proteins into the plasma membrane of the infected cells is the basis for the "social behavior" of these cells (Spear *et al.*, 1970; Keller *et al.*, 1970). The rationale for this hypothesis is as follows: Infection of cells with different strains of HSV give rise to differences in the social behavior of the infected cells. The two strains which show the greatest difference in this respect are strain F, which produces cell clumping, and strain MP, which induces fusion of the cells. As discussed above, these two strains of HSV also differ significantly with respect to the glycoproteins they induce that become associated with the smooth membranes of the infected cells.

There is, however, no direct correlation between the type of viral glycoproteins in the membranes and the social behavior of the cells. The relative amounts, as well as the degree of glycosylation, of the proteins that become associated with the smooth membrane differ in different cell lines infected with these two virus strains. Thus, the relatively large differences in electrophoretic profiles of the glycoproteins that become associated with the smooth membranes observed when HEp-2 cells are infected with either of these two strains of virus is not observed when Vero cells are infected with the same two virus strains (Keller *et al.*, 1970). Both cell lines, however, respond to infection with the MP virus strain by fusion and to F virus strain by clumping.

The most convincing evidence available at the present time that the type of structural viral glycoprotein which becomes associated with the cellular membranes of the infected cells may determine the social behavior of these cells comes from the following experiment (Roizman, 1970): When HEp-2 cells are doubly infected with the F and the MP strains, the genotype of both strains is reproduced. However, the glycoproteins present in the envelope of the virions produced by these cells, as well as those inserted into the smooth membranes of the infected cells, are characteristic of the glycoproteins specified by the F strain only. Thus, the F strain is dominant with respect to the specification of viral glycoproteins. The doubly infected cells also exhibit a social behavior similar to that of cells infected with the F strain only. On the basis of these findings, Roizman concluded that the glycoproteins inserted into the smooth membranes are responsible for the behavior (clumping or fusing) of the infected cells. However, even if one assumes that the glycoproteins are indeed inserted into the plasma membrane (see above), the dominance of the F strain over the MP strain with respect to both the type of glycoproteins that become associated with the smooth membrane and the social behavior of the infected cell does not necessarily indicate a direct correlation between the two phenomena. It is by no means clear to what degree the two virus strains are genetically related, and the F strains may be dominant not only with respect to the specification of glycoproteins but also with respect to other factors which determine the "social behavior" of the cells.

In conclusion, the type of social behavior exhibited by cells infected with different strains of the herpesviruses may reflect the integration into the plasma membrane of different types of viral envelope proteins as postulated by Roizman. Thus, differences in degree of "stickness" of the surface of the cells induced by infection with different viruses may be the basis for the differences in the behavior of the cells and may be mediated by different viral envelope glycoproteins. On the other hand, Poste has found a correlation between release of lysosomal enzyme, membrane thickness, and cell fusion. The evidence available to support either of these hypotheses is at present inconclusive.

VII. Virion Assembly

A. Capsid Formation

As discussed in detail in Section V,E, most of the structural viral proteins are synthesized in the cytoplasm of the infected cells and thereafter migrate to the nucleus where they are assembled into nucleocapsids. No information is available at present concerning the state of the proteins migrating to the nucleus, i.e., whether the viral proteins migrate as subunits or whether some form of protein subunit assembly (such as a capsomere formation) occurs in the cytoplasm.

B. Integration of Viral DNA into Virions

By use of inhibitors of DNA synthesis, such as 5-fluorodeoxyuridine (FUdR) or 1β-D-arabinofuranosylcytosine (Ara-C), it has been demonstrated that DNA synthesis precedes virus assembly. The addition of the inhibitors to the cells at various stages of the infective process does not result in an immediate arrest of virus synthesis; some infectious virus continues to be formed (Levitt and Becker, 1967; O'Callaghan *et al.*, 1968b). That viral DNA synthesized early in infection can be integrated into virions formed later was demonstrated in a more direct manner by showing that the amount of labeled viral DNA synthesized between 3 and 4 hours after infection that becomes associated with virions increases as the number of infectious viral particles produced by the cells increases (Ben-Porat and Kaplan, 1963). Thus, DNA synthesized early by the infected cells is used for the formation of viral particles assembled later in the infective process.

Viral DNA is made in excess, and about 15% of the DNA synthesized between 3 and 4 hours after infection becomes associated with virions (Ben-Porat and Kaplan, 1963). This finding raised the question of whether DNA synthesized at different times after infection has an equal chance to be integrated into viral particles. Figure 7 illustrates the results of an experiment designed to answer this question. In this experiment, cells were pulse labeled at different times after infection, and the amount of labeled DNA integrated into viral particles released from the cells at various times of the infective process was determined. If withdrawal of DNA from the pool of DNA for the formation of particles is a random process, the fractions of the viral DNA that have been synthesized at different times postinfection (i.e., DNA that has been labeled during the different pulse times) that become integrated into viral particles should be the same. The results in Fig. 7 show that this is indeed the case and that DNA molecules synthesized at different times after infection have an equal chance to become part of the virions. Thus, in the

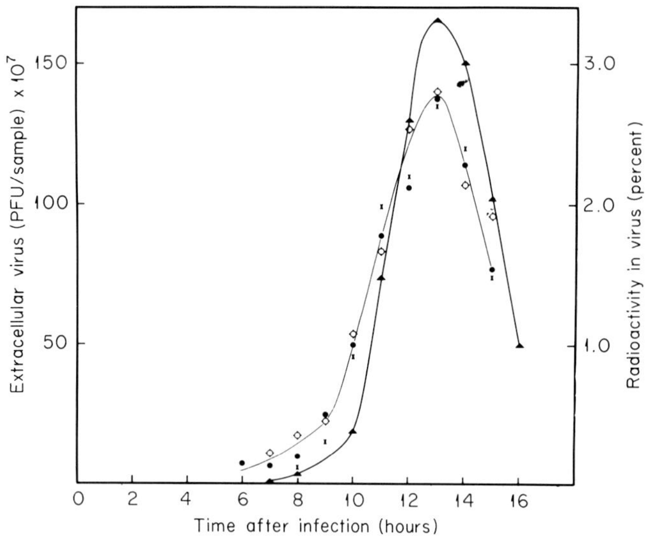

FIG. 7. The fractions of DNA synthesized at different time intervals that become integrated into virus released at various times during the infective process. The DNA synthesized by infected cells during different time intervals after infection was labeled with [2-^{14}C]thymidine. The virus released from the different cultures during 1 hour intervals was harvested. The amount of labeled DNA integrated into virus released during the hour preceding the indicated time was determined. PFU, heavy line and closed triangles. Radioactivity in released virus, light line; DNA labeled between 3 and 4 hours, closed circles; between 5 and 6 hours, open knobbed circles; between 7 and 8 hours, crosses. (From Ben-Porat and Kaplan, 1963.)

infected cells, there is a pool from which precursor DNA is withdrawn at random for the formation of viral particles released by the cells (Ben-Porat and Kaplan, 1963).

Quite soon after its formation and before it becomes part of mature virions, viral DNA can be demonstrated in structures that are insensitive to the action of DNase. These structures have not been characterized, but they bear a precursor relationship to the mature virions (Kaplan, 1964).

The mechanism of assembly of nucleocapsids is not well understood at present. It is interesting that electron microscopic observations indicate that empty capsids, i.e., capsids containing no DNA, appear first in the nuclei of the infected cells. Thereafter, the nucleocapsids (capsids containing DNA cores) make their appearance (see Chapter 5). Thus, empty capsids could be the precursors of the nucleocapsids observed later, indicating that the viral DNA may become integrated into viral capsids which have been at least partially assembled. However, the empty capsids that accumulate in infected cells in which viral DNA synthesis is reduced by FUdR (Reissig and Kaplan, 1962; O'Callaghan *et al.*, 1968b) cannot serve as precursors for mature virions (J. R. Griffin and A. S. Kaplan, unpublished results). The mature virions formed after the addition of thymidine to cultures in which empty capsids have accumulated consist only of those proteins made subsequent to the release of the inhibition of DNA synthesis. It is possible, however, that capsids which accumulate in the cells under conditions of limited DNA synthesis are not identical to the capsids observed in the early stages of normal infection.

C. *Is There More than One Type of Viral Envelope?*

Roizman and co-workers (Spring and Roizman, 1968; Roizman, 1970) have postulated that in addition to the outer envelope which the virions acquire by budding from cellular membranes, the herpesviruses are surrounded by an electron-translucent inner membrane. Essentially the same view has also been expressed by Asher *et al.* (1969). The experimental basis for this conclusion is the following:

Electron microscopic studies show that early in infection naked nucleocapsids are restricted to the nucleus, whereas enveloped nucleocapsids may be observed only in the cytoplasm. However, significant amounts of naked nucleocapsids (capsids containing DNA but devoid of a lipid-containing envelope) have not yet been isolated from nuclei of HSV-infected cells. Instead, both Spring and Roizman (1968) and Asher *et al.* (1969) have reported that particles can be isolated from the nuclei of infected cells that sediment in sucrose gradients faster than capsids but more slowly than mature virions. These particles are infectious and are sensitive to deoxycholate and phospholipase, as are mature virions; they are, however, more unstable in CsCl. Asher *et al.* (1969) advanced the hypothesis that lipids may be integrated into the coat of the nucleocapsids, the viral envelope being completed during passage of the virus through the nuclear membrane. Roizman *et al.* (1969) postulated that the virions are made up of at least two envelopes: (1) an inner envelope, which is sufficient for infectivity, is electron translucent, and may enable the nucleocapsid to adhere to the inner lamella of the nuclear membrane and (2) an outer envelope which the virus acquires by budding from this inner lamella. Preliminary evidence that the inner nuclear membrane may not be just a portion of the outer membrane was given by Roizman *et al.* (1969), who showed that infectious virus isolated from nuclear and cytoplasmic fractions may not be antigenically identical.

Infectious nuclear particles with properties similar to those of HSV have also been isolated from PRV-infected cells (Ben-Porat and Kaplan, 1970; Ben-Porat *et al.*, 1970; Sydiskis, 1970). These particles contain DNA, have a lower sedimentation value, a fourfold lower specific infectivity, and a higher density in CsCl than mature cytoplasmic virus. Electrophoretic analysis of the proteins of these particles revealed that they contain all the envelope glycoproteins, but in lesser amounts than do mature virions. These particles also contain phospholipids with a composition similar to that of the phospholipids present in mature virus which is shown in Table II (A. S. Kaplan, unpublished results).

The finding that the nuclear particles are associated with viral envelope similar to that of mature virus argues against their being surrounded by an "inner viral envelope" which cannot be visualized in the electron microscope. Since the membranes associated with the nuclear and with the mature viral particles have similar compositions, it is difficult to understand why the membrane associated with the nuclear particles should (in contrast to that associated with mature virus) be translucent to the electron beam. Furthermore, under certain conditions, NP-40-treated, infected nuclei freed of all viral glycoproteins but containing other viral proteins can be obtained (Spear and Roizman, 1970). The nuclear membrane has presumably been removed by this method, indicating that it is unlikely that glycoproteins are found in the interior of the nucleus. Since the infectious viral particles isolated from the nuclear fractions are associated with glycoproteins, they cannot, therefore, represent the intranuclear nucleocapsids visualized by electron microscopy, and one is led to the conclusion that the latter are unstable under the conditions of isolation used in the experiments described above.

The isolation of nuclear particles entails the disruption of the nuclei, a procedure which may rupture the intranuclear "tubules" encasing non-enveloped particles (Nii *et al.*, 1968a; Shipkey *et al.*, 1967) and it is conceivable that fragments of these membranes (the broken ends of which may fuse around the particles in some cases) may remain associated with the virus. The nuclear particles would be thus surrounded by an incomplete envelope. One would expect such particles to be less infectious and less stable, but as sensitive to desoxycholate or to phospholipase as are mature particles. The infectious particles isolated from the nuclei have all these characteristics, and it seems likely that these particles are artifacts of isolation. The only indication that this may not be so comes from preliminary data (Roizman *et al.*, 1969), indicating that one of three herpesvirus-specific antisera was more active in inhibiting the infectivity of the cytoplasmic virus than of nuclear virus, a finding that suggests that the envelope surrounding the nuclear particles may contain antigenic determinants which differ from those present in the envelope surrounding mature virus. This observation was, however, not confirmed by Andonov *et al.* (1971) who reported that nuclear and cytoplasmic virus shared common antigens.

D. Envelopment

The virions of the herpesviruses bud from areas of cellular membranes which have been "modified" in the sense that they do not contain cellular proteins. The question of the biogenesis of these membranes is discussed in detail in Section VI,B. It is interesting that only the nucleocapsids acquire an outer envelope; envelopment of empty capsids is a rare event. This has been demonstrated mainly by electron microscopy (Felluga, 1963; Nii *et al.*, 1968b; Spring *et al.*, 1968) but is also supported by biochemical analyses of the different types of the viral particles produced by the cells. The mechanism which ensures the envelopment of nucleocapsids only is not clearly understood, but it seems likely that the empty and full capsids differ in some respects in their surface structure.

E. Virus Release

Information relating to the mechanisms which ensure the release from the cells of mature virions has been adduced mainly from electron microscopic observations and is discussed in detail in Chapter 5 of this book.

VIII. Abortive Infection

Infection of cells does not always result in the formation of infectious virus. If virus adsorbs to a cell, penetrates it, and, although one or more viral components are synthesized, no infectious virus is produced, this type of infection may be considered abortive. This definition excludes nonsusceptible cells which do not adsorb virus. Many cases of abortive infection have been reported.

The causes for abortive infection differ, as would be expected, in different systems. An example of a host-dependent abortive infection is provided by the interaction of the MP strain of HSV with canine kidney cells (Aurelian and Roizman, 1964, 1965; Roizman and Aurelian, 1965). Infection of these cells with HSV leads to cell death with the production of viral antigens and viral DNA but not of infectious virus. Since the canine kidney cells will support the replication of PRV, it was concluded that the MP strain of HSV cannot code correctly in the canine kidney cells for some element required for its synthesis. Subsequent studies revealed that naked nucleocapsids are assembled but envelopment does not take place during the abortive infection, probably as a result of the lack of reduplication of the nuclear membrane which usually characterizes productively infected cells. The abortively infected cells also contain at least ten times less of the surface antigens (Spring *et al.*, 1968). Thus, the block in the formation of the MP strain of HSV in canine kidney cells appears to be due to a failure of envelopment because of a defect in the formation of virus-specific membrane material.

Another instance of host-dependent abortive infection is the case of HSV type I which, in contrast to HSV type II, cannot grow in chick embryo cells (Figueroa and Rawls, 1969). Type I virus adsorbs to chick embryo cells and produces cytoplasmic, as well as nuclear, antigens. However, viral DNA synthesis does not occur, and the production of surface antigens is greatly reduced. (It is interesting that the lack of surface antigen production in this system is related to the absence of viral DNA synthesis). Particle formation was also inhibited in the abortively infected cells; particles were seen only rarely in a small percentage of cells (Lowry *et al.*, 1971).

Abortive infection occurs also at elevated temperatures (Lust and Carmichael, 1971; Stevens, 1966; Stevens and Jackson, 1967) and by deprivation of the infected cells of arginine (see Section V,F). Temperature-sensitive mutants also give rise to abortive infection as exemplified by the mutant described by Schaffer *et al.* (1971) that is defective in the synthesis of viral DNA and viral glycoproteins at nonpermissive temperatures. Abortive infection may also be induced by preventing, with a variety of inhibitors, the formation in the infected cells of macromolecules essential to virus replication.

It has recently been reported that infection of cells with ultraviolet-irradiated virus may, under certain conditions, lead to the acquisition by the cells of virus-induced functions, as well as to their transformation (Munyon *et al.*, 1971; Duff and Rapp, 1971). Thus, some viral functions are expressed in some cells infected with the virus, and this is certainly one of the more interesting instances of an abortive infection. However, under the conditions of these experiments, most of the cells do not respond to infection. Thus, for example, syncytia formation and disaggregation of cellular polysomes, as well as virus-induced formation of enzymes, do not occur in the majority of the cells infected with ultraviolet-irradiated virus (Ogino and Rapp, 1972; Sydiskis and Roizman, 1967). The phenomenon, therefore, is at present not amenable to biochemical analysis.

IX. Enzymology of the Infected Cells

The early studies on the effect of infection on the enzymes involved in the synthesis of DNA revealed that there is a marked increase in the level of activity of several of these enzymes, an increase that is dependent upon the synthesis of RNA and protein in the infected cells.

Recent evidence indicates that different members of the herpes group of viruses induce enzymes that differ with respect to physicochemical characteristics, differences which probably reflect the distant genetic relatedness of these viruses (see Chapter 3). Furthermore, different strains of the same virus may induce enzymes which show varying degrees of activity and which exhibit different antigenic characteristics. Although a systematic study of the response of different host cells to the same virus has not been performed, quantitative differences in the levels of enzyme activity induced by the same virus have been reported, and these differences may be host-dependent.

Keir and Gold (1963) were first to report that after infection of BHK 21 cells with HSV there is, after an initial decline in the activity of DNA polymerase, an increase in activity of this enzyme of about sevenfold by 7 hours after infection; later (8–16 hours after infection) the activity is reduced. Most of the enzyme activity was associated with the nuclei of the infected cells. In RK cells infected with PRV, there is also an increase in the activity of DNA polymerase, which starts between 1.5 and 2 hours and continues up to about 6 hours after infection (Nohara and Kaplan, 1963; Kamiya *et al.*, 1964, 1965). In both systems, the increase in activity of DNA polymerase precedes the formation of infectious virus.

Infection with HSV and with PRV results also in an increase in the activity of thymidine kinase and thymidylate (dTMP) kinase (Nohara and Kaplan, 1963; Kit and Dubbs, 1963a; Hamada *et al.*, 1966; Kaplan *et al.*, 1967; Newton, 1964; Kamiya *et al.*, 1965). In mouse fibroblasts infected with HSV, the activity of the enzymes starts to increase about 2 hours after infection and increases rapidly over the next 6 hours. The increase in the activity of thymidine kinase and of dTMP kinase in RK cells infected with

PRV parallels that of DNA polymerase, i.e., the increase is detectable about 1–2 hours and reaches a maximum 6 hours after infection.

Increases in the level of dCMP deaminase (Diwan and Prusoff, 1968; McGeoch and Keir, 1968) and deoxycytidine kinase (Perera and Morrison, 1970; Hay *et al.*, 1971) have also been reported for HSV-infected cells. Cohen (1972) showed also that there is an increase in reductase activity after infection of cells with HSV. The reductase activity induced by infection is less sensitive to feedback inhibition by dTTP than is the enzyme activity present in uninfected cells.

Increases in the activity of uridine kinase and of choline kinase in cells infected with some strains of HSV have also been reported (Dundaroff and Falke, 1972). The level of activity of the other kinases involved in DNA synthesis remains the same in infected and in uninfected cells (Hamada *et al.*, 1966; Hay *et al.*, 1971). Other enzymes on the pathway of DNA synthesis which do not increase in activity after infection of cells with HSV are thymidylate synthetase (Frearson *et al.*, 1965) and dihydrofolate reductase (Frearson *et al.*, 1966).

A. Characteristics of the Virus-Induced Enzymes

1. Thymidine Kinase

The induction of this enzyme is most pronounced after infection of cells with the herpesviruses (Nohara and Kaplan, 1963; Kit and Dubbs, 1963a; Frearson *et al.*, 1965; Kamiya *et al.*, 1965; Klemperer *et al.*, 1967). However, the degree of induction of thymidine kinase varies with the different strains of the virus. It has been recently clearly shown by Dundaroff and Falke (1972) that RK cells infected with different strains (including both type I and type II) of HSV have different levels of thymidine kinase activity. As a rule, HSV type II induces a lower level of thymidine kinase activity than does type I (Rawls *et al.*, 1971; Thouless and Skinner, 1971).

Hamada *et al.* (1966) showed that the thymidine kinase produced in RK cells infected with PRV is immunologically distinct from the enzyme present in uninfected cells. This was also found to be the case for the enzyme present in BHK 21 cells infected with HSV (Klemperer *et al.*, 1967). The thymidine kinase present in the virus-infected cells also differs from the enzyme present in uninfected cells with respect to K_m value and to sensitivity to the inhibitory effect of trifluoromethyl-2′-deoxyuridine (Kit *et al.*, 1967). Furthermore, the virus-induced enzyme has a lower pH optimum and is relatively insensitive to inhibition by dTTP. The enzyme may also be more thermostable than the host cell enzyme, the relative thermostability of the virus-induced enzyme being lost upon filtration on Sephadex columns

(Klemperer *et al.*, 1967). However, this is not always the case, and Prusoff *et al.* (1965) found no difference in thermostability between the enzymes from HSV-infected and uninfected BSC_1 cells.

The differences between the thymidine kinases present in infected and uninfected cells with respect to antigenic determinants and physicochemical characteristics may be the result of allosteric alterations in the enzyme which may be caused by changes in the intracellular milieu resulting from infection. Alternatively, the virus could activate the synthesis of an isozyme which is normally synthesized only in small amounts in uninfected cells. However, there are some lines of evidence demonstrating that thymidine kinase may be a new enzyme coded for by the viral genome. Kit and his associates (Kit and Dubbs, 1963a,b, 1965; Dubbs and Kit, 1964, 1965) have isolated a mutant of mouse fibroblast cells (strain $LMTK^-$) that lacks (or has very low levels of) thymidine kinase. Infection of these mutant cells with HSV leads to a considerable increase of thymidine kinase activity. Mutants of HSV have been isolated that induce in the $LMTK^-$ cells only low levels of thymidine kinase activity. Although the thymidine kinaseless mutants both of the cells and of the virus are "leaky," the above results provide reasonable support for the view that the thymidine kinase induced in cells by infection is a new protein coded by the virus. This is also indicated by the finding that the enzyme produced in BHK cells infected with HSV is antigenically similar to that found in RK13 cells infected with the same virus (Klemperer *et al.*, 1967) and is different when induced by vaccinia virus and HSV in $LMTK^-$ cells (Kit *et al.*, 1967).

Another indication that thymidine kinase induced by infection is virus-coded has been provided by Buchan and Watson (1969) who compared the antigenic determinants of the thymidine kinase induced by infection of BHK 21 cells either with PRV or with HSV. They found that the enzymes induced by infection with these two viruses were serologically distinct and concluded, therefore, that each of the enzymes are probably coded by the genome of the respective virus. The enzymes induced by HSV types I and II also differ with respect to their stability and serologic specificity (Thouless and Skinner, 1971).

In addition to antigenic differences, thymidine kinase induced by PRV differs also in other properties from the enzyme induced by HSV. Herpes simplex virus-induced thymidine kinase can use deoxyuridine as a substrate (Kit *et al.*, 1967), whereas the enzyme induced by PRV cannot (Kaplan and Ben-Porat, 1970). Thymidine kinase induced by some strains of HSV may also function as a deoxycytidine kinase (Subak-Sharpe *et al.*, 1971). In cells infected with PRV, on the other hand, there is a large increase in the activity of thymidine kinase but no change in the activity of deoxycytidine kinase (Kaplan and Ben-Porat, 1970).

2. DNA Polymerase

DNA polymerases present in BHK 21 cells or in HEp-2 cells infected with HSV appear to be more thermostable than the enzymes present in uninfected cells. Furthermore, the enzymes from infected and uninfected cells display different ionic and primer requirements for *in vitro* activity (Keir *et al.*, 1966). Deoxyribonucleic acid polymerase present in the infected cells also differs in its antigenic properties from the enzyme present in uninfected cells.

Deoxyribonucleic acid polymerases present in PRV-infected and uninfected cells, on the other hand, cross react, under certain conditions, with heterologous sera, indicating that the enzymes from the two sources have some antigenic determinants in common (Hamada *et al.*, 1966). The difference in the results obtained with HSV and PRV may be due to differences in the method of preparation of the specific antisera used in the two sets of experiments.

3. DNase

An increase in the level of DNase activity in HSV-infected cells was first described by Keir and Gold (1963). The DNase from infected cells can be differentiated serologically from the enzyme from uninfected cells. Furthermore, in infected cells this activity is due mainly to an exonuclease; exonuclease activity is usually low in uninfected cells. The exonuclease activity in infected cells seems to be associated with two proteins, one of these being the virus-induced DNA polymerase (Paton and Morrison, 1969).

4. dTMP Kinase

After infection of RK cells with PRV and HSV, there is an apparent increase in the level of activity of dTMP kinase (Nohara and Kaplan, 1963; Newton, 1964). The dTMP kinase present in PRV-infected cells is more thermostable than the enzyme from uninfected cells and, in contrast to the latter, does not require substrate for stabilization (Nohara and Kaplan, 1963). The stability of dTMP kinase from infected cells in the absence of added substrate is not due to a larger pool of thymidine derivatives in these cells because the enzyme remains stable even after dialysis (Kaplan *et al.*, 1967). The increase in the level of activity of dTMP kinase, although prevented by inhibitors of protein synthesis, is not due to the synthesis of new enzyme protein; instead, the enzyme present in uninfected cells, which is normally unstable *in vitro*, seems to acquire new properties after infection that confer stability upon it *in vitro*. Protein synthesis is required for the creation of the conditions that favor the stabilization of the enzymes and that change their characteristics. The identity of these proteins is not known (Kaplan *et al.*, 1967).

B. The Effects of the Changes in Enzyme Activities Resulting from Infection upon the Patterns of DNA Synthesis

The changes induced by infection on the level of activity and in the properties of enzymes involved in the synthesis of DNA, as determined by *in vitro* experiments, affect several aspects of DNA synthesis *in vivo* in the infected cells. Thus, for instance, both HSV- and PRV-infected cells are not susceptible to concentrations of thymidine or deoxyadenosine which inhibit DNA synthesis in uninfected cells (Kaplan and Ben-Porat, 1970; Cohen, 1972). The resistance of the infected cells to the nucleosides is probably due to the induction by infection of a ribonucleotide diphosphate reductase which is less susceptible to feedback inhibition than is the enzyme performing the same function in uninfected cells.

The differences in the levels of activity of different enzymes, as well as differences in the characteristics of these enzymes, in infected and uninfected cells also affect the relative level of utilization of different nucleosides (Kaplan and Ben-Porat, 1970). This observation is pertinent to the question of the chemotherapeutic effectiveness of analogues of nucleosides in suppressing viral growth. To be effective, a nucleoside analogue must be taken up by the cells where it may have to be phosphorylated, and perhaps reduced, as well as incorporated into DNA. There are complex interactions within the cells that control the rates of any one of these reactions, all of which may or may not be changed by infection. These interactions will control the degree to which an externally supplied nucleoside will be used by the cells. A nucleoside analogue which is used to a greater extent by infected than by uninfected cells should, theoretically, be a good candidate for viral chemotherapy. Thus, cells infected with PRV and exposed to relatively low concentrations of iododeoxyuridine (IUdR) substitute a greater proportion of IUdR for thymidine in DNA than do uninfected cells (Kaplan and Ben-Porat, 1967, 1970), indicating that IUdR is in this case a so-called specific antiviral agent. On the other hand, Ara-C is more effective in inhibiting DNA synthesis in uninfected cells than it is in PRV- or HSV-infected cells. The relative resistance of PRV-infected cells to Ara-C is due to the low level of activity of deoxycytidine kinase *in vivo* and the consequent low level of phosphorylation of the inhibitor in cells infected with these viruses.

A systematic analysis of the changes in the ability of cells to use nucleosides after infection is of practical importance, since such an analysis could, in principle, provide a rational approach to the chemotherapy of the herpesviruses. However, as discussed above, infection of cells with different strains of herpesvirus leads to quantitative as well as to qualitative, differences in the enzymes that are involved in the synthesis of DNA. Thus, for example, whereas Ara-C is not an effective antiviral agent for PRV, it may be effective in the treatment of some cases of infection with HSV, since infection of cells with some strains of this virus have been reported to induce an increase in the activity of deoxycytidine kinase (see above). The effectiveness of a nucleoside analogue in inhibiting the growth of different strains of a virus may thus differ. One may also expect, therefore, differences in the effectiveness of nucleoside analogues in the treatment of disease caused by the herpesviruses, depending on the strain of virus involved.

C. *Role of Virus-Induced Enzymes in the Infective Process*

A key step in the control of the synthesis of DNA may be the level of activity of one of the enzymes leading to the formation of dTTP, a possibility that has been discussed extensively. The level of activity of these enzymes is low in cells in the stationary phase, so that an increase in their activity after infection could be essential to the survival of the infecting virus. Indeed, most strains of HSV and of PRV that have been studied are not dependent on a specific stage of the growth cycle of the host cell for replication, probably because these viruses are able to induce the enzymes required for the synthesis of viral DNA. The only herpesvirus which has been demonstrated to depend on a specific state of the cell cycle for replication is EAV; it replicates only in cells in the S phase of their growth cycle. This is true also for many of the smaller DNA-containing viruses which probably cannot code for enzymes required for DNA synthesis (Kaplan and Ben-Porat, 1968).

The possible role of thymidine kinase in various systems has been the subject of much speculation. The function of this enzyme may be explained in terms of competition between anabolic and catabolic enzymatic pathways as suggested by Potter (1958, 1960) and Cannellakis *et al.* (1959). An increase in the level of activity of this enzyme provides an alternative pathway for dTMP synthesis. However, Kit and Dubbs (1969) have pointed out that the synthesis of virus is not inhibited by a lack of thymidine kinase in the infected cells. This was shown by growing a mutant of HSV which is deficient in the ability to induce the enzyme in cells which are also deficient in that enzyme. Furthermore, the high level of activity of thymidine kinase observed in extracts of infected cells is not accompanied by a similar increase in the rate of phosphorylation of thymidine *in vivo*. The pools of phosphorylated thymidine are about the same in PRV-infected and uninfected, actively growing RK cells, despite a great difference of enzyme activity present in extracts of the cells (Kaplan *et al.*, 1967).

It is well established that actively growing cells contain lower levels of phosphatase than do nongrowing cells (Maley and Maley, 1961; Beltz, 1962; Fiala *et al.*, 1962; Eker, 1965), and although thymidine kinase may have no survival value if infection occurs in growing cells, it may be of importance if viral DNA synthesis is to occur in resting cells. To overcome the effect of the catabolic enzymes present in the stationary phase cells, the infecting virus must establish a mechanism to ensure the accumulation of the deoxyribonucleotide triphosphates necessary for the synthesis of DNA. Thymidine kinase induced by infection with PRV may indeed be essential if DNA synthesis is to occur in cells having a high level of phosphatase activity (Kaplan *et al.*, 1967). This function of thymidine kinase has also been suggested as one reason for the increased activity of this enzyme in polyomavirus-infected cells (Kit *et al.*, 1966).

X. Control of the Infective Process

The infective process follows a well-ordered sequence of events in the virus-infected cells. The virion attaches to the cells and penetrates them, and, after the virion has been uncoated, different parts of the viral genome are transcribed sequentially and translated into proteins. Structural viral components accumulate and are assembled into the infectious virus which is then released from the cells. Certain processes of infection become operative and others inoperative at critical junctures of the virus growth cycle. The basis for the molecular control of all these events is at present unknown. The information available on the subject is summarized below.

A. Mechanism of Inhibition of the Synthesis of Cell-Specific Macromolecules

One of the consequences of infection of cells with the herpesviruses is a gradual inhibition of the synthesis of cellular macromolecules (see above). The process of inhibition of the synthesis of cellular DNA, RNA, and protein in the infected cells seems to be distinct and to be regulated, at least in part, by positive control factors.

1. DNA

The following possible mechanisms have been invoked to account for the virus-induced inhibition of cellular DNA synthesis: (1) Cellular DNA cannot act as a template for replication in the infected cells. (2) Regulatory histone-like molecules that act as inhibitors of cellular DNA replication are formed in the infected cells. (3) There is an inhibition in the infected cells of the synthesis of cellular proteins, such as histones or enzymes which are required for the synthesis of cellular DNA but not of viral DNA. The information available about the mechanism of inhibition of cellular DNA synthesis in the infected cells, which is summarized below, shows that any or all of these possibilities may play a role.

1. The inhibition of the synthesis of cellular DNA by infection is not due to viral interference with the entrance of the cells into the S-phase of their growth cycle (Kaplan and Ben-Porat, 1963; O'Callaghan *et al.*, 1968b). This inhibition is also not due to a successful competition of viral DNA with cellular DNA to act as a template for DNA replication, nor to a greater affinity of the DNA polymerase present in virus-infected cells for viral DNA than for cellular DNA (Ben-Porat and Kaplan, 1965). However, although cellular DNA does not become acid-soluble in the infected cells, it may in some cases be cleaved to relatively small molecules (20 S–30 S) (Nonoyama and Pagano, 1972). Furthermore, the location of cellular DNA within the nucleus of the infected cell is changed by infection (Munk and Sauer, 1964).

2. Proteins synthesized in the infected cells are directly or indirectly responsible for the inhibition of the synthesis of cellular DNA. These proteins do not act catalytically (Ben-Porat and Kaplan, 1965). Stevens *et al.* (1969) have reported that arginine-rich, acid-extractable nuclear proteins are synthesized in the infected cells and are found associated with cellular DNA.

3. Histone synthesis is inhibited in virus-infected cells (Shimono and Kaplan, 1968; Stevens *et al.*, 1969). Robbins and Borun (1967) have shown that the synthesis of DNA and histones is normally coordinated, so that the inhibtion of DNA synthesis could be the result of the inhibition of cellular proteins in the infected cells. Since the gradual interference of infection with cellular protein synthesis itself requires the synthesis of a protein (Ben-Porat *et al.*, 1971), the dependence of the inhibition of DNA synthesis, discussed above, on protein synthesis could be indirect and due to its effect on cellular protein synthesis.

2. RNA

Evidence presently available does not indicate that infection interferes preferentially with the transcription of one of the types of cellular RNA; the rate of inhibition after infection of the synthesis of precursor rRNA and of C-RNA are approximately the same and roughly equal to the rate of inhibition of total RNA synthesis. The more rapid decrease in the synthesis of mature rRNA can be ascribed to the interference by infection with the proper processing of these RNA molecules (Wagner and Roizman, 1969a; Rakusanova and Kaplan, 1970). This is probably also the case for the relatively rapid decrease in synthesis of functional cellular mRNA (Rakusanova *et al.*, 1972).

The rate of inhibition of RNA synthesis after infection of cells with the herpesviruses is dependent on the multiplicity of infection (Aurelian and Roizman, 1965). This inhibition is mediated (directly or indirectly) by a virus-induced protein (Rakusanova *et al.*, 1971).

Sasaki *et al.* (1972) have recently reported that the RNA polymerases present in infected cells effectively use HSV DNA as a primer even in the absence of the stimulating factors normally required for the transcription of cellular DNA. In addition, the infected cells contain factors which inhibit the transcription of cellular DNA but not of viral DNA. These findings suggest that the decrease in the rate of transcription of cellular DNA in the infected cells is due to the formation of factors favorable to the transcription of viral but not of cellular DNA.

3. Proteins

The inhibition in infected cells of cell-specific protein synthesis is due to the synthesis of factors which prevent the association of cellular mRNA with ribosomes and the consequent formation of cell-specific polyribosomes. This conclusion was first drawn by Sydiskis and Roizman (1967) on the basis of the following observation: In HEp-2 cells productively infected with HSV, inhibitors of the synthesis of RNA and of protein were ineffective in preventing the virus-induced disaggregation of polysomes that occurs during the early stages of infection. However, these inhibitors were effective in preventing disaggregation in abortively infected canine kidney cells. The authors' interpretation of these results was that a virus-induced factor which inhibits cell-specific protein synthesis is formed in the infected cells. This factor is required only in trace amounts and may act catalytically; therefore, its formation cannot be effectively prevented in productively infected cells. On the other hand, this protein is faulty in abortively infected cells, and in order to be effective, it is required in relatively large amounts. Consequently, disaggregation of host polysomes in the abortively infected cells can be prevented by the inhibitors of RNA and protein synthesis.

The synthesis in PRV-infected cells of a protein which interferes with the formation of cell-specific polysomes was demonstrated as follows (Ben-Porat *et al.*, 1971): In this system, inhibition of cell-specific protein synthesis occurs only if RNA synthesis is allowed to proceed in the infected cells. The gradual inhibition of cell-specific protein synthesis requires continuous RNA synthesis. If the infected cells are allowed to synthesize RNA but not protein during the first few hours after infection, cell-specific polysomes remain intact in the infected cells; furthermore, the attachment of cellular mRNA to ribosomes and the formation of new cell-specific polyribosomes are unaffected. However, within several minutes after these cells are allowed to resume protein synthesis, cell-specific polysomes disappear. Thus, RNA responsible for the formation of the inhibitory protein has accumulated in the infected cells in the absence of protein synthesis and is translated soon after protein synthesis is allowed to proceed (Ben-Porat *et al.*, 1971; Rakusanova *et al.*, 1972).

The ability of cellular mRNA to function has been shown to be impaired in bacteriophage-infected bacteria. In this system, proteins are induced in the infected cells which confer restrictive properties on the ribosomes. It seems likely that this is also the mechanism by which cellular protein synthesis is inhibited in herpesvirus-infected cells.

B. Regulation of Enzyme Activity in the Infected Cells

As discussed above, an increase in the activity of several enzymes occurs in cells infected with either HSV or PRV. The level of activity of these enzymes starts rising during the early stages of infection, reaches a maximum, and remains unchanged thereafter until the end of the infective process when the level of activity drops. This sequence of events is analogous to that observed in bacteriophage-infected bacteria. In case of bacteriophage, the synthesis of the so-called "early" enzymes has been shown to occur in a variety of systems for a limited period of time only, unless there is interference with a mechanism which normally regulates the level of the enzymes. This interference can be achieved by ultraviolet irradiation of the infecting virus (Dirksen *et al.*, 1960; Delihas, 1961) or when the bacteria are infected with certain amber mutants of T4 phage which do not allow the synthesis of viral DNA to proceed at a normal rate (Wiberg *et al.*, 1962). Thus, the control of the synthesis of the early enzymes seems to be correlated with the level of progeny viral DNA.

A lack of regulation of enzyme activity can also be obtained in cells infected with the herpesviruses, if cells infected with these viruses are incubated with BUdR or IUdR, so that most of the thymidine present in the viral DNA is replaced by the halogenated analogues. Under these conditions, the increase in activity of the "early" enzymes occurs, but the normal cut off of enzyme activity becomes inoperative (Kaplan *et al.*, 1965; Kamiya *et al.*, 1964, 1965). The interference in the regulation of enzyme activity is probably due to the presence of IUdR or BUdR in progeny viral DNA, and it seems, therefore, that the cut off of enzyme activity is controlled by this DNA. Since progeny viral DNA accumulates in the infected cells incubated either with BUdR or with IUdR, and there is, nevertheless, interference with the regulation of the level of enzyme activity, it seems that regulation is not dependent upon the replication of parental viral DNA but upon the presence of *competent* progeny viral DNA.

C. *Cell Necrosis and the End of the Infective Cycle*

The end of the infective cycle is due to the cessation in the infected cells of macromolecular synthesis. Several factors may contribute to it: (1) The inhibition of cell-specific RNA and protein syntheses could be a major factor, since the synthesis of viral components is dependent on at least some cell-specific products, for example, products such as ribosomes, tRNA, and probably some enzymes. Some of these molecules may have a relatively short half-life, and since their synthesis is inhibited in the infected cells, their absence could cause macromolecular synthesis to come to a halt. (2) The accumulation of viral products within the infected cells could also interfere with continued macromolecular synthesis. (3) Changes in the cellular membranes wrought by infection could impair the ability of the membranes to function in maintaining cellular integrity.

Although factors (1) and (2) may play a role in determining the end of the infective cycle, evidence indicating that these factors are not critical comes from the following findings: The substitution of IUdR or BUdR for thymidine into the progeny viral DNA results in defective transmission of information with respect to mechanisms controlling the infective process. Thus, the normal shut off of enzyme synthesis does not occur (see Section X,B), and the accumulation of viral components (DNA and proteins) continues well beyond the normal level (Kaplan *et al.*, 1965; Kamiya *et al.*, 1965). Whereas, under conditions of normal infection, viral DNA and proteins are synthesized between 2 and ~ 10 hours postinfection, in infected cells treated with BUdR or IUdR, viral products accumulate at a normal rate up to 10 hours postinfection and their synthesis is extended for several hours thereafter.

The synthesis of cell-specific macromolecules (DNA and proteins) is inhibited in infected cells treated with IUdR or BUdR (A. S. Kaplan, unpublished results), as it is under conditions of normal infection. Thus, in these cells, there is an inhibition of cell-specific macromolecular synthesis, as well as an accumulation of viral components, and yet infected cells treated with the analogues are able to continue synthesizing viral DNA and proteins for an extended period of time. It seems unlikely, therefore, that during the course of normal infection, the end of the infective process is due to the cessation of synthesis of cellular macromolecules or to the accumulation of viral products.

Present evidence indicates that changes in the cellular membrane and consequent leakage of proteins from the cells may be responsible for the termination of the infective process. During the later stages of infection (between 10 and 16 hours), there is, in PRV-infected cells, a decrease in enzyme activity which is correlated with a leakage of proteins from the cells. This is shown by the fact that enzymes bound to cellular organelles are retained by the infected cells to a greater extent than are so-called "soluble" enzymes (Zemla *et al.*, 1967). Furthermore, both leakage of proteins and of enzymes from the cells is dependent upon the synthesis of a protein(s), 80% of which is synthesized between 5 and 7 hours after infection. Progeny viral DNA plays a role in the formation of the proteins responsible for leakage of macromolecules from the cells; leakage is retarded when either IUdR or BUdR is substituted for thymidine in progeny viral DNA. As mentioned above, viral components continue to accumulate under these conditions well beyond the time at which infected cells normally have ceased macromolecular synthesis.

It is reasonable to believe that the extensive leakage of proteins and enzymes essential to macromolecular synthesis is responsible for the cessation of the latter. The correlation between the extension of macromolecular synthesis in these cells with the lack of leakage of proteins lends further support to the conclusion that there is probably a causal relationship between the two.

The proteins which cause the leakage of macromolecules from the infected cells may be only indirectly responsible. Thus, these proteins may perform an essential function in virus growth (such as in the release of mature virions or in the establishment of other viral-induced cytopathic changes) which, in turn, cause the leakage of proteins from the cells and the consequent cessation of macromolecular synthesis.

Acknowledgment

Our work has been supported by the U.S. National Institutes of Health (AI-10947).

References

Andonov, P., Dundarov, S., Kavaklova, L., and Karabasheva, V. (1971). *Proc. Int. Congr. Virol., 2nd, 1972.* p. 99.
Asher, Y., Heller, M., and Becker, Y. (1969). *J. Gen. Virol.* **4**, 65.
Aurelian, L., and Roizman, B. (1964). *Virology* **22**, 452.
Aurelian, L., and Roizman, B. (1965). *J. Mol. Biol.* **11**, 539.
Bachenheimer, S. L., and Roizman, B. (1972). *Abstr. 72nd. Annu. Meet. Amer. Soc. Microbiol.* p. 221.
Becker, Y., Olshevsky, U., and Levitt, J. (1967). *J. Gen. Virol.* **1**, 471.
Bell, D., Wilkie, N. M., and Subak-Sharpe, J. H. (1971). *J. Gen. Virol.* **13**, 463.
Beltz, R. E. (1962). *Arch. Biochem. Biophys.* **99**, 304.
Ben-Porat, T., and Kaplan, A. S. (1963). *Virology* **20**, 310.
Ben-Porat, T., and Kaplan, A. S. (1965). *Virology* **25**, 22.
Ben-Porat, T., and Kaplan, A. S. (1970). *Virology* **41**, 265.
Ben-Porat, T., and Kaplan, A. S. (1971). *Virology* **45**, 252.

Ben-Porat, T., and Kaplan, A. S. (1972). *Nature* (*London*) **235**, 164.
Ben-Porat, T., Reissig, M., and Kaplan, A. S. (1961). *Nature* (*London*) **190**, 33.
Ben-Porat, T., Shimono, H., and Kaplan, A. S. (1969). *Virology* **37**, 56.
Ben-Porat, T., Shimono, H., and Kaplan, A. S. (1970). *Virology* **41**, 256.
Ben-Porat, T., Rakusanova, T., and Kaplan, A. S. (1971). *Virology* **46**, 890.
Buchan, A., and Watson, D. H. (1969). *J. Gen. Virol.* **4**, 461.
Canellakis, E. S., Jaffee, J. J., Mantsavinos, R., and Krakow, J. S. (1959), *J. Biol. Chem.* **234**, 2096.
Chen, J. H., and Purchase, H. G. (1970). *Virology* **40**, 410.
Cocuzzo, G., and Russo, G. (1966). *Boll. Ist. Sieroter. Milan.* **45**, 228.
Cohen, G. H. (1972). *J. Virol.* **9**, 409.
Cohen, G. H., Vaughan, R. K., and Lawrence, W. C. (1971a). *J. Virol.* **7**, 783.
Cohen, G. H., Atkinson, P. H., and Summers, D. F. (1971b). *Nature* (*London*), *New Biol.* **231**, 212.
Cohen, S. S. (1949). *Bacteriol. Rev.* **13**, 1.
Courtney, R. J., McCombs, R. M., and Benyesh-Melnick, M. (1970). *Virology* **40**, 379.
Courtney, R. J., McCombs, R. M., and Benyesh-Melnick, M. (1971). *Virology* **43**, 356.
Delihas, N. (1961). *Virology* **13**, 242.
Dirksen, M. L., Wiberg, J. S., Koerner, J. F., and Buchanan, J. M. (1960). *Proc. Nat. Sci. U.S.* **46**, 1425.
Diwan, A., and Prusoff, W. H. (1968). *Virology* **34**, 184.
Dubbs, D. R., and Kit, S. (1964). *Virology* **22**, 493.
Dubbs, D. R., and Kit, S. (1965). *Virology* **25**, 256.
Duff, R., and Rapp, F. (1971). *J. Virol.* **8**, 469.
Dundarov, S., and Falke, D. (1972). *Arch. Gesamte Virusforsch.* **38**, 56.
Eker, P. (1965). *J. Biol. Chem.* **240**, 419.
Falke, D. (1967). *Z. Med. Mikrobiol. Immunol.* **153**, 175.
Falke, D., and Peterknecht, W. (1968). *Arch. Gesamte Virusforsch.* **24**, 267.
Falke, D., Bittner-Suermann, D., and Clauss, T. (1969). *Arch. Gesamte Virusforsch.* **27**, 317.
Felluga, B. (1963). *Ann. Sclavo* **5**, 412.
Fiala, S., Fiala, A., Tobar, G., and McQuilla, H. (1962). *J. Nat. Cancer Inst.* **28**, 1269.
Figueroa, M. E., and Rawls, W. E. (1969). *J. Gen. Virol.* **4**, 259.
Fine, D. L., Lake, R. S., and Ludwig, E. H. (1970). *J. Virol.* **5**, 226.
Flanagan, J. F. (1967). *J. Virol.* **1**, 583.
Frearson, P. M., Kit, S., and Dubbs, D. R. (1965). *Cancer Res.* **25**, 737.
Frearson, P. M., Kit, S., and Dubbs, D. R. (1966). *Cancer Res.* **26**, 1643.
Frenkel, N., and Roizman, B. (1971). *J. Virol.* **8**, 591.
Fujiwara, S., and Kaplan, A. S. (1967). *Virology* **32**, 60.
Gerber, P., and Hoyer, B. H. (1971). *Nature* (*London*) **231**, 46.
Gergely, L., Klein, G., and Ernberg, I. (1971a). *Int. J. Cancer* **7**, 293.
Gergely, L., Klein, G., and Ernberg, I. (1971b). *Virology* **45**, 22.
Gold, E., Wildy, P., and Watson, D. H. (1963). *J. Immunol.* **91**, 666.
Greenham, L. W., and Poste, G. (1971). *Microbios* **3**, 97.
Hamada, C., and Kaplan, A. S. (1965). *J. Bacteriol.* **89**, 1328.
Hamada, C., Kamiya, T., and Kaplan, A. S. (1966). *Virology* **28**, 271.
Hay, J., and Low, M. (1970). *Biochem J.* **117**, 21P.
Hay, J., Köteles, G. J., and Keir, H. M. (1966). *Nature* (*London*) **210**, 387.
Hay, J., Perera, P. A. J., Morrison, J. M., Gentry, G. A., and Subak-Sharpe, J. H. (1971). *Strategy Viral Genome Ciba Founda. Symp.* pp. 355–376.
Heine, J. W., Spear, P. G., and Roizman, B. (1972). *J. Virol.* **9**, 431.
Heine, U., Ablashi, D. V., and Armstrong, G. R. (1971). *Cancer Res.* **31**, 1019.

Hershey, A. D. (1956). *In* "Currents of Biochemical Research." (David E. Green, ed.), pp. 1–28. Wiley (Interscience), New York.
Huang, H. L., Szabocsik, J. M., Randall, C. C., and Gentry, G. A. (1971). *Virology* **45**, 381.
Kamiya, T., Ben-Porat, T., and Kaplan, A. S. (1964). *Biochem. Biophys. Res. Commun.* **16**, 410.
Kamiya, T., Ben-Porat, T., and Kaplan, A. S. (1965). *Virology* **26**, 577.
Kaplan, A. S. (1957). *Virology* **4**, 435.
Kaplan, A. S. (1959). "Virology Monographs." S. Gard, C. Hallaver, and K. F. Meyer, eds. Vol. 5, Springer, New York.
Kaplan, A. S. (1962). *Virology* **16**, 305.
Kaplan, A. S. (1964). *Virology* **24**, 19.
Kaplan, A. S., and Ben-Porat, T. (1960). *Virology* **11**, 12.
Kaplan, A. S., and Ben-Porat, T. (1963). *Virology* **19**, 205.
Kaplan, A. S., and Ben-Porat, T. (1964). *Virology* **23**, 90.
Kaplan, A. S., and Ben-Porat, T. (1966). *Symposia Int. Cong. Microbiol. 9th, 1966.* p. 409.
Kaplan, A. S., and Ben-Porat, T. (1967). *Virology* **31**, 734.
Kaplan, A. S., and Ben-Porat, T. (1968). *In* "Medical and Applied Virology" (M. Sanders and E. H. Lennette, eds.) pp. 56–76. Warren H. Green, St. Louis, Missouri.
Kaplan, A. S., and Ben-Porat, T. (1970). *Ann. N. Y. Acad. Sci.* **173**, 346.
Kaplan, A. S., Ben-Porat, T., and Kamiya, T. (1965). *Ann. N. Y. Acad. Sci.* **130**, 226.
Kaplan, A. S., Ben-Porat, T., and Coto, C. (1967). *In* "The Molecular Biology of Viruses" (S. J. Colter and W. Paranchych, eds.), pp. 527–545. Academic Press, New York.
Kaplan, A. S., Shimono, H., and Ben-Porat, T. (1970). *Virology* **40**, 90.
Keir, H. M., and Gold, E. (1963). *Biochim. Biophys. Acta* **72**, 263.
Keir, H. M., Subak-Sharpe, H., Shedden, W. I. H., Watson, D. H., and Wildy, P. (1966). *Virology* **30**, 154.
Keller, J. M., Spear, P. G., and Roizman, B. (1970). *Proc. Nat. Acad. Sci. U.S.* **65**, 865.
Kieff, E. D., Bachenheimer, S. L., and Roizman, B. (1971). *J. Virol.* **8**, 125.
Kit, S., and Dubbs, D. R. (1963a). *Biochem. Biophys. Res. Commun.* **11**, 55.
Kit, S., and Dubbs, D. R. (1963b). *Biochem. Biophys. Res. Commun.* **13**, 500.
Kit, S., and Dubbs, D. R. (1965). *Virology* **26**, 16.
Kit, S., and Dubbs, D. R. (1969). "Enzyme Induction by Viruses" (Monographs in Virology) (J. L. Melnick, ed.). Karger, Basel.
Kit, S., Dubbs, D. R., Frearson, P. M., and Melnick, J. L. (1966). *Virology* **29**, 69.
Kit, S., Dubbs, D. R., and Anken, M. (1967). *J. Virol.* **1**, 238.
Klemperer, H. G., Haynes, G. R., Shedden, W. I. H., and Watson, D. H. (1967). *Virology* **31**, 120.
Lawrence, W. C. (1971). *J. Virol.* **7**, 736.
Lee, L. F. (1972). *J. Virol.* **10**, 167.
Levitt, J., and Becker, Y. (1967). *Virology* **31**, 129.
Lowry, S. P., Bronson, D. L., and Rawls, W. E. (1971). *J. Gen. Virol.* **11**, 47.
Lust, G., and Carmichael, L. E. (1971) *J. Infec. Dis.* **124**, 572.
McGeoch, D. J., and Keir, H. M. (1968). *Symp. Soc. Gen. Microbiol.* **18**, 85.
Maley, F., and Maley, G. F. (1961). *Cancer Res.* **21**, 1421.
Mark, G. E., and Kaplan, A. S. (1971). *Virology* **45**, 53.
Mark, G. E., and Kaplan, A. S. (1972). *Virology* **49**, 102.
Morris, V. L., Wagner, E. K., and Roizman, B. (1970). *J. Mol. Biol.* **52**, 247.
Munk, K., and Sauer, G. (1963). *Z. Naturforsch. B* **18**, 211.
Munk, K., and Sauer, G. (1964). *Virology* **22**, 153.
Munyon, W., Kraiselburd, E., Davis, D., and Mann, J. (1971). *J. Virol.* **7**, 813.
Newton, A., and Stoker, M. G. P. (1958). *Virology* **5**, 549.

Newton, A., Dendy, P. P., Smith, C. L., and Wildy, P. (1962), *Nature* (*London*) **194**, 886.
Newton, A. A. (1964). *In* "Acidi nucleici e loro Funzione Biologica" (A. Baselli, ed.), pp. 109–128. Tipografia Successori Fusi, Pavia.
Nii, S., Morgan, C., and Rose, H. M. (1968a). *J. Virol.* **2**, 517.
Nii, S., Rosenkranz, H. S., Morgan, C., and Rose, H. M. (1968b). *J. Virol.* **2**, 1163.
Nii, S., Morgan, C., Rose, H. M., and Hsu, K. C. (1968c). *J. Virol.* **2**, 1172.
Nohara, H., and Kaplan, A. S. (1963). *Biochem. Biophys. Res. Commun.* **12**, 189.
Nonoyama, M., and Pagano, J. S. (1972). *J. Virol.* **9**, 714.
O'Callaghan, D. J., Cheevers, W. P., Gentry, G. A., and Randall, C. C. (1968a). *Virology* **36**, 104.
O'Callaghan, D. J., Hyde, J. M., Gentry, G. A., and Randall, C. C. (1968b). *J. Virol.* **2**, 793.
Ogino, T., and Rapp, F. (1972). *Proc. Soc. Exp. Biol. Med.* **139**, 783.
Olshevsky, U., and Becker, Y. (1970). *Nature* (*London*) **226**, 851.
Olshevsky, U., Levitt, J., and Becker, Y. (1967). *Virology* **33**, 323.
Paton, R. D., and Morrison, J. M. (1969). *Biochem. J.* **144**, 1.
Pearson, G., Dewey, F., Klein, G., Henle, G., and Henle, W. (1970). *J. Nat. Cancer Inst.* **45**, 989.
Perera, P. A. J., and Morrison, J. M. (1970). *Biochem. J.* **117**, 21P.
Poste, G. (1970). *Advan. Virus Res.*. **16**, 303.
Poste, G. (1971a). *Microbios* **3**, 55.
Poste, G. (1971b). *Microbios* **3**, 105.
Potter, V. R. (1958). *Fed. Proc., Fed. Amer. Soc. Exp. Biol.* **17**, 691.
Potter, V. R. (1960). "Nucleic Acid Outlines," Vol. 1. Burgess, Minneapolis, Minnesota.
Prusoff, W. H., Bakhle, Y. S., and Sekely, L. (1965). *Ann. N. Y. Acad. Sci.* **130**, 135.
Rakusanova, T., and Kaplan, A. S. (1970). *Fed. Proc. Fed. Amer. Soc. Exp. Biol.* **29**, 309.
Rakusanova, T., Ben-Porat, T., and Kaplan, A. S. (1971). *Virology* **46**, 877.
Rakusanova, T., Ben-Porat, T., and Kaplan, A. S. (1972). *Virology* **49**, 537.
Rawls, W. E., Lowry, S. P., and Bresnick, E. (1971). *Proc. Int. Congr. Virol., 2nd 1972*; p. 103.
Reissig, M., and Kaplan, A. S. (1962). *Virology* **16**, 1.
Roane, P. R., Jr., and Roizman, B. (1964). *Virology* **22**, 1.
Robbins, E., and Borun, T. W. (1967). *Proc. Nat. Acad. Sci. U.S.* **57**, 409.
Roizman, B. (1965). *Virology* **27**, 113.
Roizman, B. (1970). *In* "Viruses Affecting Man and Animals" (M. Sanders, ed.), pp. 37–71. Green, St. Louis, Missouri.
Roizman, B., and Aurelian, L. (1965). *J. Mol. Biol.* **11**, 528.
Roizman, B., and Roane, P. R., Jr. (1964). *Virology* **22**, 262.
Roizman, B., and Spear, P. G., (1971). *Science* **171**, 298.
Roizman, B., and Spring, S. B. (1967). *In* "Cross-Reacting Antigens and Neoantigens." (J. J. Trentin, ed.), pp. 85–97, Williams & Wilkins, Baltimore, Maryland.
Roizman, B., Borman, G. S., and Rousta, M. K. (1965). *Nature* (*London*) **206**, 1374.
Roizman, B., Spring, S. B., and Roane, P. R., Jr. (1967). *J. Virol.* **1**, 181.
Roizman, B., Spring, S. B., and Schwartz, J. (1969). *Fed. Proc., Fed. Amer. Soc. Exp. Biol.* **28**, 1890.
Roizman, B., Bachenheimer, S., Wagner, E. K., and Savage, T. (1970). *Cold Spring Harbor Symp. Quant. Biol.* **35**, 753.
Russell, W. C., Gold, E., Keir, H. M., Omura, H., Watson, D. H., and Wildy, P. (1964). *Virology* **22**, 103.
Sasaki, Y., Sasaki, R., Cohen, G. H., and Pizer, L. I. (1972). *Abstr. 72nd Annu. Meet. Amer. Soc. Microbiol.* p. 221.
Saxton, R. E., and Stevens, J. G., (1972). *Virology* **48**, 207.
Schaffer, P. A., Courtney, R. J., McCombs, R. M., and Benyesh-Melnick, M. (1971). *Virology* **46**, 356.

Sharon, N. (1966). *Proc. Int. Congr. Microbiol. 9th, 1966* p. 508.
Shimono, H., and Kaplan, A. S. (1968). *Fed. Proc., Fed. Amer. Soc. Exp. Biol.* **27**, 615.
Shimono, H., Ben-Porat, T., and Kaplan, A. S. (1969). *Virology* **37**, 49.
Shipkey, F. H., Erlandson, R. A., Bailey, R. B., Babcock, V. I., and Southam, C. M. (1967). *Exp. Mol. Pathol.* **6**, 39.
Siekevitz, P. (1972). *Annu. Rev. Physiol.* **34**, 117.
Spear, P. G., and Roizman, B. (1968). *Virology* **36**, 545.
Spear, P. G., and Roizman, B. (1970). *Proc. Nat. Acad. Sci. U.S.* **66**, 730.
Spear, P. G., and Roizman, B. (1972). *J. Virol.* **9**, 143.
Spear, P. G., Keller, J. M., and Roizman, B. (1970). *J. Virol.* **5**, 123.
Spring, S. B., and Roizman, B. (1968). *J. Virol.* **2**, 979.
Spring, S. B., Roizman, B., and Schwartz, J. (1968). *J. Virol.* **2**, 384.
Spring, S. B., Roizman, B., and Spear, P. G. (1969). *Virology* **38**, 710.
Stevens, J. G. (1966). *Virology* **29**, 570.
Stevens, J. G., and Jackson, N. L. (1967). *Virology* **32**, 654.
Stevens, J. G., Kado-Boll, G. J., and Haven, C. B. (1969). *J. Virol.* **3**, 490.
Subak-Sharpe, H., and Hay, J. (1965). *J. Mol. Biol.* **12**, 924.
Subak-Sharpe, H., Shepherd, W. M., and Hay, J. (1966). *Cold Spring Harbor Symp, Quant. Biol.* **31**, 583.
Subak-Sharpe, J. H., Gentry, G. A., and Jamison, A. (1971). *Proc. Int. Congr. Virol., 2nd 1972* p. 97.
Sydiskis, R. J. (1970). *J. Virol.* **6**, 280.
Sydiskis, R. J., and Roizman, B. (1966). *Science* **153**, 76.
Sydiskis, R. J., and Roizman, B. (1967). *Virology* **32**, 678.
Sydiskis, R. J., and Roizman, B. (1968). *Virology* **34**, 562.
Szabocsik, J. M., Huang, H. L., Gentry, G. A., and Randall, C. C. (1972). *Abstr. 72th Annu. Meet. Amer. Soc. Microbiol.* p. 221.
Tankersley, R. W., Jr. (1964). *J. Bacteriol.* **87**, 609.
Tevethia, S. S., Lowry, S. P., Rawls, W. E., Melnick, J. L., and McMillan, V. (1972). *J. Gen. Virol.* **15**, 93.
Thouless, M. E., and Skinner, G. R. B. (1971). *J. Gen. Virol.* **12**, 195.
Tokumaru, T. (1965). *J. Immunol.* **95**, 189.
Tokumaru, T. (1968). *Arch. Gesamte Virusforsch.* **24**, 104.
Wagner, E. K. (1972). *Virology* **47**, 502.
Wagner, E. K., and Roizman, B. (1969a). *J. Virol.* **4**, 36.
Wagner, E. K., and Roizman, B. (1969b). *Proc. Nat. Acad. Sci. U.S.* **64**, 626.
Watkins, J. F. (1964). *Nature (London)* **202**, 1364.
Watson, D. H., Shedden, W. I. H., Elliot, A., Tetsuka, T., Wildy, P., Bourgaux-Ramoisy, D., and Gold, E. (1966). *J. Immunol.* **11**, 399.
Wiberg, J. S., Dirksen, M. L., Epstein, R. H., Luria, S. E., and Buchanan, J. M. (1962). *Proc. Nat. Acad. Sci. U.S.* **48**, 293.
Winters, W. D., and Russell, W. C. (1971). *J. Gen. Virol.* **10**, 181.
Zemla, J., Coto, C., and Kaplan, A. S. (1967). *Virology* **31**, 736.

Chapter 7
Immunological Relationships

Berge Hampar and Lidia M. Martos

Serological analyses serve two purposes in virology. First, they serve as a tool for detecting virus-associated products in infected cell, and, secondly, they serve as a means of measuring a host's response to virus infection. This chapter is accordingly divided into two major parts. The first part deals with serological tests and the second with the antigenic relationships among herpesviruses.

I. Serological Tests

A. Complex Nature of Herpesvirus Antigens

The successful application of serological techniques to virus studies is influenced by the number and spatial arrangement of the antigenic components comprising the virion. In this regard, the complex nature of the herpes virion (Becker and Olshevsky, 1972) has proved a formidable obstacle in the carrying out of meaningful studies.

Electrophoretic studies in polyacrylamide gels have demonstrated the diverse nature of the proteins associated with herpesviruses; including herpes simplex virus (HSV) (Spear and Roizman, 1968; Watson, 1969; Olshevsky and Becker, 1970; Robinson and Watson, 1971), pseudorabies virus (PRV) (Shimono *et al.*, 1969; Kaplan and Ben-Porat, 1970), Epstein-Barr Virus (EB virus) (Weinberg and Becker, 1969), equine abortion virus (EAV) (Abodeely *et al.*, 1971), and Marek's disease virus (MDV) (Chen *et al.*, 1972). While the procedures employed for the isolation of peptides may alter their native antigenic specificities, there is no doubt that the diversity of peptides isolated from herpesviruses reflects the antigenic diversity of the virion, as demonstrated immunologically by agar gel immunodiffusion *in vitro* (Tokumaru, 1965b; Watson *et al.*, 1966) and by immunoferritin *in situ* (Nii *et al.*, 1968b; Miyamoto *et al.*, 1971).

Serological studies with herpesviruses must take into consideration the temporal sequence of antigen synthesis and virus assembly. The sequence of herpesvirus antigen production has been followed immunologically by immunofluorescence (Roizman *et al.*, 1967; Ross *et al.*, 1968; Wildy, 1972) and has been correlated with virus assembly by complement-fixation and infectivity assays (Gold *et al.*, 1963) and by immunoferritin (Miyamoto *et al.*, 1971). The temporal sequence of herpesvirus antigen synthesis has particular relevance with respect to the possible role of these viruses in oncogenesis. Since productive infection with herpesviruses invariably leads to cell death, any oncogenic capability of these viruses would require persistence in cells of a repressed viral genome. This is seen with EB virus in human lymphoblastoid cells (Zur Hausen and Schulte-Holthausen, 1970) where activation of the repressed viral genome occurs either spontaneously (Hampar *et al.*, 1971b) or after exposure to DNA analogues in "virus-negative" cells (Hampar *et al.*, 1972a; Gerber, 1972). It remains to be established unequivocally whether cells carrying a repressed complete herpesvirus genome can express any viral functions, such as viral coded antigens, which could serve as immunologic markers.

Closely related to the questions of diversity and temporal sequence of antigen production is the question of efficiency of virus replication, which determines the spectrum of antigens available for study. The more permissive the cell, the more efficient is virus replication, and this favors synthesis of the entire spectrum of viral antigens. Conversely, the less permissive the cell, the less efficient is virus replication, and this may result in a deficiency in one or more of the antigens required for infectious virus synthesis. Some herpesviruses, even under the best conditions, replicate relatively inefficiently (e.g., EB virus), as evidenced by high particle–infectivity ratios and the accumulation of defective particles.

The efficiency of herpesvirus replication and its effects on serological studies are best demonstrated by specific experimental conditions. Curtailment of biosynthetic pathways in infected cells may inhibit virus synthesis, resulting in the accumulation of defective particles and "abnormal" intracellular structures (Chitwood and Bracken, 1964). Similarly, when cells are grown in the presence of DNA analogues, herpesvirus antigens may be synthesized, although the particles produced are defective due to faulty transcription of the analogue substituted DNA (Kaplan *et al.*, 1965). With high concentration of DNA analogues, such as 5-bromodeoxyuridine (BUdR), EB viral antigen synthesis as measured by immunofluorescence is reduced significantly, and virus particle synthesis as detected by electron microscopy is inhibited (Hampar *et al.*, 1971b). Infection of nonpermissive cells with HSV results in abortive infections, with synthesis of defective particles due to the absence of functional proteins required for envelopment of the nucleocapsids (Spring *et al.*, 1968). When infected cells are maintained on a medium which is deficient in arginine, an amino acid which is required for herpesvirus replication (Tankersley, 1964), the immunofluorescent staining pattern is altered (Roizman *et al.*, 1967), and the intensity of nuclear fluorescence and the amount of nuclear complement-fixing antigens are reduced (Courtney *et al.*, 1970). This effect of arginine deprivation on herpesvirus replication is due to reduced migration of cytoplasmic viral structural proteins into the nucleus (Mark and Kaplan, 1971; Courtney *et al.*, 1971). Finally, when a temperature-sensitive mutant of HSV is maintained at the nonpermissive temperature, the major envelope glycoprotein is not synthesized, the immunofluorescent staining pattern is altered, and infectious virus is not made (Schaffer *et al.*, 1971).

Virus-infected cells synthesize proteins which are virus-specific, and which are structural or nonstructural in nature. The physical state of a protein in infected cells, however, is not evidence, *a priori*, of its structural or nonstructural nature (Kaplan, 1969). Proteins which appear early in the infectious cycle may subsequently become incorporated into mature virions. Conversely, a structural protein which is made in excess may remain in the soluble phase throughout the infectious cycle. Finally, the physical state of an antigen may determine its ability to react with an antibody. In the case of cells infected with PRV, for example, some antibodies react only with antigens in an aggregated state (Fujiwara and Kaplan, 1967).

B. Serological Procedures

1. Source of Antiserum

The efficiency of any serological test procedure is dependent on the properties of the antiserum employed, since the detection of antigens is limited by the spectrum of available antibodies. Serological studies with herpesviruses have employed antisera prepared in experimental animals and sera from the naturally infected host.

One of the most perplexing problems in serological studies with viruses is the variability in properties of antibodies from different experimental animals (intra- and interspecies), even when identical immunization procedures and the same antigen preparations are employed. The degree of variability between antisera preparations is often accentuated with more sensitive assay procedures. As a result, it is difficult to compare the properties of antisera prepared in the same or in different laboratories, and interpretation of results should be limited to the experimental procedures employed. Obviously, sera from the naturally infected host may show significantly more variability in properties than experimental antisera which have been prepared under controlled conditions.

The selection of a suitable host for immunization with herpesviruses is dependent on a number of factors. First, the widespread nature of herpesviruses makes it imperative that precautions be taken to minimize the possibility that the animal used may already have antibodies to an indigenous virus which cross reacts with the virus under study. There is probably no way in which this can be completely avoided, however, since the detection of antibodies is limited by the sensitivity of the assay procedure, and immunization with virus may elicit antibodies to an indigenous virus (Kapsenburg, 1964; Svedmyr, 1965; Schmidt *et al.*, 1969) or to a virus to which the host was previously exposed (Davenport and Hennessy, 1957). Further, indigenous herpesviruses have yet to be isolated from all species used for immunization, and even when such viruses are available, detailed serological studies for cross reactivity may not have been carried out (Rivers and Tillett, 1923; Nesburn, 1969). At the very minimum, the selection of a suitable host for immunization should be predicated on the absence of preexisting herpesvirus antibodies, and animals whose indigenous herpesvirus(es) is known to cross react with the immunizing virus should be avoided.

Second, the selection of a suitable host is often limited by its response to the immunizing virus or antigen. Pseudorabies virus (PRV), for example, is invariably fatal to rabbits (Kaplan, 1969), as are certain strains of herpes simplex virus (HSV) (Goodpasture and Teague, 1923). Other factors, such as age (Andervont, 1929; Shope, 1931), route of inoculation, and immunizing dose (Johnson, 1964a,b) may affect an animal's response to virus infection. Finally, the possibility must be considered that the type or class of antibody elicited to the same antigen may differ according to the species used for immunization (Dixon *et al.*, 1966; Oroszlan *et al.*, 1972).

The choice of antigen for immunization obviously depends on the specificity of antibodies one wishes to elicit. Immunization with certain infectious herpesviruses may lead to a chronic infection with periodic virus shedding (Kaufman *et al.*, 1967). Under these conditions, the spectrum of antibodies elicited is not limited by the spectrum of antigens used for immunization. This problem can be circumvented by first inactivating the viral nucleic acid and infectivity without affecting the antigenicity of the virion (Wallis *et al.*, 1967). Measures should be taken to optimize the homogeneity of a virus preparation used for immunization, since injection of a mixed virus population may elicit antibody populations of multiple specificities (Hampar and Keehn, 1967). Even when homogeneous virus populations are employed for immunization, however, a host in which a chronic infection is formed may synthesize virus antigenically distinct from the immunizing virus, and this may lead to heterogeneity in the specificity of the antibodies elicited. Measures should be taken to ensure the purity of a virus preparation in order to avoid antibody synthesis to other than virus-specific antigens (Watson *et al.*, 1966). Under ideal conditions, immunizations should be carried out with purified antigens so as to elicit monospecific antisera (Watson and Wildy, 1969). Alternatively, antigens can be prepared which elicit antibodies of limited specificity (Roane and Roizman, 1966; Martin *et al.*, 1972).

Special precautions are required when absorptions are employed for narrowing the specificity of an antiserum. One cannot conclude, for example, that absorption of an antiserum with intact herpes virions removes antibodies to all structural antigens, since this would not remove antibodies to internal antigens associated with the nucleocapsid or envelope (Olshevsky and Becker, 1970; Miyamoto *et al.*, 1971). Interpretation of results with absorbed sera may be particularly difficult when attempts are made to remove antibodies to cross-reacting antigens. While absorption may remove neutralizing activity against the isologous or heterologous herpesvirus strain, one cannot conclude, *a priori*, that any remaining neutralizing activity represent antibodies to type-specific antigens. Common or cross-reacting antigens may be present in different amounts or in different spatial configurations on the surface or within the envelope of the virions under study. This problem may also be encountered in attempts to absorb out antibodies to antigens present on the surface of herpesvirus-infected cells (O'Dea and Dineen, 1957).

The antibody response to herpesvirus infection (Berlin, 1963; Cowan and Trautman, 1965) is typical of that seen with most other antigens (Uhr, 1964) and is characterized by the appearance of IgM antibodies (primary response) followed by IgG antibodies (secondary response). With respect to herpesviruses in rabbits, the progressive appearance of IgM (19 S) and IgG (7 S) antibodies has been clearly demonstrated with HSV and SA8 virus (Yoshino and Taniguchi, 1965a; Hampar *et al.*, 1968a; Stevens *et al.*, 1968). A similar sequence of IgM and IgG antibodies has been demonstrated in human sera following primary infection with HSV (Tokumaru, 1966), cytomegalovirus (CMV) (Hanshaw *et al.*, 1968), varicella–zoster virus (V–Z virus) (Leonard *et al.*, 1970), and EB virus (Hampar *et al.*, 1971a).

Significant variations are seen in the properties of 19 S and 7 S antibodies elicited at different times after immunization with herpesvirus. This has been studied in detail with sera from rabbits immunized with HSV (types 1 and 2), SA8 virus, and simian CMV. The early antisera show a predominance of 19 S antibodies (Yoshino and Taniguchi, 1964, 1965a; Hampar *et al.*, 1968a; Stevens *et al.*, 1968). The properties of early and late 7 S and 19 S antibodies differ in several respects. First, the neutralizing titers against the immunizing virus of the early 7 S and 19 S and the late 19 S antibodies are enhanced in the presence of complement, while the effect of complement with the late 7 S antibodies is limited essentially to enhancing the rate of virus neutralization (Yoshino and Taniguchi, 1965a; Hampar *et al.*, 1968a; Stevens *et al.*, 1968). Second, virus sensitized with early 7 S and late 19 S antibodies are neutralized by anti-γ-globulin (Hampar *et al.*, 1968a). Third, late 19 S antibodies show a high degree of specificity for the immunizing virus, and can be used effectively for differentiating cross-reacting intratypic (Hampar *et al.*, 1968b) and heterotypic (Stevens *et al.*, 1968; Hampar *et al.*, 1969b, 1970a) herpesvirus strains. Finally, the specificities of early and late 7 S and 19 S antibodies for HSV-associated antigens differ, as demonstrated by immunoferritin (Miyamoto *et al.*, 1971).

Variations are also seen with time in the properties of herpesvirus antibodies in the naturally infected host. In humans, for example, the complement-fixing antibodies to HSV may decline with age while the neutralizing titers remain high (Holzel *et al.*, 1953; Yoshino *et al.*, 1962). That the spectrum of human antibodies to HSV differs in acute phase and convalescent sera is suggested by immunodiffusion studies (Tokumaru, 1965a). Differences are also apparent in the antibody specificities of convalescent and "normal" sera by complement-fixation (Martin *et al.*, 1972).

Of possible diagnostic value are findings which suggest that acute phase sera from herpetic patients contain a predominance of complement-requiring neutralizing (CRN) antibodies which are essentially absent in convalescent and "normal" sera (Yoshino and Taniguchi, 1966). Comparable findings have been reported (Lerner *et al.*, 1970) with sera from adults suffering from herpetic encephalitis. In contrast, no significant difference in CRN versus non-CRN antibodies was noted (Heineman, 1967) in acute phase and convalescent sera from young adults with primary or recurrent herpetic infection. It has been suggested (Yoshino *et al.*, 1971) that the assay for CRN antibodies may be of diagnostic value at an early stage of primary infection, whereas the detection of CRN antibodies may be difficult in adults previously exposed to HSV.

2. Neutralization Test and Tests for Antibody–Virus Interactions by Visual Observation

Many immunological procedures are available for the study of viruses, and most have been employed with herpesviruses. The discussion here will be limited to general comments concerning a few of the more widely used tests, and the reader is referred elsewhere for details of test procedures and theoretical considerations (Tokumaru and Scott, 1964; Casals, 1967; Svehag, 1968).

a. Neutralization Test. The choice of a suitable assay procedure obviously depends on the antigen(s) one wishes to study. The neutralization test, which is widely used in herpesvirus studies, is highly specific in that a positive result depends on the interaction of antibody and virus. However, the number of antigens detectable by neutralization is limited and probably includes only those which are at or near the surface of the herpesvirus envelope (Roizman, 1969; Hampar *et al.*, 1971c). An understanding of the mechanism of herpesvirus neutralization is further complicated by the relative paucity of information concerning the exact nature of the antigenic site. Here not only the primary structure of the proteins comprising the antigenic site(s) must be considered, but also the spatial or steric configuration of the antigens on the virion surface. The presence of presumably common antigens on the surface of cross-reacting herpesvirions does not preclude significant differences in the neutralizing titers of antibodies directed against these sites. These differences in neutralizing titers against isologous and heterologous virus strains may be reduced significantly in the presence of cofactors such as complement (Stevens *et al.*, 1968; Hampar *et al.*, 1969a), suggesting that the configuration or accessibility of the antigenic site may be the dominant factor in determining the efficiency and rate of neutralization. Conversely, reactivity of antibody with "noncritical" antigenic sites may sterically hinder reactivity of other antibody molecules to "critical" sites, resulting in a persistent fraction of unneutralized virus (Dulbecco *et al.*, 1956; Rappaport, 1970), as suggested for HSV (Yoshino and Morishima, 1972).

There is ample evidence with polio and other viruses that the interaction between antibody and virus which results in neutralization is not due to irreparable damage of the virus (Mandel, 1960), but rather to blockage of one or more stages in the virus replication cycle (reviewed by Svehag, 1968). The ability of the virus–antibody complex to adsorb to cells is dependent on the amount and type of antibody used and the time allowed for virus–antibody interaction (Mandel, 1967). If the complex can adsorb to cells, then blockage of virus synthesis occurs at either the stage of penetration or uncoating (Joklik, 1964).

Virus neutralization apparently requires the interaction of one antibody molecule with one "critical" virion antigenic site (Dulbecco *et al.*, 1956). To accomplish this, however, may require association of many antibody molecules with the virion surface (Amelunxen and Werder, 1960). The association of antibody with virus without resultant neutralization has been ascribed to various factors (reviewed by Svehag, 1968) which need not be considered here. What is relevant to this discussion is that the "sensitized" virus–antibody complex can be neutralized by adding certain cofactors.

The first demonstration of "sensitization" with a herpesvirus was by Yoshino and Taniguchi (1965b) who showed that herpes simplex virus (HSV) which had been irreversibly "sensitized" with antibody could be rapidly neutralized by adding complement. This finding was correlated with earlier findings by these same investigators that the neutralization titers of rabbit (Yoshino and Taniguchi, 1964), guinea pig, and human (Yoshino and Taniguchi, 1966) antibodies elicited early after infection with HSV were enhanced significantly in the presence of complement. Similar findings have been noted with early antibodies against bacteriophage (Toussaint and Muschel, 1962) and other mammalian viruses (reviewed by Iwasaki and Oguna, 1968).

The concept of complement-requiring neutralizing (CRN) antibodies (Yoshino and Taniguchi, 1964) is probably incorrect, and a better term may be complement-potentiated neutralizing antibodies (C-PNab) (Iwasaki and Oguna, 1968). The role of complement in mediating neutralization of "sensitized" virus is apparently limited to enhancing the rate of neutralization, and neutralization occurs gradually with time in the absence of complement (Yoshino and Taniguchi, 1965b). Conversely, the concept of antibody populations which are completely independent of complement for neutralization may require modification, since complement may enhance antibody titers against heterologous cross-reacting herpesviruses while not affecting the titers against isologous strains (Stevens *et al.*, 1968; Hampar *et al.*, 1969a).

Although the mechanism of complement-mediated neutralization has yet to be established, no more than the first four components of complement are required (Linscott and Levinson, 1969; Daniels *et al.*, 1970). The mechanism of complement-mediated neutralization may involve factors related to antibody affinity and specificity, since the relative amount of C-PNab decreases with time after infection, while the affinity of antibody for antigen increases with time (reviewed by Svehag, 1968). In the case of early rabbit antiserum against HSV, C-PNab is found in both the 7 S and 19 S antibody populations, while in hyperimmune sera C-PNab is found predominantly in the 19 S antibody population (Yoshino and Taniguchi, 1965a; Hampar *et al.*, 1968a). The possibility that in rabbits only 7 S antibodies show increased affinity for antigen with time may be excluded, since 19 S rabbit antibodies of low and high affinities for the same antigenic site of poliovirus have been demonstrated (Svehag, 1968). This suggests that the C-PNab found in 19 S antibody populations from early and late rabbit anti-HSV sera is not due to the inability of rabbits to produce 19 S antibodies of high affinity, but rather is related to differences in the specificity of these antibody populations for virion-associated antigens (Miyamoto *et al.*, 1971).

Neutralization of "sensitized" virus can also be affected by antibody to the sensitizing immunoglobulin (Goodman and Donch, 1965). In the case of HSV, virus "sensitized" either *in vitro* (Ashe and Notkins, 1966) or *in vivo* (Centifano and Kaufman, 1970) can be neutralized by adding anti-γ-globulin.

b. TEST FOR ANTIBODY–VIRUS INTERACTIONS BY VISUAL OBSERVATION. Visual observation of virus–antibody complexes has proved ideal for following the sequence of antigen synthesis in infected cells and for screening of sera to determine antibody activity.

The immunofluorescent test (Coons and Kaplan, 1950), which has been used extensively in herpesvirus studies, suggests that the accumulation of aggregated virus-specific antigen(s) occurs early (2–3 hours) in both the nucleus and cytoplasm of HSV-infected cells (Roizman *et al.*, 1967), and from the third hour after infection at the cell surface (Wildy, 1972). The detection of antigens by immunofluorescence obviously depends on the specificity of the antisera used. Similarly, the temporal sequence of antigen accumulation and virus replication may vary depending on the input multiplicity of infection and the cells used. Figure 1 shows the progressive accumulation of intracellular antigens (Figs. 1A–C) and infectious virus (Fig. 1E) in WI-38 cells infected with a low multiplicity (< 1) of a simian CMV (strain SA6), as detected by direct immunofluorescence using rabbit anti-SA6 neutralizing serum (Martos *et al.*, 1970). Virus-specific antigens are first detected in the nucleus prior to the appearance of infectious virus (Figs. 1A,E). The small foci of nuclear antigens increase in size and ultimately coalesce to form a large intranuclear inclusion (Fig. 1B). The appearance of antigens in the cytoplasmic inclusion (Fig. 1C) is related temporally to the detection of infectious progeny virus (Fig. 1E). Figure 1D shows staining of cytoplasmic but not nuclear inclusions by "normal" rabit serum. This cytoplasmic staining is seen readily with rabbit (Hampar, unpublished observations) and human (Jack and Wark, 1972) sera which show no other evidence of CMV antibodies and is considered nonspecific.

The immunoperoxidase test, which has been adapted for light microscopy,

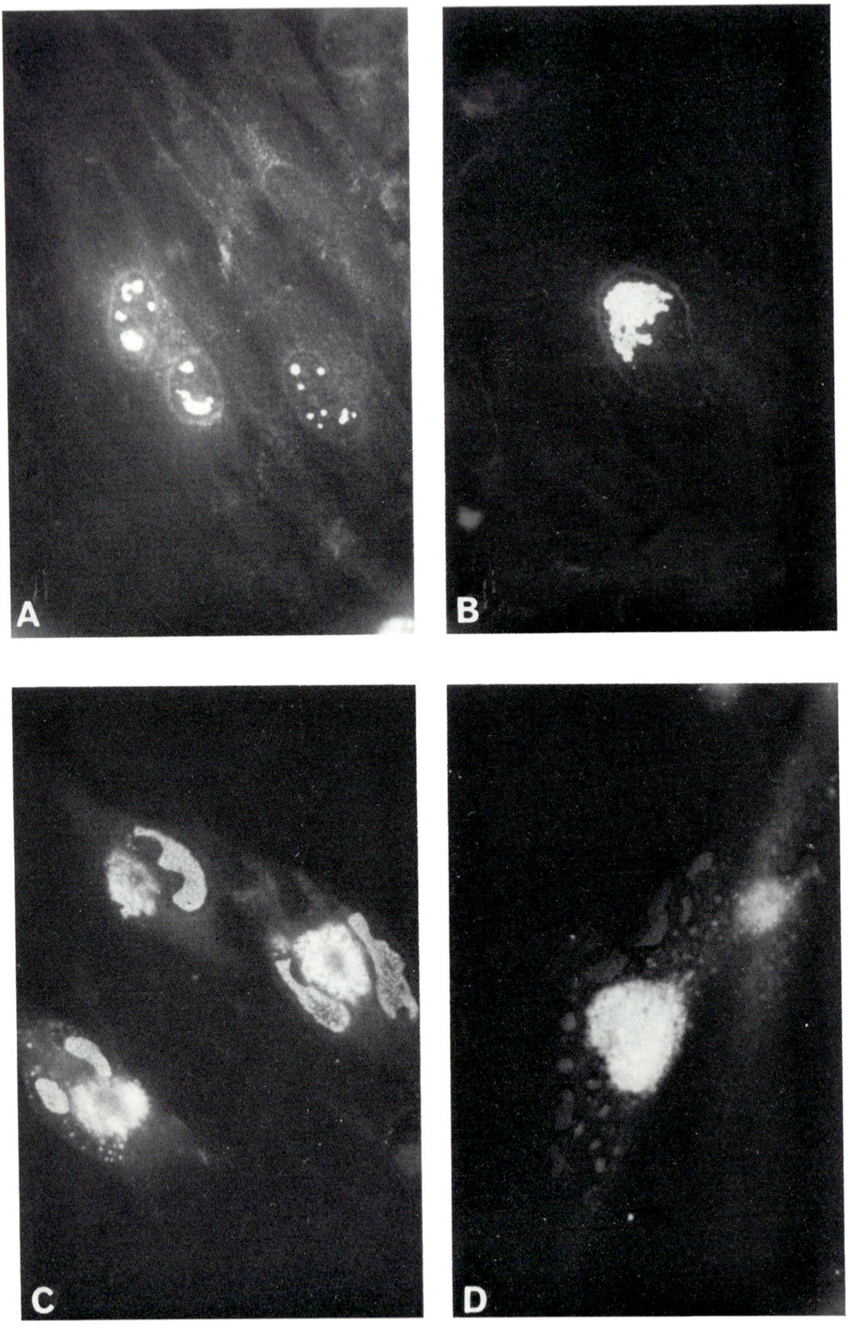

FIG. 1. (A)–(D)

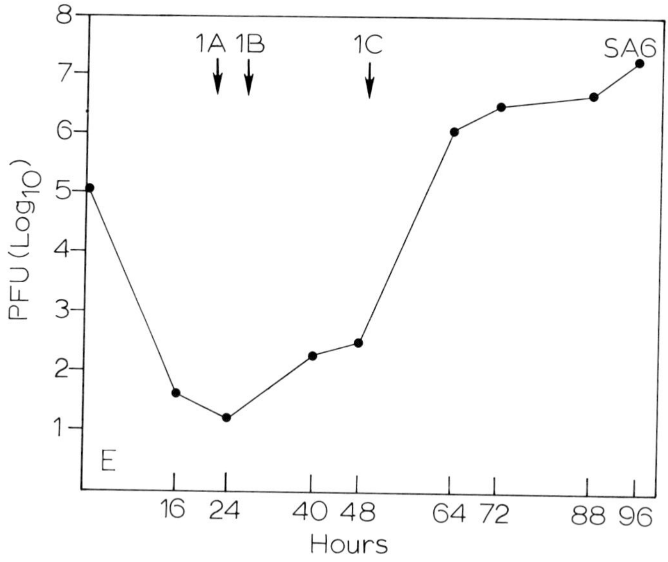

FIG. 1. (E)

FIG. 1. Appearance of intracellular antigens and infectious virus in WI-38 cells infected with a simian CMV (strain SA6). Direct immunofluorescent staining employed antiserum prepared in rabbits. (A, B) Staining of nuclear antigens. (C) Staining of nuclear and cytoplasmic antigens. (D) Nonspecific staining of cytoplasmic antigens. (E) Appearance of infectious virus in infected cells and medium.

has also been used with herpesviruses (Kurstak, 1971). Figure 2 shows immunoperoxidase staining of cells infected with a syncytium- (Fig. 2A) and a nonsyncytium-inducing strain (Fig. 2B) of HSV, varicella–zoster virus (Fig. 2C), and human CMV (Fig. 2D). The cells were stained by the indirect technique using neutralizing antisera prepared in rabbits to each virus (Hampar *et al.*, 1970a; Martos *et al.*, 1970). The immunoperoxidase test offers certain advantages over the immunofluorescent test. First, the autofluorescence seen with some cells is not a problem in the immunoperoxidase technique. Second, the amount of nonspecific staining is greatly reduced in the immunoperoxidase test. Third, the immunoperoxidase technique allows for better localization of intracellular antigens since a light microscope is used. Finally, with the immunoperoxidase technique a permanent record is obtained for future studies.

The immunoferritin technique (Breese and Hsu, 1971) is ideal for visualizing the interaction of antibody with herpesviruses and for studying the sequence of virus antigen synthesis and assembly (Nii *et al.*, 1968a; Miyamoto *et al.*, 1971). Figure 3 shows direct immunoferritin tagging of EB virus

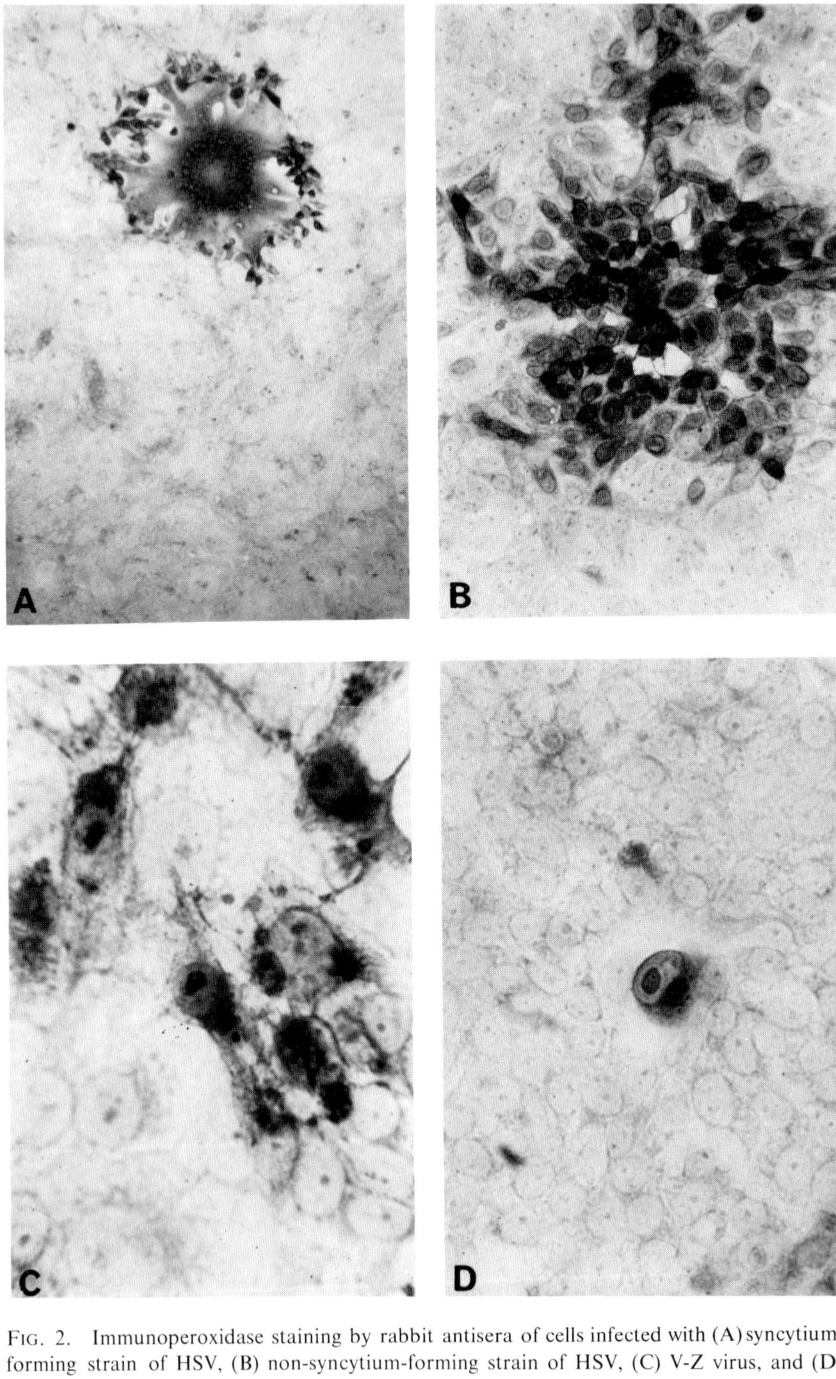

FIG. 2. Immunoperoxidase staining by rabbit antisera of cells infected with (A) syncytium-forming strain of HSV, (B) non-syncytium-forming strain of HSV, (C) V-Z virus, and (D) human CMV.

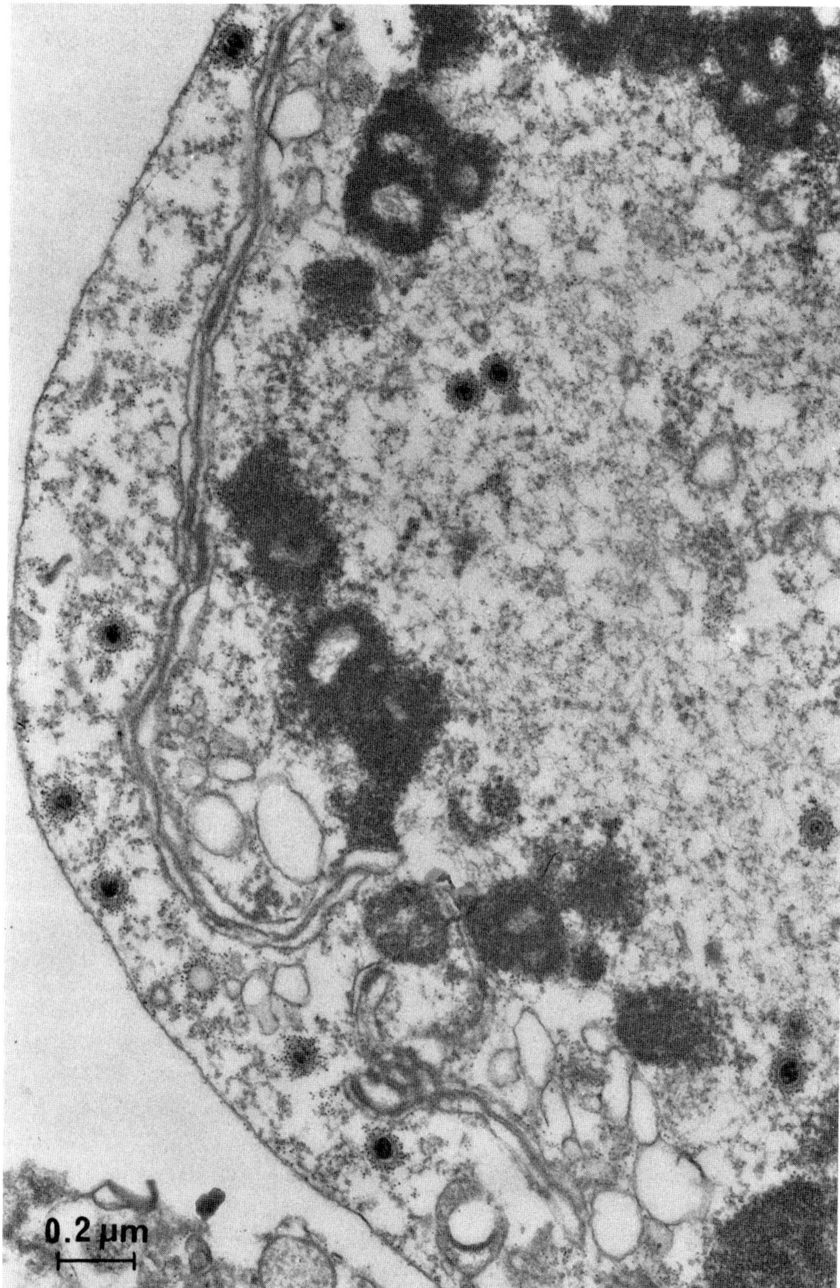

FIG. 3. Immunoferritin tagging of EB virus capsids by rabbit antiserum prepared against purified capsids. No tagging of duplicated nuclear membrane or plasma membrane. (Photograph courtesy of Mr. J. L. Walker).

capsids by rabbit antiserum prepared against partially purified capsid particles (Hampar *et al.*, 1970b). These rabbit antisera show no activity against EB virus envelope antigens by neutralization or immunofluorescence with infected cell plasma membranes (Gerber and Goldstein, 1970). Specific ferritin tagging is evident with nuclear and cytoplasmic capsids, but no tagging is seen with antigens associated with the nuclear or plasma membranes. This contrasts with antisera possessing neutralizing activity, as shown in Fig. 4, where HSV-infected human lymphoblastoid cells (EB virus "negative") reacted with a ferritin-conjugated rabbit anti-HSV neutralizing serum showing tagging of nuclear and plasma membranes, enveloped particles, and capsids.

II. Immunology of Herpesviruses

Antigenic relationships among herpesviruses have been extensively studied using various serological techniques. The possibility of antigens common to all herpesviruses within any one species or between species has been suggested, but the evidence presented thus far is too meager to allow definitive conclusions. Similarly, some studies reporting antigenic relationships between specific herpesviruses have yet to be confirmed and are not included here. Detailed discussions of the immunology of specific herpesviruses are limited essentially to the four human types and the most frequently described cross reactions between herpesviruses are summarized in Table I.

A. Herpes Simplex Virus (H. hominis)

Epidemiologic studies have demonstrated the ubiquitous nature of herpes simplex virus (HSV) in humans (Scott, 1954). The primary exposure to virus is usually uneventful, although antibodies appear which persist throughout life. Early studies employing the constant serum-varying virus method for neutralization led to the conclusion that the presence of antibodies in humans was an all-or-none event, with no fluctuations in titers between individuals (Burnet and Lush, 1939). Subsequent studies employing the more sensitive constant virus-varying serum method showed appreciable differences in the neutralizing titers of individual sera (Kilbourne and Horsfall, 1951; Rose, 1952; Buddingh *et al.*, 1953).

Serum antibody levels in children may show fluctuations associated with virus reisolation following primary infection (Buddingh *et al.*, 1953; Dascomb *et al.*, 1955), but antibody levels in adults usually remain relatively high and constant (Scott, 1957), and do not fluctuate appreciably in association with virus shedding or recurrent infections (Douglas and Couch, 1970).

Antibodies to HSV may be detected in approximately 40% of newborns up

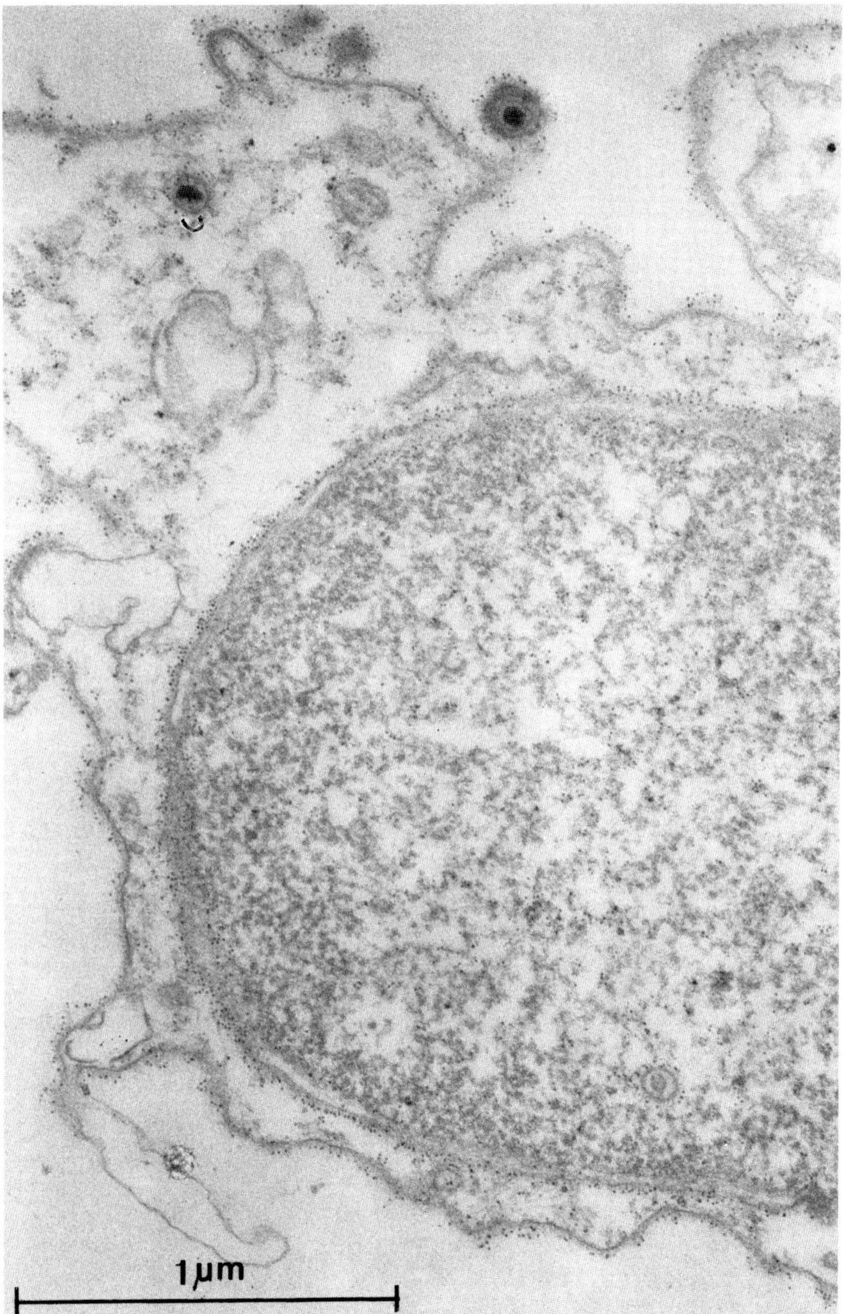

FIG. 4. Immunoferritin tagging of HSV enveloped particles and capsids and nuclear and plasma membranes by rabbit anti-HSV neutralizing serum. (Photograph courtesy of Mr. J. L. Walker).

TABLE I
CROSS-REACTIONS BETWEEN HERPESVIRUSES

Virus[a]	Test	References
HSV and B virus	Neutralization (anti-B neutralizes HSV to high titers; anti-HSV neutralizes B virus to low titers	Sabin, 1934a; Burnet *et al.*, 1939; Schneweis, 1962b; Watson *et al.*, 1967; Ueda *et al.*, 1968
	Immunofluorescence	Benda, 1966
SA8 virus	Immunodiffusion	Watson *et al.*, 1967
	Complement fixation	Martin *et al.*, 1972
	Neutralization	Hull, 1968; Stevens *et al.*, 1968
MHV	Immunofluorescence	Holmes *et al.*, 1964
PRV	Immunodiffusion	Watson *et al.*, 1967
Canine herpes	Neutralization	Aurelian, 1968
Equine herpes type 1	Complement fixation (anti-HSV and human sera fix C with equine herpes, type 1; no reaction between anti-equine herpes, type 1 and HSV	Pulmmer, 1964.
Human CMV and simian CMV	Complement fixation (simian sera fix C′ with human CMV; no reactions between human sera and simian CMV)	Black *et al.*, 1963; Dreesman and Benyesh-Melnick, 1967
EB virus and subhuman primate herpes-type virus(es)	Immunofluorescence	Goldman *et al.*, 1968; Gerber and Goldstein, 1970; Landon and Malan, 1971; Levy *et al.*, 1971
	Immunodiffusion	Stevens *et al.*, 1970
	Complement-fixation	Gerber and Birch, 1967; Gerber and Deal, 1970
	Coating of virus particles	Gerber and Birch, 1967
PRV and equine herpes type 1	Complement-fixation	Plummer, 1964
B virus	Immunodiffusion	Watson *et al.*, 1967
MDHV	Immunofluorescence	Sharma *et al.*, 1972
MDHV and turkey herpesvirus	Immunofluorescence and Immunodiffusion	Witter *et al.*, 1970
Equine herpes, type 1 and equine herpes type 2	Complement-fixation	Plummer, 1964; Plummer *et al.*, 1969
IBR	Complement-fixation (one way cross with anti-IBR)	Plummer, 1964
MHV and SMHV	Neutralization	Hull *et al.*, 1972

[a]HSV, herpes simplex virus; MHV, marmoset herpesvirus; PRV, pseudorabies virus; CMV, cytomegalovirus; MDHV, Marek's disease herpesvirus; IBR, infectious bovine rhinotracheitis virus; SMHV, spider monkey herpesvirus.

to age 4 months due to placental transfer of maternal antibodies. Approximately 10% of children between the ages of 4 months and 4 years show antibodies to HSV, but this percentage increases with age and reaches levels of 60% more in adults (Scott *et al.*, 1952; Buddingh *et al.*, 1953; Yoshino *et al.*, 1962).

1. Serological Classification

The earliest studies employed techniques which were usually too insensitive for detecting antigenic differences between HSV strains (reviewed by Nahmias and Dowdle, 1968), although some studies by neutralization and complement-fixation did suggest such differences (Slavin and Gavett, 1946; Womack and Hunt, 1954).

The classification of HSV strains into at least three antigenically distinct groups was proposed by Shubladze *et al.* (1959, 1960), based on reciprocal neutralization tests in mice with antisera prepared in rats. Schneweis (1962a) studied 30 virus strains by complement-fixation, neutralization end point, and neutralization kinetics and grouped them into two distinct types. However, reliable classification of the strains was accomplished only with antisera prepared against type 1 virus.

Ashe and Scherp (1963) studied 15 laboratory-adapted strains and classified them into four serotypes by neutralization kinetics with rabbit antisera. In subsequent studies (Ashe and Scherp, 1965), these investigators reported antigenic differences between fresh HSV isolates from recurrent labial lesions. Significantly, they also noted antigenic differences in virus isolated from the same individual following successive recurrencies.

Plummer (1964) tested a number of HSV strains by cross-neutralization and neutralization kinetics using rabbit antisera, and grouped them into two subtypes. In contrast to Schneweis (1962a), Plummer was able to classify his strains with antisera prepared against either subtype 1 or 2 virus.

Pauls and Dowdle (1967) studied a small number of strains by a micromodification of the quantal neutralization test (de St. Groth, 1961). Their preliminary findings suggested that HSV strains could be classified into two distinct types, in agreement with the findings of Schneweis (1962) and Plummer (1964). Subsequently, these investigators reported findings carried out with 91 strains of HSV obtained from various laboratories (Dowdle *et al.*, 1967). Rabbit antisera prepared against one reference type 1 strain and one reference type 2 strain were tested by microquantal neutralization against the 91 strains. By this method, they classified 49 strains as type 1 and 42 strains as type 2. When they compared the original site of virus isolation with their designated classification, they found that all type 2 strains had been isolated "from herpetic infections related directly or indirectly to involvement of the adult genital tract, both male and female." In contrast, strains classified as type 1, with one exception, had been isolated from sites other than those associated with or in proximity to the genital tract. The one exception was an isolate "from the penis of a 3-year-old boy who also yielded type 1 virus from the pharynx." Furthermore, six strains isolated from recurrent herpes labialis and shown by Ashe and Scherp (1963) to differ antigenically by neutralization kinetics were classified by Dowdle *et al.* (1967) as type 1. Although other investigators reported the isolation of type 2 strains from nongenital sites (Nahmias and Dowdle, 1968), it would appear that HSV strains associated with genital tract infections comprise a distinct antigenic group (Dowdle *et al.*, 1967; Rawls *et al.*, 1968b; Plummer *et al.*, 1970).

Most serologic studies for differentiating HSV types 1 and 2 have used experimental antisera produced in animals, although human sera have also been employed. The test procedures include end-point neutralization by plaque reduction (Wheeler *et al.*, 1969), microquantal neutralization (Pauls and Dowdle, 1967), neutralization kinetics (Plummer, 1964; Rawls *et al.*, 1968a), neutralization using artificial mixtures of different virus types (Ejercito *et al.*, 1968; Wheeler *et al.*, 1969), neutralization using highly specific rabbit late 19 S antibodies (Hampar *et al.*, 1970a), complement fixation (Schneweis, 1962a; Nahmias *et al.*, 1968; Martin *et al.*, 1972), microindirect hemagglutination (Fuccillo *et al.*, 1970), immunofluorescence of fixed cells (Nahmias *et al.*, 1969b), membrane immunofluorescence (Nahmias *et al.*, 1971; Geder and Skinner, 1971), immunodiffusion and inhibition-passive hemagglutination (Schneweis and Nahmias, 1971), *in vitro* stimulation of immune lymphocytes (Rosenberg *et al.*, 1972), and ^{51}Cr release (Smith *et al.*, 1972).

The finding that genitally transmitted strains of HSV differed antigenically from nongenitally transmitted strains led to sero-epidemiologic studies to determine the frequency of infection by these two virus types in the human population. The incidence of antibodies to types 1 and 2 virus in human sera was studied by microquantal neutralization (Nahmias and Dowdle, 1968) and neutralization kinetics (Rawls *et al.*, 1968a). The initial findings which suggested a higher incidence of antibodies to type 2 virus in women with carcinoma of the cervix than in matched controls led to intensive investigations of a possible etiologic role for HSV type 2 in cervical carcinoma. More recent studies (Adam *et al.*, 1971, 1972), however, suggest that the incidence of type 2 antibodies in cervical carcinoma patients and control women may not be significantly different in all populations used for study, and are influenced to a significant extent by the criteria employed for selecting matched controls (Rawls *et al.*, 1972).

Questions may be raised concerning the reliability of methods used for detecting antibodies to different HSV serotypes in human sera. While the detection of antibodies to the virus type responsible for a primary herpetic infection seems reliable, doubts exist as to the reliability of detection methods in cases where a human serum contains antibodies to more than one virus type. The basis of these doubts are related to findings with antisera produced in rabbits to mixed virus populations. For example, when rabbit antisera were prepared against a mixed population of HSV variants, four plaque-purified isolates from the population could be divided into only two distinct serologic groups by reciprocal neutralization kinetics (Hampar and Keehn, 1967). However, when antisera were prepared against each of the four isolates and tested by reciprocal neutralization kinetics, it was possible to show that each isolate was antigenically distinct. These findings were subsequently confirmed with rabbit antisera prepared against a mixture of HSV types 1 and 2 (Nahmias *et al.*, 1969a).

Despite the apparent clear-cut antigenic distinction between HSV types 1 and 2, the serological classification of HSV strains remains a controversial issue. The issue in question is whether HSV strains should be classified into distinct "serotypes," or whether they should be grouped into one "serotype" with variants being classified as "subtypes" (Roizman *et al.*, 1970; Hampar *et al.*, 1971c).

The basis of the argument for a "subtype" classification are findings from a number of laboratories which suggest "that a spectrum of HSV antigenic variants exist whose degree of relatedness covers a relatively wide range" (Hampar *et al.*, 1968b). Involved in the argument are two questions: the first concerning the degree of relatedness between HSV variants, and the second concerning the stability of variants in their natural environment or following laboratory manipulations.

The degree of relatedness between HSV variants must be considered from two viewpoints. The first involves the degree of relatedness as measured by various serologic tests. A "subtype" classification for HSV is suggested by findings that both HSV types 1 and 2 can be neutralized by heterologous antisera, and differentiation requires relatively sensitive neutralization procedures (Plummer, 1964; Dowdle *et al.*, 1967; Ejercito *et al.*, 1968; Rawls *et al.*, 1968b; Wheeler *et al.*, 1969; Hampar *et al.*, 1970a). Although differences between type 1 and 2 strains by neutralization are below the levels usually accepted for classification of other viruses (e.g., polio) into distinct serotypes, it may be argued that this criteria need not hold true for herpesviruses. A "serotype" classification for HSV is suggested by findings that the antigenic differences within strains of each type are relatively minor; corresponding to intratypic variants. This argument is somewhat tenous, however, since strains exist which have been classified as intermediate between types 1 and 2 (Dowdle *et al.*, 1967; Ejercito *et al.*, 1968; Plummer *et al.*, 1970). Although fresh HSV isolates have also been shown to differ antigenically

(Ashe and Scherp, 1965; Ejercito *et al.*, 1968; Plummer *et al.*, 1970), no clear-cut intermediate strains of fresh isolates have been described. One case has been reported (Terni and Roizman, 1970), however, of the isolation of viruses from simultaneous recurrent herpetic lesions of the lip and thigh. The isolate from the thigh was classified as type 2 by neutralization, while the isolate from the lip was related to, but was not identical to, type 1. In another series of studies carried out with 44 randomly collected HSV strains and employing the reciprocal neutralization kinetic test (Wildy, 1972), a clustering of oral and genital strains was observed when analyzed by the principal coordinates method (Gower, 1966), but there was overlapping of the clusters such that "the nearest genital and oral isolates are closer than the most distant isolates within each group."

The second point with respect to the degree of relatedness of HSV variants concerns the specificity of antigens coded for by different strains. There seems no doubt that antigenic differences between type 1 and 2 strains can be detected by various serologic procedures (Schneweis and Nahmias, 1971; Nahmias *et al.*, 1971; Geder and Skinner, 1971, Wildy, 1972; Rosenberg *et al.*, 1972; Smith *et al.*, 1972). In fact, the absence of "type" -specific antigens would be somewhat surprising, since type 1 and 2 strains differ in various biological, biophysical, and biochemical properties (reviewed by Nahmias and Dowdle, 1968), including the buoyant density of their respective DNA's (Goodheart *et al.*, 1968) which show only partial homology (Ludwig *et al.*, 1972; Kieff *et al.*, 1972). A rationale for the antigenic differences observed between HSV strains has been proposed by Roizman and co-workers (reviewed by Roizman, 1970) who suggest "that immunological specificity in neutralization tests, effects on the behavior of infected cells, and certain physical characteristics of the virus are covariant properties dependent on the structure of the surface of the virus" (Roizman *et al.*, 1970). The neoantigens which appear on the surface of HSV-infected cells (O'Dea and Dineen, 1957) are identical or at least serologically related to one or more envelope antigens of the virion (Roane and Roizman, 1964; Roizman and Spear, 1971), and glycoproteins associated with smooth membranes of infected cells share common electrophoretic characteristics with glycoproteins associated with virions (Keller *et al.*, 1970). As would be expected, the electrophoretic patterns of membrane-associated glycoproteins differ for type 1, type 2, and intermediate strains (Roizman *et al.*, 1970). It has also been demonstrated by immunoferritin (Miyamoto *et al.*, 1971) that late 19 S rabbit antibodies which show a high degree of specificity for isologous virus by neutralization react preferentially with antigens associated with membranes of infected cells, and these antigens ultimately appear in the virus envelope.

Although distinct differences in the various biological, biophysical, and biochemical properties of HSV variants have been demonstrated clearly only for type 1, type 2, and intermediate strains, it is probable that minor differences in certain properties have gone undetected due to the relative insensitivity of available assay procedures. Using sensitive neutralization kinetic techniques, for example, minor antigenic differences between fresh isolates and between laboratory strains have been demonstrated clearly, suggesting a continuous spectrum of antigenic variants with type 1 and 2 strains being situated at opposite extremes.

While a hypothesis has been proposed to explain why differences exist in the properties of HSV variants (reviewed by Roizman, 1970), other *in vitro* studies suggest a mechanism to explain how these differences arise. When Chinese hamster cells are infected with HSV, chronic infections are established that are characterized by recurrent cycles of cell destruction and regrowth with accompanying virus synthesis (Hampar and Copeland, 1965). The underlying mechanism responsible for these chronic infections has been attributed to continuous changes which occur with time in the susceptibility of the cells and the virulence of the virus being produced (Hampar and Keehn, 1967; Hampar and Burroughs, 1969). As a result of these changes, the cells in chronically infected cultures at any time, t, are more susceptible to the virus being produced at any time $> t$, than at any time $< t$. Conversely, the virus isolated from chronically infected cultures at any time, t, is more virulent for cells isolated at any time $< t$, than at any time $> t$. When cells are infected with a low multiplicity of virus to which they are only partially permissive, restrictive lesions are initiated which are repaired by growth of contiguous uninfected cells. Two types of virus can be isolated from these restrictive lesions. One type is similar to the input virus and shows a low degree of virulence for the cells, while the second type shows a high degree of virulence for the cells. The isolation of two dissimilar viruses from a single lesion induced by one infectious unit suggests that host cell-induced changes occurred in the properties of the virus. Accompanying these progressive changes in the infective properties of the virus are progressive changes in its antigenic properties. This has resulted in the original type 1 virus being converted after one year of chronic infection into an intermediate type (B. Hampar, unpublished data). In contrast, continuous passage of any one virus isolate in highly permissive primary rabbit kidney cells results in no appreciable change in either its infective or antigenic properties. Antigenic conversion of HSV *in vitro* has been described in other cell systems (Hoggan and Roizman, 1959; Wheeler, 1964; Dowdle *et al.*, 1967), attesting to the frequency of this event.

The studies *in vitro* indicate that HSV variants can arise readily during adaptation of the virus to new host cells. The less permissive the cells, the more radical and rapid are the changes which occur in the properties of the virus during adaptation. This ability of HSV to readily adapt to new host cells obviously has survival value and suggests a mechanism which may also be operative *in vivo*. If such is indeed the case, then any classification scheme for herpesviruses would have to be tempered by the realization that the properties being defined may only hold true for a specific time period, and the virus may acquire new properties under different experimental conditions or under different host physiologic influences. An adequate classification system to cover all of these possibilities has yet to be described.

2. Cross-Reactions with Other Herpesviruses

a. B Virus (*H. simiae*). Originally isolated from a fatal human infection (Sabin and Wright, 1934), B virus is indigenous to rhesus and other Old World monkeys. Both B virus and HSV share common antigens as demonstrated by cross-neutralization (Sabin, 1934a; Burnet *et al.*, 1939; Schneweis, 1962b; Watson *et al.*, 1967; Ueda *et al.*, 1968) and immunofluorescence (Benda, 1966). Experimental antisera to B virus neutralize HSV to the same or higher titers that they neutralize B virus. Conversely, experimental antisera to HSV neutralize B virus to low, but significant levels. Antisera from monkeys naturally infected with B virus also neutralize HSV. Similarly, human sera containing antibodies to HSV neutralize B virus (Burnet *et al.*, 1939; Melnick and Banker, 1954; Van Hoosier and Melnick, 1961; Hull *et al.*, 1962), and this has been attributed to a heterotypic response rather than to human infection with B virus.

Common antigens between B virus and HSV have also been demonstrated by agar gel immunodiffusion (Watson *et al.*, 1967), with three common precipitin bands being identified with HSV antisera, whereas B virus antisera show only one common band. Similarly, antisera prepared in rabbits to B virus (Martin *et al.*, 1972) fix complement with HSV types 1 and 2 capsid, envelope, and soluble antigens.

b. SA8 Virus. The SA8 virus was isolated from African green monkeys (Malherbe and Harwin, 1957, 1958), but some doubts exist as to the natural host of this virus owing to the paucity of isolations from these monkeys (Hull, 1968). Both SA8 virus and HSV share common antigens as demonstrated by reciprocal neutralization with guinea pig (Hull, 1968) and rabbit (Stevens *et al.*, 1968) antisera. The cross-neutralizing activity of the hyperimmune rabbit sera has been attributed to the 7 S antibodies, while the 19 S antibodies show little capacity to neutralize heterologous virus.

Neutralization of SA8 virus is also seen with human sera containing antibodies to HSV (Hampar *et al.*, 1969a), and this has been attributed to a heterotypic response rather than to human infection with SA8 virus. The neutralization of heterologous SA8 virus by human adult sera is enhanced in the presence of complement, although complement does not enhance the titers against HSV.

c. Pseudorabies Virus (*Herpesvirus suis*). The possible sharing of common antigens by pseudorabies virus (PRV) and HSV was suggested by Sabin (1934b) who reported resistance to a small, but definitely infectious dose of PRV in guinea pigs immunized with HSV. In contrast, Kaplan and co-workers (Kaplan and Vatter, 1959; Kaplan, 1969), who have carried out extensive studies with PRV, have found no evidence of shared structural antigens with HSV.

Watson *et al.* (1967) reported that rabbit antisera to HSV and B virus forms a precipitin band of identity with HSV-, B virus-, and PRV-infected cell extracts. No relationship between PRV and HSV or B virus was noted by neutralization with antisera to the latter two viruses. It was suggested that the findings by immunodiffusion may represent a nonstructural group antigen common to these three herpesviruses. The possibility that the immunodiffusion results were due to contamination was excluded, since the common precipitin band detected was not the most pronounced antigen.

B. Human Cytomegaloviruses

The cytomegalovirus (CMV) group of human herpesviruses shows a high degree of antigenic heterogeneity between virus strains. Following their initial isolation and propagation *in vitro* (Smith, 1956; Rowe *et al.*, 1956; Weller *et al.*, 1957), extensive serological studies were carried out by complement-fixation (Rowe *et al.*, 1956; Weller *et al.*, 1960), neutralization using the end-point dilution (Rowe *et al.*, 1956; Weller *et al.*, 1957) and plaque-reduction (Plummer and Benyesh-Melnick, 1964; Wentworth and French, 1970) methods, and immunofluorescence (Hanshaw *et al.*, 1968). A platelet aggregation test (Penttinen *et al.*, 1970) and an indirect hemagglutination test (Bernstein and Stewart, 1971; Fucillo *et al.*, 1971) have been described which may prove more sensitive than complement fixation for detecting low antibody levels. Soluble and virion-associated CMV antigens have been distinguished by agar gel immunodiffusion (Furukawa *et al.*, 1972) and complement fixation (Benyesh-Melnick *et al.*, 1966).

Human CMV antibodies appear in the absence of obvious disease. Sera from children and young adults usually contain both complement-fixing and neutralizing antibodies, while adult sera usually show a predominance of neutralizing antibodies (Rowe *et al.*, 1956). The properties of newborn sera are similar to those of adult sera (Weller *et al.*, 1960), suggesting placental transfer of maternal antibodies. Seroconversion with or without accompanying disease following the initial antigenic exposure to CMV in newborns or adults is characterized by antibodies of the IgM class, as detected by immunofluorescence (Hanshaw *et al.*, 1968; Lang and Hanshaw, 1969; Chiang *et al.*, 1970; Langenhuysen *et al.*, 1970), indirect hemagglutination (Bernstein and Stewart, 1971; Fuccillo *et al.*, 1971), and neutralization. The complement-fixation is relatively insensitive for the detection of IgM antibodies (Lang and Noren, 1968). A high incidence of anti-CMV-like IgM antibodies have been observed by indirect immunofluorescence in heterophile-positive infectious mononucleosis patients, although failure to isolate CMV and the absence of complement-fixing antibodies raises doubts as to the specificity of these antibodies for CMV (Hanshaw *et al.*, 1972).

SEROLOGICAL CLASSIFICATION AND CROSS REACTIONS

Sera from African green monkeys (Black *et al.*, 1963; Dreesman and Benyesh-Melnick, 1967) and rhesus monkeys (Dreesman and Benyesh-Melnick, 1967) naturally infected with simian CMV react by complement-fixation with some strains of human CMV. However, this cross reactivity occurs in only one direction, and human complement-fixing antibodies do not react with simian CMV.

Human CMV strains can be differentiated to some extent by complement-fixation using human sera (Medearis, 1964; Hanshaw, 1966), although the specificity of human complement-fixing antibodies broadens with the individual's age (Medearis, 1964; Stern and Elek, 1965). Differentiation of human CMV by complement-fixation is better accomplished with sera from naturally infected African green monkeys or rhesus monkeys (Dreesman and Benyesh-Melnick, 1967). In one study (Dreesman and Benyesh-Melnick, 1967), 100% of African green monkey sera which fixed complement with simian CMV antigens also reacted with human strain AD 169 (Rowe *et al.*, 1956), but none of the sera reacted with human strain C 87 (Benyesh-Melnick *et al.*, 1964). Other human strains were intermediate between strains AD 169 and C 87 in their reactivity with monkey sera. The broad reactivity of strain AD 169 complement-fixing antigens compared to other human CMV strains is also seen with human sera (Hanshaw, 1966).

Although human and simian CMV share complement-fixing antigens, they apparently possess antigenically distinct virion antigens, since human and monkey sera show species specificity when tested by neutralization (Dreesman and Benyesh-Melnick, 1967). One possible exception involves the neutralization of human CMV strain C 87 by African green monkey sera (Graham *et al.*, 1969). Baboon sera, which neutralized simian CMV, did not neutralize stran C 87. It is of interest that the neutralization titers of African green monkey sera against strain C 87 were enhanced in the presence of complement. This effect of complement to enhance the neutralization titers against heterologous herpesvirus strains is also seen with human (Hampar *et al.*, 1969a) and rabbit antisera (Hampar *et al.*, 1968b; Stevens *et al.*, 1968).

Antisera to human CMV have been prepared in monkeys, baboons, (Plummer and Benyesh-Melnick, 1964; Graham *et al.*, 1969), rabbits (Vaczi *et al.*, 1965; Mantyjarvi, 1968; Martos *et al.*, 1970; Andersen, 1971), guinea pigs (Krech and Jung, 1969; Wentworth and French, 1970), and goats (Haines *et al.*, 1971). Neutralization titers (based on final antibody dilutions) of 1:640 to 1:1280 have been obtained with rabbit antisera (Martos *et al.*, 1970) to strain AD 169 in the presence or absence of complement. This contrasts with neutralization titers of 1:100 to 1:200 in the absence of complement, and 1:900 to 1:1800 in the presence of complement with goat antisera to strain AD 169 (Haines *et al.*, 1971). The reason for the difference in the neutralization titers against isologous virus of the rabbit and goat antisera in the presence and absence of complement is probably due to the host's response to the particular virus strain employed, as demonstrated in rabbits immunized with various strains of CMV (Andersen, 1972).

Differentiation of human CMV strains by neutralization has been accomplished with human sera (Weller *et al.*, 1960) and with hyperimmune sera prepared in monkeys (Plummer and Benyesh-Melnick, 1964), guinea pigs (Krech and Jung, 1969; Wentworth and French, 1970), rabbits (Andersen, 1971), and goats (Haines *et al.*, 1971). Neither goat (Haines *et al.*, 1971) nor rabbit (B. Hampar, unpublished observations) anti-human-CMV sera neutralize simian CMV; conversely, anti-simian-CMV sera do not neutralize human CMV.

C. Simian Cytomegaloviruses

Cytomegaloviruses (CMV) have been isolated from African green monkeys (Malherbe and Harwin, 1957; Black *et al.*, 1963), rhesus monkeys (Smith *et al.*, 1969), and owl monkeys (Chopra *et al.*, 1972). Natural antibodies to simian CMV are found in sera from African green monkeys, rhesus monkeys, and baboons (Dreesman and Benyesh-Melnick, 1967).

Neutralizing antisera to simian CMV have been prepared in rabbits (Ablashi *et al.*, 1969), monkeys, baboons (Graham *et al.*, 1969), and goats (Haines *et al.*, 1971). The neutralization titers (based on final antibody dilutions) of rabbit and goat antisera are comparable (1:1290 to 1:1800). In the case of hyperimmune rabbit antisera (Hampar *et al.*, 1969b), the 19 S antibodies show a high degree of specificity for the immunizing virus, and have been used for differentiating closely related strains.

D. *Varicella–Zoster Virus*

The viruses associated with varicella (chicken pox) and zoster (shingles) are considered identical and are classified into one herpesvirus group. Varicella–zoster virus (V–Z virus) for serologic studies can be obtained either from vesicular fluids or from infected tissue cultures (Weller, 1953).

Complement-fixation tests using human sera reveal no antigenic differences between the viruses isolated from varicella and zoster lesions (Brain, 1933; Weller and Witton, 1958; Taylor-Robinson and Downie, 1959; Caunt *et al.*, 1961; Schmidt *et al.*, 1964; Gold and Godek, 1965). Neutralization studies with V–Z virus were hampered initially by the lack of suitable virus preparations, since infectious virus is not readily found in the nutrient fluids from infected cultures. However, infectious virus can be obtained from sonically disrupted human or African green monkey (vero) infected cells (Caunt, 1963; Caunt and Taylor-Robinson, 1964; Gold, 1965; Caunt and Shaw, 1969). In contrast to the cell association of tissue culture grown virus, cell-free virus which is neutralizable can be obtained from vesicular fluids (Taylor-Robinson, 1959). Neutralization studies by plaque reduction (Rapp and Vanderslice, 1964) or tube dilution, immunofluorescent studies (Weller and Coons, 1954), and indirect hemagglutination tests (Furukawa and Plotkin, 1972) with human sera reveal no antigenic differences between the viruses of varicella and zoster, and there is no evidence of antigenic heterogeneity (intratypic variants) among various isolates.

The primary infection with V–Z virus (varicella) is characterized by the appearance of both IgM and IgG antibodies, while in secondary infections (zoster) only IgG antibodies are demonstrable (Leonard *et al.*, 1970). Significant differences have been noted (Leonard *et al.*, 1970) in the IgG antibodies following varicella and zoster infections, which are related to their electrophoretic mobilities. The "slow" migrating IgG antibodies in both varicella and zoster infections neutralize V–Z virus and react with infected cells by immunofluorescence. In contrast, the "fast" migrating IgG antibodies in varicella infections react weakly by immunofluorescence but show no neutralizing activity, while comparable antibodies in zoster infections react by both neutralization and immunofluorescence. Differences in the properties of antibodies produced in response to primary and secondary V–Z virus infections have also been detected by the indirect hemagglutination (IHA) test (Furukawa and Plotkin, 1972). In secondary zoster infections, the serum IHA titers correlate well with the complement-fixing and neutralization titers, while in primary varicella infections the IHA titers are low or absent despite significant complement-fixing titers and variable neutralization titers. Antibodies detected by IHA are limited to the IgG class even though anti-V–Z virus IgM antibodies may be present in the same serum.

It appears that the complement-fixing and precipitating antigens of V–Z virus differ from both vesicular fluids (Taylor-Robinson and Rondle, 1959) and tissue culture prepared antigens (Caunt *et al.*, 1961). In the tissue culture system, for example, optimal complement-fixing antigen is obtained at 36°–38°C, while precipitating antigen is more readily demonstrated in cultures incubated at 27°–31°C (Caunt *et al.*, 1961). Multiple precipitin bands have been detected with human convalescent sera using antigens from vesicular fluids (Brunell *et al.*, 1971) and infected tissue cultures (Brunell *et al.*, 1972).

Experimental antisera to V–Z virus have been prepared in rhesus monkeys (Schmidt *et al.*, 1965), guinea pigs (Kissling *et al.*, 1968), and rabbits (Kissling *et al.*, 1968; Martos *et al.*, 1970).

Using human sera, no antigenic relationship has been observed between V–Z virus and HSV by immunofluorescence (Weller and Coons, 1954) or between V–Z virus and HSV (Weller and Witton, 1958) or human CMV (Rowe *et al.*, 1956; Weller *et al.*, 1957) by complement fixation or indirect hemagglutination (Furukawa and Plotkin, 1972). However, numerous studies have suggested a relationship between V–Z virus and HSV based on a rise in antibody titers to the heterologous virus following human infection with either virus. This anamnestic response is dependent upon a preexisting infection with the heterologous virus. Following infection with HSV, for example, the antibody titers to V–Z virus may increase as detected by complement fixation (Kapsenburg, 1964; Svedmyr, 1965; Schmidt *et al.*, 1969), neutralization, and immunofluorescence (Schmidt *et al.*, 1969). Conversely, infection with V–Z virus may be followed by increased antibody titers to HSV by complement fixation (Ross *et al.*, 1965; Schmidt *et al.*, 1969), but apparently not by neutralization (Schmidt *et al.*, 1969). It is of interest that increased antibody titers to heterologous HSV are more apt to occur following the onset of varicella than zoster, which may be a reflection of the more systemic character of varicella in comparison to the more circumscribed pattern of zoster (Schaap and Huisman, 1968). One preliminary report (Trlifajova *et al.*, 1970) also suggests partial or complete identity of V–Z virus and HSV precipitin antigen(s) in agar gel.

Despite the proposed antigenic relationship between V–Z virus and HSV, no such relationship has been observed by immunofluorescence with monkey antisera (Schmidt *et al.*, 1965). Similarly, guinea pig antisera prepared against HSV types 1 or 2 capsid and enveloped particles do not fix complement with V–Z virus-associated antigens, and guinea pig antisera to V–Z virus antigens do not fix complement with HSV types 1 or 2 capsid, envelope, or soluble antigens (Kissling *et al.*, 1968; Martin *et al.*, 1972). Furthermore, high titered rabbit antisera to V–Z virus (Martos *et al.*, 1970) at a 1:4 dilution in the presence or absence of complement show no neutralizing activity against HSV types 1 or 2 (B. Hampar, unpublished observations). Conversely, high-titered rabbit antisera to HSV types 1 and

2 (Hampar *et al.*, 1970a) do not neutralize V–Z virus at 1:4 dilutions in the presence or absence of complement. The same rabbit antisera by direct immunofluorescence show no cross reactivity between V–Z virus and HSV.

Based on the apparent discrepancies between the findings with human sera and animal antisera, the question of common antigens between V–Z virus and HSV remains unanswered. It may be that the anamnestic rise in antibody titers to heterologous virus seen in human infections is a reflection of antibody stimulation resulting from these two viruses affecting the same target cells, rather than a reflection of common or cross-reacting antigens.

E. Epstein-Barr Virus (Human Herpes-Type Virus)

The discovery of a herpes-type virus (EB virus) in human lymphoblastoid cells derived from Burkitt's lymphoma (Epstein *et al.*, 1964) has led to intensive studies to determine a possible etiologic role for this virus in human tumors. The interest in EB virus was further heightened by evidence, discovered using different techniques, of a repressed viral genome in "virus-negative" cells (Hinuma and Grace, 1968; Zur Hausen and Schulte-Holthausen, 1970; Hampar *et al.*, 1971b) which could be activated by treatment with 5-bromodeoxyuridine (Hampar *et al.*, 1972a; Gerber, 1972). This is the first human herpesvirus shown capable of persisting in human cells in a repressed but inducible state.

Serologic studies with EB virus were initiated by Henle and co-workers who demonstrated by direct and indirect immunofluorescence (Henle and Henle, 1966) and by complement fixation (Armstrong *et al.*, 1966) the reactivity of virus-containing cells with human sera from "healthy" individuals and from individuals suffering from either Burkitt's lymphoma or other nonrelated diseases. The incidence of antibodies to EB virus, or a serologically related virus, in the United States, is approximately 30% in children and 90% in adults as shown by immunofluorescence (Armstrong *et al.*, 1966), attesting to the widespread nature of this virus. In African children with lymphomas, the incidence of antibodies to EB virus is 100% as shown by immunofluorescence (Armstrong *et al.*, 1966), while "healthy" African children show an incidence level of approximately 50% (Levy and Henle, 1966). Comparable results have been obtained by complement fixation, with 100% of African children with lymphomas showing antibodies (Armstrong *et al.*, 1966), while 45–70% of American children and 90% of adults having complement-fixing antibodies (Gerber and Rosenblum, 1968; Porter *et al.*, 1969). Sero-epidemiologic studies indicate that complement-fixing antibodies to EB virus appear before comparable antibodies to herpes simplex or human cytomegalovirus (Gerber and Rosenblum, 1968; Porter *et al.*, 1969).

An etiologic role for EB virus, or a serologically related virus, in the onset of heterophile-positive infectious mononucleosis (I.M.) was proposed by the Henle's (Henle and Henle, 1968; Diehl *et al.*, 1968) based on observations that (a) the appearance of antibodies to EB virus coincided with the onset of I.M.; (b) the onset of I.M. coincided with the ability of buffy coat cells to undergo spontaneous blastoid transformation *in vitro*, which apparently requires the presence of the EB virus genome (Pope *et al.*, 1969b; Gerber *et al.*, 1969); and (c) EB virus was present in lymphoblastoid cell lines derived from I.M. patients. The serologic findings with I.M. were confirmed (Gerber *et al.*, 1968; Niederman *et al.*, 1968; Evans *et al.*, 1968) and were extended by immunoferritin studies (Hampar *et al.*, 1971a) which showed that antibodies to EB virus capsids in acute I.M. sera (heterophile antibody-positive) were of the IgM class, whereas antibodies of similar specificity in "normal" adult human sera were of the IgG class. Antibodies to EB virus of the IgM class have also been detected in I.M. patient sera by immunofluorescence (Blacklow *et al.*, 1971; Banatvala *et al.*, 1972), and it has been suggested that detection of IgM antibodies may be enhanced by fractionating the sera to avoid possible inhibition by cross-reacting IgG antibodies (Banatvala *et al.*, 1972). The presence of IgM antibodies in I.M. patient sera suggest a primary immunogenic exposure to this virus (Uhr, 1964).

A possible relationship between EB virus and other malignancies has been suggested on the basis of sero-epidemiologic studies. Although the number and types of studies carried out are still not sufficient to allow definitive conclusions, there does seem to be a high incidence of antibodies to EB virus in patients with carcinoma of the postnasal spaces (de Schryver *et al.*, 1969; Old *et al.*, 1966) and with Hodgkins disease (Johansson *et al.*, 1970; Levine *et al.*, 1971).

Most studies with EB virus and associated antigens have been carried out with human sera, although some studies have employed antisera prepared in rabbits against partially purified virus. The difficulties in attempting to draw conclusions with such sera should be obvious, since the human sera contain antibodies of diverse specificities and the rabbit antisera were made against virus preparations of questionable purity. Despite these short-comings, some progress has been made in delineating the spectrum of antigens associated with EB virus particles and infected cells. However, caution is advisable before accepting the conclusions drawn with these reagents concerning the specificity of the antigen(s) being detected.

The antigens used for serologic studies with EB virus have come from three major sources. The first two sources, which have been used in most of the studies to date, have employed either carrier cultures of EB virus or "virus-negative" lymphoblastoid cells which have been infected with

EB virus derived from carrier cultures. The third source, which has only recently been described (Hampar *et al.*, 1972a; Gerber, 1972), employs "virus-negative" cells in which the virus genome has been activated by treatment with 5-bromodeoxyuridine or 5-iododeoxyuridine.

Immunofluorescent studies using human sera suggest at least three major antigen complexes associated with EB virus-infected cells. The first is an "early" antigen (EA) complex (Henle *et al.*, 1970) which appears in "virus-negative" cells infected with EB virus prior to virus synthesis and which also appears in cells where infection is aborted. The EA complex, which appears first in the nucleus, apparently consists of at least two components (Henle *et al.*, 1971b). The antigen(s) responsible for the diffuse staining resists fixation in ethanol and methanol, while staining of the restricted antigen(s) is substantially reduced with these fixatives. Conversely, fluorescent staining of the restricted antigen(s) is more resistant to treatment with proteolytic enzymes than is staining of the diffuse antigen(s). The EA complex is the only one seen by immunofluorescence following activation of the EB virus genome by short-term treatment with 5-bromodeoxyuridine or 5-iododeoxyuridine (Gerber, 1972; Gerber and Lucas, 1972; Didier-Fichet and de-Thé, 1972) and is the first antigen seen in long-term treated cells prior to the appearance of virus (Hampar *et al.*, 1972a,b).

The second major EB virus–antigen complex apparently involves "virus-associated" (VCA) antigens. Human sera which show specificity for this antigen complex react as shown by immunofluorescence, with fixed cells which contain virus particles (zur Hausen *et al.*, 1967; Epstein and Achong, 1968) and possess antibodies which either coat cell-free virus particles (Mayyasi *et al.*, 1967; Hinuma *et al.*, 1967; de Schryver *et al.*, 1969) or react, by immunoferritin, with intracellular virus (Hampar *et al.*, 1970b). All human sera which react with the EA complex also react with the VCA antigen complex, while the converse is not true (Henle *et al.*, 1971a). It has been suggested that the intracellular VCA complex detected by immunofluorescence consists of EB virus capsid antigens (Henle *et al.*, 1970). This conclusion has been questioned, however, by findings with rabbit antisera prepared by intravenous immunization with partially purified virus where reaction with intracellular virus capsids is observed by immunoferritin (Fig. 3), although the sera do not react by immunofluorescence with virus-containing cells (Hampar *et al.*, 1970b). Alternatively, rabbit antisera prepared against partially purified virus by a combination of intramuscular and intravenous injections (Epstein and Achong, 1968) do react by immunofluorescence with virus-containing cells. It is of interest that rabbit antisera prepared against partially purified virus by a combination of intramuscular, footpad, and intravenous injections (Konn *et al.*, 1969) show three precipitin bands with EB virus-infected cell extracts; only one of which contains antibody-coated virus particles by electron microscopy.

The third major EB virus–antigen complex detected by immunofluorescence is associated with cell membranes (Klein *et al.*, 1966; Goldstein *et al.*, 1969). This antigen complex is detected on the surface of viable (unfixed) cells, in contrast to EA and VCA antigen(s) which are detected in fixed cells. The membrane–antigen complex can also be detected by techniques utilizing radio-iodine-labeled globulins (Inoue and Klein, 1970; Hewetson *et al.*, 1972). The specificity of the membrane antigen(s) and VCA and EA complexes, apparently differ (Pearson *et al.*, 1969; Henle *et al.*, 1971a). The membrane-associated complex probably consists of more than one antigen (Pearson *et al.*, 1969; Svedmyr *et al.*, 1970) and apparently includes at least one antigen which is also present in the EB virus envelope (Gerber and Goldstein, 1970; Pearson *et al.*, 1970; Silvestre *et al.*, 1971). This is analogous to HSV, where envelope antigen(s) appear on the surface of infected cells (Roane and Roizman, 1964). The synthesis of membrane-associated antigen(s) in experimentally infected cells follows the synthesis of EA and may occur before or simultaneously with the synthesis of VCA (Pearson *et al.*, 1971). Similarly, in "virus-negative" cells where the viral genome has been activated by short-term treatment with 5-bromodeoxyuridine, synthesis of EA occurs in the absence of VCA or membrane antigen(s) synthesis (Gerber and Lucas, 1972).

Activation of the EB viral genome in lymphoblastoid cells occurs during the "normal" cell cycle, and recruitment of additional activated cells is inhibited by the DNA inhibitors, 1β-D-arabinofuranosylcytosine (ara-C) and hydroxyurea (HU) (Hampar *et al.*, 1972b). Once the activation step has been initiated, synthesis of EA, but not VCA, occurs in the presence of ara-C (Gergely *et al.*, 1971) or HU. Synthesis of EA is followed by synthesis of new DNA which bands in neutral cesium chloride at densities corresponding to normal human DNA and EB virus DNA. Synthesis of this new DNA is inhibited by ara-C but not HU and is followed by synthesis of VCA (Hampar *et al.*, 1972b).

Three major antigen complexes have also been detected by complement fixation in EB virus infected cells. One complex is associated with virus particles (probably capsids) and is heat resistant (Gerber and Birch, 1967; Walters and Pope, 1971). The second complex, which is heat labile, is separable from virus particles but is sedimentable at 70,000 *g* for 2 hours (Walters and Pope, 1971) and may represent a subviral component. The third complex is heat resistant and soluble (Gerber and Deal, 1970; Vonka *et al.*, 1970b; Walters and Pope, 1971). A comparable soluble complex has been detected in "virus-negative" cells (Pope *et al.*, 1969a; Gerber and Deal, 1970; Vonka *et al.*, 1970a). Whether this complex is virus specific and whether it is identical to the soluble complex from the virus-positive cells have not been established unequivocally.

A recently described fluorescent complement-fixation test (Floyd *et al.*,

1971) may also prove useful in studies relating to EB virus. This test apparently detects intracellular antigen–antibody complexes.

CROSS REACTIONS WITH OTHER HERPESVIRUSES

The EB virus is apparently unrelated serologically to other human herpesviruses (Henle and Henle, 1966). However, a herpes-type virus in subhuman primates is closely related, if not identical, to EB virus in man. Cultures of chimpanzee peripheral cells show a herpes-type virus (Landon *et al.*, 1968) which react with human and simian sera as demonstrated with immunofluorescence (Goldman *et al.*, 1968) and immunodiffusion (Stevens *et al.*, 1970). Conversely, complement-fixing antibodies to EB virus are detected readily in sera from chimpanzees, cynomologous, rhesus, and African green monkeys, but rarely in baboons (Gerber and Birch, 1967). Chimpanzee sera react with EB virus particles as demonstrated by the antibody-coating test (Gerber and Birch, 1967) and with EB "virus-associated (Goldman *et al.*, 1968; Levy *et al.*, 1971) and membrane-associated antigens (Gerber and Goldstein, 1970) as shown by immunofluorescence. Sera from macaques monkeys also react with EB virus-infected human cells as demonstrated by immunofluorescence (Landon and Malan, 1971), with the incidence of antibodies being related to the age and the containment conditions of the animals. Sera from African green monkeys have also been shown to react with the soluble complement-fixing antigen complex from human "virus-negative" lymphoblastoid cells (Gerber and Deal, 1970). Although some studies suggest antigenic differences between EB virus and the herpes-type virus in subhuman primates (Goldman *et al.*, 1968; Stevens *et al.*, 1970), conclusive proof will require more sensitive procedures using purified reagents.

Acknowledgments

The studies cited from our laboratory were supported in part by Contract No. NIH-NCI-E-71-2097 from the Special Virus-Cancer Program of the National Cancer Institute. We thank Mr. J. L. Walker for the electron micrograph and Mr. David Coates for photographic work. Our special thanks to Nancy Tucker, without whom this chapter would not have been completed.

References

Ablashi, D. V., Martos, L. M., Gilden, R. V., and Hampar, B. (1969). *J. Immunol.* **102**, 263.
Abodeely, R. A., Palmer, E. L., Lawson, L. A., and Randall, C. C. (1971). *Virology* **44**, 146.
Adam, E., Levy, A. H., Rawls, W. E., and Melnick, J. L. (1971). *J. Nat. Cancer Inst.* **47**, 941.
Adam, E., Sharma, S. D., Zeigler, O., Iwamoto, K., Melnick, J. L., Levy, A. H., and Rawls, W. E. (1972). *J. Nat. Cancer Inst.* **48**, 65.

Amelunxen, R. E., and Werder, A. A. (1960). *J. Bacteriol.* **80**, 271.
Andersen, H. K. (1971). *Arch. Gesamte Virusforsch.* **33**, 187.
Andersen, H. K. (1972). *Arch. Gesamte Virusforsch.* **36**, 133.
Andervont, H. B. (1929). *J. Infec. Dis.* **44**, 383.
Armstrong, D., Henle, G., and Henle, W. (1966). *J. Bacteriol.* **91**, 1257.
Ashe, W. K., and Notkins, A. L. (1966). *Proc. Nat. Acad. Sci. U.S.* **56**, 447.
Ashe, W. K., and Scherp, H. W. (1963). *J. Immunol.* **91**, 658.
Ashe, W. K., and Scherp, H. W. (1965). *J. Immunol.* **94**, 385.
Aurelian, L. (1968). *Proc. Soc. Exp. Biol. Med.* **127**, 485.
Banatvala, J. E., Best, J. M., and Waller, D. K. (1972) *Lancet* **2**, 1205.
Becker, Y., and Olshevsky, U. (1972). *In* "Oncogenesis and Herpesviruses" (P. M. Biggs, G. de-Thé, and L. N. Payne, eds.), pp. 420–427. Int. Agency Res. Cancer, Lyon.
Benda, R. (1966). *Acta Virol. (Prague), Engl. Ed.* **10**, 348.
Benyesh-Melnick, M., Rosenberg, H. S., and Watson, P. (1964). *Proc. Soc. Exp. Biol. Med.* **117**, 452.
Benyesh-Melnick, M., Vonka, V., Probstmeyer, F., and Wimberly, I. (1966). *J. Immunol.* **96**, 261.
Berlin, B. S. (1963). *Proc. Soc. Exp. Biol. Med.* **113**, 1013.
Bernstein, M. T., and Stewart, J. A. (1971). *Appl. Microbiol.* **21**, 84.
Black, P. H., Hartley, J. W., and Rowe, W. P. (1963). *Proc. Soc. Exp. Biol. Med.* **112**, 601.
Blacklow, N. R., Watson, B. K., Miller, G., and Jacobson, B. M. (1971). *Amer. J. Med.* **51**, 549.
Brain, R. T. (1933). *Brit. J. Exp. Pathol.* **14**, 67.
Breese, S. S., Jr., and Hsu, K. C. (1971). *In* "Methods in Virology" (K. Maramorosch and H. Koprowski, eds.), Vol 5, pp. 399–422. Academic Press, New York.
Brunell, P. A., Cohen, B., and Granat, M. (1971). *Bull. WHO* **44**, 811.
Brunell, P. A., Granat, M., and Gershon, A. A. (1972). *J. Immunol.* **108**, 731.
Buddingh, G. J., Schrum, D. I., Lanier, J. C., and Guidry, D. J. (1953). *Pediatrics* **11**, 595.
Burnet, F. M., and Lush, D. (1939). *Lancet* **1**, 629.
Burnet, F. M., Lush, D., and Jackson, A. V. (1939). *Aust. J. Exp. Biol. Med. Sci.* **17**, 41.
Casals, J. (1967). *In* "Methods in Virology" (K. Maramorosch and H. Koprowski, eds.), Vol. 3, pp. 113–193. Academic Press, New York.
Caunt, A. E. (1963). *Lancet* **2**, 982.
Caunt, A. E., and Shaw, D. G. (1969). *J. Hyg.* **67**, 343.
Caunt, A. E., and Taylor-Robinson, D. (1964). *J. Hyg.* **62**, 413.
Caunt, A. E., Rondle, C. J. M., and Downie, A. W. (1961). *J. Hyg.* **59**, 249.
Centifano, Y. M., and Kaufman, H. E. (1970). *Infec. Immunity,* **2**, 778.
Chen, J. H., Lee, L. F., Nazerian, K., and Burmester, B. R. (1972). *Virology* **47**, 434.
Chiang, W.-T., Wentworth, B. B., and Alexander, E. R. (1970). *J. Immunol.* **104**, 992.
Chitwood, L. A., and Bracken, E. C. (1964). *Virology* **24**, 116.
Chopra, H. C., Lloyd, B. J., Jr., Ablashi, D. V., and Armstrong, G. R. (1972). *J. Nat. Cancer Inst.* **48**, 1333.
Coons, A. H., and Kaplan, M. H. (1950). *J. Exp. Med.* **91**, 1.
Courtney, R. J., McCombs, R. M., and Benyesh-Melnick, M. (1970). *Virology* **40**, 379.
Courtney, R. J., McCombs, R. M., and Benyesh-Melnick, M. (1971). *Virology* **43**, 356.
Cowan, K. M., and Trautman, R. (1965). *J. Immunol.* **94**, 858.
Daniels, C. A., Borsos, T., Rapp, H. J., Snyderman, R., and Notkins, A. L. (1970). *Proc. Nat. Acad. Sci. U.S.* **65**, 528.
Dascomb, H. E., Adair, C. V., and Rogers, N. (1955). *J. Lab. Clin. Med.* **46**, 1.
Davenport, F. M., and Hennessy, A. V. (1957). *J. Exp. Med.* **106**, 835.
de Schryver, A., Friberg, S., Jr., Klein, G., Henle, W., Henle, G., de Thé, G., Clifford, P., and Ho, H. H. (1969). *Clin. Exp. Immunol.* **5**, 443.
de St. Groth, F. (1961). *Nature (London)* **191**, 891.
Didier-Fichet, M-L., and de-Thé, G. (1972). *C. R. Acad. Sci. Paris* **274**, 2549.

Diehl, V., Henle, G., Henle, W., and Kohn, G. (1968). *J. Virol.* **2**, 663.
Dixon, F. L., Jacot-Guillarmod, J., and McConahey, P. J. (1966). *J. Immunol.* **97**, 350.
Douglas, R. G., Jr., and Couch, R. B. (1970). *J. Immunol.* **104**, 289.
Dowdle, W. R., Nahmias, A. J., Harwell, R. W., and Pauls, F. P. (1967). *J. Immunol.* **99**, 974.
Dreesman, G. R., and Benyesh-Melnick, M. (1967). *J. Immunol.* **99**, 1106.
Dulbecco, R., Vogt, M., and Strickland, A. G. R. (1956). *Virology* **2**, 162.
Ejercito, P. M., Kieff, E. D., and Roixman, B. (1968). *J. Gen. Virol.* **2**, 357.
Epstein, M. A., and Achong, B. G. (1968). *J. Nat. Cancer Inst.* **40**, 593.
Epstein, M. A., Achong, B. G., and Barr, Y. M. (1964). *Lancet* **1**, 702.
Evans, A. S., Niederman, J. C., and McCollum, R. W. (1968). *N. Engl. J. Med.* **279**, 1121.
Floyd, R., Vonka, V., and Benyesh-Melnick, M. (1971). *J. Nat. Cancer Inst.* **46**, 383.
Fuccillo, D. A., Moder, F. L., Catalano, L. W., Jr., Vincent, M. M., and Sever, J. L. (1970). *Proc. Soc. Exp. Biol. Med.* **133**, 735.
Fuccillo, D. A., Moder, F. L., Traub, R. G., Hensen, S., and Sever, J. L. (1971). *Appl. Microbiol.* **21**, 104.
Fujiwara, S., and Kaplan, A. S. (1967). *Virology* **32**, 60.
Furukawa, T., and Plotkin, S. A. (1972). *Infec. Immunity.* **5**, 835.
Furukawa, T., Jensen, F., Fioretti, A., and Plotkin, S. A. (1972). *ASM Abstr*, **v-364**, 226.
Geder, L., and Skinner, G. R. B: (1971). *J. Gen. Virol.* **12**, 179.
Gerber, P. (1972). *Proc. Nat. Acad. Sci. U.S.* **69**, 83.
Gerber, P., and Birch, S. M. (1967). *Proc. Nat. Acad. Sci. U.S.* **58**, 478.
Gerber, P., and Deal, D. R. (1970). *Proc. Soc. Exp. Biol. Med.* **134**, 748.
Gerber, P., and Goldstein, G. (1970). *J. Immunol.* **105**, 793.
Gerber, P., and Lucas, S. (1972). *Proc. Soc. Exp. Biol. Med.* **141**, 431.
Gerber, P., and Rosenblum, E. N. (1968). *Proc. Soc. Exp. Biol. Med.* **128**, 541.
Gerber, P., Hamre, D., Moy, R. A., and Rosenblum, E. N. (1968). *Science* **161**, 173.
Gerber, P., Whang-Peng, J., and Monroe, J. H. (1969). *Proc. Nat. Acad. Sci. U.S.* **63**, 740.
Gergely, L., Klein, G., and Ernberg, I. (1971). *Int. J. Cancer* **7**, 293.
Gold, E. (1965). *J. Immunol.* **95**, 683.
Gold, E., and Godek, G. (1965). *J. Immunol.* **95**, 692.
Gold, E., Wildy, P., and Watson, D. H. (1963). *J. Immunol.* **91**, 666.
Goldman, M., Landon, J. C., and Reisher, J. I. (1968). *Cancer Res.* **28**, 2489.
Goldstein, G., Klein, G., Pearson, G. R., and Clifford, P. (1969). *Cancer Res.* **29**, 749.
Goodheart, C. R., Plummer, G., and Waner, J. L. (1968). *Virology* **35**, 473.
Goodman, J. W., and Donch, J. J. (1965). *Immunochemistry* **2**, 351.
Goodpasture, E. W., and Teague, O. (1923). *J. Med. Res.* **44**, 121.
Gower, J. C. (1966). *Biometrika* **53**, 325.
Graham, B., Minamishima, Y., and Benyesh-Melnick, M. (1969). *Bacteriol. Proc.* **69**, 198.
Haines, H. G., von Essen, R., and Benyesh-Melnick, M. (1971). *Proc. Soc. Exp. Biol. Med.* **138**, 846.
Hampar, B., and Burroughs, M. A. K. (1969). *J. Nat. Cancer Inst.* **43**, 621.
Hampar, B., and Copeland, M. L. (1965). *J. Bacteriol.* **90**, 205.
Hampar, B., and Keehn, M. A. (1967). *J. Immunol.* **99**, 554.
Hampar, B., Notkins, A. L., Mage, M., and Keehn, M. A. (1968a). *J. Immunol.* **100**, 586.
Hampar, B., Mage, M., and Keehn, M. A. (1968b). *J. Immunol.* **101**, 256.
Hampar, B., Stevens, D. A., Martos, L. M., Ablashi, D. V. Burroughs, M. A. K., and Wells, G. A. (1969a). *J. Immunol.* **102**, 397.
Hampar, B., Martos, L. M., Ablashi, D. V., Siguenza, R. F., and Wells, G. A. (1969b). *J. Immunol.* **103**, 1155.
Hampar, B., Martos, L. M., Chakrabarty, M., and Burroughs, M. A. K. (1970a). *J. Immunol.* **104**, 593.

Hampar, B., Gerber, P., Hsu, K. C., Martos, L. M., Walker, J. L., Siquenza, R. F., and Wells, G. A. (1970b). *J. Nat. Cancer Inst.* **45**, 75.
Hampar, B., Hsu, K. C., Martos, L. M., and Walker, J. L. (1971a) *Proc. Nat. Acad. Sci. U.S.* **68**, 1407.
Hampar, B., Derge, J. G., Martos, L. M., and Walker, J. L. (1971b). *Proc. Nat. Acad. Sci. U.S.* **68**, 3185.
Hampar, B., Miyamoto, K., and Martos, L. M. (1971c). *J. Immunol.* **106**, 580.
Hampar, B., Derge, J. G., Martos, L. M., and Walker, J. L. (1972a). *Proc. Nat. Acad. Sci. U.S.* **69**, 78.
Hampar, B., Derge, J. G., Martos, L. M., Tagamets, M. A., and Burroughs, M. A. (1972b). *Proc. Nat. Acad. Sci. U.S.* **69**, 2589.
Hanshaw, J. B. (1966). *Pediat. Clin. N. Amer.* **13**, 279.
Hanshaw, J. B., Steinfeld, H. J., and White, C. J. (1968). *N. Engl. J. Med.* **279**, 566.
Hanshaw, J. B., Neiderman, J. C., and Chessin, L. N. (1972). *J. Infec. Dis.* **125**, 304.
Heineman, H. S. (1967). *J. Immunol.* **99**, 214.
Henle, G., and Henle, W. (1966). *J. Bacteriol.* **91**, 1248.
Henle, G., and Henle, W. (1968). *Proc. Nat. Acad. Sci. U.S.* **59**, 94.
Henle, G., Henle, W., Klein, G., Gunven, P., Clifford, P., Morrow, R. H., and Ziegler, J. L. (1971a). *J. Nat. Cancer Inst.* **46**, 861.
Henle, G., Henle, W., and Klein, G. (1971b). *Int. J. Cancer* **8**, 272.
Henle, W., Henle, G., Zajac, B. A., Pearson, G. R., Waubke, R., and Scriba, M. (1970). *Science* **169**, 188.
Hewetson, H. F., Gothoskar, B., and Klein, G. (1972). *J. Nat. Cancer Inst.* **48**, 87.
Hinuma, Y., and Grace, J. T., Jr. (1968). *Cancer* **22**, 1089.
Hinuma, Y., Konn, M., Yamaguchi, J., Wurdarski, D. J., Blakeslee, J. R., Jr., and Grace, J. T. Jr. (1967). *J. Virol.* **1**, 1045.
Hoggan, M. D., and Roizman, B. (1959). *Amer. J. Hyg.* **70**, 208.
Holmes, A. W., Caldwell, R. G., Dedmon, R. E., and Deinhardt, F. (1964). *J. Immunol.* **92**, 602.
Holzel, A., Feldman, G. U., Tobin, J. O., and Harper, J. (1953). *Acta Pediat.* **42**, 206.
Hull, R. N. (1968). *Virol. Monogr.* **2**, 2–66.
Hull, R. N., Peck, F. B., Jr., Ward, T. G., and Nash, J. C. (1962). *Amer. J. Hyg.* **76**, 239.
Hull, R. N., Dwyer, A. C., Holmes, A. W., Nowakowski, E., Deinhardt, F., Lennette, E. H., and Emmons, R. W. (1972). *J. Nat. Cancer Inst.* **49**, 225.
Inoue, M., and Klein, G. (1970). *Clin. Exp. Immunol.* **7**, 39.
Iwasaki, T., and Oguna, R. (1968). *Virology* **34**, 46.
Jack, I., and Wark, M. C. (1972). *In* "Oncogenesis and Herpesviruses" (P. M. Biggs, G. de-Thé, and L. N. Payne, eds.), pp. 339–340. Int. Agency Res. Cancer, Lyon.
Johansson, B., Klein, G., Henle, W., and Henle, G. (1970). *Int. J. Cancer.* **6**, 450.
Johnson, R. T. (1964a). *J. Exp. Med.* **119**, 343.
Johnson, R. T. (1964b). *J. Exp. Med.* **120**, 359.
Joklik, W. K. (1964). *Virology* **22**, 620.
Kaplan, A. S. (1969). "Herpes Simplex and Pseudorabies Viruses." Springer-Verlag, New York.
Kaplan, A. S., and Ben-Porat, T. (1970). *Proc. Nat. Acad. Sci. U.S.* **66**, 799.
Kaplan, A. S., and Vatter, A. E. (1959). *Virology* **7**, 394.
Kaplan, A. S., Ben-Porat, T., and Kamiya, T. (1965). *Ann. N. Y. Acad. Sci.* **130**, 226.
Kapsenburg, J. G., (1964). *Arch. Gesamte Virusforsch.* **15**, 67.
Kaufman, H. E., Brown, D. C., and Ellison, E. D. (1967). *Science* **156**, 1628.
Keller, J. M., Spear, P. G., and Roizman, B. (1970). *Proc. Nat. Acad. Sci. U.S.* **65**, 865.
Kieff, E. D., Hoyer, B., Bachenheimer, S., and Roizman, B. (1972). *J. Virol.* **9**, 738.

Kilbourne, E. D., and Horsfall, F. L. (1951). *J. Immunol.* **67**, 321.
Kissling, R. E., Casey, H. L., and Palmer, E. L. (1968). *Appl. Microbiol.* **16**, 160.
Klein, G., Clifford, P., Klein, E., and Stjernsward, J. (1966). *Proc. Nat. Acad. Sci. U.S.* **55**, 1628.
Konn, M., Yohn, D. S., Hinuma, Y., Yamaguchi, J., and Grace, J. T., Jr., (1969). *Cancer* **23**, 990.
Krech, U., and Jung, M. (1969). *Arch. Gesamte Virusforsch.* **28**, 248.
Kurstak, E. (1971). *In* "Methods in Virology" (K. Maramorosch and H. Koprowski, eds.), Vol. 5, pp. 423–444. Academic Press, New York.
Landon, J. C., and Malan, L. B. (1971). *J. Nat. Cancer Inst.* **46**, 881.
Landon, J. C., Ellis, L. B., Zeve, V. H. and Fabrizio, D. P. A. (1968). *J. Nat. Cancer Inst.* **40**, 181.
Lang, D. J., and Hanshaw, J. B. (1969). *N. Engl. J. Med.* **280**, 1145.
Lang, D. J., and Noren, B. (1968). *J. Pedia.* **73**, 812.
Langenhuysen, M. M. A. C., The, T. H., Nieweg, H. O., and Kapsenberg, J. G. (1970). *Clin. Exp. Immunol.* **6**, 387.
Leonard, L. L., Schmidt, N. J., and Lennette, E. H. (1970). *J. Immunol.* **104**, 23.
Lerner, A. M., Bailey, E. J., and Nolan, D. C. (1970). *J. Immunol.* **104**, 607.
Levine, P. H., Ablashi, D. V., Berard, C. W., Carbone, P. P., Waggoner, D. E., and Malan, L. B. (1971). *Cancer* **27**, 416.
Levy, J. A., and Henle, G. (1966). *J. Bacteriol.* **92**, 275.
Levy, J. A., Levy, S. B., Hirshaut, Y., Kafuko, G., and Prince, A. (1971). *Nature (London)* **233**, 559.
Linscott, W. D., and Levinson, W. E. (1969). *Proc. Nat. Acad. Sci. U.S.* **64**, 520.
Ludwig, H. O., Biswal, N., and Benyesh-Melnick, M. (1972). *Virology* **49**, 95.
Malherbe, H., and Harwin, R. (1957). *Brit. J. Exp. Pathol.* **38**, 539.
Malherbe, H., and Harwin, R. (1958). *Lancet* **2**, 530.
Mandel, B. (1960). *Ann. N. Y. Acad. Sci.* **83**, 515.
Mandel, B. (1967). *Virology* **31**, 238.
Mantyjarvi, R. (1968). *Acta Pathol. Microbiol. Scand.* **72**, 345.
Mark, G. E., and Kaplan, A. S. (1971). *Virology* **45**, 53.
Martin, M. L., Palmer, E. L., and Kissling, R. E. (1972). *Infec. Immunity* **5**, 248.
Martos, L. M., Ablashi, D. V., Gilden, R. V., Siguenza, R. F., and Hampar, B. (1970). *J. Gen. Virol.* **7**, 169.
Mayyasi, S. A., Schidlovsky, G., Bulfone, L. M., and Buscheck, F. T. (1967). *Cancer Res.* **27**, 2020.
Medearis, D. N., Jr. (1964). *Bull. Johns Hopkins Hosp.* **114**, 181.
Melnick, J. L., and Banker, D. D. (1954). *J. Exp. Med.* **100**, 181.
Miyamoto, K., Morgan, C., Hsu, K. C., and Hampar, B. (1971). *J. Nat. Cancer Inst.* **46**, 629.
Nahmias, A. J., and Dowdle, W. R. (1968). *Progr. Med. Virol.* **10**, 110.
Nahmias, A. J., Dowdle, W. R., Naib, Z. M., Josey, W., and Luce, C. F. (1968). *Pediatrics* **42**, 659.
Nahmias, A. J., Dowdle, W. R., Kramer, J. H., Luce, C. F., and Mansour, S. C. (1969a). *J. Immunol.* **102**, 956.
Nahmias, A. J., Chiang, W.-T., Del Buono, I., and Duffey, A. (1969b). *Proc. Soc. Exp. Biol. Med.* **132**, 386.
Nahmias, A. J., Del Buono, I., Schneweis, K.-E., Gordon, D. S., and Thies, D. (1971). *Proc. Soc. Exp. Biol. Med.* **138**, 21.
Nesburn, A. B. (1969). *J. Virol.* **3**, 59.
Niederman, J. C., McCollum, R. W., Henle, G., and Henle, W. (1968). *J. Amer. Med. Ass.* **203**, 205.
Nii, S., Morgan, C., and Rose, H. M. (1968a). *J. Virol.* **2**, 517.
Nii, S., Morgan, C., Rose, H. M., and Hsu, K. C. (1968b). *J. Virol.* **2**, 1172.
O'Dea, J. F., and Dineen, J. K. (1957). *J. Gen. Microbiol.* **17**, 19.

Old, L. J., Boyse, E. A., Oettgen, H. F., De Harven, E., Geering, G., Williamson, B., and Clifford, P. (1966). *Proc. Nat. Acad. Sci. U.S.* **56**, 1699.
Olshevsky, U., and Becker, Y. (1970). *Virology* **40**, 948.
Oroszlan, S., Bova, D., Toni, R., and Gilden, R. V. (1972). *Science* **176**, 420.
Pauls, F. P., and Dowdle, W. R. (1967). *I. Immunol.* **98**, 941.
Pearson, G. R., Klein, G., Henle, G. Henle, W., and Clifford, P. (1969). *J. Exp. Med.* **129**, 707.
Pearson, G. R., Dewey, F., Klein, G., Henle, G., and Henle, W. (1970). *J. Nat. Cancer Inst.* **45**, 989.
Pearson, G. R., Henle, G., and Henle, W. (1971). *J. Nat. Cancer Inst.* **46**, 1243.
Penttinen, K., Kaarianen, L., and Myllyla, G. (1970). *Arch. Gesamte Virusforsch.* **29**, 189.
Plummer, G. (1964). *Brit. J. Exp. Pathol.* **45**, 135.
Plummer, G., and Benyesh-Melnick, M. (1964). *Proc. Soc. Exp. Biol. Med.* **117**, 145.
Plummer, G., Bowling, C. P., and Goodheart, C. R. (1969). *J. Virol.* **4**, 738.
Plummer, G., Waner, J. L., Phuangrab, A., and Goodheart, C. R. (1970). *J. Virol.* **5**, 51.
Pope, J. H., Horne, M. K., and Wetters, E. J. (1969a). *Nature (London)* **222**, 186.
Pope, J. H., Horne, M. K., and Scott, W. (1969b). *Int. J. Cancer* **4** 255.
Porter, D. D., Wimberly, I., and Benyesh-Melnick, M. (1969). *J. Amer. Med. Ass.* **208**, 1675.
Rapp, F., and Vanderslice, D. (1964). *Virology* **22**, 321.
Rappaport, I. (1970). *J. Gen. Virol.* **6**, 25.
Rawls, W. E., Tompkins, W. A. F., Figueroa, M. E., and Melnick, J. L. (1968a). *Science* **161**, 1255.
Rawls, W. E., Laurel, D., Melnick, J. L., Glicksman, J. M., and Kaufman, R. H. (1968b). *Amer. J. Epidemiol.* **87**, 647.
Rawls, W. E., Adam, E., and Melnick, J. L. (1972). *In* "Oncogenesis and Herpesviruses" (P. M. Biggs, G. de-Thé, and L. N. Payne, eds.), pp. 424–427. Int. Agency Res. Cancer, Lyon.
Rivers, T. M., and Tillett, W. S. (1923). *J. Exp. Med.* **38**, 673.
Roane, P. R., Jr., and Roizman, B. (1964). *Virology* **22**, 1.
Roane, P. R., Jr., and Roizman, B. (1966). *Virology* **29**, 668.
Robinson, D. J., and Watson, D. H. (1971). *J. Gen. Virol.* **10**, 163.
Roizman, B. (1969). *Curr. Top. Microbiol. Immunol.* **49**, 1.
Roizman, B. (1970). *In* "Viruses Affecting Man and Animals" (M. Sanders, ed), pp. 37–72. Green, St. Louis, Missouri.
Roizman, B., and Spear, P. G. (1971). *Science* **171**, 298.
Roizman, B., Spring, S. B., and Roane, P. R., Jr. (1967). *J. Virol.* **1**, 181.
Roizman, B., Keller, J. M., Spear, P. G., Terni, M., Nahmias, A. J., and Dowdle, W. R. (1970). *Nature (London)* **227**, 1253.
Rose, H. M. (1952). *J. Immunol.* **68**, 687.
Rosenberg, G. L., Wohlenberg, C., Nahmias, A. J., and Notkins, A. L. (1972). *J. Immunol.* **109**, 413.
Ross, C. A. C., Subak-Sharp, J. H., and Ferry, P. (1965). *Lancet* **2**, 708.
Ross, L. J. N., Watson, D. H., and Wildy, P. (1968). *J. Gen. Virol.* **2**, 115.
Rowe, W. P., Hartley, J. W., Waterman, S., Turner, H. C., and Huebner, R. J. (1956). *Proc. Soc. Exp. Biol. Med.* **92**, 418.
Sabin, A. B. (1934a). *Brit. J. Exp. Pathol.* **15**, 321.
Sabin, A. B. (1934b). *Brit. J. Exp. Pathol.* **15**, 372.
Sabin, A. B., and Wright, A. (1934). *J. Exp. Med.* **59**, 115.
Schaap, G. J. P., and Huisman, J. (1968). *Arch. Gesamte Virusforsch.* **25**, 52.
Schaffer, P. A., Courtney, R. J., McCombs, R. M., and Benyesh-Melnick, M. (1971). *Virology* **46**, 356.

Schmidt, N. J., Lennette, E. H., Shon, C. W., and Shinomoto, T. T. (1964). *Proc. Soc. Exp. Biol. Med.* **116**, 144.
Schmidt, N. J., Lennette, E. H., Woodie, J. D., and Ho, H. H. (1965). *J. Lab. Clin. Med.* **66**, 403.
Schmidt, N. J., Lennette, E. H., and Magoffin, R. L. (1969). *J. Gen. Virol.* **4**, 321.
Schneweis, K.-E. (1962a). *Z. Immunitaetsforsch.* **124**, 24.
Schneweis, K.-E. (1962b). *Z. Immunitaetsforsch.* **124**, 337.
Schneweis, K.-E., and Nahmias, A. J. (1971). *Z. Immunitaetsforsch.* **141**, 471.
Scott, T. F. McN. (1954). *N. Engl. J. Med.* **250**, 183.
Scott, T. F. McN. (1957). *Amer. J. Ophthalmol.* **43**, 134.
Scott, T. F. McN., Coriell, L., Blank, H., and Burgeon, C. F. (1952). *J. Pediat.* **41**, 835.
Sharma, J. M., Burger, D., and Kenzy, S. G., (1972). *Infec. Immunity* **5**, 406.
Shimono, H., Ben-Porat, T., and Kaplan, A. S. (1969). *Virology* **37**, 49.
Shope, R. E., (1931). *J. Exp. Med.* **45**, 233.
Shubladze, A. K., and Chzhu-Shan, K. (1959). *Vopr. Virusol.* **4**, 80.
Shubladze, A. K., Maevskaia, T. M., Ananev, V. A., and Volkova, V. N. (1960). *Vopr. Virusol.* **5**, 735.
Silvestre, D., Kourilsky, F. M., Klein, G., Yata, Y., Neauport-Sautes, C., and Levy, J. A. (1971). *Int. J. Cancer* **8**, 222.
Slavin, H. B., and Gavett, E. (1946). *Proc. Soc. Exp. Biol. Med.* **63**, 343.
Smith, J. W., Adam, E., Melnick, J. L., and Rawls, W. E. (1972). *J. Immunol.* **109**, 554.
Smith, K. O., Thiel, J. F., Newman, J. T., Harvey, E., Trousdale, M. D., Gehle, W. D., and Clark, G. (1969). *J. Nat. Cancer Inst.* **42**, 489.
Smith, M. G. (1956). *Proc. Soc. Exp. Biol. Med.* **92**, 424.
Spear, P. G., and Roizman, B. (1968). *Virology* **36**, 545.
Spring, S. B., Roizman, B., and Schwartz, J. (1968). *J. Virol.* **2**, 384.
Stern, H., and Elek, S. D. (1965). *J. Hyg.* **63**, 79.
Stevens, D. A., Pincus, T., Burroughs, M. A. K., and Hampar, B. (1968). *J. Immunol.* **101**, 979.
Stevens, D. A., Pry. T. W., Blackman, E. A., and Manaker, R. A. (1970). *Proc. Soc. Exp. Biol. Med.* **133**, 678.
Svedmyr, A. (1965). *Arch. Gesamte Virusforsch.* **17**, 495.
Svedmyr, A., Demissie, A., Klein, G., and Clifford, P. (1970). *J. Nat. Cancer Inst.* **44**, 595.
Svehag, S.-E. (1968). *Progr. Med. Virol.* **10**, 1.
Tankersley, R. W., Jr. (1964). *J. Bacteriol.* **97**, 609.
Taylor-Robinson, D. (1959). *Brit. J. Exp. Pathol.* **40**, 521.
Taylor-Robinson, D., and Downie, A. W. (1959). *Brit. J. Exp. Pathol.* **40**, 398.
Taylor-Robinson, D., and Rondle, C. J. M. (1959). *Brit. J. Exp. Pathol.* **40**, 517.
Terni, M., and Roizman, B. (1970). *J. Infec. Dis.* **121**, 212.
Tokumaru, T. (1965a). *J. Immunol.* **95**, 181.
Tokumaru, T. (1965b). *J. Immunol.* **95**, 189.
Tokumaru, T. (1966). *J. Immunol.* **97**, 248.
Tokumaru, T., and Scott, T. F. McNair (1964). *In* "Diagnostic Procedures for Viral and Rickettsial Diseases" (E. H. Lennette and J. N. Schmidt, eds.), pp. 381–433. Amer. Pub. Health Ass., New York.
Toussaint, A. J., and Muschel, L. H. (1962). *J. Immunol.* **89**, 35.
Trlifajova, J., Sourek, J., and Ryba, M. (1970). *Acta Virol. (Prague), Engl. Ed.* **14**, 25.
Ueda, Y., Tagaya, I., and Shiroki, K. (1968). *Arch. Gesamte Virusforsch.* **24**, 231.
Uhr, J. (1964). *Science* **145**, 457.
Vaczi, L., Gonozol, E., Lehel, F., and Geder, L. (1965). *Acta Microbiol.* **12**, 115.

Van Hoosier, G. L., Jr., and Melnick, J. L. (1961). *Tex. Rep. Biol. Med.* **19**, 376.

Vonka, V., Benyesh-Melnick, M., and McCombs, R. M. (1970a). *J. Nat. Cancer Inst.* **44**, 865.

Vonka, V., Benyesh-Melnick, M., Lewis, R. T., and Wimberly, I. (1970b). *Arch. Gesamte Virusforsch.* **31**, 113.

Wallis, C., Scheiris, C., and Melnick, J. L. (1967). *J. Immunol.* **99**, 1134.

Walters, M. K., and Pope, J. H. (1971). *Int. J. Cancer* **8**, 32.

Watson, D. H. (1969). *J. Gen. Virol.* **4**, 15.

Watson, D. H., and Wildy, P. (1969). *J. Gen. Virol.* **4**, 163.

Watson, D. H., Shedden, W. I. H., Elliot, A., Titsuka, T., Wildy, P., Bourgauz-Ramoisy, D., and Gold, E. (1966). *Immunology* **11**, 399.

Watson, D. H., Wildy, P., Harvey, B. A. M., and Shedden, W. I. H. (1967). *J. Gen. Virol.* **1**, 139.

Weinberg, A., and Becker, Y. (1969). *Virology* **39**, 312.

Weller, T. H. (1953). *Proc. Soc. Exp. Biol. Med.* **83**, 340.

Weller, T. H., and Coons, A. H. (1954). *Proc. Soc. Exp. Biol. Med.* **86**, 789.

Weller, T. H., and Witton, H. M. (1958). *J. Exp. Med.* **108**, 869.

Weller, T. H., Macaulay, J. C., Craig, J. M., and Wirth, P. (1957). *Proc. Soc. Exp. Biol. Med.* **94**, 4.

Weller, T. H., Hanshaw, J. B., and Scott, D. E. (1960). *Virology* **12**, 130.

Wentworth, B. B., and French, L. (1970). *Proc. Soc. Exp. Biol. Med.* **135**, 253.

Wheeler, C. E., Jr. (1964). *J. Immunol.* **93**, 749.

Wheeler, C. E., Jr., Briggaman, R. A., and Henderson, R. R. (1969). *J. Immunol.* **102**, 1179.

Wildy, P. (1972). *In* "Oncogenesis and Herpesviruses" (P. M. Biggs, G. de-Thé, and L. N. Payne, eds.), pp. 409–419. Int. Agency Res. Cancer, Lyon.

Witter, R. L., Nazerian, K., Purchase, H. G., and Burgoyne, G. H. (1970). *Amer. J. Vet. Res.* **31**, 525.

Womack, C. R., and Hunt, B. P. (1954). *Science* **120**, 227.

Yoshino, K., and Morishima, T. (1972). *Jap. J. Microbiol.* **16**, 125.

Yoshino, K., and Taniguchi, S. (1964). *Virology* **22**, 193.

Yoshino, K., and Taniguchi, S. (1965a). *Virology* **26**, 44.

Yoshino, K., and Taniguchi, S. (1965b). *Virology* **26**, 61.

Yoshino, K., and Taniguchi, S. (1966). *J. Immunol.* **96**, 196.

Yoshino, K., Taniguchi, S., Furasi, R., Nojima, T., Fujii, R., Minamitani, M., Tada, R., and Kubota, H. (1962). *Jap. J. Med. Sci. & Biol.* **15**, 235.

Yoshino, K., Morishima, T., and Aoki, Y. (1971). *Jap. J. Microbiol.* **15**, 53.

zur Hausen, H., and Schulte-Holthausen, H. (1970). *Nature (London)* **227**, 245.

zur Hausen, H., Henle, W., Hummeler, K., Diehl, V., and Henle, G. (1967). *J. Virol.* **1**, 830.

Chapter 8

Interference and Interferon with Respect to Herpesviruses

R. Z. Lockart, Jr.

I. Introduction

When a cell (or animal) is infected with more than one virus, there are two possible outcomes: (1) the primary infecting virus may prevent or depress the replication of the second virus or (2) both viruses may replicate in the same cell. The first phenomenon is termed interference, and the second, dual infection. Both phenomena have been recognized for some time, but interference, because of the medical importance, has had a far greater impact on virology. The early studies on interference soon established the fact that the interfering virus may be active or inactive, that both viruses may be related or unrelated, and that interference may occur with or without the intervention of interferon (Schlesinger, 1959; Wagner, 1963).

The purpose of this chapter is to discuss currently available information pertinent to interference and interferon as well as to dual infections which involve the herpesviruses.

II. Interference—Possibly Mediated by Interferon

A. *"Magrassi Phenomenon"*

One of the earliest reported examples of viral interference is the "Magrassi phenomenon" (Magrassi, 1935, 1936; Doerr and Kon, 1937; Doerr and Seidenberg, 1937; Hallauer, 1937). These workers showed that the inoculation of a nonencephalitogenic strain of herpes simplex virus into the cornea of eyes of rabbits prevented the development of encephalitis by the intracerebral inoculation a few days later of an encephalitogenic strain of herpesvirus. Perhaps even more striking was the demonstration that an encephalitogenic strain of herpesvirus when inoculated either subcutaneously or into the rabbits corneas protected animals from death after a subsequent intracerebral inoculation with the encephalitogenic strain of virus. Under the experimental conditions chosen, there was a peculiar prerequisite for a 7-day period between inoculations for the protective effect of the first to occur. Intracerebral inoculation earlier or later than 7 days after the subcutaneous inoculation resulted in death. The resistance could have resulted from interferon, specific immunity, or an as yet unknown type of viral interference. The earlier workers did not resolve the possibilities.

B. *Homologous Interference in Mice*

The above phenomenon was quite closely repeated in mice in a number of recent experiments by Catalano *et al.* (1970). Their results differed slightly however, as they found a later protective effect (after 6 days) which they showed was due to a specific antibody. However, they also found an early protective effect ($\sim 50\%$ protection at 3–6 days) of the subcutaneous inoculation of virus which was probably not due to antibody, since no antibody could be demonstrated in the sera or tissues of the animals while the mice resisted the intracerebral inoculation of a large dose of the unrelated encephalomyocarditis virus.

1. Role of Interferon

Interferon was considered the most likely possibility especially because of the report by Bostandzhyan and Bikbulatov (1967) in which they reported that mice inoculated with herpes simplex virus made interferon and that the highest titers were found in the brain tissue. However, Catalano *et al.*

(1970) were unable to conclude that the protective effect was due to interferon in the brain, as they could find none there. Furthermore, with but one exception, they could not find interferon in any of several other types of mouse tissues examined. Casting further doubt on the role of interferon in the interference was the results of another study (Catalano and Baron, 1970). In that study, the authors showed that they could induce high titers of circulating interferon in mice by use of complexed polyriboinosinic and polyribocytidylic acids (poly rI:poly rC). Yet mice so induced were not spared when inoculated intracerebrally with the same amount of the same strain of herpesvirus as was used in the previous study. However, if the amount of challenge virus was reduced to one $TCID_{50}$, some increase in survival could be demonstrated in the mice induced to make interferon. In a study in guinea pigs, Tokumaru (1967) found that local or systemic injections of interferon protected animals against herpes simplex virus injected cutaneously, peritoneally, or intravenously but gave no protection to animals inoculated by the intracerebral, intranasal, or corneal routes. These findings would seemingly explain the foregoing results by indicating the importance of the route of viral administration. The routes of the two inoculations of the virus also appears to be quite important as the study by Hamilton *et al.* (1969) suggested. They found that mice which had received herpesvirus intraperitioneally could be protected by the intraperitoneal inoculation of poly rI:poly rC given even 24 hours after the virus. Presumably, effective concentrations of interferon could be brought to bear at the site of infection. However, other effects of the poly rI.poly rC were not ruled out in that study.

After consideration of all the foregoing studies, there is some doubt as to the extent that experimental infections with herpesvirus have predictive value for natural infections. Also, we are still left without definite proof that interferon is responsible for the protective effect seen in the "Magrassi phenomenon," the classic case of interference with herpesvirus, even though it still appears to be the best explanation. If interferon is responsible, two points seem to emerge from these data. Herpes simplex virus must be considerably more resistant to the antiviral state in brain tissues than encephalomyocarditis virus (Catalano and Baron, 1970), and herpesvirus which can reach the brain from more peripheral sites brings about more effective concentrations of interferon in the brain than that obtained from circulating interferon and thus provides better protection.

2. Role of Macrophages

An interesting possibility is that peritoneal macrophages stimulated by poly rI:poly rC or the initial virus inoculation were responsible for the instances of increased resistance. The involvement of macrophages in such a mechanism was shown by Hirsch *et al.* (1970). They showed that macrophages from adult mice when stimulated by a protease–peptone solution and injected intraperitoneally into otherwise susceptible suckling mice were capable of protecting them from an otherwise fatal infection resulting from the intraperitoneal injection of herpes simplex virus. The authors showed, additionally, that the macrophages stimulated with protease–peptone produced more interferon after infection with herpesvirus, displayed enhanced phagocytosis, attached to tissue surfaces and spread more rapidly, and released less infectious virus than unstimulated macrophages. The role of macrophages cannot be discounted in the studies in which poly rI:poly rC were employed and even leave the possibility that both interferon and macrophages were involved. This concept holds especially true in those cases where both the route of infection and the dose of challenge virus are highly significant determinants of whether or not one sees protection.

III. Interference Not Mediated by Interferon

A. Homologous

In addition to those instances attributed to interferon, there are several reports of interference of an intracellular nature in which either homologous herpes or another virus interferes with herpesviruses. In a unique example of homologous interference, Roizman (1965) demonstrated that a strain of herpes simplex that produced few, if any, infectious virions in dog kidney cells greatly inhibited the multiplication of a mutant of that same strain which could reproduce in these cells. His analysis of the mechanism of the inhibition led him to conclude that nonfunctional proteins or peptides of the deficient virus formed aggregates by polymerizing with potentially functional subunits of the multiplying strain, thus rendering them nonfunctional and bringing about the observed interference.

B. Heterologous

Johnson *et al.* (1964) showed that poliovirus could interfere with plaque formation by herpes simplex virus on human amnion cells. They ruled out both interferon and altered adsorption of herpesvirus as being responsible. The excellent series of experiments by Saxton and Stevens (1972) provided the explanation. They found that HeLa cells infected with herpes simplex virus and superinfected 5 or 10 hours later with poliovirus promptly stopped making herpesvirus proteins. Herpesvirus DNA and RNA were not affected. They showed that the superinfection with poliovirus brought about a rapid disaggregation of polysomes containing herpesvirus RNA, and thus translation of herpesvirus mRNA into protein was prevented. They even went a step further and showed that poliovirus RNA replication was not required (but gene expression was) for the inhibition to be manifest. They did this by showing that poliovirus could inhibit herpesvirus in the presence of 1.5 m*M* guanidine, but poliovirus was unable to inhibit the herpesvirus if it had been inactivated by ultraviolet irradiation. In another study in which interferon was not implicated, Van der Noordaa *et al.* (1966) showed that herpes simplex virus multiplication was greatly reduced in either hamster or human cells which had been transformed by SV40 virus. After ruling out that reduced viral adsorption was responsible, they concluded that some yet unknown mechanism, owing to the presence in the nucleus of the SV40 genome, was responsible. Interestingly both Sindbis virus, an RNA virus, and vaccinia, another DNA virus but one which multiplies in the cytoplasm, multiplied normally in the transformed cells. Frankel and Groupé (1971) recently reported similarly that cells from a flock of pathogen-free chickens when first infected with the avian leukosis virus, Rous-associated virus 2, were considerably reduced in their ability to support the multiplication of Marek's disease herpesvirus. The authors could find no interferon, and they showed there was no effect on the multiplication of herpes simplex and vesicular stomatitis viruses. Thus while the authors feel otherwise, and I agree with them, the latter two cases could have conceivably been due to an interferonlike inhibition brought about by undetectable amounts of interferon. Downie and Oxford (1969) arrived at just that conclusion in order to explain their findings that hamster lung cells persistently infected with rubella virus were somewhat resistant to herpes simplex virus. In this case, however, the cells were resistant to vaccinia virus. However, it is possible that truly another type of interference is occasionally encountered, and it is hoped that additional work will be done to determine the mechanisms. For instance, cytomegalovirus was demonstrated to induce intrinsic interference to Newcastle disease virus in human fibroblast cells under conditions in which the cytomegalovirus caused no cytopathological effect (Seto and Carver, 1969). Undoubtedly other examples will emerge.

IV. Relative Resistance of Herpesviruses to Interferon and Poly rI:Poly rC

Several studies in cell cultures have been done which bear out the relative resistance of herpesviruses to interferon or poly rI:poly rC. Perhaps the earliest example was provided in the work by Isaacs *et al.* (1958). They showed that interferon inoculated on the chick chorion *in ovo* diffused and inhibited influenza virus reproduction in neighboring allantoic cells. Pock production by vaccinia virus was also inhibited on these cells, but pock development by herpes simplex virus was not significantly affected.

Brown (1966) determined the sensitivity to interferon of herpes simplex virus compared to that of western equine encephalomyelitis (WEE) virus in chick embryo cells. She found, by the plaque-reduction assay method or the inhibition of virus yields, that about 100 times more interferon was required to obtain an amount of inhibition equivalent to that for WEE virus. No amount of interferon prevented cytopathologic effects from herpesvirus infection, She further found that inhibition could be obtained only by prior addition of interferon. Hilleman (1970) reported that it took 100-fold greater concentrations of poly rI:poly rC to inhibit herpes simplex virus on rabbit kidney cells than it took to inhibit vesicular stomatitis and vaccinia viruses. Glasgow *et al.* (1967) also found herpesvirus considerably more resistant than vescular stomatitis and sindbis virus to interferon in human cells. These authors also tested the comparative sensitivity of human cytomegalovirus and found it even more resistant than the herpesvirus which they had tested. Youngner *et al.* (1972) have found that whereas pseudorabies virus is relatively resistant to the action of interferon when tested in primary rabbit kidney cells and in a continuous line (RK-13) of rabbit kidney cells, it is susceptible to interferon in chicken or mouse cells. Others (Osborn and Meadaris, 1967a; Rabson *et al.*, 1969; Easton *et al.*, 1970) also have reported cytomegalovirus to be relatively resistant to inhibition by interferon in mouse and human cells. Still another herpesvirus, herpes saimiri was recently shown to be relatively resistant to interferon in monkey cells (Barahona and Melendez, 1971).

V. Induction of Interferon

Herpesvirus infections have been shown to cause the production of interferon in tissue cultures of mouse (Glasgow and Habel, 1963), chick (Lampson *et al.*, 1965), and dog cells (Aurelian and Roizman, 1964). Herpesvirus infections have also been held responsible for interferons from various organs of mice (Bostandzhyan and Bikbulatov, 1967), from ocular tissues of rabbits (Oh, 1970), and for the nonimmunological resistance of hamsters to polyoma virus (Barski, 1963). Also Rosenquist and Loan (1969) found that infectious bovine rhinotracheitis virus-induced interferon which was recoverable in the sera of infected calves. Interferon is considered to be a product of the genome of the cell which produces it. In this respect, Lampson *et al.* (1965) showed that chicken interferon was the same whether stimulated by herpesvirus or RNA viruses. Even herpesvirus that was rendered noninfectious by ultraviolet irradiation will stimulate interferon production in embryonated eggs as demonstrated by Fruitstone *et al.* (1964). A mouse cytomegalovirus was also reported to produce what was probably interferon in an early study by Henson and Smith (1964). The authors found that low dilutions of the fluid from mouse embryo cultures infected with cytomegalovirus inhibited the reproduction of encephalomyocarditis virus. On the other hand, Osborn and Meadaris (1967a,b) were unable to detect interferon in cell cultures infected with cytomegalovirus or to find interferon in the livers and salivary glands of infected suckling and weanling mice. In fact, they found that mice infected with cytomegalovirus displayed a marked inhibition of the capacity to produce interferon in response to the intravenous injection of Newcastle disease virus. However, mice similarly infected still produced interferon in response to endotoxin. The authors were unable to provide a definitive explanation for their results. One explanation in light of the intrinsic interference alluded to earlier (p. 265) (Seto and Carver, 1969) might be that the cytomegalovirus inhibited the Newcastle disease virus from accomplishing those steps required to induce interferon. If this is the case, however, the intrinsic interference must have been in only the population of those cells which produce interferons, since Osborn and Meadaris (1967b) also showed that Newcastle disease virus underwent an increased rate of replication in the spleens of cytomegalovirus-infected mice. The overwhelmingly clear results of their study was the failure to find interferon in mice infected with cytomegalovirus and their inability to alter the course of the disease with either endogenous or exogenous interferon. The study of Glasgow *et al.* (1967) offers another explanation. Using a human cytomegalovirus they found first little or no interferon resulted after the infection of either WI38 or human foreskin fibroblasts with the virus. Furthermore, they showed that the latter cells, which produced considerable interferon in response to chikungunya and Newcastle disease virus, had inhibited interferon production when already infected with cytomegalovirus. This is another instance in which the cytomegalovirus was shown to affect the induction of interferon by the cell, but again, no real explanation could be deduced.

VI. Dual Infections

It should also be pointed out that owing to the characteristic appearance of infections by the intranuclear herpesvirus, it has provided some of the best examples of simultaneous dual infections in the same cell. Thus, Syverton and Berry (1947) and Anderson (1942) showed that cells infected with herpesviruses could support the multiplication of fowl pox, vaccinia, and rabies viruses. More recently, Bell *et al.* (1968) reported that human embryo fibroblasts persistently infected with reovirus type 3 showed no signs of interference when the cells were doubly infected with the two viruses.

VII. Conclusion

In conclusion, herpesviruses stimulate interferon in a number of *in vivo* and *in vitro* situations but not in all. The virus is inhibited by interferon, but in all the studies carried out it has been found to be comparatively more difficult to inhibit than most other viruses. Interestingly, the most promising therapeutic possibility, so far, for interferon and its double-stranded RNA inducers has been found in the treatment of herpetic keratoconjunctivitis, a special, localized condition. There seems to be little evidence that generalized infections with the herpesviruses respond favorably to interferon. It seems that the lack of promise for interferon, and its inducers for use in combating the diseases resulting from herpesviruses should not be surprising in light of the poor ability of the herpesviruses to induce interferon and their relative resistance to its effects. A sidelight of potential interest to emerge from these studies, however, is the suggestion that macrophages and lymphocytes bear a major role in the control of herpes infections, and these are probably stimulated to greater effectiveness by some of the interferon inducers. Thus, perhaps serendipity will prevail and a means of treating the frequently stubborn herpes infections will yet emerge.

References

Anderson, K. (1942). *Amer. J. Pathol.* **18**, 577–583.

Aurelian, L., and Roizman, B. (1964). *Virology* **22**, 452–461.

Barahona, H. H., and Melendez, L. V. (1971). *Proc. Soc. Exp. Biol. Med.* **136**, 1163–1167.

Barski, G. (1963). *C. R. Acad. Sci.* **256**, 5459–5462.

Bell, T. M., Munube, G. M. R., and Griffin, E. R. (1968). *Int. J. Cancer* **3**, 751–759.

Bostandzhyan, M. G., and Bikbulatov, R. (1967). *Acta Virol. (Prague), Engl. Ed.* **11**, 159–160.

Brown, R. M. (1966), M. S., Thesis, University of Texas, Austin.

Catalano, L. W., Jr., Moossy, J., and Sell, S. (1970). *Proc. Soc. Exp. Biol. Med.* **135**, 509–514.

Catalano, L. W., Jr., and Baron, S. (1970). *Proc. Soc. Exp. Biol. Med.* **133**, 684–687.

Doerr, R., and Kon, M. (1937). *Z. Hyg. Infektionskr.* **119**, 679–705.

Doerr, R., and Seidenberg, S. (1937). *Z. Hyg. Infektionskr.* **119**, 135–165.

Downie, J. C., and Oxford, J. S. (1969). *J. Gen. Virol.* **5**, 11–17.

Easton, J. M., Ablashi, D. V., Oie, H. K., Baron, S., and Manaker, R. A. (1970). *Fed. Proc., Fed. Amer. Soc. Exp. Biol.* **29**, 636.

Frankel, J. W., and Groupé, V. (1971). *Nature (London), New Biol.* **234**, 125–126.

Fruitstone, M. J., Waddell, G. H., and Sigel, M. M. (1964). *Proc. Soc. Exp. Biol. Med.* **117**, 804–807.

Glasgow, L. A., and Habel, K. (1963). *Virology* **19**, 328–339.

Glasgow, L. A., Hanshaw, J. B., Merigan, T. C., and Petralli, J. K. (1967). *Proc. Soc. Exp. Biol. Med.* **125**, 843–849.

Guerra, R., Frezzotti, R., Bonanni, R., Dianzani, F., and Rita, G. (1970). *Ann. N. Y. Acad. Sci.* **173**, 823–830.

Hallauer, C. (1937). *Z. Hyg. Infektionskr.* **119**, 213–224.
Hamilton, L. D., Babcock, V. I., and Southam, C. M. (1969). *Proc. Nat. Acad. Sci. U.S.* **64**, 878–883.
Henson, D., and Smith, R. D. (1964). *Proc. Soc. Exp. Biol. Med.* **117**, 517–520.
Hilleman, M. R. (1970). *Ann. N. Y. Acad. Sci.* **173**, 623–628.
Hirsch, M. S., Zisman, B., and Allison, A. C. (1970). *J. Immunol.* **104**, 1160–1165.
Isaacs, A., Burke, D. C., and Fadeeva, L. (1958). *Brit. J. Exp. Pathol.* **39**, 447–458.
Johnson, T. C., Anderson, D. C., and McLaren, L. C. (1964). *Fed. Proc., Fed. Amer. Soc. Exp. Biol.* **23**, 508.
Kaufman, H. E., Ellison, E. D., and Waltman, S. R. (1969). *Amer J. Ophthalmol.* **68**, 486–491.
Lampson, G. P., Tytell, A. A., Nemes, M. M., and Hilleman, M. R. (1965). *Proc. Soc. Exp. Biol. Med.* **118**, 441–448.
Magrassi, F. (1935). *Z. Hyg. Infektionskr.* **117**, 501–508.
Magrassi, F. (1936). *Z. Hyg. Infektionskr.* **117**, 573–620.
Negoro, Y. (1970). *Folia Ophthalmol. Jap.* **21**, 133–140.
Oh, J. O. (1970). *J. Immunol.* **104**, 1359–1363.
Osborn, J. E., and Meadaris, D. N., Jr. (1967a). *Proc. Soc. Exp. Biol. Med.* **121**, 819 (1966).
Osborn, J. E., and Meadaris, D. N., Jr. (1967b). *Proc. Soc. Exp. Biol. Med.* **124**, 347.
Park, J. H., and Baron, S. (1968). *Science* **162**, 811.
Rabson, A. S., Tyrrell, S. A., and Levy, H. (1969). *Proc. Soc. Exp. Biol. Med.* **131**, 495–497.
Roizman, B. (1965). *Virology* **27**, 113–117.
Rosenquist, B. D., and Loan, R. W. (1969). *Amer. J. Vet. Res.* **30**, 1305–1312.
Saxton, R. E., and Stevens, J. G. (1972). *Virology* **48**, 207–220.
Schlesinger, R. W. (1959). *In* "The Viruses" (F. M. Burnet and W. M. Stanley, eds.), Vol. 3, pp. 157–194. Academic Press, New York.
Seto, D. S., and Carver, D. H. (1969). *J. Virol.* **4**, 12–14.
Syverton, J. T., and Berry, G. P. (1947). *J. Exp. Med.* **86**, 145–152.
Tokumaru, T. (1967) *Arch. Gesamte Virusforsch.* **21**, 61–70.
Van der Noordaa, J., Enders, J. F., and Diamandopoulos, G. T. (1966). *Proc. Soc. Exp. Biol. Med.* **122**, 915–920.
Wagner, R. R. (1963). *Amer. J. Med.* **38**, 726–737.
Youngner, J. S., Thacore, H. R., and Kelly, M. E. (1972). *J. Virol.* **10**, 171–178.

Chapter 9

Persistent and Latent Infections

Fred Rapp and Mary Ann Jerkofsky

I. Introduction and Definition of Terms

The focus of attention of researchers and clinicians has long been on acute virus infections. However, this emphasis is now changing. Prevention of acute virus diseases with the aid of vaccines is now being coupled with the emergence of a few compounds useful in chemotherapy of virus infections. This reduction in incidence of the acute diseases has served to unmask other conditions and virus infections which were always present but were previously hidden by more overwhelming symptoms. The use of antimetabolites in cancer chemotherapy and immunosuppressive therapy in tissue and organ transplantation have clearly revealed a precarious balance between host and virus in latent or persistent infections. As a result, these conditions are becoming a pressing problem for the clinician.

In these more silent infections, the virus is present in the cells but there is no gross sign of disease for long periods of time. However, a change in the internal environment of the body can trigger a sudden activation of the previously quiescent virus. The virus then expresses itself, assumes control of the cell, often with resultant cell destruction and disease. This type of infection is particularly characteristic of the herpesviruses and most are capable of producing at least one manifestation of such an infection.

There are two major classes of these silent infections: *persistent infections* and *latent infections*. A *persistent infection* is one in which infectious virus is continually released, even in the presence of circulating antibody and in the absence of symptoms of disease. A *latent infection* is one in which at least the genome of the virus is present but infectious virions cannot be recovered except during episodes of overt disease.

It is obvious that these two classes of infection are not really completely distinct entities but rather represent the two extremes of a gradient of infections. Many intermediate forms exist, and the boundaries between the two classes merge. Since the distinction between these two conditions rests on the ability to detect infectious virus, the assignment of a particular virus or infection into one class or the other is based upon the techniques used to detect infectious virus. Thus, the classification is not static. Figure 1 schematically presents these complex interactions.

These conditions can be studied at the level of the organism or at the level of the individual infected cell. In this chapter, we will first discuss conditions in the organism and then turn to model systems devised in attempts to study the events at the cellular level.

II. *In Vivo* Studies

A. Persistent Infections

The primary exposure of a susceptible individual to herpes simplex virus occurs early in life and in the absence of circulating antibodies. Although most of these primary infections are subclinical, the principal clinical manifestation is a gingivostomatitis. In one study (Scott, 1954), 38 of 5000 children (0.8%) under 5 years of age were observed to have the typical primary her-

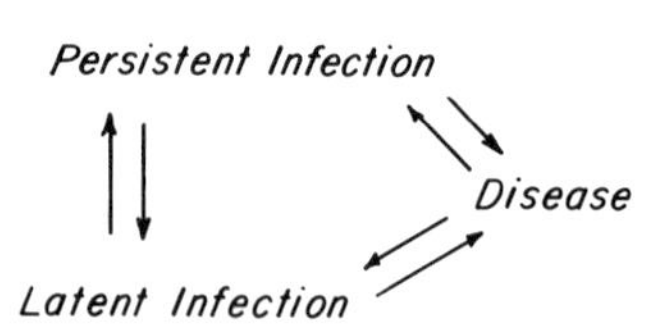

FIG. 1. Complex relationship of herpesviruses and disease.

petic gingivostomatitis; based upon surveys of antibody development, 60% were expected to have become infected within that period. Therefore, greater than 80% of the primary infections were not noticed clinically.

During the acute stage of the primary illness, herpes simplex virus can readily be isolated from the mouth and from rectal swabs. The virus appears to be replicating in the oropharynx but since virus can be so readily isolated from the stool, large quantities of virus are presumably swallowed. After clinical recovery from the primary infection, herpes simplex virus can still be isolated from saliva and stools for long periods of time. Thus, these children are persistently infected and serve as "healthy carriers" at times when they show no clinical evidence of infection (Buddingh *et al.*, 1953).

Virus can also be reisolated from these children at various intervals following cessation of the original shedding (Buddingh *et al.*, 1953). The children produce neutralizing antibodies after the primary infection but the serum titer soon drops. Antibody production often increases each time virus can be recovered but this is not always the case. Therefore, it appears that the first exposure of a susceptible individual to herpes simplex virus does not result in the establishment of a balance between latent herpes simplex virus and antibody levels; a number of reinfections are required for the establishment of such an equilibrium. However, once the equilibrium is established, antibody titers remain the same no matter how many recurrent attacks occur (Scott, 1954) (see below for discussion of latent infections by herpes simplex virus).

Normal healthy individuals have also been screened to see if persistent infection with herpes simplex virus is a common event. In one study, 571 healthy individuals were surveyed (Buddingh *et al.*, 1953). Virus could be recovered from 15 of 72 (21%) of the individuals between 7 months and 2 years of age, from 18 of 199 (9%) of the individuals 3–14 years of age, and from 5 of 185 (2.7%) of the individuals over 15 years of age. Therefore, a persistent infection with herpes simplex virus in the absence of any symptoms of disease is quite frequent early in life. These persistent infections decline in frequency later in life and can only be detected by screening apparently healthy individuals for recovery of infectious virus.

Cytomegalovirus can also frequently establish a persistent infection. The most common disease produced by cytomegalovirus is congenital cytomegalic inclusion disease. The infant is infected *in utero* and has the disease at birth. Although the condition is usually fatal, some infants recover. These infants demonstrate hepatosplenomegaly, mental retardation, persistent viruria, and virus has been isolated from liver biopsies (Weller *et al.*, 1957; Weller and Hanshaw, 1962; Medearis, 1964). Virus continues to be excreted by these children for at least 2 years, even in the presence of significant levels of neutralizing antibodies (Kluge *et al.*, 1960).

Older children can also have a chronic or persistent infection with cytomegalovirus. Virus was recovered from the mouth of 13 of 21 children with antibodies to cytomegalovirus and from the urine of 7 of 8 virus positive children (Rowe *et al.*, 1958). No virus was detected in 26 children without antibodies to cytomegalovirus. Virus was isolated for periods of 2–5 months and from 8–24 months after neutralizing antibodies were detected in their serum. In another survey (Hanshaw *et al.*, 1965), human cytomegalovirus was isolated from 1% of 200 well children and 100 nonselected pediatric patients. Institutionalized children and close contacts of children harboring the virus had rates of virus recovery of 23 and 28%. Twenty of the clinically well children received a more careful clinical evaluation. Fourteen had hepatomegaly; five had splenomegaly; and abnormal values in liver function tests were six times as frequent as in children who did not excrete virus. Almost all of the virus-positive children had antibodies to human cytomegalovirus.

In adults, certain debilitating conditions seem to activate latent cytomegalovirus infections (see Section II, B below). However, no difference in the rate of urinary excretion of cytomegalovirus was found when children with leukemia were compared with children suffering from chronic illness and with normal children of comparable age in the same community (Benyesh-Melnick *et al.*, 1964). In this study, approximately 15% of the 515 children studied were excreting virus, and more children were virus-positive when repeated urine samples were tested. Thus, persistent infections with this virus are also found in the presence of circulating antibodies and in the absence of manifest clinical disease.

B. Latent Infections

Latent viral infections have been characteristic for herpesviruses almost from the moment of their discovery. Even before the causative agent for herpetic fever blisters was identified as a virus, its ability to establish a latent infection was postulated (Goodpasture, 1929). Since that time, although much work has been done with these viruses, the actual mechanisms involved in these complex virus–cell interactions remain elusive. However, recent work with *in vitro* systems may soon clarify the situation (see Section III below).

Latent infections are characterized by the presence of virus in a host in a latent or masked form. Infectious virus is neither released nor can it be detected or recovered. However, certain changes in internal environment and certain apparent nonspecific stimuli can trigger induction of virus production. Generally, this is followed by shedding of the virus and subsequently by clinical illness. Therefore, it is important to define and to study these triggering stimuli in order to determine how the virus exists during its masked or latent state.

Numerous stimuli are known to cause an eruption of fever blisters in man due to herpes simplex virus. These include ultraviolet light, fever, hormonal changes associated with the menstrual cycle, and emotional upsets. However, there are also some experimentally controlled studies of induction of latent infections in experimental animals in which the stimuli have been partially defined.

1. Activation by Specific Stimuli

The best example of activation of a latent virus by a specific stimulus is found in the Lucké adenocarcinoma of frogs. Rafferty (1964) has summarized the early observations of this virus–tumor system. An epithelial tumor of the kidney is frequently found in the frog species *Rana pipiens* from Vermont, Wisconsin, and Michigan. The tumor appears to have two phases: a "winter phase" and a "summer phase." "Winter phase" tumors are detected in frogs from mid-October to late May, and especially as the frogs emerge from hibernation. The cells of the tumor have enlarged nuclei, marginated chromatin, and Cowdry type A inclusion bodies, and these cells produce herpes virions. Tumors detected in frogs in late spring, summer, and early fall lack inclusions and produce no virus particles; these are "summer phase" tumors. It appears that prolonged low temperature is the principal factor favoring inclusion formation and virus production.

Therefore, Rafferty proposed the following life cycle for the tumor: Field tumors arise in the summer of approximately the third year of life of the frog. Of the adult frogs, 3% enter hibernation with small tumors. In response to the prolonged cold, the tumor cells form inclusions; at least half of the tumors of hibernating frogs contain inclusions. As the tumor cells form the inclusions, their mitotic rate decreases but virus production increases. The virus is excreted in the urine and contaminates the water as the frogs emerge from hibernation and spawn. Young fertilized embryos or tadpoles become infected through the contaminated water. This original infection is latent in the young frogs but will cause tumor formation 2–3 years later. Virus-producing cells in the tumor die but other tumor cells respond to warm weather by increasing their mitotic rate and soon become dominant. The frog will die with a large virus-free tumor the following summer. Mizell and Zambernard (1965) suggest a similar life cycle but propose that infection occurs during gametogenesis. Other workers (McKinnell and Duplantier, 1970) suggest that temperature fluctuation may be inadequate as the only stimulus, and they suggest other factors such as crowding, environmental stress, and pollution as contributing factors.

However, it does seem to be well established that temperature is the major factor controlling the production of herpesvirus by the tumor cells. Frogs maintained at 20°–25° C die of large tumors which produce no virus, whereas frogs maintained at 5° C with no feeding for 2 months to simulate hibernation yield only virus-producing tumors (Roberts, 1963). "Summer phase" tumors producing no virus become virus producers following incubation at 4°C for several months (Rafferty, 1965).

Since most primary tumors are multicentric in origin, they cannot be used to test for time of induction of virus following treatment with low temperatures. Therefore, more controlled studies have used transplanted tumor sections grown in the anterior chamber of the frog eye. Frogs containing such virus-negative transplanted tumors were maintained originally at 20°–26°C, then shifted to 7.5° ± 5°C and the tumors checked for virus production. The first virus production was detected 8 weeks later, with the plateau of virus production in 20% of the cells by the 14th–16th week (Mizell *et al.*, 1968, 1969; Stackpole, 1969). These first studies were carried out in *R. pipiens*, but could not be used to rule out migration of the virus from the host if the virus was a passenger virus which preferentially grew in tumor cells. Therefore, the experiments were repeated with two species in which the tumor is never found, *R. clamitans* and the toad *Bufo americimus* (Mizell *et al.*, 1969). The results were similar to those obtained with *R. pipiens*. However, these experiments do not rule out the possibility of levels of virus production that are not detectable by electron microscopy in the "summer phase" cells; specific immunofluorescence tests may help to clarify that point.

One possibility for inhibition of virus production is that host antibodies keep virus production in check. However, the delayed appearance of virus in the eye chamber transplants seems to argue against this. Therefore, the low temperatures seem to act directly on the tumor cells to activate a temperature-sensitive step, possibly enzymatic, in virus production. These results also suggest that the complete viral genome is present in the tumor cells. Recent results (Breidenbach *et al.*, 1971) confirm this. "Summer phase" tumors maintained *in vitro* at 7.5°C for 13–14 weeks induce the formation of herpesvirus. Therefore, the factors regulating virus production reside in the tumor cells themselves and not in the frog as a whole. The actual mechanism of induction and the reason for the delay in virus production are still unclear.

2. Activation by Nonspecific Stimuli

In most systems, no one principal triggering stimulus is known; numerous stimuli with no known common denominator produce induction. One of the first experimental systems used was the development of a latent encephalitis in rabbits with herpes simplex virus (Perdrau, 1938). A rabbit injected into the testicle with one strain of herpes simplex virus (H4), resisted challenge with an even more virulent strain (E.L.I.) injected intracerebrally. However, 6 months later, the rabbits developed a herpetic encephalitis. The virus recovered from these animals was the H4 strain of virus used in the original immunization and not the challenge virus; this virus apparently had been dormant in the brain until unknown factors triggered its expression.

Anaphylactic shock was found to be a good stimulus for the induction of herpetic encephalitis in a previously sensitized animal. Rabbits were injected intramuscularly and intracerebrally with herpes simplex virus and suffered no apparent infection (Good and Campbell, 1945). They were then sensitized to ovalbumin and put into anaphylactic shock. A herpetic encephalomyelitis developed 7 days later. Sensitized animals which were put into anaphylactic shock but which had not been injected previously with herpes simplex virus did not develop encephalitis.

Other studies (Good, 1947) confirmed the observation that anaphylactic shock could precipitate latent herpesvirus encephalitis, even if the herpesvirus was injected into a previously sensitized animal (Good and Campbell, 1948). Herpes simplex virus could be recovered from the central nervous system of animals during a fatal or spontaneous activation, during periods of quiescence after the precipitation, and during chronic renewal of the essential disease process. The anaphylactic shock appeared to upset the previous balance between virus and host so that a persistent infection or carrier state developed; herpes simplex virus could be recovered between periods of disease.

An Arthus reaction could also precipitate a latent herpesvirus infection (Anderson *et al.*, 1961). A herpetic keratitis was induced in both eyes of a rabbit by the injection of herpes simplex virus into the cornea. After the initial keratitis had healed, an Arthus reaction induced in one healed cornea would precipitate a recurrent keratitis whereas the unchallenged eye remained normal.

Other investigators (Schmidt and Rasmussen, 1960) found that the injection of adrenalin into a rabbit that had no signs of disease, but which had been previously injected with herpes simplex virus could transform a quiescent, inapparent herpetic focus of infection into an acute fatal encephalitis. Neutralization tests showed that the virus recovered was the same as the virus originally inoculated. None of the animals that had been injected with virus but not with the drug developed a spontaneous encephalitis. The authors postulated that since many of the conditions in man that predispose him to activation of a latent herpesvirus infection also stimulate the secretion of adrenaline, perhaps the adrenaline acted as the controlling factor. Perdrau (1931) had shown that the infectivity of herpes simplex virus destroyed by oxidation could be restored by subsequent reduction. Therefore, the temporary vasoconstriction caused by the increased adrenalin could produce a local anoxia and reactivate residual herpes simplex virus.

All of these studies have used experimental model systems in which a latent infection was induced deliberately. Man has natural latent infections, and some accidental conditions have helped to determine some of the stimuli which induce virus production.

One surgical procedure which frequently induced herpetic lesions of the face is the sensory section of the trigeminal nerve. In the original study (Carton and Kilbourne, 1952), 17 patients with classical trigeminal neuralgia were treated therapeutically by sectioning the posterior root of the affected trigeminal nerve. In all but one (or 94%), labial herpes vesicles appeared 48–96 hours after the operation. Lesions were usually restricted to the areas of skin supplied by the sectioned portion of the trigeminal sensory root, although lesions did not always appear in a denervated area. Herpes simplex virus could be isolated from the lesions, although virus could not be isolated from removed ganglion tissue of a patient who would later develop the labial lesions. The patients had antibodies before the operation and at the time of appearance of the lesion, although the one patient who did not develop lesions also had antibodies. This system appeared to be a good model because (unlike other stimuli such as fever that produce profound and widespread physiological changes) these effects did not extend beyond the innervated area. Carton and Kilbourne (1952) suggested that the latent herpesvirus did not reside in the Gasserian ganglion and spread from there after inactivation because the lesions were limited to one section of the trigeminal nerve; the second and third sections were frequently involved whereas the first section was not. Johnson (1964) had previously shown, by immunofluorescence techniques in suckling mice injected subcutaneously and intranasally, the centripetal spread of herpesvirus along peripheral and cranial nerves through endoneural cells such as Schwann cells but not through axons. Instead, Carton and Kilbourne postulated activation of residual islands of latent virus in the regions of the skin and mucosa where fever blisters usually occur.

Since the vesicles appeared simultaneously over the affected area rather than starting at one site and spreading from there, other workers (Ellison *et al.*, 1959) decided that the herpesvirus appeared to be widely distributed in the skin and oral mucosal epithelium before the activation. In 5 of 8 patients subjected to a secondary operative procedure, herpes lesions appeared, but never in the sensory area denervated by the original procedure (Carton, 1953). The author postulated that damage to the ganglion cells secondary to the surgical procedure produced an increased irritability to the respective sensory nerve fibers and therefore changes in the skin that reactivated the latent herpesvirus. A previous interruption of the sensory pathways would prevent this sequence.

Various debilitating conditions in man seem to activate latent infections, although the mechanisms involved are not known. In analyzing deaths in 60 cases of kidney, liver, or spleen transplant operations (Hill *et al.*, 1967), an unavoidable chain of events appears to occur early in the postoperative period. A violent immunological reaction by the allograph recipient necessitates a correspondingly rigorous regimen of immunosuppressive therapy; this regimen so damages the host defense mechanisms that the patient is unable to resist infection with previously ambient, saprophytic, or latent organisms. Death in the first 3 weeks after surgery is rare but later deaths are almost always due to infection. In liver homotransplant patients, the types of infection are similar to those in renal transplants but appear to be greater in severity (Fulginiti *et al.*, 1968).

In one series of renal transplant operations, the bacterial infections were analyzed to determine if the infection was derived from the donor or was already present in the recipient (Rifkind *et al.*, 1964a). In at least 26 of 30 patients studied, the infection appeared to be endogenous in the recipient; the patient was a preoperative carrier of the organism which would cause a serious illness later. *Staphylococcus* phage typing of bacterial strains determined this in several cases. One donor consistently carried *E. coli* but the recipient developed an infection with *Pseudomonas*. Since all patients were kept in strict isolation, person-to-person transmission was not likely. These considerations seem to point to endogenous flora as the major cause of infection of patients receiving immunosuppressive therapy. This seems to apply to viral infections as well. Therefore, the viral infections which appear in patients receiving immunosuppressive therapy or suffering from other debilitating conditions such as malignancy seem to be due to endogenous or latent viruses, although spread from a donor to a patient in a debilitated state cannot be completely ruled out.

Cytomegalovirus infection is one of the disease manifestations frequently detected following immunosuppressive therapy in homotransplantation. Cytomegalovirus was detected in the lungs of 10 of 17 renal transplant patients at autopsy, although only 4 had clinically recognized pneumonia before death (Rifkind *et al.*, 1964b). The longer a patient survived the transplantation operation, the more frequent was the isolation of the virus or the symptoms of disease (Hill *et al.*, 1964; Kanich and Craighead, 1966). Since the detection of antibodies to cytomegalovirus in normal populations increases from 15% in infancy to 81% in persons over 35 years of age (Rowe *et al.*, 1956), the recovery of virus in 50% of renal transplant patients does not conflict with the hypothesis of activation of a latent infection. Spread of the virus from the transplanted kidney could be ruled out conclusively in one particular case, since the donor of the kidney had no detectable antibodies to cytomegalovirus, no virus could be detected in his throat or urine, and no viral inclusion bodies were detected at autopsy (Hedley-Whyte and Craighead, 1965). An increase in antibody titer with or without the accompanying recovery of virus was possible in greater than 91% of patients with serological evidence of previous infection with cytomeglovirus at the time of surgery, whereas this occurred in only 47% of those with no serological evidence of previous infection (Craighead *et al.*, 1967; Craighead, 1969). These latter patients, who were younger and were ruled virus-negative on the basis of antibody development, had probably not yet received their initial exposure to cytomegalovirus. Since all of the transplant patients were maintained in a separate ward, spread from patients excreting virus was possible. Therefore, it appears that a combination of factors may influence cytomegalovirus infection following immunosuppressive therapy; activation of latent virus occurs in patients with previous exposure to the virus, while those with no previous exposure develop a primary and perhaps a persistent infection.

Herpes zoster infection also occurs following renal transplantation operations but at a much lower frequency. In one study (Rifkind, 1966), 6 of 73, or 8.2%, of the patients developed zoster in a dermatome with no dissemination. All of the patients had previous varicella infection and had complement-fixing antibodies to the varicella-zoster virus. Although there was no relation between the dose of immunosuppressive drug used, there was a significant temporal association between the use of local X-irradiation and the onset of the lesion; the lesions occurred in close proximity to the area irradiated.

Infections with herpes simplex virus are noted but not particularly troublesome following transplantation operations (Montgomerie *et al.*, 1969). However, typical labial herpes does progress to involve adjacent areas of the face, eye, nares, mouth, and esophagus (Montgomerie *et al.*, 1969), and to the lung in one reported case (Douglas *et al.*, 1969).

The presence of leukemia and other malignancies also appears to stimulate activation of latent viruses, possibly through the mediation of immunosuppressive and X-ray therapy. The activation of cytomegalovirus appears to follow the disease process, since the virus is not detected during episodes of clinical remission but is present during exacerbation of the leukemia (Hanshaw and Weller, 1961). In Hodgkin's disease, the lesions of cytomegalovirus are found where there is extensive replacement of the normal structures of the spleen and lymph nodes by neoplastic tissue. Similar results are detected with herpes zoster in that either tumor foci were detected near the involved ganglia or X-ray therapy had been used in the affected area (Sokal and Firat, 1965). The majority of the patients with zoster have a history of varicella, and the peak of zoster occurs at a time when varicella is at a low level in the community. These facts favor the hypothesis of reactivation, although some cases have documented exposure to varicella.

3. Theoretical Considerations

The overwhelming amount of evidence suggests that herpesviruses are frequently harbored by individuals who show no sign of disease. It is possible that this involves an equilibrium or balance between host and parasite so that the virus is unable to produce disease and yet the host is not able to rid itself of the virus infection. Or perhaps the virus has developed a specialized function, such as integration into the host cell genome, which permits it to exist in harmony with the cell. Certain as yet not completely defined factors can apparently upset the equilibrium in favor of the virus and disease results. By studying these factors and how they influence virus expression, it may be possible to control latent infections by forcing them to remain latent. As yet, we do not know if a virus during a latent infection is really inactive or if its influence on the host is so subtle that we do not yet know how to measure it. It does appear that the use of some recently developed *in vitro* model systems may help clarify the parameters involved in latent infections.

C. Recurrent Disease

Certain of the disease states produced by the herpesviruses are characterized by recurrences. Herpes zoster is a disease caused by varicella virus which has remained dormant for long periods of time. Zoster never occurs in epidemic form and only occurs in individuals with a previous history of varicella infection. One physician summarized all the cases of zoster that he had seen during a general practice of 16 years (Hope-Simpson, 1965). In all cases, those who developed zoster had had varicella previously, even a 2-year-old boy who had had varicella at 6 months of age. This author postulated that the varicella virus goes to sensory ganglia through the sensory nerve endings. A latent infection is then established in the nuclei of the neurons in the sensory ganglia. Thus, each individual would have approximately 50 foci of latent virus infection. Each focus of latent virus reverts to virulence at a certain frequency but circulating antibodies localize the infection. Occasionally some factor will cause depression of antibody level as one focus produces virus. The virus can then multiply freely. It moves down the nerve fiber and produces the disease symptoms in the skin and mucous membranes supplied by that single sensory ganglion. This could explain why zoster attacks only the area supplied by one ganglion; if more than one ganglion is affected, they are widely separated. This could also explain the fact that zoster mainly affects the area supplied by the fifth cranial nerve and the thoracic area supplied by the dorsal root ganglia from the third dorsal to the second lumbar region; varicella lesions have centripetal spread and occur mainly on the trunk. However, zoster can also be stimulated by chemical means, such as arsenic poisoning (Jacob, 1931).

Herpes simplex virus infections are recurrent fever blisters at almost exactly the same cutaneous site at fairly definite intervals. As early as 1929, Goodpasture postulated that the diversity of conditions which would initiate such an attack necessitate the assumption of a wide dissemination of the herpesvirus or a very readily spontaneous generation of virus, and the observations suggested a latent infection between outbreaks of the lesion. There are cases of known self-inoculation of herpesviruses, especially among nurses, with repeated recurrences at the same site (Findlay and MacCallum, 1940; Stern *et al.*, 1959). Therefore, all of these states of recurrent disease may really be the activation of a latent infection by unrecognized stimuli.

III. Latency *in Vitro*

Many studies have been performed in attempts to produce *in vitro* a model system which would mimic the latent infections detected *in vivo*. The first series of studies sought to establish a persistent infection in cultured cells with herpes simplex virus. This was most frequently done by introducing antibodies to herpes simplex virus into the culture fluids (Wheeler and Canby, 1959, 1960a; Fernandez, 1960; Szanto, 1963). The antibodies were required for the maintenance of the persistent infection. If antibodies were removed, the cultures were destroyed by viral cytopathic effects. However, since antibodies do not prevent cell-to-cell passage of the herpesviruses (Andrews, 1930; Black and Melnick, 1955; Stoker, 1958), the infection persisted. Other workers were later able to obtain a persistent infection *in vitro* without antibodies, but other conditions, such as decreasing cellular metabolism by low-temperature incubation (Wheeler and Canby, 1960b; Coleman and Jawetz, 1961), depletion of certain nutrients in culture fluids (Pelmont and Morgan, 1959), or the presence of interferon (Glasgow and Habel, 1963) or an interferonlike factor (Blackmore and Morgan, 1967), had to be manipulated carefully for the effect to be observed.

Hampar and Copeland (1965) were then able to establish a persistent infection in Chinese hamster cells without antibodies or other known supportive measures. This system was characterized by cycles of virus synthesis and cell destruction followed by regrowth of the cultures. The infection was maintained by cell-to-cell passage of the virus, by extracellular virus, and by reattachment of infectious material (Hampar, 1966a). The cycle of infection was initiated in a few localized areas. These lesions expanded and the infected cells detached. New foci of infection arose through the reattachment of infectious cell material as well as by the spread of extracellular virus. As the infection spread to new areas, cell regrowth occurred in the original focus. Thus, cell regrowth occurred in some areas simultaneously with virus growth and cytopathic effects in other areas (Hampar, 1966b).

However, certain changes did occur with time in culture. The original virus was the NP variant (Hampar, 1966c). Less than 1% of the virus produced was infectious. Therefore, all of the susceptible cells were not killed. Then the GC variant of the virus arose. With this virus, 10% of the virus in the medium was infectious. Thus, the infection spread rapidly. After several cycles of replication, the susceptible cells were eliminated and reduced to the level of the control cells. This, in turn, reduced the severity of the infection. Changes had been detected previously in cells persistently infected with herpes simplex virus, but such changes were only detected in the presence of antibody (Hoggan and Roizman, 1959; Hinze and Walker, 1961); these changes of virus properties occurred in cells never exposed to antibody. The virus acquired new antigenic determinants, but retained others (Hampar and Keehn, 1967). With time, the cells showed a progressive decrease in susceptibility to herpes simplex virus, and the virus showed an increasing virulence for the cells (Hampar and Burroughs, 1969). The host cell appeared to induce the change in virus properties, but the selective pressure of virus more adapted to grow in the cells probably also occurred. The observed changes in the virus were stable through passage in other cells so that a true genetic change, probably a mutation, had occurred. The authors suggested that this may be the normal sequence of events as a virus adapts to grow in a less permissive cell. They also postulated a model for latent human infections with herpes simplex virus. A virus–cell equilibrium causes localized human infections to remain at a low level during remission. There is a slow rate of change in the properties of the virus and of the cells. Unknown stimuli can produce a severe change in the virus or in the cell. The level of virus replication is increased to the point where excerbations occur in the presence of circulating antibodies. The virus and cell then reestablish a new equilibrium, and active virus production ceases until something again upsets the balance. Some antigenic heterogeneity has been detected in some but not all herpes simplex virus isolates from the same individual (Ashe and Scherp, 1965).

A persistent infection of Earle's L cells by herpes simplex virus also results in an infection characterized by a cyclic rise and fall in virus infection that is accompanied by cell destruction followed by regrowth (Nii, 1969). The cycles in this system are much more irregular, and it appears that physiological conditions of the cells influence the cycles (Nii, 1970). This author suggests that virus could be harbored in physiologically inactive cells, such as Schwann cells or satellite cells, in a latent infection for long periods of time.

The use of organ cultures has recently lead to the recovery of infectious herpes simplex virus from mice and rabbits with latent herpetic infections (Stevens and Cook, 1971, 1972; Stevens *et al.*, 1972). When the spinal ganglia from mice which had recovered from a posterior paralysis produced by the injection of herpes simplex virus were explanted and maintained *in vitro* in organ culture, infectious virus was recovered. Since these animals were not shown to have recurrent herpetic disease, similar experiments were performed with rabbits with known cases of recurrent herpetic eye disease. Again, virus was recovered only from the trigeminal ganglia maintained in organ culture; no virus could be isolated from cell extracts of the ganglia at the time of explant or from explants of nerves peripheral to the ganglia or nerve nuclei in the medulla oblongata. In experimentally infected animals, virus is initially detected in neurons and spreads from there to satellite cells and other supporting cells. In an immune environment, virus can be detected in the neurons, but there is no spread to supporting cells. Although nerves without neural somas can synthesize virus if infected in tissue culture, they do not appear to harbor latent virus in the intact animal; virus can be isolated only from ganglia with neural somas. How the virus is maintained in the ganglia has yet to be determined. The study of the mechanisms of virus maintenance and activation in this system should produce a model system for the study of latent infections in intact animals.

The DNA inhibitor, cytosine arabinoside, has been used to set up a latent infection *in vitro* (O'Neill *et al.*, 1972). Human embryonic lung cells infected with herpes simplex virus type 2 were maintained in the presence of cytosine arabinoside for 3–4 weeks. This treatment prevented the synthesis of infectious virus and the development of virus cytopathic effects. After the removal of the drug, infectious herpes simplex virus reappeared but only after a delay of 5–6 days. No infectious virus could be detected in the cultures before that time, although the cells could be superinfected with either vesicular stomatitis virus or additional herpes simplex virus type 2. However, infectious center assays demonstrated that the virus was present in a noninfectious form in at least 1 in 800 cells. Again, the reason for the delay in the appearance of infectious virus is not known. Perhaps the cell must repair damage produced by the cytosine arabinoside. Perhaps the virus information had been integrated into the cell genome, and dissociation occurs only as the cell can resume normal DNA synthesis. In either case, resolution of the exact mechanisms involved should increase our understanding of latent infections.

IV. Transformation of Cells *in Vitro*

There is also some recent evidence to suggest that herpesviruses are capable of interacting with the cell genome to induce new properties in progeny cells. Ultraviolet-irradiated herpes simplex virus type 1 can change the phenotype of thymidine kinase-less mouse L cells to thymidine kinase-positive cells (Munyon *et al.*, 1971). This thymidine kinase had a thermal stability similar to that of the thymidine kinase from cells infected with herpes simplex type 1 but different from that of the thymidine kinase isolated from normal L cells. This is suggestive evidence that the gene for thymidine kinase production has been transferred in a permanent state from the herpesvirus to the cell, since the cell phenotype has been stable for 8 months.

Ultraviolet-irradiated herpes simplex virus type 2 has been shown to transform morphologically normal hamster embryo fibroblasts exposed to the virus *in vitro* (Duff and Rapp, 1971a,b; Rapp and Duff, 1971, 1972). Virus-specific antigens were detected, usually in the cytoplasm, in 1–5% of fixed, transformed cells by the indirect immunofluorescence test, and antigens have also been detected at the surface of viable (unfixed) cells. However, no virus has been recovered from these cells. These morphologically tranformed cells were capable of inducing tumors when inoculated into newborn hamsters. The sera of tumor-bearing animals reacted with the virus-specific antigens of the transformed cells in indirect immunofluorescence tests and also contained herpes simplex virus-specific neutralizing antibodies. As of yet, no virus-specific transplantation antigens have been detected. Preliminary attempts to detect virus-specific nucleic acid in the transformed cells by using nucleic acid hybridization methodology suggest that virus-specific mRNA is present (E. Kieff and B. Roizman, personal communication). Therefore, following exposure to ultraviolet-irradiated herpes simplex virus type 2, these hamster embryo fibroblast cells appear to retain markers characteristic for herpes simplex virus and to behave in a similar manner to cells transformed by other DNA viruses.

Another herpesvirus, Epstein-Barr (EB) virus, has long been associated with the malignant Burkitt lymphoma of African children. Epstein *et al.* (1964) originally detected a herpes-like virus in a line of lymphoblasts established in cell culture from a Burkitt tumor. Later studies demonstrated that a small percentage of cells in established cell lines contained virus particles (Epstein *et al.*, 1965) and viral antigens as detected by indirect immunofluorescence tests (Henle and Henle, 1966). The percentage of cells releasing virus particles could be increased by cocultivation of the cells with a continuous line of African green monkey kidney cells (Hampar *et al.*, 1971). Nucleic acid hybridization studies then revealed that EB virus DNA was present in cell lines not producing virus particles (Zur Hausen and Schulte-Holthausen, 1970; Nonoyama and Pagano, 1971). These virus-negative cells could be stimulated to produce virus particles and viral antigens by treatment with the DNA analogue, bromodeoxyuridine (Gerber, 1972; Hampar *et al.*, 1972); this same treatment had been used previously to activate mammalian C-type virus genomes (Lowy *et al.*, 1971; Aaronson *et al.*, 1971).

The Burkitt lymphoblastoid cells can also be fused and hybridized to both mouse and human cells (Glaser and O'Neill, 1972). Although the hybrid cells contain neither virus particles nor viral antigens, treatment with iododeoxyuridine (IUdR) stimulates production of both (Glaser and Rapp, 1972). Nucleic acid hybridization studies also suggest that the EB virus DNA is present (R. Glaser and M. Nonoyama, personal communication). Therefore, the EB virus genome appears to be carried in the tumor cells but is rarely expressed. How it is maintained and what triggers its occasional expression has yet to be determined.

Herpes simplex virus type 2 has also been associated with human cervical carcinoma. Most of the early studies were based upon epidemiological methods; increased incidences of antibodies to herpes simplex virus type 2 were detected in women with cervical carcinoma as compared to women without this disease (Rawls *et al.*, 1969; Royston and Aurelian, 1970a; Nahmias *et al.*, 1970; Aurelian *et al.*, 1970). Exfoliative cells from these patients contain specific antigens associated with herpes simplex virus type 2 as determined by immunofluorescence tests (Royston and Aurelian, 1970b). A herpesvirus has recently been isolated from spontaneously degenerating cultures of cervical tumor cells grown *in vitro*; duplicate cultures of viable cells did not release virus. The virus was identified as herpes simplex virus type 2 on the basis of biological properties and immunologic specificity. Therefore, there are at least two cases in which herpesviruses are associated with human neoplasia. The role of the viruses in the etiology of these diseases remains unknown but is the subject of extensive investigation in many laboratories.

V. Recapitulation

In a review of persistent infections with herpes simplex viruses, Roizman (1965) suggested two possible mechanisms for the persistence of the viral genome. In the "dynamic state" he postulated a slow but constant replication accompanied by release of the virus. This would be similar to persistent infections *in vivo* and to the carrier cultures which have been established *in vitro*. The main criterion in defining such a system is the sensitivity of the techniques used to detect the infectious virus; the technique must be sensitive enough to detect minute quantities of virus. The other suggested state of the virus genome was a "static state." This hypothesis called for reversible interruption of the replication of the virus in certain "virogenic cells." Latent infections, both *in vivo* and *in vitro*, would fall into this classification. Since virus multiplication is interrupted, no infectious virus is produced. However, this condition is reversible, and a number of factors can stimulate the virus–cell complex into one capable of supporting virus synthesis. Certain observations with *in vitro* systems have begun to establish conditions allowing manipulation of cells from the nonvirogenic to virogenic state. The Lucké frog adenocarcinoma cells will release virus following maintenance at low temperatures; spinal ganglia grown in organ culture release virus; cervical carcinoma cells sometimes release virus after cultivation *in vitro*; BUdR and IUdR cause Burkitt lymphoma cells to produce virus; and exposure to ara-C has been used to establish a reversible latent infection with herpes simplex virus *in vitro*. However, in all these systems, there is a delay between the activating stimulus and the production of virus. What must occur during this delay in order to activate virus synthesis has yet to be determined. However, the continued study of the various systems may reveal a common factor or mechanism underlying the ability of herpesviruses to establish latent infections. In turn, this will hopefully yield clues concerning the oncogenic potential of these viruses and conditions required to turn a persistent infection into a latent state, with transformation of the cell a possible sequela.

References

Aaronson, S. A., Todaro, G. J., and Scolnick, E. M. (1971). *Science* **174**, 157.
Anderson, W. A., Margruder, B., and Kilbourne, E. D. (1961). *Proc. Soc. Exp. Biol. Med.* **107**, 628.
Andrews, C. H. (1930). *J. Pathol. Bacteriol.* **33**, 301.
Ashe, W. K., and Scherp, H. W. (1965). *J. Immunol.* **94**, 385.
Aurelian, L., Royston, I., and Davis, H. J. (1970). *J. Nat. Cancer Inst.* **45**, 455.
Benyesh-Melnick, M., Dessy, S., and Fernbach, D. J. (1964). *Proc. Soc. Exp. Biol. Med.* **117**, 624.
Black, F. L., and Melnick, J. L. (1955). *J. Immunol.* **74**, 236.
Blackmore, R. V., and Morgan, H. R. (1967). *Acta Virol.* (*Prague*). *English Ed.* **11**, 1.
Breidenbach, G. P., Skinner, M. S., Wallace, J. H., and Mizell, M. (1971). *J. Virol.* **7**, 679.
Buddingh, G. J., Schrum, D. I., Lanier, J. C., and Guidry, D. J. (1953). *Pediatrics* **11**, 595.
Carton, C. A. (1953). *J. Neurosurg.* **10**, 463.
Carton, C. A., and Kilbourne, E. D. (1952). *N. Engl. J. Med.* **246**, 172.
Coleman, V., and Jawetz, E. (1961). *Virology* **13**, 375.
Craighead, J. E. (1969). *Amer. J. Epidemiol.* **90**, 506.
Craighead, J. E., Hanshaw, J. B., and Carpenter, C. B. (1967). *J. Amer. Med. Ass.* **201**, 725.
Douglas, R. G., Jr., Anderson, S., Weg, J. G., Williams, T., Jenkins, D. E., Knight, V., and Beall, A. C., Jr. (1969). *J. Amer. Med. Ass.* **210**, 902.
Duff, R., and Rapp, F. (1971a). *Nature* (*London*) (*New Biol.*) **233**, 48.
Duff, R., and Rapp, F. (1971b). *J. Virol.* **8**, 469.
Ellison, S. A., Carton, C. A., and Rose, H. M. (1959). *J. Infec. Dis.* **105**, 161.
Epstein, M. A., Achong, B. G., and Barr, Y. M. (1964). *Lancet* **1**, 702.
Epstein, M. A., Henle, G., Achong, B. G., and Barr, Y. M. (1965). *J. Exp. Med.* **121**, 761.
Fernandez, C. G. (1960). *Nature* (*London*) **185**, 268.
Findlay, G. M., and MacCallum, F. O. (1940). *Lancet* **1**, 259.
Fulginiti, V. A., Scribner, R., Groth, C. G., Putnam, C. W., Brettschneider, L., Gilbert, S., Porter, K. A., and Starzl, T. E. (1968). *N. Engl. J. Med.* **279**, 619.

Gerber, P. (1972). *Proc. Nat. Acad. Sci. U.S.* **69**, 83.
Glaser, R., and O'Neill, F. J. (1972). *Science* **176**, 1245.
Glaser, R., and Rapp, F. (1972). *J. Virol.* **10**, 288.
Glasgow, L. A., and Habel, K. (1963). *Virology* **19**, 328.
Good, R. A. (1947). *Proc. Soc. Exp. Biol. Med.* **64**, 360.
Good, R. A., and Campbell, B. (1945). *Proc. Soc. Exp. Biol. Med.* **59**, 305.
Good, R. A., and Campbell, B. (1948). *Proc. Soc. Exp. Biol. Med.* **68**, 82.
Goodpasture, E. W. (1929). *Medicine* (*Baltimore*) **8**, 223.
Hampar, B. (1966a). *J. Bacteriol.* **91**, 1959.
Hampar, B. (1966b). *J. Bacteriol.* **91**, 1965.
Hampar, B. (1966c). *J. Bacteriol.* **92**, 1741.
Hampar, B., and Burroughs, M. A. K. (1969). *J. Nat. Cancer Inst.* **43**, 621.
Hampar, B., and Copeland, M. L. (1965). *J. Bacteriol.* **90**, 205.
Hampar, B., and Keehn, M. A. (1967). *J. Immunol.* **99**, 554.
Hampar, B., Martos, L. M., and Walker, J. L. (1971). *J. Nat. Cancer Inst.* **47**, 535.
Hampar, B., Derge, J. G., Martos, L. M., and Walker, J. L. (1972). *Proc. Nat. Acad. Sci. U.S.* **69**, 78.
Hanshaw, J. B., and Weller, T. H. (1961). *J. Pediat.* **58**, 305.
Hanshaw, J. B., Betts, R. F., Simon, G., and Boynton, R. C. (1965). *N. Engl. J. Med.* **272**, 602.
Hedley-Whyte, E. T., and Craighead, J. E. (1965). *N. Engl. J. Med.* **272**, 473.
Henle, G., and Henle, W. (1966). *J. Bacteriol.* **91**, 1248.
Hill, R. B., Jr., Rowlands, D. T., Jr., and Rifkind, D. (1964). *N. Engl. J. Med.* **271**, 1021.
Hill, R. B., Jr., Dahrling, B. E., Starzl, T. E., and Rifkind, D. (1967). *Amer. J. Med.* **42**, 327.
Hinze, H. C., and Walker, J. L. (1961). *J. Bacteriol.* **82**, 498.
Hoggan, M. D., and Roizman, B. (1959). *Amer. J. Hyg.* **70**, 208.
Hope-Simpson, R. E. (1965). *Proc. Roy. Soc. Med.* **58**, 9.
Jacob, F. M. (1931). *Arch. Dermatol. Syphilol.* **24**, 280.
Johnson, R. T. (1964). *J. Exp. Med.* **119**, 343.
Kanich, R. E., and Craighead, J. E. (1966). *Amer. J. Med.* **40**, 874.
Kluge, R. C., Wicksman, R. S., and Weller, T. H. (1960). *Pediatrics* **25**, 35.
Lowy, D. R., Rowe, W. P., Teich, N., and Hartley, J. W. (1971). *Science* **174**, 155.
McKinnell, R. G., and Duplantier, D. P. (1970). *Cancer Res.* **30**, 2730.
Medearis, D. N., Jr. (1964). *Bull. Johns Hopkins Hosp.* **114**, 181.
Mizell, M., and Zambernard, J. (1965). *Ann. N.Y. Acad. Sci.* **126**, 146.
Mizell, M., Stackpole, C. W., Halperen, S., and Isaacs, J. (1968). *Proc. Soc. Exp. Biol. Med.* **127**, 808.
Mizell, M., Stackpole, C. W., and Isaacs, J. J. (1969). *Recent Results Cancer Res. Spec. Suppl. Biology of Amphibian Tumors*, p. 337.
Montgomerie, J. Z., Becroft, D. M. O., Croxson, M. C., Doak, P. B., and North, J. D. K. (1969). *Lancet* **2**, 867.
Munyon, W., Kraiselburd, E., Davis, D., and Mann, J. (1971). *J. Virol.* **7**, 813.
Nahmias, A. J., Josey, W. E., Naib, Z. M., Luce, C. F., and Guest, B. A. (1970). *Amer. J. Epidemiol.* **91**, 547.
Nii, S. (1969). *Biken J.* **12**, 45.
Nii, S. (1970). *Biken J.* **13**, 339.
Nonoyama, M., and Pagano, J. S. (1971). *Nature* (*London*) (*New Biol.*) **233**, 103.
O'Neill, F. J., Goldberg, R. J., and Rapp, F. (1972). *J. Gen. Virol.* **14**, 189.
Pelmont, J., and Morgan, H. R. (1959). *Ann. Inst. Pasteur Paris* **96**, 448.
Perdrau, J. R. (1931). *Proc. Roy. Soc.* **109**, 304.
Perdrau, J. R. (1938). *J. Pathol. Bacteriol.* **47**, 447.

Rafferty, K. A., Jr. (1964). *Cancer Res.* **24**, 169.
Rafferty, K. A., Jr. (1965). *Ann. N.Y. Acad. Sci.* **126**, 3.
Rapp, F., and Duff, R. G. (1971). *Perspect. Virol.* **7**, 37.
Rapp, F., and Duff, R. (1972). *Fed. Proc., Fed. Amer. Soc. Exp. Biol.* **31**, 1660.
Rawls, W. E., Tompkins, W. A. F., and Melnick, J. L. (1969). *Amer. J. Epidemiol.* **89**, 547.
Rifkind, D. (1966). *J. Lab. Clin. Med.* **68**, 463.
Rifkind, D., Marchioro, T. L., Waddell, W. R., and Starzl, T. E. (1964a). *J. Amer. Med. Ass.* **189**, 397.
Rifkind, D., Starzl, T. E., Marchioro, T. L., Waddell, W. R., Rowlands, D. T., Jr., and Hill, R. B., Jr. (1964b). *J. Amer. Med. Ass.* **189**, 808.
Roberts, M. E. (1963). *Cancer Res.* **23**, 1709.
Roizman, B. (1965). *Perspect. Virol.* **4**, 283.
Rowe, W. P., Hartley, J. W., Waterman, S., Turner, H. C., and Huebner, R. J. (1956). *Proc. Soc. Exp. Biol. Med.* **92**, 418.
Rowe, W. P., Hartley, J. W., Cramblett, H. G., and Mastrota, F. M. (1958). *Amer. J. Hyg.* **67**, 57.
Royston, I., and Aurelian, L. (1970a). *Amer. J. Epidemiol.* **91**, 531.
Royston, I., and Aurelian, L. (1970b). *Proc. Nat. Acad. Sci. U.S.* **67**, 204.
Schmidt, J. R., and Rasmussen, A. F., Jr. (1960). *J. Infec. Dis.* **106**, 154.
Scott, T. F. McN. (1954). *N. Engl. J. Med.* **250**, 183.
Sokal, J. E., and Firat, D. (1965). *Amer. J. Med.* **39**, 452.
Stackpole, C. W. (1969). *J. Virol.* **4**, 75.
Stern, H., Elek, S. D., Millar, D. M., and Anderson, H. F. (1959). *Lancet* **2**, 871.
Stevens, J. G., and Cook, M. L. (1971). *Science* **173**, 843.
Stevens, J. G., and Cook, M. L. (1973). *Perspect. Virol.* **8**, 171.
Stevens, J. G., Nesburn, A. B., and Cook, M. L. (1972). *Nature* (*London*), (*New Biol.*) **235**, 216.
Stoker, M. G. P. (1958). *Nature* (*London*) **182**, 1525.
Szanto, J. (1963). *Acta Virol.* (*Prague*) *English Ed.* **7**, 385.
Weller, T. H., and Hanshaw, J. B. (1962). *N. Engl. J. Med.* **266**, 1233.
Weller, T. H., Macauley, J. C. Craig, J. M., and Wirth, P. (1957). *Proc. Soc. Exp. Biol. Med.* **94**, 4.
Wheeler, C. E., and Canby, C. M. (1959). *AMA Arch. Dermatol.* **79**, 86.
Wheeler, C. E., and Canby, C. M. (1960a). *J. Immunol.* **84**, 394.
Wheeler, C. E., and Canby, C. M. (1960b). *J. Bacteriol.* **79**, 657.
Zur Hausen, H., and Schulte-Holthausen, H. (1970). *Nature* (*London*) **227**, 245.

Chapter 10
Herpes Simplex Virus

William E. Rawls, M.D.

I. Introduction

A standard nomenclature for members of the Herpesvirus group has not been uniformly accepted. Synonyms for the virus of herpes simplex include herpes simplex virus, herpesvirus hominінis and herpesvirus. Recently, it has become apparent that isolates of this virus from humans can be separated into two groups by antigenic and biological differences (Dowdle *et al.*, 1967; Parker and Banatvala, 1967; Ejercito *et al.*, 1968; Nahmias and Dowdle, 1968; Figueroa and Rawls, 1969; Kleger and Prier, 1969; Plummer *et al.*, 1970; Lowry *et al.*, 1971; Smith *et al.*, 1971; Docherty *et al.*, 1971a,b; Geder and Skinner, 1971; Longson, 1971; Ratcliff, 1971; Kieff *et al.*, 1972). The distinguishing characteristics of the two groups of virus are not always dramatic and may vary with laboratory conditions (Lowry *et al.*, 1971; Stubbs *et al.*, 1971), and within each group strain differences can be found

(Amstey and Balduzzi, 1970a; Terni and Roizman 1970; Wentworth and Zablatney, 1972). Therefore, there is not uniform agreement as to whether the groups constitute separate types (Goodheart *et al.*, 1968); some authors have suggested that they should be considered subtypes (Roizman *et al.*, 1970; Hampar *et al.*, 1971). In this chapter, the term herpesvirus type 1 will be used for viruses which are normally responsible for oral lesions, and the term herpesvirus type 2 will be used for viruses which are normally responsible for genital lesions.

The contents of this chapter are not necessarily proportionate to the problems caused by the herpesviruses which are encountered in medical practice. Descriptions of the acute manifestations commonly associated with herpesvirus infections have appeared repeatedly in medical literature and are not detailed in this review; detailed descriptions of these diseases can be found in standard medical textbooks. Topics which have received recent attention by investigators in the field are reviewed in greater detail.

Recovery from infections with herpesviruses, unlike recovery from infections with many other viruses, is not associated with complete immunity. The virus may remain latent after the initial infection, and later in life virus replication and excretion may occur. Lesions caused by the viruses have been classified as primary or recurrent. Primary infections have been defined as those infections occurring in individuals who did not have antibodies to the virus. Lesions occurring in individuals with antibodies to the virus have been considered recurrent (Burnet and Williams, 1939). With the awareness of two types of herpesviruses, these definitions are no longer adequate. Theoretically, each type of virus may infect the host for the first time, and each virus may produce a recurrent lesion. Arbitrarily, the term *initial* infection will be used to designate the first infection of a patient with either herpesvirus type. The term primary infection would then apply to the first infection with one type of virus, and a subsequent disease associated with that type of virus would be recurrent. Thus, a patient could have a primary infection and recurrent lesions with type 1 virus and a primary infection and recurrent lesions with type 2 virus. Since the antibodies produced during an infection with either type of virus will cross react with the heterologous virus, the presence or absence of neutralizing antibodies cannot be used as a sole criterion for a lesion being primary or recurrent.

Controversy exists regarding recurrent disease. The lesions may be caused by a chronic infection which is periodically activated, or the lesions may result from reinfection by virus from exogenous sources. The prevailing theory is that most recurrent lesions are produced by latent virus, although, the mechanisms of latency are speculative (Paine, 1964; Roizman, 1965). Most likely the virus remains latent in nerve tissue and is reactivated under conditions of fever, emotional stress, menstruation, or exposure to sunlight.

Herpetic eruptions of the face commonly develop 3–4 days after surgical sectioning of the sensory root of the trigeminal nerve ganglion; however, herpetic lesions do not follow sectioning of the nerves peripheral to the ganglion nor after the ganglion is injected with alcohol. These observations suggest that the virus remains latent in the sensory cells of the ganglion.

Recently, the results of experiments in animals have supported the concept of the virus remaining latent in ganglion cells. Stevens and Cook (1971a) infected the foot pads of the hindlegs of mice, and after the animals had recovered from the acute illness, the spinal root ganglia were examined for herpesvirus. Virus was not found in the ganglion at the time of autopsy; however, if the ganglia were cultured *in vitro* herpesvirus could be demonstrated. Similar experiments were performed in rabbits in which the conjunctiva of the eye was infected with the virus inoculum. After several months, virus could be recovered from the trigeminal ganglion but not from brain tissues or peripheral nerve tissues which were also cultivated *in vitro* (Stevens *et al.*, 1972).

However, it has been proposed that there are chronic infections of herpesvirus with multiplication of the virus in glandular structures such as the lacrimal and salivary glands; recurrent lesions develop when the virus enters a break in the integument (Kaufman *et al.*, 1967). The ability to periodically isolate the virus from lacrimal secretions in the absence of apparent disease tends to support this concept (Ashe and Rizzo, 1967; Kaufman *et al.*, 1967, 1968; Brown and Kaufman, 1969; Laibson and Kibrick, 1969). However, the parotid gland does not appear to be a source of virus during asymptomatic oral excretion of herpesvirus (Douglas and Couch, 1970). Finally, some cases of recurrent lesions appear to be reinfections, since the virus is from exogenous sources. This has been demonstrated by willful or accidental inoculation of virus into humans who possess neutralizing antibodies to the virus (Nahmias and Dowdle, 1968). Reinfection has also been demonstrated in animal studies (Nahmias *et al.*, 1971a). Because of their different modes of transmission, reinfection may be more common with herpesvirus type 2 than with herpesvirus type 1, however, this point has not been proven.

II. Pathology and Pathogenesis

Herpesviruses type 1 and 2 are cytolytic, and the basic pathologic changes are necrosis of the infected cells as well as infiltration of inflammatory cells into the infected area. The inflammatory cells are predominantly mononuclear. In the skin, the injury is confined to the parabasal and intermediate epithelial cells. As can be seen in Fig. 1, an intraepithelial vesicle forms as a result of acantholysis while the superficial cornified layer of squamous cells remains intact. The cells infected with the virus can be seen

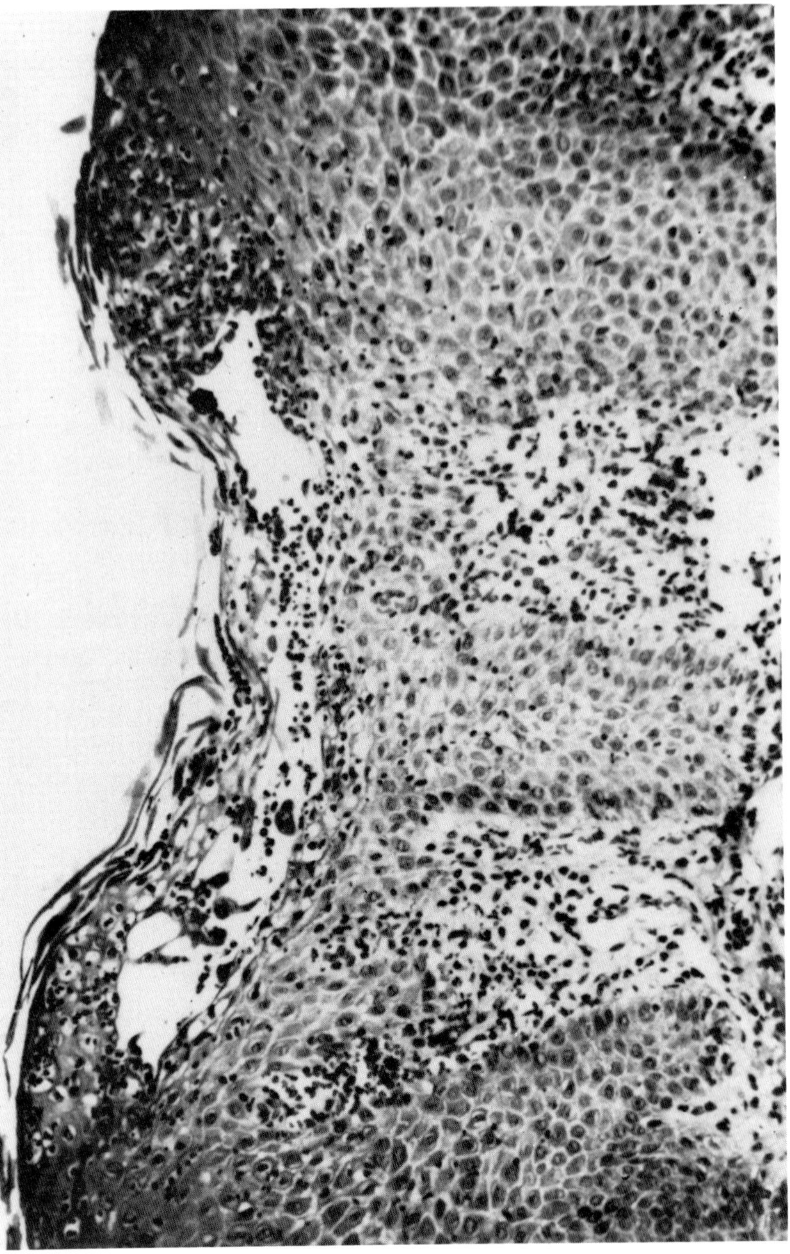

FIG. 1. Histologic section of a vesicular lesion of the vulva. The thin cornified layer is seen covering the intraepithelial vesicle. There is infiltration of inflammatory cells beneath the corium. × 100. (Illustration kindly provided by Dr. Raymond H. Kaufman.)

undergoing changes characteristic of the virus. These can be seen in Fig. 2. There are formations of multinucleated cells and balloon degeneration of the cell nuclei. Cowdry type A inclusions can be found in the nuclei of some of the infected cells. The corium beneath the lesion is infiltrated with inflammatory cells. Cells of the corium are not destroyed, and the lesion heals without scar formation.

When deeper tissues are infected, necrosis is commonly seen. Disseminated infections may be fatal, and in these cases coagulation necroses of the liver, adrenals, lungs, and spleen are frequently observed. Cells containing classic intranuclear inclusions are generally observed, especially at the periphery of the necrotic areas. Necrosis is also a characteristic finding in patients with herpetic encephalitis. The necrotic changes of the brain are most pronounced in the temporal cortex. Necroses are observed in both the gray matter and the white matter. Inclusion bodies in the nuclei of oligodendrocytes and neurons are often observed; however, they may be absent. Meningeal exudates consisting of lymphocytes and plasma cells and scattered perivascular hemorrhage are also found (Haymaker *et al.*, 1958).

Histologic examination of the lesions or examination of cells exfoliated from herpetic lesions are of diagnostic significance (Medak *et al.*, 1971). Examination of exfoliated cells has been of considerable value in detecting herpetic lesions of the female genital tract (Naib *et al.*, 1966; An, 1969; Ng *et al.*, 1970a; Wolinska and Melamed, 1970; Jordon *et al.*, 1972; Cederqvist *et al.*, 1970). Cells obtained by cervical scraping or aspiration may display the changes induced by the virus. An example is shown in Fig. 3. A most striking feature is the presence of numerous multinucleated cells. Balloon degeneration of the nuclei is observed. Initially this appears as a coarse cloudy flocculation, and later the nucleus becomes structureless and swollen giving it a "ground glass" appearance. Intranuclear inclusion bodies develop in some cells. It has been suggested that primary genital infections can be differentiated from recurrent lesions on the basis of the cytologic changes noted in the exfoliated cells. In primary infections, a high percentage of cells with "ground glass" nuclei and a low percentage of cells with intranuclear inclusions have been noted, while in recurrent infections, the cells with these two types of changes were found with about equal frequency (Ng *et al.*, 1970a).

Relatively little information is available regarding the pathogenesis of herpesvirus infections in humans. Presumably the virus, after initial entry, replicates locally in the skin or mucous membranes and spreads cell to cell. The lymph vessels and lymph nodes draining the primary site of infection become inflamed and might be sites of virus replication. A viremia may occur, and herpesvirus has been isolated from the blood of adult patients, as well as from children, with generalized infections (Baker *et al.*, 1952;

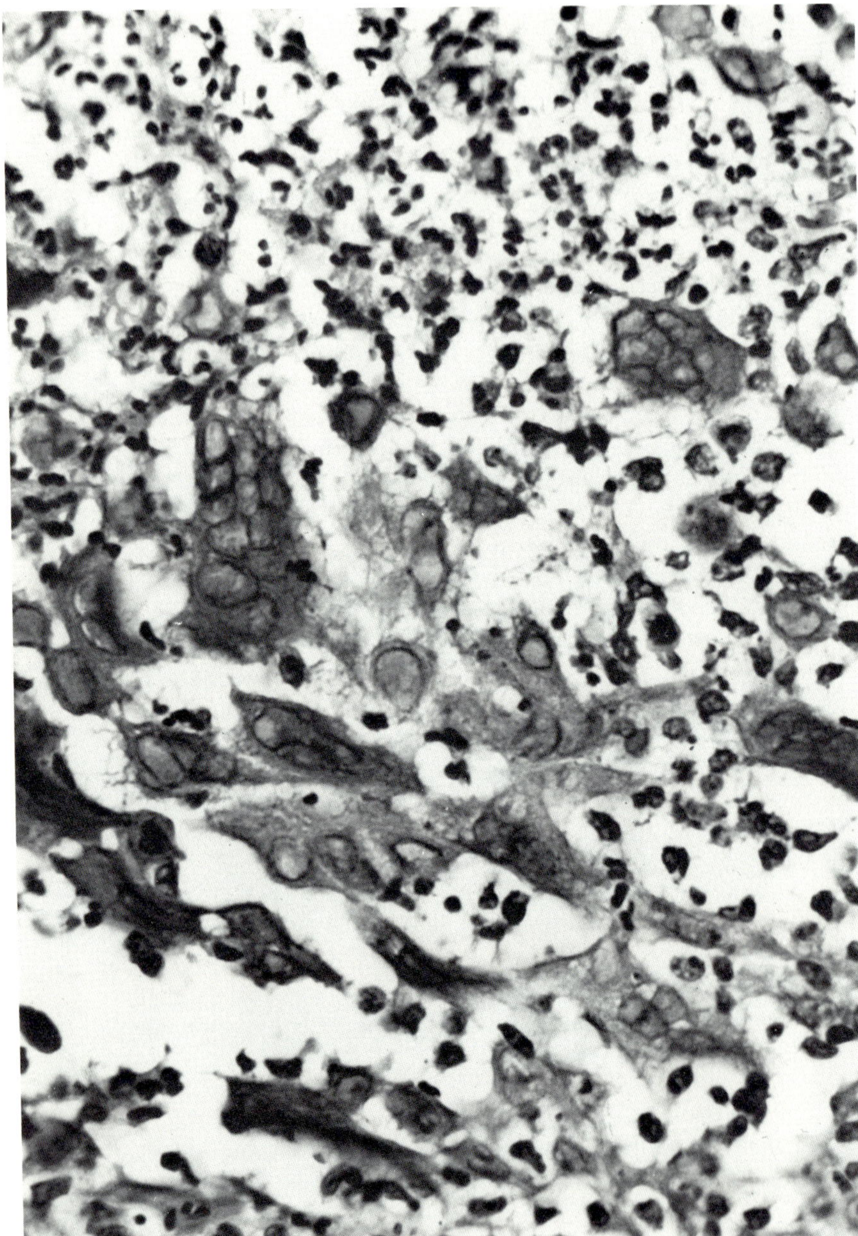

FIG. 2. Histologica section of the vulvar lesion showing multinucleated cells at the base of the vesicle. The balloon degeneration of the nuclei is also apparent. × 350. (Illustration kindly provided by Dr. Raymond H. Kaufman.)

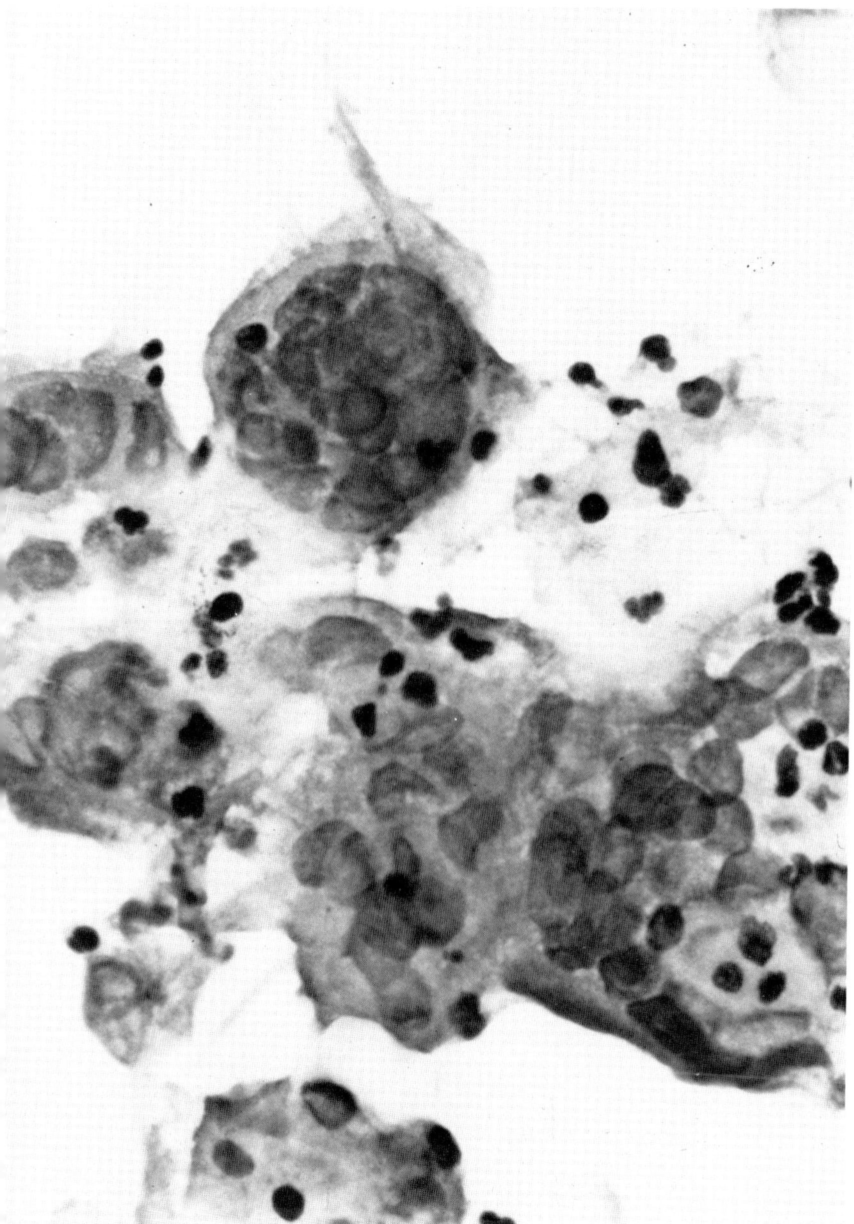

FIG. 3. Papanicolaou smear of a patient with herpes genitalis showing multinucleated cells. (Illustration kindly provided by Dr. Raymond H. Kaufman.)

Becker *et al.*, 1963). In addition, the virus has been found in the blood of patients with herpetic keratitis (Leopold, 1965) and herpetic rhinitis (Ruchman and Dodd, 1950). In neonates and in patients with severe infections, the virus may spread to various organs of the body; however, this is probably not a common occurrence in most infected persons.

Considerable experimental effort has been directed at examining the pathogenesis of herpesvirus infections in laboratory animals; this has been reviewed by Kaplan (1969). The applicability of the observations made in animals to the disease process in man is not yet clear. However, there are several findings in animals which may be comparable to the human disease process. For example, a parallel appears to exist regarding age and severity of infection. Herpesvirus acquired at birth not uncommonly results in a severe, fatal disease; this is observed in both humans and mice (Andervont, 1929; Lennette and Koprowski, 1944; Witzleben and Driscoll, 1965). In mice, infection of the central nervous system is associated with a fatal outcome, and adult or newborn mice die when inoculated intracerebrally. However, when the animals are inoculated intraperitoneally, only newborn mice die of central nervous system infection. The results of recent studies suggest that age-dependent changes in macrophages account for the differences in the severity of the illness. In newborn mice, macrophages are capable of spreading virus to the brain, while in adult animals the macrophages appear to limit the infection (Johnson, 1964b). Suppression of macrophage function with antimacrophage serum or with silica increases the severity of the infection in animals beyond the newborn period (Hirsh *et al.*, 1970). Examination of the macrophage–virus interaction in mice of different ages has demonstrated that an abortive infection occurs in the macrophages of the adult animals (Stevens and Cook, 1971b). Whether or not similar differences in the ability of herpesviruses to replicate in the macrophages of human neonates and of adults remains to be determined.

The mechanism by which herpesvirus reaches the central nervous system has received considerable attention. Subcutaneous inoculation in the hindquarters of laboratory animals not infrequently results in an ascending paralysis. In these instances, it has been demonstrated that the virus may travel along the nerve (Johnson, 1964a; Wildy, 1967). The virus probably does not ascend the axon of the nerve fiber but rather travels in the perineuronal tissues (Johnson, 1964a). When the virus is inoculated into the peritoneal cavity or into the blood stream, hematogenous spread to the central nervous system occurs. Herpes encephalitis in adult human beings could result from hematogenous spread or from spread of the virus along a cranial nerve. The predilection for involvement of the temporal lobes would suggest that virus may spread from the nasal mucosa through the olfactory nerves, olfactory bulbs, and olfactory tracts to the brain. However, herpesvirus has not been commonly isolated from the nasopharynx of patients with encephalitis. In some patients, the encephalitis may represent a recurrent infection (Leider *et al.*, 1965). Data on the distribution of virus and viral antigens in different parts of the brain and cranial nerves in patients with herpes encephalitis would be helpful in determining the mechanism by which the virus gets to the brain.

The genesis of the inflammatory response associated with herpesvirus infections may depend upon the immune status of the host. The virus in cytolytic, and it has been demonstrated *in vitro* that factors released from infected cells interact with complement to produce chemotactic factors. The factors released from the cells may be proteolytic enzymes which cleave the components of complement, the cleavage products mediating chemotaxis for polymorphonuclear leukocytes (Brier *et al.*, 1970). In the immune host, the reaction may be accelerated. Antibodies which are cytolytic *in vitro* can be found in the immune host; *in vivo* these antibodies might hasten the lysis of the infected cell (Brier *et al.*, 1971; Smith *et al.*, 1972). There is a greater production of the chemotactic substances with the interaction of viral antigens, antibody, and complement than with the interaction of the factors released from infected cells and complement (Snyderman *et al.*, 1972). Finally, sensitized lymphocytes upon interaction with antigens release soluble factors which contribute to the inflammatory response (Rocklin, 1971).

III. Epidemiology

Herpesvirus type 1 is spread primarily by the oral–respiratory route, while herpesvirus type 2 appears to be a venereally transmitted agent. The agents are labile, and exchange of contaminated secretions appears to be the major mode of host-to-host spread of both herpesvirus types 1 and 2. Infections with herpesvirus type 1 do not show marked seasonal variation in incidence, and epidemics are not common, even within families. The incubation period of both types of virus are similar; they range from 2 to 12 days with a usual incubation period of about 3 to 9 days. Man is the only natural host, and the infected patient is the only known reservoir. The virus excretion associated with asymptomatic infections probably represents the major source of the virus which infects susceptible individuals. Early studies demonstrated that herpesvirus could be readily isolated from the saliva of asymptomatic carriers (Buddingh *et al.*, 1953). This has been confirmed repeatedly, and approximately 2–5% of adults in cross-sectional epidemiologic surveys have been found to be excreting virus (Stern *et al.*, 1959; Mufson *et al.*, 1967; Lindgren *et al.*, 1968; Greenberg *et al.*, 1969; Cesario *et al.*, 1969; Kloene *et al.*, 1970). Repeat sampling of patients with antibodies to herpesvirus have demonstrated that 27% or more will have virus excreted in their saliva over the intervals studied (Greenberg *et al.*, 1969; Cesario *et al.*, 1969; Douglas and Couch, 1970). Thus, for herpesvirus type 1, asymptomatic excretion provides a major source of virus. Similar excretion patterns probably occur for herpesvirus type 2 (Centifanto *et al.*, 1971), and the contaminated genital secretions of symptomatic or asymptomatic patients provide the source of virus for herpes genitalis.

Sero-epidemiologic studies have suggested two prominent factors which influence the occurrence of herpesvirus type 1. These factors are age and socioeconomic conditions (Smith *et al.*, 1967; Gerber and Rosenblum, 1968; Porter *et al.*, 1969; Wentworth and Alexander, 1971; Black *et al.*, 1970). Although these studies were performed using methods which did not delineate between past infections with herpesvirus type 1 and herpesvirus type 2, the basic conclusions appear valid. Herpesvirus spreads more readily under lower socioeconomic conditions and less readily under upper socioeconomic conditions. Among the lower social classes, most mothers possess antibodies to herpesvirus type 1, and infection of the infant before 6 months of age is uncommon. Infection occurs most frequently between 1 and 3 years of age, and essentially all of the population has been infected by the age of puberty. Infection in the upper social classes tends to occur beyond early childhood and in some populations 40–50% of young adults do not possess antibodies to the virus.

Herpesvirus type 2 is typically acquired during sexual intercourse; thus, herpes genitalis is primarily a venereal disease (Parker and Banatvala, 1967; Josey *et al.*, 1968, 1972). Several lines of evidence support the venereal mode of transmission of the virus. The most direct evidence is the demonstration of a high risk of becoming infected among sexual contacts of patients with herpes genitalis. Female contacts of males suffering from herpes genitalis were found to be infected by herpesvirus type 2 with much greater frequency than other women of a similar social setting. It has been estimated that approximately 80% of susceptible female contacts of males with herpes genitalis will become infected by the virus (Nahmias *et al.*, 1969a; Rawls *et al.*, 1971).

The distribution of antibodies to herpesvirus type 2 in various segments of the population also supports the concept that the virus is venereally transmitted. Antibodies do not appear in the population until the age when heterosexual activity begins. The percentage of the population with antibodies to the virus then increases rather rapidly during the next two decades of life and remains relatively constant thereafter (Rawls *et al.*, 1969; Nahmias *et al.*, 1970a; Adam *et al.*, 1972a). Antibodies to the virus are rarely found among chaste women (Nahmias *et al.*, 1970b), while the occurrence of antibodies among prostitutes is high (Rawls *et al.*, 1969; Dueñas *et al.*, 1972).

The prevalence of herpesvirus type 2 infections correlates with the degree of sexual activity. This is suggested from the data presented in Fig. 4 which was taken from the report of Ng *et al.* (1970b). Infections are observed most commonly in women age 20–29 years and next most commonly in women less than 20 years of age, the ages of maximal sexual activity. Using cytologic changes or virus isolation, the prevalence of herpesvirus infections among women receiving routine cervicovaginal cytologic examination has been estimated to be between 0.09 and 0.42% (Kleger *et al.*, 1968; Naib *et al.*, 1969; Wolinska and Melamed, 1970; Jeansson and Molin, 1970; Jordon *et al.*, 1972). Among women attending venereal disease clinics, 1.6–6.7% have been found to be infected by herpesvirus type 2 (Kleger *et al.*, 1968; Beilby *et al.*, 1968; Jeansson and Molin, 1970; Rawls *et al*; 1971; Josey *et al.*, 1972), and the virus was found among 6.9% of the prostitutes examined (Dueñas *et al.*, 1972). The isolation rate in the prostitute population was age-dependent; 12% of women under 19 years of age were excreting virus, and 6% of women 20–29 years of age were excreting virus. Virus was recovered from 2.8% of prostitutes over age 30 years (Dueñas *et al.*, 1972).

Finally, it is not uncommon to find infections by herpesvirus type 2 associated with other venereal diseases. Co-infection of patients by herpesvirus and gonococcal organisms has been repeatedly observed (Beilby *et al.*, 1968; Dickie, 1969; Amstey and Balduzzi, 1970b; Jeansson and Molin, 1971b). A greater than expected incidence of trichomoniasis, condyloma accumi-

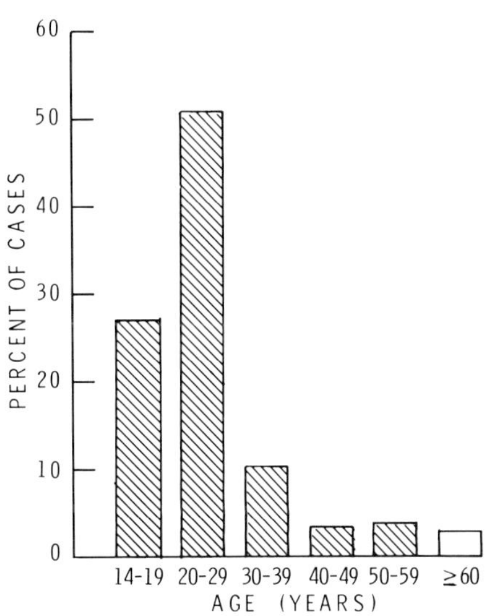

FIG. 4. Age distribution of women with herpes genitalis. (Drawn from data of Ng *et al.*, 1970b.)

natum, and *Hemophilus vaginalis* infections have also been observed among women with herpes genitalis (Nahmias *et al.*, 1969a; Rawls *et al.*, 1971). In addition, a correlation between antibodies to herpesvirus type 2 and serologic evidence of syphilis has been noted (Dueñas *et al.*, 1972).

IV. Immunity to Herpesvirus

Infection by herpesviruses results in the production of antibodies which can be detected by a number of serologic methods. Neutralizing antibodies appear about 1 week after infection and reach maximum titers in 3–4 weeks. In most individuals, antibodies to the viruses remain for many years, and significant decreases in titer in older age groups have not been consistently observed (Wentworth and Alexander, 1971). Recurrent lesions are not generally associated with an increase in antibody titers (Douglas and Couch, 1970). It is generally held that antibodies provide little protection against recurrent disease. Secretory IgA has been implicated as a possible factor in preventing local recurrence; however, neutralizing activity of IgA obtained from the oral secretions could not be demonstrated (Douglas and Couch, 1970).

In addition to a humoral immune response, there is a cellular immune response to the viruses. This can be detected by a delayed type of hypersensitivity reaction to the intradermal injection of viral antigens (Nagler, 1944, 1946; Rose and Molloy, 1947; Jawetz *et al.*, 1951; Anderson and Kilbourne, 1961; Lausch *et al.*, 1966). The blastogenic response of lymphocytes in the presence of antigen and the production of macrophage migration inhibitory factor and cytotoxin by the lymphocytes in the presence of specific antigens are thought to be *in vitro* correlates of cellular immunity. These *in vitro* correlations of cellular immunity have also been applied to measure the reaction to the herpesviruses (Wilton *et al.*, 1972; Rosenberg *et al.*, 1972). It would appear that cellular immune functions play an important role in recovery of herpesvirus infections and in preventing recurrent disease. The fact that patients with defects in cellular immune functions not uncommonly develop severe herpetic lesions supports this supposition. Recently, evidence has been presented which suggest that the susceptibility to recurrent disease by the virus is due to the impaired production of macrophage migration inhibitory factor and lymphocyte cytotoxins by sensitized lymphocytes of the patient (Wilton *et al.*, 1972).

Precise definition of the antigens of herpesvirus types 1 and 2 has not yet been accomplished. Infection with one type of virus results in the production of antibodies that will cross react with the heterologous virus, although, the degree of cross reactivity is usually less than the reactivity to the homologous virus (Royston and Aurelian, 1970a; Nahmias *et al.*, 1970a; Rawls *et al.*, 1970a). The viruses appear to share common antigens, and, in addition, each type of virus possesses one or more specific antigens (Schneweis and Nahmias, 1971). In addition to cross-reacting antibody, we have observed cross reaction of the delayed hypersensitivity response in rabbits (W. E. Rawls, unpublished observations), and cross reactivity in the stimulation of lymphocyte blastogenesis *in vitro* has also been observed (Rosenberg *et al.*, 1972). Thus, there seems to be some degree of cross immunity between herpesvirus types 1 and 2. Clinical observations support this concept; patients who have had prior infections with type 1 virus generally have less severe manifestations of the illness when they subsequently become infected with type 2 virus than patients with type 2 as their initial herpesvirus infection (Rawls *et al.*, 1971).

Prior infection with one type of virus may alter the immune response to the second virus. The ^{51}Cr release test has been used to quantitate antibodies to the specific antigens appearing on the surface of cells infected with herpesvirus type 2. Appreciable quantities of antibodies to these antigens were detected in the convalescent sera of patients who had experienced a type 2 virus infection as their initial herpesvirus infection. However, little or no antibody activity to the type 2 specific antigens was found in the convalescent sera of patients who had herpes genitalis and evidence of a prior herpesvirus type 1 infection (Smith *et al.*, 1972).

V. Clinical Manifestations of Herpesvirus Type 1

A variety of clinical entities may be produced by herpesvirus types 1 and 2. Generally, the lesions produced by the viruses occur in tissues derived from embryonic ectoderm; the skin, oral cavity, vagina, conjunctiva, and nervous system are the most frequent sites of infection. However, in newborn infants and in patients with defects of host defense mechanisms, tissues derived from other embryonic tissues may be involved. The lesions which develop in the integument characteristically begin with the formation of a painful superficial vesicle. Upon rupture of the vesicle, the lesion becomes a shallow ulcer. Virus can be readily isolated from the infected tissues.

Excellent descriptions of most of the clinical manifestations of herpesviruses can be found elsewhere (Brain, 1956; Scott and Tokumaru, 1965; Tokumaru, 1969). With the socioeconomic conditions that presently prevail in the industrialized countries, many persons reach adult life without having been infected by the virus. Manifestations of herpesvirus infections which were previously thought to occur only in children are now being seen in adults. In addition, infection with type 2 virus as an initial herpesvirus infection appears to be occurring with increasing frequency among young adults of the upper socioeconomic classes. Severe herpes genitalis is not uncommon in this group.

The clinical entities associated with infection by the herpesviruses can be arbitarily classified as those caused by type 1 virus and those caused by type 2 virus. This classification is artificial in that either virus may be associated with any of the clinical entities described. Herpes genitalis is normally caused by herpesvirus type 2, but isolates from about 1–5% of the cases have been found to be type 1 virus. Similarly, type 1 virus is normally isolated from oral lesions, but occassionally type 2 virus can be isolated from the oral secretions (Josey *et al.*, 1972; Kaufman and Rawls, 1972). No distinctive features of the clinical illness has been found between infections of the same site caused by the two types of virus.

Acute herpetic gingivostomatitis is the usual symptomatic manifestation of an initial infection by herpesvirus type 1 in children (Dodd *et al.*, 1938). About 15% of the infections are manifest in this form, and the peak occurrence of the disease has been described as being between 1 and 3 years of age. The illness is an infection of the mucous membranes of the oral cavity. At first, the lesions of the membranes are vesicular but quickly evolve into grayish-yellow plaques and ulcers. The gums are red and swollen as are the other ulcerated membranes of the mouth. There is frequently an oral fetor, drooling, and local lymphadenopathy. The child is often febrile with fever of 104–105°F not uncommonly observed. In addition, malaise, sleepiness, and diarrhea may accompany the illness. In some cases, the onset is insidious, with fever and irritability preceding the oral lesions by 2–3 days. The number and size of the lesions vary. When the lesions begin in the tonsillar region, the infection may appear as a tonsillitis or pharyngitis. The disease is self-limiting and lesions resolve in 2–3 weeks. The nose may also be the primary site of the initial infection, in which case there are vesicles in the nostrils (Ruchman and Dodd, 1950). In adults, an initial infection with herpesvirus may also produce acute gingivostomatitis. In studies of individuals beyond early childhood, predominate clinical manifestations have been those of pharyngitis and tonsillitis (Evans and Dick, 1964; Tokumaru, 1966; Sheridan and Herrmann, 1971). However, since herpesvirus can be isolated from asymptomatic patients as well as from patients with pharyngitis caused by other organisms, the etiologic role of herpesvirus in pharyngitis remains unclear.

Herpes labialis or herpes simplex is a manifestation of recurrent herpesvirus type 1. The disease usually involves the mucocutaneous junction of the lip and tends to recur at the same site time after time. As discussed above, the virus is thought to remain latent in the sensory cells of the trigeminal nerve ganglion; under conditions of stress, fever, or exposure to sunlight the virus becomes activated and descends the sensory nerve to the lip.

Burning or a sense of irritation often precedes by several hours the appearance of a series of red papules. The papules progress to vesicles within a matter of hours. Frequently there are multiple vesicles at the site. The thin-walled vesicles have an erythematous base. The clear fluid becomes cloudy within a day or so. The lesions tend to heal rapidly, and within 5–7 days healing without residual scarring is complete. In some patients, erythema multiforme may develop in association with recurrent herpes labialis.

Skin lesions of herpesvirus type 1 include primary herpetic dermatitis, eczema herpeticum, and traumatic herpes. The virus does not normally infect intact skin; however, infection can occur in diseased skin or skin broken by trauma. In *primary herpetic dermatitis*, skin manifestations appear to be a part of the initial infection. The disease is usually seen in young children and is characterized by a generalized eruption and systemic symptoms of fever and malaise. Gingivostomatitis may be associated with the cutaneous lesions. The eruption may appear in crops and resemble the rash of varicella; however, the vesicles of herpesvirus appear to be smaller. Occassionally the eruption occurs along the distribution of a sensory nerve producing a zoster-like illness (Music *et al.*, 1971; Mok, 1971).

Eczema varicelliform herpeticum Kaposi is a rather severe infection of the skin among patients with atopic eczema. The disease may also occur in patients with Darier's disease (Doeglas and Moolhuysen, 1969; Izumi and Goldschmidt, 1970). In this infection herpesvirus type 1 appears to enter by way of the diseased skin. There is an acute onset of numerous vesicles over large areas of the body. The vesicles may appear in crops for 3–4 days and may remain for as long as 9 days. The patients are usually febrile, and sometimes the illness may be severe. Large areas of epithelium may be denuded which can result in the loss of large quantities of body fluids. Death due to dehydration, secondary bacterial infection, and shock, owing to adrenal necrosis, has been described. Recurrent attacks may follow the primary infection; however, the recurrent disease is less severe, and the duration is shorter than the initial illness.

Traumatic herpes results from infection by the virus which enters through a break in the normal skin. These infections may be caused by either type 1 or 2 herpesvirus. The break in the epithelium is usually an abrasion or minor laceration. Traumatic herpes may occur anywhere on the body; however, there are special settings in which the disease is more commonly seen. For example, the fingers are common sites for infection, and lesions at this site have been called "herpetic whitlow" (Stern *et al.*, 1959). The disease may occur among wrestlers and has been called "herpetic gladiatorum" (Selling and Kibrick, 1964; Wheeler and Cabaniss, 1965). Skin which has been injured by heat is also susceptible to the infection by the virus, and a systemic herpetic infection may occur in burn patients (Foley *et al.*, 1970).

The distal segments of the fingers, especially the thumb and index finger, are the usual sites of herpetic whitlow (Stern *et al.*, 1959). At first there is erythema and tenderness at the site of trauma. Soon after the appearance of the lesion small vesicles form; the vesicles tend to enlarge and coalesce to form a large vesicle with a surrounding bright border of erythema. The lesion may be accompanied by considerable discomfort and throbbing pain. The lymphatics draining the lesion become inflamed producing lymphangitis and lymphadenitis. If the infection is the initial experience of the patient with herpesvirus, there may be systemic symptoms of fever and malaise. The disease is self-limiting and the lesion resolves in 2–3 weeks. Recurrent eruptions at the site of the initial lesion are not uncommon. Herpetic whitlow in a patient with a prior infection by the herpesviruses is usually less severe, and the course of the illness is shorter than in patients without a prior infection. Herpetic whitlow is an occupational hazard of physicians, dentists, and nurses (Stern *et al.*, 1959; Brightman and Guggenheimer, 1970; Davies and Longson, 1970; Muller and Herrmann, 1970; Nally and James, 1970; Orkin, 1970; Rosato *et al.*, 1970; Juel-Jensen, 1971; Larossa and Hamilton, 1971; Green and Levin, 1971). Accidental contamination of minor abrasions of the fingers with herpesvirus-containing secretions of patients is thought to be the mode of infection. Infections of the fingers may be associated with gingivostomatitis in both children and adults, especially among those who habitually bite their fingernails (Davies and Longson, 1970; Muller and Herrmann, 1970). The lesions may also develop on the finger of patients with herpes genitalis (Friedrich *et al.*, 1969).

The cutaneous lesions of wrestlers are located at sites of maximal abrasions incurred during wrestling. The face, scalp, ears, wrist, and forearms are the usual sites of lesions and more often appear on the right side of the body than on the left. This distribution is in keeping with the areas most commonly traumatized by standard throws used in the sport (Selling and Kibrick, 1964; Dyke *et al.*, 1965; Porter and Baughman, 1965; Wheeler and Cabaniss, 1965).

Infections of the eye by herpesvirus are not rare. Isolates from eye lesions are usually type 1 virus. Both primary and recurrent infections occur, and the severity of disease depends largely upon the depth of involvement (Brown, 1971). In the primary infection, the disease manifests itself as an acute follicular conjunctivitis with vesicle formation of the lid margin and skin. Ulcers may develop on the conjunctiva, and preauricular lymphadenopathy may be observed. Fever and gingivostomatitis may accompany the eye lesions in the initial herpesvirus infection. The lesions may remain confined to the conjunctiva or the cornea may become infected. Recurrent infections of the cornea are not usually accompanied by follicular conjunctivitis; however, cases of recurrent herpetic conjunctivitis have been described (Nauheim, 1969).

Superficial infections of the cornea produce characteristic dendritic ulcerations. Several forms of ulceration may occur which give rise to superficial punctate erosions or small dendritic ulcers. Dendritic ulcers may develop as extensions of vesicular lesions first appearing at the border of the cornea. Occasionally deep, unbranched, marginal ulcers are observed in recurrent disease, and large erosions of the cornea are also seen. The infections produce considerable pain, and the patients complain of severe photophobia and lacrimation. Resolution usually requires 2–3 weeks, and in the absence of secondary bacterial infection the herpesvirus infection does not normally damage the eye permanently.

Disciform keratitis is a deeper form of disease which follows a superficial infection. If the stromal fibers are not destroyed, the lesion heals in 2–3 months with minimal scarring. More commonly the lesion is severe, and there is necrosis of stromal fibers. Upon healing scar formation occurs which may impair vision. Hypopyon keratitis may follow large corneal ulcerations, and this lesion also may heal with scarring. Iridocyclitis may complicate keratitis and is characterized by severe pain, circumcorneal flush, and multiple keratitic precipitates. Opacification of the lens as well as formation of synechia are associated with iridocyclitis. Virus particles and viral antigens can be detected in the fluid aspirated from the anterior chamber of the eyes of patients with kerato-iritis (Pavan-Langston and Brockhurst, 1969; Patterson *et al.*, 1969; Kaufman *et al.*, 1971).

Herpetic encephalitis may occur in disseminated infections, especially in the newborn, or it may occur as an infection limited primarily to the brain. Encephalitis beyond the newborn period is caused by herpesvirus type 1 and is one of the most common causes of severe sporadic encephalitis in adults (Olson *et al.*, 1967; Miller and Ross, 1968). No consistent seasonal variation in the occurrence of the disease has been observed (Olson *et al.*, 1967), nor does there seem to be a significant difference in the incidence of the disease between males and females (Olson *et al.*, 1967; Gurwith *et al.*, 1971). At least some cases of encephalitis appear to represent recurrent lesions. Antibodies to the virus are often found in serum obtained soon after the onset of illness, and a number of patients have a past history of herpes labialis (Leider *et al.*, 1965; Rawls *et al.*, 1966). In addition, the age distribution of patients developing encephalitis does not parallel the susceptibility of the population to infection. This is illustrated in Fig. 5 which is the age distribution of 123 cases compiled by reviewing the literature (Booth *et al.*, 1961; Drachman and Adams, 1962; Itabashi *et al.*, 1966; Miller *et al.*, 1966; Rawls *et al.*, 1966; Olson *et al.*, 1967; Harland *et al.*, 1967; Miller and Ross, 1968; Welt *et al.*, 1969; Nolan *et al.*, 1970; Meyer *et al.*, 1970; Gurwith *et al.*, 1971). The disease has occurred in the reported cases with approximately equal frequency in all age groups. If the disease were the result of a primary infection, a decrease with increasing age would be expected.

Herpetic encephalitis in adults is unique in that the infection appears to involve localized areas of the brain. The virus produces an acute necrotizing lesion which involves one or both temporal lobes. There is widespread inflammation of the meninges. Typical intranuclear inclusions may be found on histologic examination of diseased tissues (Smith *et al.*, 1941). Virus particles can be found in the infected cells by electron microscopy (Roy and Wolman, 1969; Upton and Gumpert, 1970), and viral antigens can be detected by immunofluorescent techniques (Gurwith *et al.*, 1971; Johnson *et al.*, 1972).

In the prodromal period, patients may experience fever and malaise. Some patients develop symptoms of an upper respiratory tract infection, however, typical herpetic lesions of the mouth or pharynx are not usually noted. The onset of the neurologic abnormalities is often abrupt. Some patients develop peculiar behavior, hallucinations, or memory loss, while in others convulsive seizures herald the onset. Fever, headache, nuchal rigidity, coma, and generalized seizures, which are signs observed in most forms of encephalitis, are also observed in patients with herpetic encephalitis. In addition, patients with herpetic encephalitis develop signs of focal involvement of the cerebral hemispheres. These include aphasia, focal motor seizures, conjugate eye deviation, focal (usually facial) paralysis, and unilateral paralysis. The localizing features of the disease provide characteristics which permit a tentative diagnosis of herpesvirus encephalitis to be made on clinical grounds.

The course of the disease is rapid, and the majority of patients die within

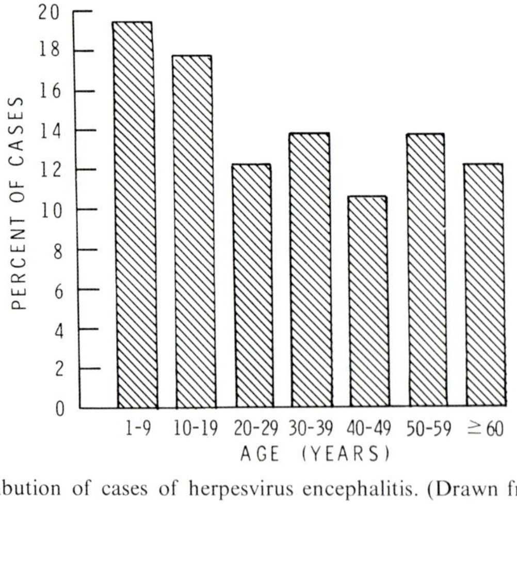

FIG. 5. Age distribution of cases of herpesvirus encephalitis. (Drawn from data obtained from literature.)

3 weeks of onset of symptoms. Of patients who become comatosed, only 30% survive, and many of these patients are left with residual neurologic abnormalities. The prognosis is better for those who do not lapse into coma; approximately 85% survive (Gurwith *et al.*, 1971). The residual neurologic abnormalities range in severity and may include partial paralysis, mental retardation, and Korsakoff's psychosis. In the latter, the memory defect appears to be due to destruction of the inferomedial portion of the cerebral cortex, and the defect may be more pronounced for verbal stimuli than for other forms of stimuli (Starr and Phillip, 1968; Victor, 1969; Silk and Roome, 1970; Johnson *et al.*, 1972).

The localized inflammation and edema of the temporal lobes are associated with changes in structures and functions that can be detected by electroencephalography, angiography, or brain scan. The electroencephalographic changes have been considered diagnostic by some authors (Scott and Prior, 1970; Upton and Gumpert, 1970) but not by others (Pelc, 1971). The changes include (a) slow wave activity which may be generalized, lateralized or focal; (b) disruption, slowing or flattening of background rhythm; and (c) sharp waves, spikes or "irritative" waves. Localized sharp waves or spike and wave complexes occurring at quasiregular intervals are seen, and these waves sometime develop into focal electrographic seizures (Drachman and Adams, 1962; Rawls *et al.*, 1966). It has been suggested that the rapid development of the periodic complexes within 2–15 days of the onset of illness followed by the disappearance of the complexes in the face of no clinical improvement may be diagnostic of herpesvirus encephalitis (Upton and Gumpert, 1970). The infected area of the brain may give the appearance of a mass lesion by angiography or by brain scan (Davis and Potchen, 1970; Halpern *et al.*, 1970; Mishkin, 1970; Radcliffe *et al.*, 1971).

Several reports have suggested that herpesviruses may somehow play a role in behavioral disorders. Periodic episodes of abnormal behavior, thought to represent recurrent inflammation of the cerebrum, have been described in patients recovering from herpesvirus encephalitis. Recently, case–control studies have demonstrated associations of certain psychiatric disorders with increased antibody activity to herpesvirus type 1. In one study in which the kinetics of neutralization was used to assay antibodies, an increased activity to the virus among patients with psychopathic disorders was demonstrated (Cleobury *et al.*, 1971). In another study more patients suffering from psychotic depression were found to have elevated complement-fixing antibody titers than control patients (Rimon *et al.*, 1971).

Serologic studies of patients have suggested that some cases of meningitis are caused by herpesvirus (Olson *et al.*, 1967). The virus has rarely been isolated from the cerebrospinal fluid. Symptoms of meningitis appear to accompany herpesvirus type 2 infections more commonly than herpesvirus type 1. The symptoms of meningitis occur shortly after the development of the genital lesions and last for 1–2 weeks. Lymphocytosis is observed in the cerebrospinal fluid, and this may persist for 1 week or so after clinical recovery. Headaches and/or neuralgia may accompany recurrence of the genital lesion (Slavin and Ferguson, 1950; Hunt and Comer, 1955; Duxbury and Lawrence, 1959; Constantine *et al.*, 1968; Terni *et al.*, 1971). Rarely, herpesvirus may be associated with progressive dysfunction of the spinal cord in the absences of signs and symptoms of encephalitis (Klastersky *et al.*, 1972).

Herpetic hepatitis is a common feature of neonatal infection and disseminated infections of adults and has been described in a woman who was apparently normal except for being pregnant (Flewett *et al.*, 1969). Hepatitis as a manifestation of a herpesvirus infection is probably an uncommon event in otherwise healthy individuals beyond the newborn period.

Herpesvirus infections in immunologically incompetent patients may behave in an unusual manner. Severe disseminated infections normally occur only in the newborn period. However, generalized herpesvirus infections have been reported among patients who have received allotransplants and who are receiving immunosuppressent drugs (Montgomerie *et al.*, 1969; Stinson *et al.*, 1971). Patients on immunosuppressive therapy and patients with hematologic malignancies have been found to have unusually severe infections by herpesvirus involving the skin (Stroud, 1961; Bean and Fusaro, 1969; Lynfield *et al.*, 1969; Merigan and Stevens, 1971; Muller *et al.*, 1972; Nishimura *et al.*, 1972) and respiratory tract (Crosby *et al.*, 1969; Douglas *et al.*, 1969; Nash and Foley, 1970). These patients also may develop chronic cutaneous herpetic ulcers (Neff and Lane, 1970; Logan *et al.*, 1971). Severe disseminated herpesvirus infections are observed in malnourished children (Brain *et al.*, 1957; Becker *et al.*, 1968; Templeton, 1970), and herpetic pneumonitis has been reported in a chronic alcoholic (Caldwell and Porter, 1971). Infection with the virus may produce a severe illness which is sometimes fatal in children with the Wiskott-Aldrich syndrome (St. Geme *et al.*, 1965; Evans and Holzel, 1970). Thus, herpesvirus infections may pose serious problems among patients with malignancies of the hematopoietic system. In addition, the viruses may produce life-threatening infections among transplant patients; however, among this group of patients all investigators have not experienced this problem (Spencer and Andersen, 1970).

VI. Clinical Manifestations of Herpesvirus Type 2

Herpes genitalis is an infection of the genitalia and is usually caused by herpesvirus type 2. The infection may produce illnesses of varying severity.

The majority of infections in women do not produce symptoms of sufficient severity to warrant medical attention. In several surveys of women, in which the presence of infection was determined through the use of the Papanicolaou smear or by virus isolation, about 40% of the infections were not associated with symptoms; lesions could not be detected at gynecological examination in about an equal percentage of infected women (Josey *et al.*, 1966; Ng *et al.*, 1970b). Lesions produced by the virus are most commonly found on the vulva, vagina, cervix, and the perineum. Less common sites are perianal, on the thighs, buttocks, and mons pubis. The lesions are characteristic of herpetic lesions located elsewhere on the body. Where the cornium is thick, a vesicle filled with clear fluid first appears on an erythematous papule. The vesicle ruptures leaving a shallow painful ulcer. On the moist membranes of the vagina and cervix, vesicular eruptions are not commonly seen. The lesions often resemble a thin membrane or mucouslike patch which may be associated with diffuse reddness. Necrotic-appearing ulcers of the cervix are sometimes observed (Gardner and Kaufman, 1969).

The chief symptoms associated with the lesions are hyperesthia, burning, itching, and pain on urination. Dyspareunia and a burning leukorrhea are commonly experienced. Initial genital infections may be associated with severe dysuria, urinary retention, inguinal lymphadenopathy, and constitutional symptoms (Dickie, 1969; McIndoe and Churchouse, 1972). Among patients with dysuria, intranuclear inclusion bodies can be detected in cells of the urinary sediment (Boyd and Nedelkoska, 1967) and virus can be readily isolated from the urine (W. E. Rawls, unpublished observations). Primary infections generally last 2 or 3 weeks before resolution. Recurrent lesions, which commonly occur, are less severe and of shorter duration than primary lesions.

Herpesvirus type 2 in the male usually produces a vesicular eruption on the glans, prepuce, or shaft of the penis. In addition to the pain and irritation associated with the lesion, the patient may also experience a scant watery urethral discharge and pain on micturition. Symptoms of urethritis and prostatitis appear to occur in the absence of an overt lesion on the penis in some patients. Virus has been isolated from cases of nonspecific urethritis and prostatitis; usually from a minority of the patients studied (Goodwin *et al.*, 1970; Morrisseau *et al.*, 1970; Jeansson and Molin, 1971a).

Neonatal herpes is an infection of infants within the first 4 weeks of life. The manifestations of infection in the newborn period may be unusually severe, and the illness can be considered as a separate clinical entity. For some time the disease was thought to be almost uniformly fatal; however, recent reports indicate that the virus produces infections of varying severity. The infection is usually acquired at birth, and the source of the virus is the infected birth canal of the mother. Consequently, herpesvirus type 2 appears to be responsible for more than 80% of the cases of neonatal herpes. A great deal of the data available in the literature regarding the disease comes from reports of fatal cases. This literature has been reviewed by Witzleben and Driscoll (1965) and Nahmias *et al.* (1970c). In recent years it has become apparent that a portion of the infections are not fatal, and some infections are virtually asymptomatic. The frequency of expression of the disease in various degrees of severity has not been established.

The severe, disseminated infection may become evident at any time from birth to 24 days of age; most illnesses begin from 3 to 14 days after birth. The signs accompanying the illness are not specific and may include poor feeding, lack of weight gain, vomiting, diarrhea, respiratory difficulty, hypoactivity, and vasomotor instability. Jaundice, conjunctivitis, or neurologic abnormalities sometimes herald the onset of the illness. The course of the disseminated infection is often characterized by rapid deterioration and death. The mean duration of illness is about 6 days. Those infants surviving may have residual damage of the central nervous system and eyes. Hypoadrenalism in a survivor has been reported (Bahrani *et al.*, 1966).

Abnormalities of multiple organs may become manifest during the disseminated infection. About half of the cases show evidence of involvement of the central nervous system. This may be expressed clinically as convulsions, opisthotonos, bulging fontanelle, changes in muscle tone, and coma. The cerebrospinal fluid is abnormal in most cases of disseminated herpesvirus infection of the newborn, and virus can be readily isolated from this fluid. Evidence of hepatic involvement has been found in almost all cases; however, in about 30% of the cases neither jaundice nor hepatomegaly are observed. The indirect bilirubin is often elevated, and the SGOT and SGPT levels may also be high. Vesicular eruptions of the skin have been reported in about one-third of the patients. Herpetic lesions may be seen on the mucous membranes of the oral cavity and conjunctiva. Pneumonitis, splenomegaly, pericarditis, and involvement of the adrenal glands may be observed. Terminally, a bleeding diathesis may develop which is manifest as bleeding from the gastrointestinal tract, hematuria, and circulatory collapse. In some cases the bleeding diathesis appears to result from disseminated intravascular coagulation (Haynes *et al.*, 1968; Shershaw *et al.*, 1969; Hathaway *et al.*, 1969; Miller *et al.*, 1970; Ekert, 1970; Catalano *et al.*, 1971).

Infection by the virus in some infants appears to be localized; clinical or pathologic evidence of visceral involvement cannot be found. The infections are generally confined to the central nervous system, skin, eyes, or oral cavity. Infections of the central nervous system are the most common, and about half of the reported cases terminated fatally. The clinical signs are those of meningoencephalitis; the spinal fluid contains abnormal numbers of cells, which are predominately lymphocytes, and elevated quantities of protein. Survivors of the illness are often left with sequalae such as microcephaly, hydrocephaly, porencephalic cysts, and varying degrees of psychomotor retardation. Eye involvement may be seen alone or in combination with infection of the central nervous system. Conjunctivitis and keratitis may lead to corneal scarring with blindness. Chorioretinitis has been reported to develop in several infants with herpesvirus infection of the eye (Cogan, 1964; Young *et al.*, 1965; Golden *et al.*, 1969; Hagler *et al.*, 1969). Isolated vesicular eruptions have been the only apparent manifestation in some infants. Herpetic eruptions, commonly at the same site, may recur repeatedly for at least the first 2 years of life. Some of the infants with only skin manifestations noted at birth have, on follow-up, been found to have evidence of psychomotor retardation, suggesting undetected neurologic involvement by the virus in the neonatal period.

Infection of the newborn can occur without producing detectable clinical manifestations. In following infants born to mothers with herpes genitalis, we have observed an infant with serologic evidence of type 2 infection without clinical disease. Herpesvirus type 2 has also been isolated from infants without apparent symptoms attributable to the virus (Sanders and Cramblett, 1968). The frequency of asymptomatic type 2 infections in the newborn period remains to be determined.

The conditions required for neonatal infection have not been clearly elucidated. Premature infants are disproportionally represented among those with severe disseminated disease; approximately half of the reported cases of severe neonatal herpes were noted to have low birth weight or were premature according to gestational age. Whether the virus contributes to the prematurity or the prematurity contributes to the severity of the virus infection has not been clearly established (Amstey, 1971; Nahmias *et al.*, 1971b). Relatively few infants born to mothers with herpes genitalis appear to develop severe neonatal herpes. It has been estimated that the incidence of clinically recognized infections of the newborn is about 1 per 7500 births in the lower socioeconomic classes (Nahmias *et al.*, 1969b). Evidence of herpesvirus infections of the genital tract, in a similar social setting, has been found in about 1 per 100 to 1 per 280 pregnant women (Ng *et al.*, 1970b; South and Rawls, 1970; Nahmias *et al.*, 1971b). Of the women with virus present in the genital tract at delivery, the risk of infection of the newborn appears to be greater with a primary maternal infection than with a recurrent disease. In one study, 3 (50%) of 6 infants born to mothers with primary disease became infected, while only 1 (4%) of 23 infants born to mothers with recurrent disease became infected (Nahmias *et al.*, 1971b). An initial infection with herpesvirus type 2 may create an even greater risk to the newborn than a primary type 2 infection in a woman with a previous type 1 infection. Thus, the type of infection experienced by the mother may contribute significantly to the risk of neonatal infection.

In addition to infection of the newborn, herpesvirus infections during pregnancy may also contribute to abortions and congenital malformations. An increased abortion rate has been reported for women with herpes genitalis in the first 20 weeks of pregnancy, and an increase in prematurity rate was noted among children of women with herpes genitalis after 30 weeks of pregnancy (Nahmias *et al.*, 1971b). This was not observed in another study (Ng *et al.*, 1970b). Congenital malformations associated with maternal herpesvirus infections have been recorded as case reports (Shaffer, 1965; South *et al.*, 1969) and are probably uncommon events (Korones *et al.*, 1970).

VII. Herpesvirus Type 2 and Cervical Cancer

There is an association between herpesvirus type 2 and squamous cell carcinoma of the cervix. The results of epidemiologic studies of cervical cancer suggest that women with the malignancy have attributes which would have placed them at a higher risk of acquiring venereal diseases than other women (Rotkin, 1967; Martin, 1967; Priden and Lilienfeld, 1971). Thus, the association between the venereally transmitted virus and the cancer may be one of covariability of sexual promiscuousness. However, the virus may be etiologically related to the malignancy. Data conclusively distinguishing between these possibilities are not yet available.

The bulk of the evidence related to the association of the virus and the cancer has been supplied by sero-epidemiologic studies. Generally, antibodies to herpesvirus type 2 have been found more frequently among women with cervical cancer than among control women of similar race, age, and socioeconomic level. However, the absolute percentage of women with antibodies to the virus was found to vary in different racial groups and with different techniques used for antibody assay. Among Negro women, a strong association between antibodies to the virus and cervical cancer has been repeatedly observed. In Houston, Texas, 72% of Negro women suffering from cancer were found to have antibodies to the virus, while antibodies were found in only 22% of control women (Rawls *et al.*, 1969). Antibodies to the virus were found among 83% of Negro women with cervical cancer and 35% of control women in Atlanta, Georgia (Nahmias *et al.*, 1970b). All women with cancer and 67% of control women in Baltimore, Maryland, were reported to have antibodies to the virus (Royston and Aurelian, 1970a). A high percentage of both cancer cases and control women were found to have antibodies to type 2 virus in Uganda (Adam *et al.*, 1972a).

Considerable variation in the occurrence of antibodies to herpesvirus type 2 has been reported among Caucasian women. The highest occurrence was found in Belgium, where 83% of women with cancer and 33% of control woman had antibodies (Sprecher-Goldberger *et al.*, 1970). Similarly, antibodies to type 2 virus was found among 85% of Danish women with cervical cancer while only 47% of control women had antibodies (Vestergaard *et al.*, 1972). About one-third to one-half of women with cancer were found to have antibodies to the virus in most other studies reported. In Chicago, Illinois, 48% of women with cancer and 18% of control women, respectively, had antibodies (Plummer and Masterson, 1971). Only 31% of women in New Zealand with cancer possessed antibodies to the virus while 23% of control women had antibodies (Rawls *et al.*, 1970b). In a study of Jewish women with cancer in Israel, 38% were found to have antibodies. Two control groups were examined; one was selected from women with gynecological disorders and 51% were found to have antibodies. Only 13% of a control group drawn from the general population had antibodies (Priden and Lilienfeld, 1971).

Antibodies to herpesvirus type 2 have been examined among women with the preinvasive cervical lesions of dysplasia and carcinoma *in situ*. A summary of the results is presented in Table I. It is evident that considerable variation in the occurrence of antibodies to the virus was found in different populations using different serologic techniques. Generally, a greater occurrence of antibodies has been observed among women with preinvasive lesions than among control women. In addition, the occurrence of antibodies has been noted to increase according to the increase in severity of the lesion; the lowest occurrences were found among women with dysplasia, and the highest occurrences were found among women with invasive cancer.

The incongruities in the results of the sero-epidemiologic studies may, in part, be related to technical difficulties in assaying for antibodies to herpesvirus type 2. As described above, the antibody response to the specific antigens of type 2 virus may be diminished or absent when a type 2 virus infection occurs in an individual who has previously experienced a type 1 infection (Smith *et al.*, 1972). In most serologic techniques used to detect antibodies to type 2 virus, the relative antibody activity to the two viruses have been compared (Nahmias *et al.*, 1970a; Rawls *et al.*, 1970a; Royston and Aurelian, 1970a). The criteria accepted as an antibody pattern indicating a past infection by herpesvirus type 2 have been empirically derived. Since the relative amounts of antibody activity to the two viruses may depend upon the total experiences of the individual to the two viruses, in different social and cultural settings the empirically derived criteria may not accurately reflect the actual number of women with a past infection by herpesvirus type 2.

Case control studies have been analyzed by absolute titers of antibody activity to herpesvirus types 1 and 2. No differences between cases and

TABLE I
ANTIBODIES TO HERPESVIRUS TYPE 2 AMONG WOMEN WITH PREINVASIVE CERVICAL LESIONS AND CONTROL WOMEN

Dysplasia				Carcinoma *in situ*				
Cases		Controls		Cases		Controls		
No. positive / No. tested	Percent positive	No. positive / No. tested	Percent positive	No. positive / No. tested	Percent positive	No. positive / No. tested	Percent positive	Reference
34/36	95	16/36	44	32/32	100	17/32	57	Royston and Aurelian (1970a)
23/45	56	8/45	18	26/38	70	9/38	24	Nahmias *et al.* (1970b)
5/21	24	—	—	8/23	35	11/51	22	Rawls *et al.* (1969)
—	—	—	—	13/31	42	11/62	18	Catalano and Johnson (1971)
—	—	—	—	14/44	32	12/53	23	Rawls *et al.* (1970b)

controls in mean antibody titers to herpesvirus type 1 were observed; however, patients with cervical disease were found to have higher mean antibody titers to type 2 virus than control women (Skinner *et al.*, 1971; Adam *et al.*, 1972b). The antibody activity to herpesvirus type 2 was found to be age-dependent among control women but not among women with cancer (Royston and Aurelian, 1970a; Adam *et al.*, 1972b). This suggests that women with cancer are infected by type 2 virus earlier in life than control women. Higher mean titers among cancer cases than among control women was observed in both Negroes and Caucasians; however, the mean antibody titers to both type 1 and type 2 virus were higher among Negro women than among Caucasian women. Thus, the case–control difference in antibodies was found in both races, but the differences appeared to exist at different absolute levels of antibody activity (Adam *et al.*, 1972b).

Data have been presented which suggest that the association between herpesvirus type 2 and cervial cancer may not simply represent one of covariability of sexual promiscuousness. Infection by the virus appears to precede the epithelial changes of the cervix. In a group of women who were being followed prospectively for the development of cervical epithelial abnormalities, antibodies to type 2 virus were present among 36% of the patients who subsequently developed carcinoma *in situ*; antibodies to the virus were only found among 7% of control women who did not develop cervical lesions during the same period of observation (Catalano and Johnson, 1971). Women with herpetic cervicitis, confirmed by laboratory diagnosis, were found to have a greater risk of subsequently developing cervical anaplasia than control women (Naib *et al.*, 1969). This, however, has not been observed by all authors (Ng *et al.*, 1970b; Wolinska and Melamed, 1970; Jordon *et al.*, 1972). The differences in the distribution of antibodies to the virus between cancer cases and controls cannot be solely accounted for by differences in the attributes associated with an increased risk of developing cervical cancer. When controls were selected with attributes similar to the cases there was still significantly more antibodies among cases (Adam *et al.*, 1972b). In addition, cases and controls, who differed in the occurrence of antibodies to herpesvirus type 2, did not differ in the occurrence of two other venereal diseases—syphilis and trichomoniasis (Royston and Aurelian, 1970a).

Several observations have been reported which suggest that herpesvirus type 2 genetic information may be present in malignant cells of the cervix. Using immunofluorescent techniques, herpesvirus antigens have been detected in the cytoplasm of abnormal cells which were exfoliated from the cervix of women with preinvasive or invasive lesions (Royston and Aurelian, 1970b; Aurelian *et al.*, 1972). In addition, herpesvirus type 2 has been isolated from a cell line derived from a lesion of carcinoma *in situ* (Aurelian *et al.*, 1971). The virus appears to have oncogenic potential as demonstrated by the *in vitro* transformation of hamster embryo fibroblasts by ultraviolet-irradiated virus (Duff and Rapp, 1971). Confirmation and extension of the above observations will be needed to elucidate the association between herpesvirus type 2 and cervical cancer.

VIII. Laboratory Diagnosis

With the development of effective chemotherapeutic agents, rapid and accurate diagnosis of herpesvirus infections become increasingly important. This is especially true for herpesvirus encephalitis and disseminated infections. The virus can be readily isolated from the infected lesions using standard laboratory techniques (Tokumaru, 1969). Cells obtained from the lesion, on fixation and staining, display changes which are of diagnostic importance (Medak *et al.*, 1971). Viral antigens can be demonstrated by immunofluorescent techniques and detection of these antigens provide evidence that the infection is due to herpesvirus (Gardner *et al.*, 1968).

Serologic diagnosis of the initial infection by a herpesvirus can usually be accomplished without difficulty. An antigenic relationship between herpesvirus and varicella–zoster virus has been demonstrated (Trlifajova *et al.*, 1971). Patients infected with either virus may show a rise in antibodies to the other virus. This is usually seen among patients who have already had a past infection by the heterologous virus, and the rise in cross-reacting antibody is generally of lesser magnitude than the reaction to the homologous virus (Kapsenberg, 1964; Svedmyr, 1965; Ross *et al.*, 1965; Schaap and Huisman, 1968; Schmidt *et al.*, 1969). Serologic diagnosis of recurrent infections is not generally possible. Herpesvirus type 2 infections among patients who have had a prior type 1 infection can usually be detected by demonstrating an alteration in the relative antibody activity to the two types of virus (Nahmias *et al.*, 1970a; Rawls *et al.*, 1970a).

In the febrile patient with acute encephalitis, demonstration of a localized process in the temporal lobes by electroencephalography, brain scan, or angiography are indications for a brain biopsy which can provide a definitive diagnosis (Gurwith *et al.*, 1971). It has been suggested that the diagnosis of herpesvirus encephalitis can be made on a single serum sample by measuring the complement-requiring neutralizing antibody. Patients with encephalitis were found more frequently to have a significant increase in antibody titers to the virus in the presence of complement than other patients (Lerner *et al.*, 1970). In humans, however, the presence of complement-requiring antibodies following infection has not been demonstrated by all investigators (Heineman, 1967), and the validity of diagnosing encephalitis by serologic means has been questioned (Johnson *et al.*, 1968). Additional investigation regarding a means of diagnosing herpesvirus encephalitis other than by brain biopsy appears warranted.

IX. Conclusion

The acute manifestations of infections by herpesviruses have been known for many years. The viruses are ubiquitous, and once an infection occurs the agents probably remain, in latent form, with the host for life. Person-to-person spread is the major mode of transmission; contagium is relatively poor in that contact with contaminated secretions is usually required for effective transmission. Recently, it has become apparent that there are two types of herpesvirus. Type 1 virus is spread by the oral–respiratory route and is responsible for acute gingivostomatitis, herpes labilias, keratoconjunctivitis, eczema herpeticum, traumatic herpes, and encephalitis occurring beyond the newborn period. Type 2 virus is a venereally transmitted agent and is usually responsible for herpes genitalis and neonatal herpes.

Immunity to herpesvirus reinfection or recurrence appears to reside mainly with the cellular defense mechanisms rather than with the humoral defense mechanisms. Severe forms of cutaneous herpes and generalized infections are seen among patients with immune deficiencies. Infection with one type of herpesvirus results in the production of antibodies that will cross react with the other type of virus, indicating an antigenic relationship between these viruses. Infections by the second virus after primary infection with type 1 appear to be modified in that they are often asymptomatic and are rarely severe.

The role of the herpesviruses in chronic diseases remains to be resolved. Several authors have suggested a possible connection between herpesvirus type 1 and behavioral disorders. There is a relation between herpesvirus type 2 and squamous cell carcinoma of the cervix. This relation could be a causal one or one of covariability of sexual promiscuousness. These and other possible manifestations of the chronic presence of the virus will, perhaps, become clear as studies on this interesting group of agents continue.

Acknowledgments

This work was supported in part by Contract No 1 CP 33257, within the Special Virus Cancer Program of the National Cancer Institute, National Institutes of Health and by Clinical Investigation Grant CI 23 from the American Cancer Society.

References

Adam, E., Sharma, S. D., Zeigler, O., Iwamoto, K., Melnick, J. L., Levy, A. H., and Rawls, W. E. (1972a). *J. Nat. Cancer Inst.* **48**, 65.

Adam, E., Kaufman, R. H., Melnick, J. L., Levy, A. H., and Rawls, W. E. (1972b). *Amer. J. Epidemiol.* **96**, 427.

Amstey, M. S. (1971). *Obstet. Gynecol.* **37**, 515.

Amstey, M. S., and Balduzzi, P. C. (1970a). *Amer. J. Obstet. Gynecol.* **106**, 924.

Amstey, M. S., and Balduzzi, P. C. (1970b). *Amer. J. Obstet. Gynecol.* **108**, 188.
An, S. H. (1969). *Acta Cytol.* **13**, 354.
Anderson, W. A., and Kilbourne, E. D. (1961). *J. Invest. Dermatol.* **37**, 25.
Andervont, H. B. (1929). *J. Infec. Dis.* **44**, 383.
Ashe, W. K., and Rizzo, A. A. (1967). *Proc. Soc. Exp. Biol. Med.* **124**, 1150.
Aurelian, L., Standberg, J. D., Melendez, L. V., and Johnson, L. D. (1971). *Science* **174**, 704.
Aurelian, L., Strandberg, J. D., and Davis, H. J. (1972). *Proc. Soc. Exp. Biol. Med.* **140**, 404.
Bahrani, M., Boxerbaum, B., Gilger, A. P., Rosenthal, M. S., and Teree, T. M. (1966). *Amer. J. Dis. Child.* **111**, 437.
Baker, W. H., Lawton, A. M., and McCarthy, K. (1952). *Brit. Med. J.* **2**, 1334.
Bean, S. F., and Fusaro, R. M. (1969). *Acta Dermato-Venereol.* **49**, 94.
Becker, W. B., DuNaudé, T., Kipps, A., and McKenzie, D. (1963). *S. Afr. Med. J.* **37**, 74.
Becker, W. B., Kipps, A., and McKenzie, D. (1968). *Amer. J. Dis. Child.* **115**, 1.
Beilby, J. O. W., Cameron, C. H., Catterall, R. D., and Davidson, D. (1968). *Lancet* **1**, 1065.
Black, F. L., Woodall, J. P., Evans, A. S., Liebhaber, H., and Henle, G. (1970). *Amer. J. Epidemiol.* **91**, 430.
Booth, C. B., Okazaki, H., and Gaulin, J. C. (1961). *Neurology* **11**, 619.
Boyd, J. F., and Nedelkoska, N. (1967). *J. Clin. Pathol.* **20**, 835.
Brain, R. T. (1956). *Brit. Med. J.* **1**, 1061.
Brain, R. T., Pugh, R. C. B., and Dudgeon, J. A. (1957). *Arch. Dis. Childhood* **32**, 120.
Brier, A. M., Snyderman, R., Mergenhagen, S. E., and Notkins, A. L. (1970). *Science* **170**, 1104.
Brier, A. M., Wohlenberg, C., Rosenthal, J., Mage, M., and Notkins, A. L. (1971). *Proc. Nat. Acad. Sci. U.S.* **68**, 3073.
Brightman, V. J., and Guggenheimer, J. G. (1970). *J. Amer. Dent. Ass.* **80**, 112.
Brown, D. C. (1971). *Invest. Ophthalmol.* **10**, 210.
Brown, D. C., and Kaufman, H. E. (1969). *Arch. Ophthalmol.* **81**, 837.
Buddingh, G. J., Schrum. D. I., Lanier, J. C., and Guidry, D. J. (1953). *Pediatrics* **11**, 595.
Burnet, F. M., and Williams, S. W. (1939). *Med. J. Aust.* **1**, 637.
Caldwell, J. E., and Porter, D. D. (1971). *J. Amer. Med. Ass.* **217**, 1703.
Catalano, L. W., Jr., and Johnson, L. D. (1971). *J. Amer. Med. Ass.* **217**, 447.
Catalano, L. W., Jr., Safley, G. H., Museles, M., and Jarzynski, D. J. (1971). *J. Pediat.* **79**, 393.
Cederqvist, L., Eliasson, G., Lindell, L., and Stormby, K. (1970). *Acta Obstet. Gynecol. Scand.* **49**, 13.
Centifanto, Y. M., Hilderbrandt, R. J., Held, B., and Kaufman, H. E. (1971). *Amer. J. Obstet. Gynecol.* **110**, 690.
Cesario, T. C., Poland, J. D., Wulff, H., Chin, T. D., and Wenner, H. A. (1969). *Amer. J. Epidemiol.* **90**, 416.
Chang, T. W. (1971). *N. Engl. J. Med.* **284**, 765.
Cleobury, J. F., Skinner, G. R. B., Thouless, M. E., and Wildy, P. (1971). *Brit. Med. J.* **1**, 438.
Cogan, D. G. (1964). *Arch. Ophthalmol.* [N.S.] **72**, 641.
Constantine, V. S., Francis, R. D., and Montes, L. F. (1968). *J. Amer. Med. Ass.* **205**, 181.
Crosby, D., Jones, J. H., and Sussman, M. (1969). *Lancet* **2**, 1191.
Davies, R. M., and Longson, M. (1970). *Oral Surg. Oral Med. Oral Pathol.* **30**, 41.
Davis, D. O., and Potchen, E. J. (1970). *Radiology* **95**, 345.
Dickie, E. G. (1969). *Obstet. Gynecol.* **34**, 434.
Docherty, J. J., Goldberg, R. J., and Rapp, F. (1971a). *Proc. Soc. Exp. Biol. Med.* **136**, 328.
Docherty, J. J., O'Neill, F. J., and Rapp, F. (1971b). *J. Gen. Virol.* **13**, 377.
Dodd, K., Johnston, L. M., and Buddingh, G. J. (1938). *J. Pediat.* **12**, 95.
Doeglas, H. M., and Moolhuysen, T. M. (1969). *Arch, Dermatol.* **100**, 529.
Douglas, R. G., Jr., and Couch, R. B. (1970). *J. Immunol.* **104**, 289.

Douglas, R. G., Jr., Anderson, M. S., Weg, J. G., Williams, T., Jenkins, D. E., Knight, V., and Beall, A. C., Jr. (1969). *J. Amer. Med. Ass.* **210**, 902.
Dowdle, W. R., Nahmias, A. J., Harwell, R. W., and Pauls, F. P. (1967). *J. Immunol.* **99**, 974.
Drachman, D. A., and Adams, R. D. (1962). *Arch. Neurol. (Chicago)* **7**, 45.
Dueñas, A., Adam, E., Melnick, J. L., and Rawls, W. E. (1972). *Amer. J. Epidemiol.* **95**, 483.
Duff, R., and Rapp, F. (1971). *J. Virol.* **8**, 469.
Duxbury, A. E., and Lawrence, J. R. (1959). *Med. J. Aust.* **2**, 250.
Dyke, L. M., Merkawgas, V. M., Burton, O. C., Trask, S. G., and Hetrick, F. M. (1965). *J. Amer. Med. Ass.* **194**, 1001.
Ejercito, P. M., Kieff, E. D., and Roizman, B. (1968). *J. Gen. Virol.* **2**, 357.
Ekert, H. (1970). *Lancet* **2**, 775.
Evans, A. S., and Dick, E. C. (1964). *J. Amer. Med. Ass.* **190**, 699.
Evans, D. I., and Holzel, A. (1970). *Arch. Dis. Childhood* **45**, 527.
Figueroa, M. E., and Rawls, W. E. (1969). *J. Gen. Virol.* **4**, 259.
Flewett, T. H., Parker, R. G. F., and Philip, W. M. (1969). *J. Clin. Pathol.* **22**, 60.
Foley, F. D., Greenawald, K. A., Nash, G., and Pruitt, B. A., Jr. (1970). *N. Engl. J. Med.* **282**, 652.
Friedrich, E. R., Cole, W., and Middlekamp, J. N. (1969). *Amer. J. Obstet. Gynecol.* **104**, 758.
Gardner, H. L., and Kaufman, R. H. (1969). *In* "Benign Diseases of the Vulva and Vagina," pp. 236–243. Mosby, St. Louis, Missouri.
Gardner, P. S., McQuillin, J., Black, M. M., and Richardson, J. (1968). *Brit. Med. J.* **4**, 89.
Geder, L., and Skinner, G. R. B. (1971). *J. Gen. Virol.* **12**, 179.
Gerber, P., and Rosenblum, E. N. (1968). *Proc. Soc. Exp. Biol. Med.* **128**, 541.
Golden, B., Bell, W. E., and McKee, A. P. (1969). *J. Amer. Med. Ass.* **209**, 1219.
Goodheart, C. R., Plummer, G., and Waner, J. L. (1968). *Virology* **35**, 473.
Goodwin, C. S., Gostling, J. V. T., Pead, P. J., and Sims, E. H. (1970). *Brit. Med. J.* **4**, 558.
Green, L. H., and Levin, M. P. (1971). *J. Periodontol.* **42**, 170.
Greenberg, M. S., Brightman, V. J., and Skip, I. I. (1969). *J. Dent. Res.* **48**, 385.
Gurwith, M. J., Harman, C. E., and Merigan, T. C. (1971). *Calif. Med.* **115**, 63.
Hagler, W. S., Walters, P. V., and Nahmias, A. J. (1969). *Arch. Ophthalmol.* [N.S.] **82**, 169.
Halpern, S. E., Smith, C. W., Jr., and Ficken, V. (1970). *J. Nucl. Med.* **11**, 548.
Hampar, B., Miyamoto, K., and Martos, L. M. (1971). *J. Immunol.* **106**, 580.
Harland, W. A., Adams, J. H., and McSweney, D. (1967). *Lancet* **2**, 581.
Hathaway, W., Mull, M., and Pechet, G. S. (1969). *Pediatrics* **43**, 233.
Haymaker, W., Smith, M. G., Van Bogaert, L, and de Chenar, C. (1958). *In* "Viral Encephalitis," pp. 95–204. Thomas, Springfield, Illinois.
Haynes, R. E., Azimi, P. H., and Gramblett, H. G. (1968). *J. Amer. Med. Ass.* **206**, 312.
Heineman, H. S. (1967). *J. Immunol.* **99**, 214.
Hirsh, M. S., Zisman, B., and Allison, A. C. (1970). *J. Immunol.* **104**, 1160.
Hunt, B. P., and Comer, E. O. (1955). *Amer. J. Med.* **19**, 814.
Itabashi, H. H., Bass, D. M., and McCulloch, J. R. (1966). *Arch. Neurol. (Chicago)* **14**, 493.
Izumi, A., and Goldschmidt, H. (1970). *Arch. Dermatol.* **102**, 650.
Jawetz, E., Coleman, V., and Allende, M. F. (1951). *J. Immunol.* **67**, 197.
Jeansson, S., and Molin, L. (1970). *Lancet* **1**, 1064.
Jeansson, S., and Molin, L. (1971a). *Brit. Med. J.* **3**, 247.
Jeansson, S., and Molin, L. (1971b). *Lakartidiningen* **68**, 467.
Johnson, R. T. (1964a). *J. Exp. Med.* **119**, 343.
Johnson, R. T. (1964b). *J. Exp. Med.* **120**, 359.
Johnson, R. T., Olson, L. C., and Buescher, E. L. (1968). *Arch. Neurol. (Chicago)* **18**, 260.
Johnson, K. P., Rosenthal, M. S., and Lerner, P. I. (1972). *Arch. Neurol. (Chicago)* **27**, 103.

Jordon, S. W., Evangel, E., and Smith, N. L. (1972). *Acta Cytol.* **16**, 363.
Josey, W. E., Nahmias, A. J., Naib, Z. M., Utley, P. M., McKenzie, W. J., and Coleman, M. T. (1966). *Amer. J. Obstet. Gynecol.* **96**, 493.
Josey, W. E., Nahmias, A. J., and Naib, Z. M. (1968). *Amer. J. Obstet. Gynecol.* **101**, 718.
Josey, W. E., Nahmias, A. J., and Naib, Z. M. (1972). *Obstet. Gynecol. Surv.* **27**, 295.
Juel-Jensen, B. E. (1971). *Brit. J. Med.* **4**, 681.
Kaplan, A. S. (1969). *Virol. Monogr.* **5**, 1.
Kapsenberg, J. G. (1964). *Arch. Gesamte Virusforsch.* **15**, 67.
Kaufman, H. E., Brown, D. C., and Ellison, E. M. (1967). *Science* **156**, 1628.
Kaufman, H. E., Brown, D. C., and Ellison, E. M. (1968). *Amer. J. Ophthalmol.* **65**, 32.
Kaufman, H. E., Kanai, A., and Ellison, E. D. (1971). *Amer. J. Ophthalmol.* **71**, 465.
Kaufman, R. H., and Rawls, W. E. (1972). *Amer. J. Obstet. Gynecol.* **112**, 866.
Kieff, E., Hoyer, B., Bachenheimer, S., and Roizman, B. (1972). *J. Virol.* **9**, 738.
Klastersky, J., Cappel, R., Snoeck, J. M., Flament, J., and Thiry, L. (1972). *N. Engl. J. Med.* **287**, 182.
Kleger, B., and Prier, J. E. (1969). *J. Infec. Dis.* **120**, 376.
Kleger, B., Prier, J. E., Rosato, D. J., and McGinnis, A. E. (1968). *Amer. J. Obstet. Gynecol.* **102**, 745.
Kloene, W., Bang, F. B., Chakraborty, S. M., Cooper, M. R., Kulemann, H., Shah, K. V., and Ota, M. (1970). *Amer. J. Epidemiol.* **92**, 307.
Korones, S. B., Todaro, J., Roane, J. A., and Sever, J. L. (1970). *J. Pediat.* **77**, 245.
Laibson, P. R., and Kibrick, S. (1969). *Invest. Ophthalmol.* **8**, 346.
Larossa, D., and Hamilton, R. (1971). *Arch. Surg.* (*Chicago*) **102**, 600.
Lausch, R. N., Swyers, J. S., and Kaufman, H. E. (1966). *J. Immunol.* **96**, 981.
Leider, W., Magoffin, R. L., Lennette, E. H., and Leonards, L. N. R. (1965). *N. Engl. J. Med.* **273**, 341.
Lennette, E. H., and Koprowski, H. (1944). *J. Immunol.* **49**, 175.
Leopold, I. H. (1965). *Ann. N.Y. Acad. Sci.* **130**, 181.
Lerner, A. M., Bailey, E. J., and Nolan, D. C. (1970). *J. Immunol.* **104**, 607.
Lindgren, K. M., Douglas, R. G., Jr., and Couch, R. B. (1968). *N. Engl. J. Med.* **278**, 517.
Logan, W. S., Tindall, J. P., and Elson, M. L. (1971). *Arch. Dermatol.* **103**, 606.
Longson, M. (1971). *Ann. Inst. Pasteur, Paris* **120**, 699.
Lowry, S. P., Melnick, J. L., and Rawls, W. E. (1971). *J. Gen. Virol.* **10**, 1.
Lynfield, Y. L., Farhangi, M., and Runnels, J. L. (1969). *J. Amer. Med. Ass.* **207**, 944.
McIndoe, W. A., and Churchouse, M. J. (1972). *Aust. N. Z. J. Obstet. Gynecol.* **12**, 14.
Martin, C. E. (1967). *Amer. J. Pub. Health Nat. Health* **57**, 803.
Medak, H., Burlakow, P., McGrew, E. A., Cohen, L., and Tiecke, R. (1971). *Oral Surg. Oral Med. Oral Pathol.* **32**, 204.
Merigan, T. C., and Stevens, D. A. (1971). *Fed. Proc., Fed. Amer. Soc. Exp. Biol.* **30**, 1858.
Meyer, J. S., Bauer, R. B., Rivera-Olmos, V. M., Nolan, D. C., and Lerner, A. M. (1970). *Arch. Neurol.* (*Chicago*) **23**, 438.
Miller, D. R., Hanshaw, J. B., O'Leary, D. S., and Hnilicka, J. V. (1970). *J. Pediat.* **76**, 409.
Miller, J. D., and Ross, C. A. C. (1968). *Lancet* **1**, 1121.
Miller, J. K., Hesser, F., and Tompkins, V. N. (1966). *Ann. Intern. Med.* **64**, 92.
Mishkin, F. S. (1970). *J. Nucl. Med.* **11**, 608.
Mogabgab, W. T. (1968). *Amer. Rev. Resp. Dis.* **98**, 359.
Mok, C. H. (1971). *N. Engl. J. Med.* **285**, 294.
Montgomerie, J. Z., Becroft, D. M. O., Croxson, M. C., Doak, P. B., and North, J. D. K. (1969). *Lancet* **2**, 867.
Morrisseau, P. M., Phillips, C. A., and Leadbetter, G. W., Jr. (1970). *J. Urol.* **103**, 767.

Mufson, M. A., Chang, V., Gell. V., Wood, S. C., Romansky, M. J., and Chanock, R. M. (1967). *Amer. J. Epidemiol.* **86**, 526.
Muller, S. A., and Herrmann, E. C., Jr. (1970). *Arch. Dermatol.* **101**, 396.
Muller, S. A., Herrmann, E. C., Jr., and Winklemann, R. K. (1972). *Amer. J. Med.* **52**, 102.
Music, S. I., Fine, E. M., and Togo, Y. (1971). *N. Engl. J. Med.* **284**, 24.
Nagler, F. P. O. (1944). *J. Immunol.* **48**, 213.
Nagler, F. P. O. (1946). *Aust. J. Exp. Biol. Med. Sci.* **24**, 103.
Nahmias, A. J., and Dowdle, W. R. (1968). *Progr. Med. Virol.* **10**, 110.
Nahmias, A. J., Dowdle, W. R., Naib, Z. M., Josey, W. E., McLone, D., and Domescik, G. (1969a). *Brit. J. Vener. Dis.* **45**, 294.
Nahmias, A. J., Dowdle, W. R., Josey, W. E., Naib, Z. M., Painter, L. M., and Luce, C. (1969b). *J. Pediat.* **75**, 1194.
Nahmias, A. J., Josey, W. E., Naib, Z. M., Luce, C. F., and Duffey, C. (1970a). *Amer. J. Epidemiol.* **91**, 539.
Nahmias, A. J., Josey, W. E., Naib, Z. M., Luce, C. F., and Guest, B. A. (1970b). *Amer. J. Epidemiol.* **91**, 547.
Nahmias, A. J., Alford, C. A., and Korones, S. B. (1970c). *Advan. Pediat.* **17**, 185.
Nahmias, A. J., London, W. T., Catalano, L. W., Fuccillo, D. A., Sever, J. L., and Graham, C. (1971a). *Science* **171**, 297.
Nahmias, A. J., Josey, W. E., Naib, Z. M., Freeman, M. G., Fernandez, R. J., and Wheeler, J. H. (1971b). *Amer. J. Obstet. Gynecol.* **110**, 825.
Naib, Z. M., Nahmias, A. J., and Josey, W. E. (1966). *Cancer* **19**, 1026.
Naib, Z. M., Nahmias, A. J., Josey, W. E., and Kramer, J. H. (1969). *Cancer* **23**, 940.
Nally, F. F., and James, J. D. (1970). *Oral Surg., Oral Med. Oral Pathol.* **29**, 680.
Nash, G., and Foley, F. D. (1970). *Amer. J. Clin. Pathol.* **54**, 857.
Nauheim, J. S. (1969). *Arch. Ophthalmol.* [N.S.] **81**, 592.
Neff, J. M., and Lane, J. M. (1970). *J. Amer. Med. Ass.* **213**, 123.
Ng, A. B. P., Reagin, J. W., and Lindner, E. (1970a). *Acta Cytol.* **14**, 124.
Ng, A. B. P., Reagin, J. W., and Yen, S. S. C. (1970b). *Obstet. Gynecol.* **36**, 645.
Nishimura, K., Nagamoto, A., and Igarashi, M. (1972). *Pediatrics* **49**, 294.
Nolan, D. C., Carruthers, M. M., and Lerner, A. M. (1970). *N. Engl. J. Med.* **282**, 10.
Olson, L. C., Buescher, E. L., Artenstein, M. S., and Parkman, P. D. (1967). *N. Engl. J. Med.* **277**, 1271.
Orkin, F. K. (1970). *Anesthesiology* **33**, 671.
Paine, T. F. (1964). *Bacteriol. Rev.* **28**, 472.
Parker, J. D. J., and Banatvala, J. E. (1967). *Brit. J. Vener. Dis.* **43**, 212.
Patterson, A., Sommerville, R. G., and Jones, B. R. (1969). *Trans. Ophthalmol. Soc. U.K.* **89**, 243.
Pavan-Langston, D., and Brockhurst, R. J. (1969). *Arch. Ophthalmol.* [N.S.] **81**, 783.
Pelc, S. (1971). *Lancet* **2**, 320.
Plummer, G., and Masterson, J. G. (1971). *Amer. J. Obstet. Gynecol.* **111**, 81.
Plummer, G., Waner, J. L., Phuangsab, A., and Goodheart, C. R. (1970). *J. Virol.* **5**, 51.
Porter, D. D., Wimberly, I., and Benyesh-Melnick, M. (1969). *J. Amer. Med. Ass.* **208**, 1675.
Porter, P. S., and Baughman, R. D. (1965). *J. Amer. Med. Ass.* **194**, 998.
Priden, H., and Lilienfeld, A. M. (1971). *Isr. J. Med. Sci.* **7**, 1465.
Radcliffe, W. B., Guinto, F. C., Jr., Adcock, D. F., and Krigman, M. R. (1971). *Amer. J. Roentgenol., Radium. Ther. Nucl. Med.* **112**, 263.
Ratcliff, H. (1971). *J. Gen. Virol.* **13**, 181.
Rawls, W. E., Dyck, P. J., Klass, D. W., Greer, H. D., III, and Herrmann, E. C., Jr. (1966). *Ann. Intern. Med.* **64**, 104.
Rawls, W. E., Tompkins, W. A. F., and Melnick, J. L. (1969). *Amer. J. Epidemiol.* **89**, 547.

Rawls, W. E., Iwamoto, K., Adam, E., and Melnick, J. L. (1970a). *J. Immunol.* **104**, 599.
Rawls, W. E., Iwamoto, K., Adam, E., Melnick, J. L., and Green, G. H. (1970b). *Lancet* **2**, 1142.
Rawls, W. E., Gardner, H. L., Flanders, R. W., Lowry, S. P., Kaufman, R. H., and Melnick, J. L. (1971). *Amer. J. Obstet. Gynecol.* **110**, 682.
Rimon, R., Halonen, P., Attinen, E., and Evola, K. (1971). *Dis. Nerv. Syst.* **32**, 822.
Rocklin, R. E. (1971). *J. Reticuloendothel. Soc.* **10**, 50.
Roizman, B. (1965). *Perspect. Virol.* **4**, 283.
Roizman, B., Keller, J. M., Spear, P. G., Terni, M., Nahmias, A. J., and Dowdle, W. (1970). *Nature* (*London*) **227**, 1253.
Rosato, F. E., Rosato, E. F., and Plotkin, S. A. (1970). *N. Engl. J. Med.* **283**, 804.
Rose, H. M., and Molloy, E. (1947). *J. Immunol.* **56**, 287.
Rosenberg, G. L., Wohlenberg, C., Nahmias, A. J., and Notkins, A. L. (1972). *J. Immunol.* **109**, 413.
Ross, C. A. C., Subak-Sharpe, J. H., and Ferry, P. (1965). *Lancet* **2**, 708.
Rotkin, I. D. (1967). *Amer. J. Pub. Health Nat. Health* **57**, 815.
Roy, S., and Wolman, L. (1969). *J. Clin. Pathol.* **22**, 51.
Royston, I., and Aurelian, L. (1970a). *Amer. J. Epidemiol.* **91**, 531.
Royston, I., and Aurelian, L. (1970b). *Proc. Nat. Acad. Sci. U.S.* **67**, 204.
Ruchman, I., and Dodd, K. (1950). *J. Lab. Clin. Med.* **35**, 434.
St. Geme, J. W., Jr., Prince, J. T., Burke, B. A., Good, R. A., and Krivet, W. (1965). *N. Engl. J. Med.* **273**, 229.
Sanders, D. Y., and Cramblett, H. G. (1968). *Amer. J. Dis. Child.* **116**, 251.
Schaap, G. J., and Huisman, J. (1968). *Arch. Gesamte Virusforsch.* **25**, 52.
Schmidt, N. J., Lennette, E. H., and Magoffin, R. L. (1969). *J. Gen. Virol.* **4**, 321.
Schneweis, K. E., and Nahmias, A. J. (1971). *Z. Immunitaetsforsch., Allerg. Klin. Immunol.* **141**, 479.
Scott, D. F., and Prior, P. F. (1970). *Lancet* **2**, 525.
Scott, T. F. McN., and Tokumaru, T. (1965). *In* "Viral and Rickettsial Infections of Man" (F. L. Horsfall, Jr. and I. Tamm, eds.), 4th ed., pp. 892–914. Lippincott, Philadelphia, Pennsylvania.
Selling, B., and Kibrick, S. (1964). *N. Engl. J. Med.* **270**, 979.
Shaffer, A. J. (1965). *In* "Diseases of the Newborn," 2nd ed., p. 733. Saunders, Philadelphia, Pensylvania.
Sheridan, P. J., and Herrmann, E. C., Jr. (1971). *Oral Surg. Oral Med. Oral Pathol.* **32**, 390.
Shershaw, L. W., Ekert, H., and Swanson, V. L. (1969). *Acta Paediat. Scand.* **58**, 535.
Silk, B. R., and Roome, A. P. (1970). *Lancet* **1**, 411.
Skinner, G. R. B., Thouless, M. E., and Jordon, J. A. (1971). *J. Obstet. Gynecol. Brit. Commonw.* **78**, 1031.
Slavin, H. B., and Ferguson, J. J. (1950). *Amer. J. Med.* **8**, 457.
Smith, I. W., Pentherer, J. F., and MacCallum, F. O. (1967). *J. Hyg.* **65**, 395.
Smith, J. W., Rodriguez, J. E., and McKee, A. P. (1971). *Appl. Microbiol.* **21**, 350.
Smith, J. W., Adam, E., Melnick, J. L., and Rawls, W. E. (1972). *J. Immunol.* **109**, 554.
Smith, M. A., Lennette, E. M., and Reames, H. R. (1941). *Amer. J. Pathol.* **17**, 55.
Snyderman, R., Wohlenberg, C., and Notkins, A. L. (1972). *J. Infec. Dis.* **126**, 207.
South, M. A., and Rawls, W. E. (1970). *J. Pediat.* **76**, 497.
South, M. A., Tompkins, W. A. F., Morris, C. R., and Rawls, W. E. (1969). *J. Pediat.* **75**, 13.
Spencer, E. S., and Andersen, H. K. (1970). *Brit. Med. J.* **3**, 251.
Sprecher-Goldberger, S., Thiry, L., Cattoor, J. P., Hooghe, R., and Pestiau, J. (1970). *Lancet* **2**, 266.
Starr, A., and Phillip, L. (1968). *Trans. Amer. Neurol. Ass.* **93**, 286.

Stern, H., Elek, S. D., Millar, D. M., and Anderson, H. F. (1959). *Lancet* **2**, 871.
Stevens, J. G., and Cook, M. L. (1971a). *Science* **173**, 843.
Stevens, J. G., and Cook, M. L. (1971b). *J. Exp. Med.* **133**, 19.
Stevens, J. G., Nesburn, A. B., and Cook, M. L. (1972). *Nature (London) New Biol.* **235**, 216.
Stinson, E. B., Griepp, R. B., Dong, E., Jr., and Shumway, N. E. (1971). *Transplant. Proc.* **3**, 337.
Stroud, G. M. (1961). *Arch. Dermatol.* **84**, 396.
Stubbs, K. G., Snider, M. E., and Alford, C. A., Jr. (1971). *J. Infec. Dis.* **123**, 169.
Svedmyr, A. (1965). *Arch. Gesamte Virusforsch.* **17**, 495.
Templeton, A. C. (1970). *J. Clin. Pathol.* **23**, 24.
Terni, M., and Roizman, B. (1970). *J. Infec. Dis.* **121**, 212.
Terni, M., Carccialanza, P., Cassai, E., and Kieff, E. (1971). *N. Engl. J. Med.* **285**, 503.
Tokumaru, T. (1966). *J. Immunol.* **97**, 248.
Tokumaru, T. (1969). *In* "Diagnostic Procedures for Viral and Riskettsial Infections" (E. H. Lennette and N. J. Schmidt, eds.), 4th ed., pp. 641–676. Amer. Pub. Health Ass. New York.
Trlifajova, J., Sourek, J., and Ryba, M. (1971). *Acta Virol. (Prague), English Ed.* **15**, 293.
Upton, A., and Gumpert, J. (1970). *Lancet* **1**, 650.
Vestergaard, B. F., Hornsleth, A., and Pedersen, S. N. (1972). *Cancer* **30**, 68.
Victor, M. (1969). *Can. Med. Ass. J.* **100**, 1115.
Welt, J. C., Hendey, J., and Stackew, W. (1969). *Can. Med. Ass. J.* **101**, 411.
Wentworth, B. B., and Alexander, E. R. (1971). *Amer. J. Epidemiol.* **94**, 496.
Wentworth, B. B., and Zablatney, S. L. (1972). *Infection Immunity* **5**, 377.
Wheeler, C. E., and Cabaniss, W. H. (1965). *J. Amer. Med. Ass.* **194**, 993.
Wildy, P. (1967). *J. Hyg.* **65**, 173.
Wilton, J. M. A., Ivanyi, L., and Lekner, T. (1972). *Brit. Med. J.* **1**, 723.
Witzleben, C. L., and Driscoll, S. G. (1965). *Pediatrics* **36**, 192.
Wolinska, W. H., and Melamed, M. R. (1970). *Acta Cytol.* **14**, 239.
Young, G. F., Knox, D. L., and Dodge, P. R. (1965). *Arch. Neurol. (Chicago)* **13**, 15.

Chapter 11
Varicella–Zoster Viruses

Eli Gold and George A. Nankervis

I. Introduction

Varicella, the only major childhood disease for which a vaccine is not yet available, was originally considered to be a mild variety of smallpox, with smaller or "chick-pea"-sized skin lesions. These two diseases—chicken pox and smallpox—were clinically differentiated by Heberden in 1767, and it was over a century later before Tyzzer (1906) described the histology of the skin lesions, emphasizing the presence of intranuclear inclusions in varicella.

Von Bokay (1909), toward the latter part of the nineteenth century, observed that chicken pox occurred in children exposed to a patient with herpes zoster and suggested that the two diseases might be due to the same infectious agent. Transmission studies (Kundratitz, 1925; Bruusgaard, 1932) using vesicle fluid from patients with zoster provided credence to this hypothesis, but it was not until the comparatively recent studies in tissue culture (Weller, 1953; Weller and Witton, 1958) that the virus of chicken pox was shown to be indistinguishable from that of zoster. This has led to the now common appelation of "varicella–zoster or V–Z virus."

II. Clinical Features and Diagnosis (see Table I)

A. Varicella

1. Clinical

a. General. Varicella is an acute viral disease, characterized by sudden onset of fever and mild constitutional symptoms followed by a skin eruption which progresses rapidly from the transient maculopapular stage, to clear vesicles surrounded by a delicate erythematous areola, to pustules, and finally to scabs. The rash (see Fig. 1) appears first on the back of the head and over the ears and then spreads from scalp to the face, neck, trunk, and extremities; it is typically most dense centrally with fewer lesions on the extremities. The mucus membranes of the upper respiratory, genital–urinary, and gastrointestinal tracts may also be involved. The rash of varicella may be more intense in areas of skin irritation or trauma, such as

TABLE I
Contrasting Clinical and Epidemiological Characteristics of Varicella and Herpes Zoster

Varicella	Zoster
Primary infection	Past history of varicella
Disease of childhood	Disease of older age groups
Epidemic, peaks in late winter and early spring	Endemic, no seasonal peaks
Highly contagious	Less contagious
Generalized	Usually localized
Spreads via blood	Spreads via nerve fibers
Commonly occurs in normal host	Occurs with greater frequency in host with "impaired immunity"
Generalized pruritis, no paresthesia or burning	Sensory symptoms common in area of skin eruption

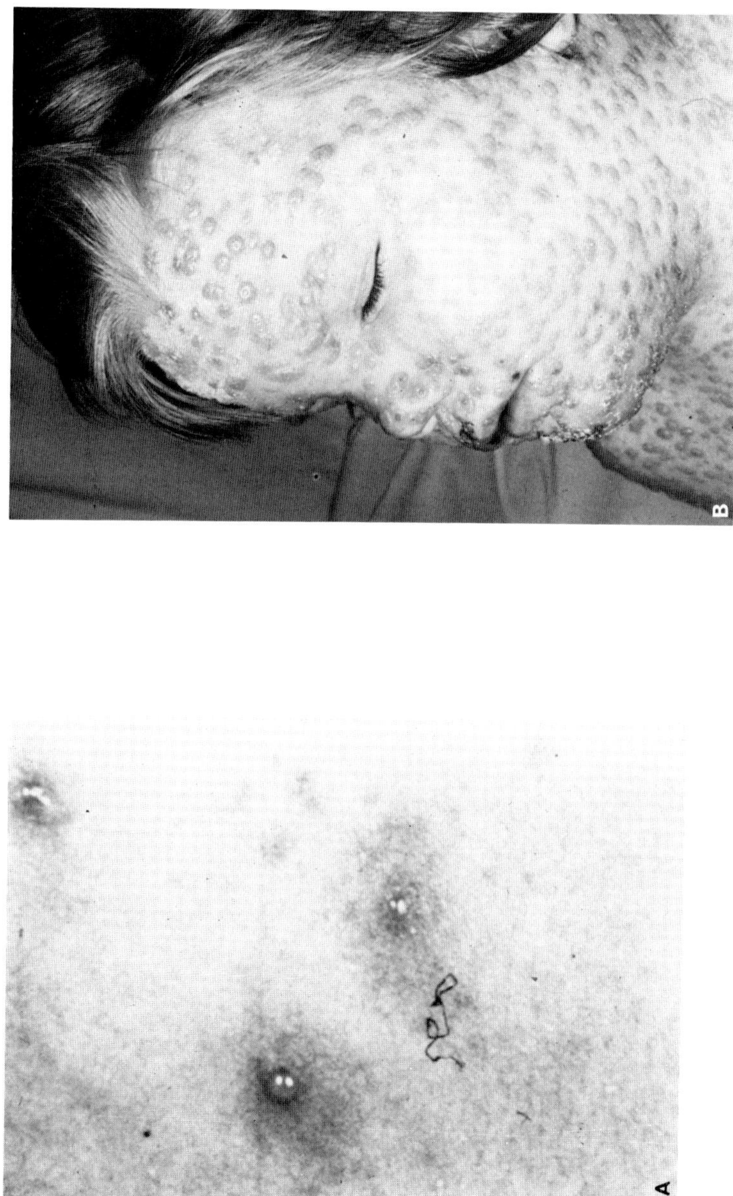

FIG. 1. (A) Very early varicella vesicle appearing as "dew on a rose petal." (B) Extensive varicella rash illustrating lesions in various stages of development.

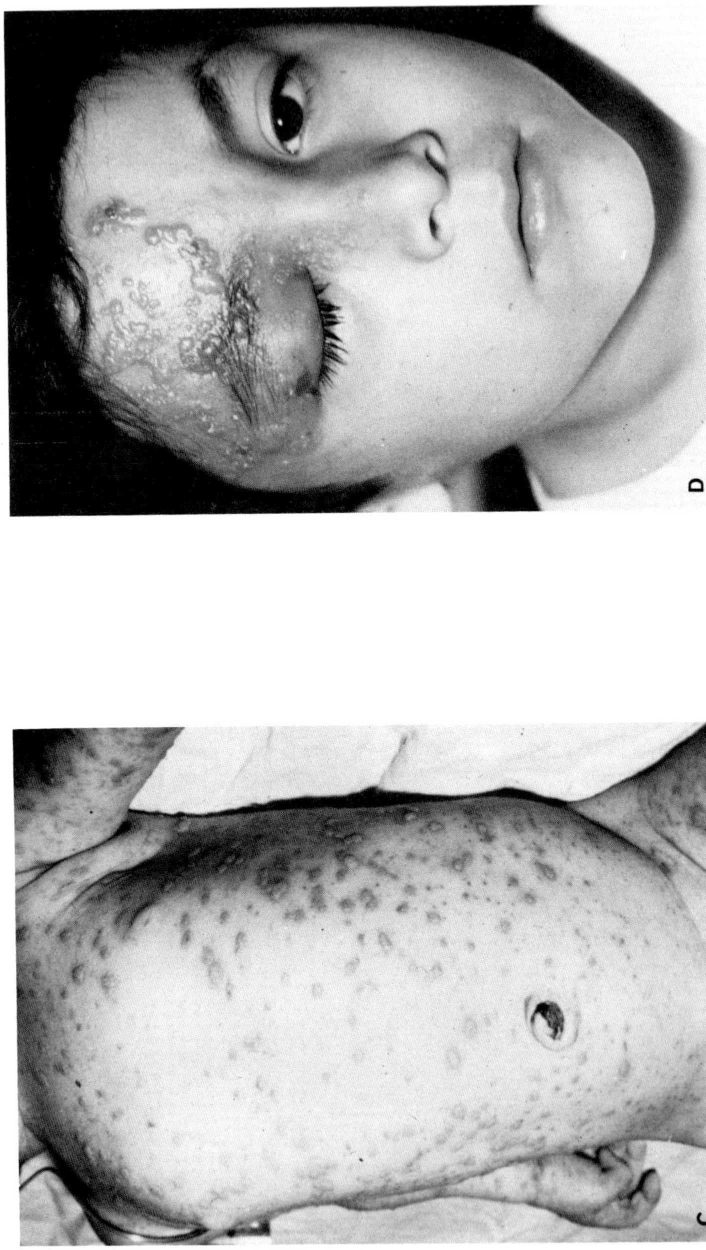

FIG. 1. (C) Neonatal varicella rash in a 12-day-old who eventually died. (D) Herpes zoster of ophthalmic branch of trigeminal nerve. Notice that the rash does not transverse the midline.

produced by burns, adhesive tape, or diapers. Repeated crops of lesions appear on the same portions of the body over a period of 2–4 days so that vesicles, pustules, and crusts may be observed simultaneously in any particular location. The lesions heal rapidly unless secondarily infected, and recovery is usually complete by the end of the second week following onset of the rash. The disease varies in severity, and mild cases with little rash may go unidentified.

Varicella is more likely to be severe or accompanied by complications when it occurs in adults. The reason for this is unknown. Adults or children with altered immunity because of underlying disease or administration of immunosuppresive drugs are not only particularly vulnerable to V–Z infection, but they also have an increased risk of a prolonged, complicated, or even fatal disease.

b. DURING PREGNANCY (SEE FIG. 2). Varicella occurs in about 1 in 1000 pregnancies (Sever and White, 1968), and although congenital malformations, maternal death, or abortion have all been described, their frequency of occurrence is extremely low. The major risk of varicella during pregnancy is the same as for any adult: varicella pneumonia.

Reports of mothers with a history of chicken pox within the final 2 weeks of pregnancy, gathered from the literature (Freud, 1958; Abler, 1964; Pearson, 1964; Brunell, 1967) plus personal experiences, provide the basis for several generalizations:

1. Less than half of the infants born to mothers who have varicella in the 2 week period prior to delivery develop varicella.
2. Generally, the interval between onset of the rash in mother and infant, in cases where neonatal chicken pox occurs, is 9–15 days, or a little shorter than the normal incubation period.
3. Infants exposed to mothers who develop chicken pox during the puerperium uniformly become infected.
4. The course in the full term infant with neonatal varicella is usually benign.

The placenta does not readily permit passage of V–Z virus, possibly because the virus is cell-associated. In most cases when a pregnant woman has varicella, insufficient virus reaches the fetus to cause infection. The repeated observation that the skin rash in mother and the congenitally affected infant usually does not occur concurrently but rather with an interval of 9–15 days suggests that when virus passes across the placenta it does so during the "secondary viremia" of the mother. The relatively small amount of infectious virus that reaches the infant initiates multiple cycles of replication, and eventually when high titers are achieved, there is dissemination of virus via the bloodstream to skin and various tissues and the development of typical

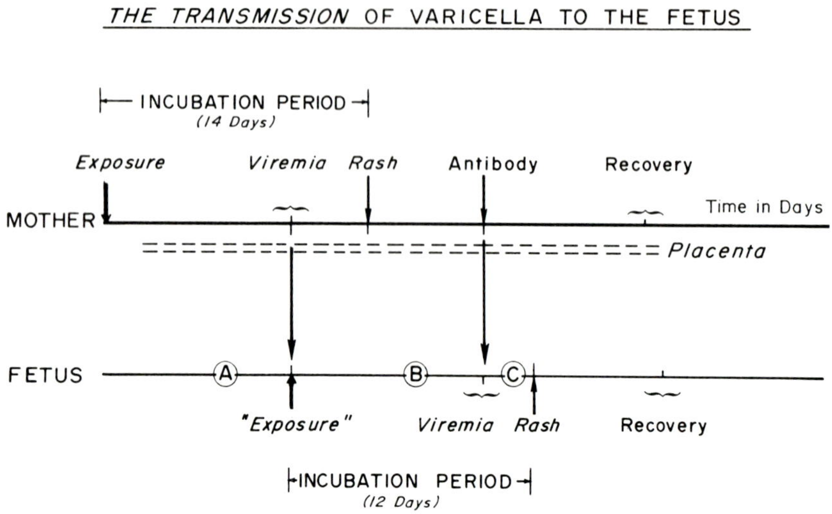

FIG. 2. The various theoretical considerations which may influence the probability of varicella occurring in the offspring of a mother who has varicella within 2 weeks of term. Infant born at time (A) or earlier is not infected *in utero* but could contract varicella after birth from his mother, who is contagious for 1–3 days before onset of rash until 3–6 days after. Infant born at time (B) who acquired infection transplacentally will develop varicella. Infant born at time (C) or later may receive transplacental V–Z antibody which can modify or prevent clinical varicella.

disease. In the rare situation, presumably when there is a massive passage of virus into the infant's circulation, the development of rash in mother and infant is concurrent.

Transfer of V–Z antibody across the placenta may influence the probability of an infant developing congenital varicella. Infants born 6 or more days following the onset of maternal V–Z infection have V–Z antibody titers in their cord sera similar to that of their mothers. This report by Brunell (1966) shows that pregnant women make 7 S antibody within 5–6 days after onset of varicella rash and that this antibody is shared with the infant *in utero*. It has already been stated that most frequently the rash of the infant follows that of the mother by a period of approximately 2 weeks. If maternal antibody reaches the infant's circulation in the middle of this interval, there may be inhibition of viral replication and modification or even termination of the developing chicken pox. This may explain the observation that infants who develop varicella within 5 days after birth generally have a milder form of disease than those who develop their illness in the second week of life (Freud, 1958).

Any infant born to a mother who had chicken pox within 14 days prior to delivery should be kept in isolation; the newborn may be incubating varicella. The infant should also be separated from the mother if she developed the rash of varicella or herpes zoster 6 days or less prior to the birth of the infant. The mother is contagious for a period of 5–6 days after onset of rash and may transmit chicken pox to her offspring. The infant who does not get varicella either by transplacental route or by direct exposure is, thereafter, just as vulnerable to chicken pox as any other nonimmune child.

2. Complications of Varicella

a. Pyogenic. Secondary infection of skin lesions often progressing to cellulitis or suppurative lymphadenitis is the most common complication of chicken pox. In cases when appropriate treatment is not provided, the pyogenic process may progress to bacteremia, epidural abscess, osteomyelitis, or meningitis.

In rare cases, individual vesciles may develop into large bullae measuring up to 3 cm in diameter. Such lesions may result from secondary infection with β hemolytic *Streptococci* or *Staphylococci* but lesions similar in appearance (Saslaw *et al.*, 1960) may occur as a rare form of varicella, called "varicella bullosa." Smears and cultures of the fluid aspirated from the bullae will aid in the differential diagnosis between superinfection and varicella bullosa. The latter if uncomplicated by secondary infection normally runs a benign course.

b. Purpura. The infrequent case of chicken pox is characterized by hemorrhagic lesions. Charkes (1961) reported a 26-year-old soldier with purpuric chicken pox and thrombocytopenia whose course was benign. The author reviewed other cases gathered from the literature and separated them into syndromes depending on several clinical and laboratory correlates. Malignant chicken pox developing with the appearance of the rash was associated with the highest mortality rate. Anaphylactoid purpura (nonthrombocytopenic) or infectious purpura (thrombocytopenic), both generally benign in course, may follow varicella. Any patient with varicella showing evidence of bleeding should be studied to determine the adequacy of various clotting factors and treated as indicated by these findings.

c. Central Nervous System. Neurologic complications of varicella occur in 1 to 2 cases per 1000 generally 4–10 days following the eruption of the rash. The list includes cerebellar ataxia, meningoencephalitis, disseminated or transverse myelitis, acute ascending spinal paralysis, polyneuritis, optic neuritis, and paralysis of cranial nerves. Acute cerebellar ataxia is the most common of these complications; it accounted for one-third of 59 cases with CNS complications reported by Appelbaum *et al.* (1962) and one-fourth of 120 cases reviewed by Underwood (1935). There was no correlation between the severity of rash and the ultimate prognosis of the neurologic complication. Generally patients with signs of cerebellar dysfunction had a complete recovery, although the convalescent period occasionally extended over an interval of several weeks. Patients who had meningoencephalitis with seizures or coma had a poorer prognosis, the mortality rate being 30–40%. An average of 80 cases of "encephalitis associated with chicken pox" have been reported yearly for the past 6 years to the National Center for Disease Control (NCDC) (1972), with a death–case ratio of 27.6:100. In all probability the more severe cases were selectively reported. In 1970, 12 of the 15 individuals who died with chicken pox encephalitis were less than 9 years of age, and 3 were 70 years or older in age. Included among these cases were children with a clinical syndrome characterized by acute cerebellar edema and fatty infiltration of the liver, referred to as Reye's syndrome. Among 62 cases of Reye's syndrome, collected over a 30 month period in an NCDC case detection program (Glick *et al.*, 1970a,b), seven, including two siblings, were associated with chicken pox; six of these children died. The interval between onset of rash and encephalopathy was 4 days in six cases and 3 days in one case. The association of chicken pox with Reye's syndrome appears to be a relatively new, but increasingly common, severe complication.

d. Pneumonia. The frequency with which pulmonary lesions, either of bacterial or viral etiology, occur in varicella was the subject of a report by Weinstein and Meade (1956). In a group of 453 patients with chicken pox, disease of the respiratory tract was noted in 41; 20 were less than 7 years old and 21 were over the age of 19 years. The authors, using defined criteria to distinguish "viral" and "bacterial" infections, concluded that primary varicella pneumonia occurred only in adults. Further studies by others (Krugman *et al.*, 1957; Knyvett, 1966) have confirmed the more frequent but not exclusive occurrence of varicella pneumonia in those over 15 years of age.

Varicella pneumonia occurs within 1–5 days after the appearance of rash, with rapid onset of cough, chest pain, dyspnea, tachypnea, possibly cyanosis, and hemoptysis. It is rarely diagnosed in the asymptomatic patient. Chest X-ray (Fig. 3) reveals extensive, nodular densities throughout all lung fields. Alveolar–capillary gas exchange is abnormal (Bocles *et al.*, 1964), and this defect may persist long beyond clinical recovery. The use of positive pressure breathing devices (Harper *et al.*, 1969) may be life saving. The course is variable, but in the usual case, clinical resolution of the pneumonia occurs in 2–3 weeks, although it may require twice as long for the radiological lesions to disappear. Occasionally the pulmonary chicken pox lesions become calcified and persist for years (A. Segel and E. Gold, unpublished). Pneumonia is frequently associated with hepatitis and other signs of general-

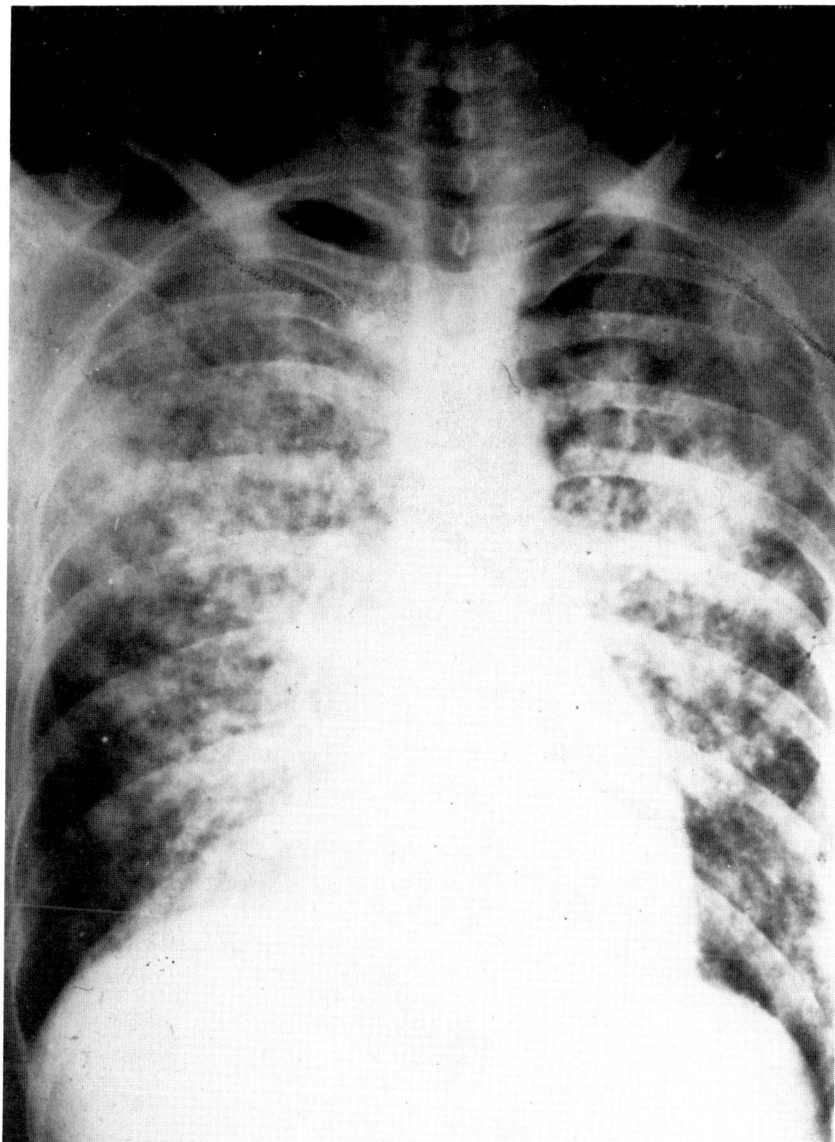

FIG. 3. Varicella pneumonia in an adult.

ized virus infection. Typical intranuclear inclusions found in cells included in sputum (Williams and Capers, 1959) may help confirm the clinical and radiological impression of varicella pneumonia.

e. Depression of Tuberculin Reactivity. Of a group of 17 children who developed chicken pox while in the hospital for treatment of tuberculosis (Starr and Berkovich, 1963), 7 who previously had reacted strongly to intradermal PPD, developed a negative tuberculin reaction in the interval—2 days before to 6 days after–onset of rash. The diminished response to tuberculin was transient and in no case persisted beyond 2 weeks. Whether the change in reactivity to tuberculin reflects an altered state of cell-mediated immunity or a change in end organ (skin) response is unknown. There was no indication that the chicken pox affected the course of tuberculosis or altered susceptibility to other infections in these children. Skin tests with PPD or other intradermal antigens should not be applied to children with acute varicella because of the probability of invalid results.

f. Other. The list of less common complications observed with varicella includes gastrointestinal bleeding, appendicitis, pancreatitis, cardiac and circulatory disorders (Moore *et al.*, 1969), nephritis, orchitis, and arthritis (Ward and Bishop, 1970).

B. Herpes Zoster

1. Clinical

The rash of herpes zoster is a linear array of vesicles or large irregular bullae on an erythematous base restricted to an area of skin supplied by the sensory nerves of a single or small group of dorsal root ganglia. The sequence of change from papule, to vesicle, to pustules, and to scabs is similar to that of varicella but the process may be slower. Lesions may occur in crops, but generally those in a cluster are in the same stage of development. Prodromal, constitutional symptoms are uncommon in zoster, but the adult patient may complain of burning or tingling in the area 24–48 hours before the appearance of the rash. A history of pain is not typically obtained from the child. Herpes zoster involves the thorax in approximately half of the cases (Burgoon *et al.*, 1957) and is less frequently ophthalmic, lumbar, cervical, or sacral in distribution. The duration and severity of herpes zoster is age-related. Younger adults and children generally have mild illness of short duration. In the older individual the course of zoster may be prolonged and complicated. New crops of lesions may continue appearing over a period of several days and persist for several weeks.

2. Complications

Among the more common complications, most of which appear following the eruption of the rash, are neuralgia (which occurs in approximately 10% of patients over 40 years of age), facial or occulomotor palsy, paralysis of motor nerves, and myelitis. Meningoencephalitis most commonly has its onset during or 2–4 days after the appearance of rash, but nervous system manifestations may precede skin manifestations (Appelbaum *et al.*, 1962). The zoster eruption in patients with meningoencephalitis frequently involves cranial nerves or the cervical or upper thoracic segments of the cord, rather than the lower levels. The spinal fluid in such patients is clear, under slightly increased pressure, has a minimally increased protein content and a normal sugar level, and contains a moderate mononuclear pleocytosis (300–400/mm^3 or less). The disease process is presumably due to direct invasion of the meninges and adjacent structures by virus originating in the dorsal root ganglia. The isolation of virus from the spinal fluid of two patients with clinical meningoencephalitis and pleocytosis is evidence of virus invasion (Gold and Robbins, 1958), but the pathogenesis of the process is uncertain.

The prognosis or course of the neurologic complications of zoster is related to the age of the patient and the presence of underlying disease, but even the selected experiences which reach the literature indicate a generally favorable outcome. In the occasional normal individual, but more frequently in the patient with a deficient immune system, herpes zoster may progress from the typical, localized process to a generalized disease that clinically resembles varicella. The majority of patients with disseminated zoster have a predisposing cause which is most frequently a malignant disease involving the hematopoietic system (Merselis *et al.*, 1964). Such patients lack the ability to confine the virus process, and extensive viral replication and dissemination results. The prognosis in generalized zoster plus varicella as it is also called, is generally poor.

C. Laboratory Characteristics

1. Tissue Culture

Within 1 week or less following the inoculation of human fibroblast tissue cultures with vesicle fluid or other infectious material from V–Z patients, foci of irregularly rounded refractile and occasional multinucleated giant cells appear. Typical intranuclear inclusions can be readily identified by staining. The focus of virus effect gradually increases in size by the involvement of adjacent cells by a process that involves cell-to-cell transmission of virus. Varicella–zoster virus propagated in tissue culture remains cell-associated and is rapidly inactivated when the host cell is disrupted (Gold and Godek, 1965), but in the human host, infectious cell-free V–Z virus is present in high titer in vesicles less than 4 days old. The direct inoculation of even a drop of such fluid will produce many foci of virus effect in tissue cultures. Virus cannot be grown from the lesions of varicella patients who have detectable levels of complement-fixing (C-F) antibodies, but the lesions of zoster yield virus as late as 7 days (Gold, 1966) after the appearance of rash, even when the patient has a high level of C-F antibody. The virus in vesicle fluid is very labile at room temperature, especially if diluted. Subculture of V–Z tissue cultures requires the transfer of whole cells; the use of the fluid phase of the culture alone is inadequate. Isolation of virus from sources other than vesicle fluid may be accomplished by the inoculation of freshly prepared cell suspensions of infected tissue such as lung, liver, or lymph node. Isolation of virus from pharyngeal secretion, blood, or spinal fluid has been reported, but this is uncommon either because there is little or no infectious virus in the inocula used or because the assay system is very insensitive. Both of these explanations may be valid. The prolonged storage of cultured strains of V–Z or infected tissues frequently results in loss of infectivity presumably because active virus persists only in cells which survive freezing and thawing. Low-temperature storage of virus material under conditions which preserve cell viability is recommended.

Laboratory methods, in the absence of an experimental animal, have not provided evidence that there are variants of V–Z which differ antigenically. However occasional reports of family outbreaks suggest that virulent variants exist. Hook *et al.* (1968), reported a family outbreak of varicella involving five children, ages 2–9 years, all of whom developed chicken pox within a 2 week period. Two children died, and one who was autopsied had a severe virus pneumonia. The two fatal cases plus two others had experienced an illness clinically typical of rubella 4–6 weeks prior to the onset of chicken pox. An explanation for this unusual event or others similar to it cannot be provided, but "host factors" are usually cited.

2. Serology

Specific complement-fixing or neutralizing antibodies develop within 6–7 days after the initiation of the varicella rash, and demonstration of a rise in antibody by the complement-fixation reaction is a generally available method to make the retrospective diagnosis of infection. Complement-fixing antibody disappears relatively rapidly following recovery from V–Z, and in most individuals is not detectable within 3 years following infection. The complement-fixation test is thus not a useful screening method for identifying those susceptible to varicella or zoster.

Most serologic studies performed with V–Z have employed the complement-fixation test because of the difficulty in preparing and maintaining the stocks of cell-free infectious virus required for neutralization tests.

3. Host Range

Tyzzer (1906), who first described the intranuclear inclusions in skin biopsies of patients with varicella, also carried out systematic attempts to isolate the causative agent in monkeys, rabbits, and other animals. He was unsuccessful, as were subsequent investigators because of the high degree of specificity of the V–Z virus for the human host. The single or isolated report of varicella in anthropoid apes (Heuschele, 1960) could not be confirmed by testing animal sera for V–Z antibody by the complement-fixation (C-F) test (Gold, 1966).

4. Laboratory Aids for Diagnosis

There are several laboratory aids which are useful in distinguishing chickenpox or herpes zoster from smallpox or vaccinia, but do not differentiate members of the herpesvirus family, i.e., V–Z from herpes simplex. In contrast to smallpox or vaccinia, scrapings from a fresh V–Z or herpes simplex vesicle, fixed and stained with hematoxylin and eosin, giemsa, or any of the other common multicolored stains, contain typical balloon cells, multinucleated giant cells, and occasionally cells with intranuclear inclusions. Biopsies of early skin lesions are more likely to contain typical intranuclear inclusions. If the use of an electron microscope is available, direct observation of vesicle fluid by the phosphotungstic acid (PTA) (Watson *et al.*, 1963) method may permit identification of the symmetrical herpes nucleocapsid which can be readily distinguished from the bricklike smallpox or vaccinia. The presumptive identification of V–Z virus may be made by the typical cytopathic effect which appears 2–3 days after the direct inoculation of specimens into cultures of human diploid fibroblast cells (see Section II, C, 1). In addition, varicella causes no grossly visible effect on the chorioallantoic membranes of embryonated chick eggs, while smallpox and vaccinia cause typical pock formation. Final identification of virus isolates, especially when members of the herpesvirus family must be separated, is made by determining the host range of the agent and by serological techniques, such as fluorescent antibody staining, neutralization test, or precipitin reaction.

D. Differential Diagnosis (see Section II,C,4 and Table II)

The characteristic appearance of the skin rash, its typical metamorphosis, the presence of various stages of the lesions in the same anatomic area, and the sequential appearance of lesions progressing from head to foot are the

TABLE II

CLINICAL AND LABORATORY CHARACTERISTICS[a] USEFUL IN DIFFERENTIATING V–Z INFECTION FROM OTHER DISEASES

	Clinical				Laboratory	
		Rash				
	Prodromal symptoms	Progression	Characteristic distribution	Stage in local area	Chorioallantoic membrane lesion	Intranuclear inclusion and giant cells
Varicella	Mild or absent	Rapid	Centripital	Varied	–	+
Variola	Severe	Slow	Centrifugal	Same	+	–
Disseminated herpes simplex	Usually absent	Moderate	None	Same	+	+
Generalized vaccinia	Usually absent	Slow	None	Varied	+	–
Hand, foot, mouth disease	Mild or absent	Moderate	Hand and/or feet and/or mouth	Same	–	–

[a]See Section II,D.

clinical manifestations that generally permit one to make a diagnosis of varicella. However several disease entities should be considered in the differential diagnosis of varicella; the following are among more confusing.

i. Smallpox. The discontinuation of routine smallpox immunization in the United States and the increasing mobility of the world's population makes the differentiation of varicella from smallpox particularly important. While varicella has a short or absent prodrome, the rash of smallpox is usually preceded by a 2–4 day illness characterized by severe constitutional symptoms. The varicella rash appears in crops which are distributed centripetally, unlike smallpox lesions which have centrifugal distribution. The latter are also in the same stage of development in any given anatomic area, develop more slowly than chicken pox lesions, and are characterized by deeper involvement of the skin. History of a recent successful smallpox vaccination makes classic smallpox unlikely; but smallpox modified by a vaccination in the distant past may be difficult to distinguish from varicella clinically.

ii. Disseminated herpes simplex. This infection usually has no prodrome, and the rash usually has no particular distribution. Ocasssionally herpes simplex vesicles may occur in a zosteriform distribution involving one or more dermatomes and creating some degree of confusion. Laboratory methods are necessary for definitive differentation (see Section II, C, 4).

iii. Generalized vaccinia. Persons who have had a primary vaccination 1–2 weeks previously may, but not usually, develop generalized vaccinia. The rash lesions appear in crops over a period of 2–6 days and resemble a series of primary vaccination lesions in various stages of development. Thus they are usually significantly larger than the classic lesions of varicella. The complicating lesions together with the primary lesion usually persist beyond the usual time of healing in the average person with a primary vaccination. History of vaccination is of course very important diagnostically. Laboratory methods are useful in making a specific diagnosis. (See Section II, C, 4.)

iv. Enterovirus infections. During the warm weather from late spring to early fall, the coxsackieviruses and occasionally the echoviruses may cause vesicular eruptions. These enterovirus rash diseases are most characteristically accompanied by mild or no prodromal symptoms, and the vesicles are usually superficial and small. There is no characteristic rash distribution except for coxsackie A-16 induced hand, foot, and mouth disease. The latter disease takes its name from the areas usually involved by the vesicular rash. The enteroviruses may be readily grown in tissue culture except for most coxsackie A viruses which require the use of suckling mice.

v. Other. Other rash diseases which may have vesicular components and be confused with varicella are impetigo, insect bites, scabies, dermatitis herpetiformis, rickettsialpox, eczema herpeticum or vaccinatum, drug eruptions, secondary lues, and erythema multiforme.

III. Pathology and Pathogenesis

A. Pathology

1. Varicella

a. Dermal and Mucous Membrane. Microscopically the early skin lesions consist of minute, unilocular vesicles involving the corium and overlying epidermis (Cheatham *et al.*, 1956). The epithelial cells within the lesions as well as those bordering the involved area undergo ballooning degeneration and frequently contain moderately basophilic, homogeneous, intranuclear inclusion bodies. Similar intranuclear inclusions may be present in the endothelial cells of capillaries adjacent to the lesions and in surrounding fibroblasts.

The more mature cutaneous lesions also contain intranuclear inclusions in various cell types, but these consist of a central, acidophilic, irregular mass, surrounded by a clear halo and finally by a ring of marginated chromatin. Large, multinucleated giant cells with multiple inclusions are numerous in these more mature lesions. Under certain circumstances there may be destruction of the germinal layer with necrosis and hemorrhage into the upper portion of the dermis. Alteration of cutaneous nerves has not been observed.

As the lesions in the skin develop, the small pools of exudate that collect around the damaged cells coalesce to form the macroscopically visible varicella vesicle (Johnson, 1940). The fluid rapidly becomes cloudy with degenerated cells, fibrin, and invading polymorphonuclear leukocytes. Finally the fluid is absorbed and a scab forms which eventually becomes detached.

Varicella lesions of mucous membranes develop histologically in a similar manner to the skin lesions. However they do not progress to scab formation, but rather the vesicles rupture resulting in the formation of shallow ulcers. The latter usually heal rapidly. In individuals with fatal forms of varicella the focal lesions in skin, mucous membrane, or tissues may become hemorrhagic or necrotic.

b. Pneumonia. At autopsy, the lungs are congested and the alveoli are filled with fluid composed of fibrin, red blood cells, and large numbers of mononuclear cells, some of which contain intranuclear inclusions (Nemir, 1967). There is proliferation of the septal cells, alveolar necrosis, and numerous hemorrhagic areas secondary to vascular damage. The patchy lobular lesions radiate from the hilus into the lungs and may show considerable coalescence.

c. HERPES ZOSTER. The microscopic pathology of the zoster skin lesions is similar to that of the varicella lesion (Head and Campbell, 1900; Cheatham *et al.*, 1956). The lesions within the dorsal root ganglion consist of round cell infiltration, focal hemorrhage, and finally neuronal destruction. Acidophilic intranuclear inclusions may be seen in satellite and ganglion cells. Approximately 2 weeks after onset of the dermal lesions, the posterior nerve root shows a maximum of degeneration, and similar alterations may be noted in the sensory nerves as well as the posterior cord columns. Occasionally this destructive process may result in a localized meningitis and rarely expand to involve areas of the anterior horn. The final result may be the replacement of the normal ganglion by scar tissue.

B. Pathogenesis

Initial infection of a susceptible young host with the V–Z virus results in dissemination of the agent and the typical general illness known as chicken pox. There is an appropriate response by the immune system of the host, one parameter of which is development of specific complement-fixing antibody which falls to nondetectable levels within 2–3 years. Most individuals, even in the absence of detectable antibody, have no further illness related to the V–Z agent but some develop zoster many years later.

Over a century ago, von Baerensprung described the association of the cutaneous rash of zoster with histologic lesions of the dorsal root ganglia. Head and Campbell (1900) later carried out extensive anatomic studies which substantiated that report. These anatomic findings plus the epidemiologic data which indicated that zoster followed varicella, that zoster was a disease of older age groups, and that zoster occurred endemically and independently of varicella epidemics, all led to the hypothesis that zoster is the manifestation of reactivation of varicella infection in a "partially immune" host. The later laboratory evidence that virus isolates from patients with varicella or zoster are indistinguishable supported this concept. The prodromal burning pain or other unpleasant sensations, occurring over the distribution of the same sensory nerves suggests that V–Z virus persists in cells of the dorsal root ganglia in a latent or dormant state and is activated. Although V–Z virus has not been cultured from the ganglia, characteristic intranuclear inclusions and typical virus particles (Evans and Melnick, 1949) have been demonstrated in ganglia supplying the involved skin segment. Virus propagated in the dorsal root ganglia then passes centrifugally down the nerve to the skin. The manner by which the varicella virus initially reaches the dorsal root ganglion, the mechanism of persistence, and the process by which the dormant virus is induced to replicate and move down to the skin are all uncertain. Varicella–zoster virus may spread to the dorsal root ganglia via the hematogenous route, or the virus may gain access to visceral nerve endings in the esophogus and pass to the dorsal root ganglia via the white ramus as proposed by Cheatham *et al.* (1956).

A history of an event which precedes the development of herpes zoster and is conceivably responsible for viral activation can be obtained from some patients with herpes zoster. The report of trauma, such as contusions, fractures, or intramuscular injections is common. The most striking association, however, is with "immune deficiency" resulting from malignant disease, therapy for malignant disease, or treatment with immunosuppressive drugs.

It has been demonstrated recently (Stevens and Cook, 1971, 1973) that another member of the herpesvirus family, herpes simplex can persist in an inactive form in dorsal root ganglia of the mouse and later be detected by growing the nerve cells in tissue culture. These experiments, however, fall short of serving as a model for the pathogenesis of herpes zoster in man, since attempts to reactivate virus in the living mouse by a multiplicity of agents, including immunosuppressive drugs, γ radiation, steroids, heat, and transplantation of tumor tissue, have been thus far unsuccessful.

IV. Immunity

A. Normal Host

Specific complement-fixing (C-F) or neutralizing antibodies develop within 6–7 days after the appearance of the varicella rash and fall to nondetectable levels during the following 2–3 years. While immunity to the common childhood exanthems, especially rubella and rubeola, may be maintained following either natural infection or immunization by repeated contact with the infectious agent which acts as "booster" immunizations, this does not appear to be the case with varicella. Serial serum samples obtained from individuals with a remote history of chicken pox and a recent history of exposure to varicella were tested (Gold, 1965) to detect rises in antibody. The subjects in this study were children or medical personnel exposed to active cases of varicella in hospitals or schools under conditions where similarly exposed, susceptible individuals contracted the disease. In none of these subjects could a booster response be detected.

The rise in C-F antibody observed in patients with zoster appears to be more rapid and to a higher level than that observed with varicella. This finding may merely reflect the difficulty in dating the onset of zoster, but it may also indicate a "booster" or anamnestic response.

There is good reason to believe that specific humoral antibody can protect the host from varicella infection. The most convincing data was obtained in recent studies (Brunell *et al.*, 1969) which showed the effectiveness of zoster immune globulin (ZIG) when used for prophylaxis. However immune mechanisms other than the ability to produce circulating antibody appear to play a significant part in limiting the course of varicella as well as other viral infections. Cell-mediated immunity is probably most important and is discussed in Section IV, B below.

The production of interferon is another mechanism which may alter host susceptibility to V–Z or other viral infections. Interferon appears in serum and body fluids during the viremia stage early in infection, while antibody appears later. The amount of interferon closely parallels the titer of virus present. This sequence has been used to support a role for interferon in recovery from infection. However, a high level of interferon may not predict a favorable clinical course, nor is a low level of interferon in blood or tissue uniformly accompanied by severe illness (Baron, 1963; Cole and Wisseman, 1969). The importance of interferon in the control of virus infections in the normal individual is uncertain.

B. Host with Immune Deficit

The death from varicella of children receiving corticosteroids, reported from Boston, raised the question of the factors involved in and the relative contribution to the fatal outcome by the underlying disease and by the therapy. Among the 12 varicella deaths reported by Haggerty and Eley (1956), 1 was in a child with a malignancy; the other 11 were children treated with steroids because of a variety of nonmalignant diseases. In subsequent studies (Finkel, 1961; Pinkel, 1961; Falliers and Ellis, 1965), it was shown that although the occurrences of chicken pox in children receiving corticosteroids could result in death, a significantly higher mortality rate from varicella was found among children who were on treatment with steroids for leukemia or other diseases which "compromise" the immune system. The implication of this observation was that the "underlying malignant disease" was the major determinent of the host response. Falliers and Ellis (1965) warned that steroid treatment should not be abruptly stopped in a patient who is exposed to or develops varicella as recommended by Eley (1961); the mortality rate may be increased by "... not using steroids rather than by using them." They advised that steroid therapy should be continued at physiologic levels. Critical evaluation of this approach has not been carried out but it is the method used by the authors.

The frequency of herpes zoster in the normal population is difficult to determine; estimates are in the range of 0.2 to 2%. Nearly half a century ago,

Pancoast and Pendergrass (1924) pointed out that adults with malignant disease, especially those with the Hodgkin's form of lymphoma, were unusually susceptible to infection with the V–Z virus. Since then a number of reports have confirmed this association. Among 600 patients with Hodgkin's disease studied at Roswell Park Memorial Institute (Sokal and Firat, 1965) between 1920 and 1963, 8% had one or more episodes of V–Z disease. This experience is similar to that reported for patients with Hodgkin's disease by several other groups (Wright and Winer, 1961; Dayan *et al.*, 1964). During a 2-year follow-up of 419 patients with cancer, Schimpff *et al.* (1972) reported herpes zoster infection in 25% of the patients with Hodgkin's, in 8.7% of patients with other forms of lymphoma, but in less than 2% of patients with acute leukemia or solid tumors. The higher incidence of V–Z infection among patients with Hodgkin's disease may have resulted from their inadvertent exposure to patients who attended clinic with acute, previously nondiagnosed V–Z disease. The occurrence of herpes zoster in 6 of 73 renal transplant recipients (Rifkind, 1966) treated with immunosuppressive therapy demonstrates that the latter group is also vulnerable to zoster.

More impressive than the high incidence of H–Z infections among groups of patients with immune deficiency is the strikingly frequent occurrence in these patients of the generalized form of the disease; rates of 30–73% have been reported (Shanbron *et al.*, 1960; Merselis *et al.*, 1964; Merigan and Stevens, 1971). It is most difficult to separate the effects of therapy from the effects of the disease process for which the drugs are being given, but some groups of patients, especially those with the Hodgkin's form of lymphoma, apparently are susceptible to viral infections, such as V–Z, in the early stages of their disease, at a time when the components of the immune system can be individually examined. Several studies of this type will be reviewed.

The observation that patients with Hodgkin's disease are more likely to be tuberculin-negative than comparable controls (Parker *et al.*, 1932) has been confirmed and extended by numerous investigators (Schier *et al.*, 1956; Lamb, 1962; Aisenberg, 1964; Sokal and Firat, 1965) who have shown that the Hodgkin's patients, even when tested before the initiation of chemotherapy or irradiation (Brown *et al.*, 1967; Young *et al.*, 1972), have a high incidence of anergy to a large battery of skin test antigens but an intact ability to form humoral antibody. Diminished delayed hypersensitivity was common in patients with a variety of malignant disease who were late in their disease and in "poor clinical condition," but the rate of skin test hypoactivity was highest in the Hodgkin's group. Among patients in "good" clinical condition, those with Hodgkin's were the only group which included a significant proportion with diminished cutaneous reactivity. The percentage of patients with Hodgkin's disease who are anergic depends upon the stage of the disease; it is low in patients with stage one and approximates 25% in patients with stage four (Han and Sokal, 1970). Significantly the occurrence of varicella–zoster infections has a similar distribution (Sokal and Firat, 1965).

Conversely, the enhanced susceptibility of immunosuppressed patients to viral illnesses such as varicella or zoster is probably not the result of depression of interferon production. Interferon has been demonstrated in the vesicles of normal patients with varicella or herpes zoster. Armstrong *et al.* (1970) studied four patients with Hodgkin's disease and V–Z infection to determine if the interferon content of their skin lesions was diminished. Three of the patients studied late in the infection (day 7 or later as recovery was beginning) had "normal" levels of interferon. One patient had a low level of interferon in vesicles on day 5 of his disease and high levels on days 9 and 11. The lesions spread beyond the original site on days 7 and 8 at a time when interferon content was increasing rapidly, and healing began on day 10. The authors concluded that early interferon production was an important correlation to the outcome of the infection and thus "... may be a factor in the host resistance ..." to infection. In an editorial comment, Ho (1970) cautions that even if the interferon content of vesicle fluid is shown to be a prediction of the course of herpes zoster, "... it may not be a crucial factor in the outcome of disease."

Hodgkin's disease thus is associated with a distinct immunologic deficiency which involves the thymic-dependent system; the ability to form antibody or interferon may not be involved. This altered immune state may be aggravated by chemotherapy or radiation but is not simply the result of lymphocytopenia and illustrates and emphasizes the extreme importance of cellular immune mechanisms in defense against viral infections including V–Z. It should be emphasized that although patients with certain types of immune deficiency are prone to disseminated or prolonged V–Z infection that the course of such an illness is not necessarily fatal. Also Hodgkin's disease patients who have anergy and a diminished *in vitro* response to PHA may have benign, localized zoster. Furthermore many normal individuals, with no demonstrable impairment of cell-mediated immunity contract zoster, some even in the generalized form. Thus cell-mediated immunity may be only one of a group of factors which influence the outcome of the interaction between V–Z virus and the host.

V. Epidemiology

A. Varicella

Reporting of varicella is not obligatory, and although the data collected by NCDC suggests a declining incidence of cases from 1965 to 1970, this may merely reflect a change in notification practices. If one assumes that only 10% of cases are reported to the NCDC, then by extrapolating their figures, over two million cases of varicella occur annually!

In the large urban centers of the United States, chicken pox is principally a disease of childhood (Gordon, 1962); 90% of the cases reported occur in children less than 9 years of age, and only 3% are in individuals over the age of 15. The disease may occur sporadically throughout the year but peaks are seen most frequently in late winter and early spring. The disease is highly contagious with attack rates among exposed susceptibles running approximately 75%. The incubation period ranges from 14–21 days, but the new case who is most infectious for 24–48 hours before the rash appears and for the first 3–4 days of rash, may spread the disease before it is diagnosed.

B. Herpes Zoster

Zoster occurs in small numbers of cases throughout the year; there is no seasonal incidence and outbreaks of zoster do not coincide temporally with epidemics of varicella (Burgoon *et al.*,1957; Hope-Simpson, 1965; Miller and Brunell, 1970). Zoster occurs with equal frequency in males and females, but the attack rate is closely related to age. Zoster is uncommon in the pediatric age group, has an incidence of approximately 1 per 1000 per year in the 10–15 year age group, and 10 or more per 1000 in the 70 year and over age group. (see Table I).

C. Control

Varicella may be disseminated by the infected individual 1–2 days before the onset of rash and for 3–5 days thereafter. Spread from the infected person is via droplets usually originating from the respiratory tract, although vesicle fluid may also be a source of infection. Laboratory and epidemiologic studies both indicate that the pustular lesions or scabs of varicella are not a source of infection. Patients with zoster very clearly may transmit their V–Z virus but such individuals are less highly contagious than those with varicella. This may be related to the absence of virus in their nasopharyngeal secretions and the rather small, usually covered, localized area of rash from which virus may be shed.

Patients with either varicella or zoster should be kept in isolated rooms in the hospital, and special precautions must be taken to protect the transplant recipient and the patient with a natural or drug-induced deficiency in the thymic-dependent or cell-mediated immune system. Although zoster most frequently results from the activation of endogenous virus, the compromised host can apparently (Schimpff *et al.*, 1972) develop zoster following contact with an exogenous source of virus.

D. *Treatment*

In a carefully controlled trial (Brunell *et al.*, 1969) a 2.0 ml dose of zoster immune globulin (ZIG) with a complement-fixing antibody titer of at least 1:256 prevented varicella when administered to children within 72 hours after household exposure. The ZIG recipients had no clinical manifestations of varicella and did not develop specific antibody to V–Z, indicating that infection was prevented, not merely modified. Virus was apparently neutralized during the early viremia stage, preventing widespread infection of cells and general dissemination. The treated normal subjects presumably become susceptible to varicella once the passive antibody has decayed. This study clearly suggests a trial of ZIG for protecting children in whom varicella may be life-threatening. It may also be desirable to determine if ZIG is of any benefit in *treating* severe varicella, especially in patients with underlying disease. A program has been developed by which such a reagent is distributed from centers throughout the United States.*

Although immune globulin may be of benefit to the severely ill, immune-incompetent patient, theoretically, at least, therapy should be directed toward improving the function of cell-mediated immunity. There are no reports of the successful use of transfer factor or "immune lymphocytes," and possibly the patient with Hodgkin's disease will not accept or respond to such substances. However, this seems to be the direction in which to turn for therapeutic help.

References

Abler, C. (1964). *Amer. J. Dis. Child.* **107**, 492.
Aisenberg, A. C. (1964). *N. Engl. J. Med.* **270**, 508, 565, and 617.
Appelbaum, E., Kreps, S. I., and Sunshine, A. (1962). *Amer. J. Med.* **32**, 25.
Armstrong, R. W., Gurwith, M. J., Waddell, D., and Merigan, T. C. (1970). *N. Engl. J. Med.* **283**, 1182.
Baron, S. (1963). *Advan. Virus Res.* **10**, 39.
Bocles, J. S., Ehrenkranz, N. J., and Marks, A. (1964). *Ann. Intern. Med.* **60**, 183.
Brown, R. S., Haynes, H. A., Foley, H. T., Godwin, H. A., Berard, C. W., and Carbone, P. P. (1967). *Ann. Intern. Med.* **67**, 291.
Brunell, P. A. (1966). *Pediatrics* **38**, 1034.
Brunell, P. A. (1967). *J. Amer. Med. Ass.* **199**, 93.
Brunell, P. A., Ross, A., Miller, L. H., and Kuo, B. (1969). *N. Engl. J. Med.* **280**, 1191.
Bruusgaard, E. (1932). *Brit. J. Dermatol. Syph.* **44**, 1.
Burgoon, C. F., Jr., Burgoon, J. S., and Baldridge, G. D. (1957). *J. Amer. Med. Ass.* **164**, 265.
Charkes, N. D. (1961). *Ann. Intern. Med.* **54**, 745.

*See the *Journal of Infectious Disease*, **125**, No. 1, 1972.

Cheatham, W. J., Weller, T. H., Dolan, T. F., Jr., and Dower, J. C. (1956). *Amer. J. Pathol.* **32**, 1015.

Cole, A. G., and Wisseman, C. L., Jr. (1969). *Proc. Soc. Exp. Biol. Med.* **130**, 359.

Dayan, A. D., Morgan, H. G., Hope-Stone, H. F., and Boucher, B. J. (1964). *Amer. J. Roentgenol., Radium Ther. Nucl. Med.* **92**, 116.

Eley, R. C. (1961). *Pediatrics* **28**, 1027.

Evans, A. S., and Melnick, J. L. (1949). *Proc. Soc. Exp. Biol. Med.* **71**, 283.

Falliers, C. J., and Ellis, E. F. (1965). *Arch. Dis. Childhood* **40**, 593.

Finkel, K. C. (1961). *Pediatrics* **28**, 436.

Freud, P. (1958). *AMA J. Dis. Child.* **96**, 730.

Glick, T. H., Ditchek, N. T., Salitsky, S., and Freimuth, E. J. (1970a). *Amer. J. Dis. Child.* **119**. 68.

Glick, T. H., Likosky, W. H., Levitt, L. P., Mellin, H., and Reynolds, D. W. (1970b). *Pediatrics* **46**, 371.

Gold, E. (1965). *J. Immunol.* **95**, 683.

Gold, E. (1966). *N. Engl. J. Med.* **274**, 181.

Gold, E., and Godek, G. (1965). *J. Immunol.* **95**, 692.

Gold, E., and Robbins, F. C. (1958). *Virology* **6**, 293.

Gordon, J. E. (1962). *Amer. J. Med. Sci.* **244**, 362.

Haggerty, R. J., and Eley, R. C. (1956). *Pediatrics* **18**, 160.

Han, T., and Sokal, J. E. (1970). *Amer. J. Med.* **48**, 728.

Harper, J. R., Marshall, R. D., and Parkinson, M. S. (1969). *Brit. Med. J.* **3**, 637.

Head, H., and Campbell, A. W. (1900). *Brain* **23**, 353.

Heuschele, W. P. (1960). *J. Amer. Vet. Med. Ass.* **136**, 256.

Ho, M. (1970). *N. Engl. J. Med.* **283**, 1222 (Editorial Comment).

Hook, E. B., Orandi, M., ten Bensel, R. W., Schamber, W. F., and St. Geme, J. W. (1968). *J. Amer. Med. Ass.* **206**, 305.

Hope-Simpson, R. E. (1965). *Proc. Roy. Soc. Med.* **58**, 9.

Johnson, H. N. (1940). *Arch. Pathol.* **30**, 292.

Knyvett, A. F. (1966). *Quart. J. Med.* **35**, 313.

Krugman, S., Goodrich, C. H., and Ward, R. (1957). *N. Engl. J. Med.* **257**, 843.

Kundratitz, K. (1925). *Wien. Klin. Wochenschr.* **38**, 502.

Lamb, D. (1962). *J. Immunol.* **89**, 555.

Merigan, T. C., and Stevens, D. A. (1971). *Fed. Proc.* **30**, 1858.

Merselis, J. G., Jr., Kaye, D., and Hook, E. W. (1964). *Arch. Intern. Med.* **113**, 679.

Miller, L. H., and Brunell, P. A. (1970). *Amer. J. Med.* **49**, 480.

Moore, C. M., Henry, J., Benzing, G., and Kaplan, S. (1969). *Amer. J. Dis. Child.* **118**, 899.

National Center for Disease Control. (1972). "Neurotropic Viral Diseases. Surveillance, Encephalitis," p. 17. Nat. Cent. Dis. Contr.

Nemir, R. L. (1967). *In* "Disorders of the Respiratory Tract in Children" (E. L. Kendig, Jr., ed.), p. 315. Saunders, Philadelphia, Pennsylvania.

Pancoast, H. K., and Pendergrass, E. P. (1924). *Amer. J. Med. Sci.* **168**, 326.

Parker, F., Jr., Jackson, H., Jr., Fitzhugh, G., and Spies, T. D. (1932). *J. Immunol.* **22**, 277.

Pearson, H. E. (1964). *Obstet. Gynecol.* **23**, 21.

Pinkel, D. (1961). *J. Pediat.* **58**, 729.

Rifkind, D. (1966). *J. Clin. Med.* **68**, 463.

Saslaw, S., Kluck, C., and Prior, J. A. (1960). *J. Amer. Med. Ass.* **173**, 1214.

Schier, W. W., Roth, A., Ostroff, G., Schrift, M. H. (1956). *Amer. J. Med.* **20**, 94.

Schimpff, S., Rumack, B., and Block, J. (1972). *Ann. Intern. Med.* **76**, 241.

Sever, J., and White, L. R. (1968). *Annu. Rev. Med.* **19**, 471.

Shanbron, E., Miller, S., and Haar, H. (1960). *Ann. Intern. Med.* **53**, 523.
Sokal, J. E., and Firat, D. (1965). *Amer. J. Med.* **39**, 452.
Starr, S., and Berkovich, S. (1964). *Pediatrics* **33**, 769.
Stevens, J. G., and Cook, M. L. (1971). *Science* **173**, 843.
Stevens, J. G., and Cook, M. L. (1973). *Gustav Stern Symp. Perspect. Virol.* (in press).
Tyzzer, E. E. (1906). *Philipp. J. Sci.* **1**, 349.
Underwood, E. (1935). *Brit. J. Child. Dis.* **32**, 83.
von Bokay, J. (1909). *Wien. Klin. Wochenschr.* **22**, 1323.
Ward, J. R., and Bishop, B. (1970). *J. Amer. Med. Ass.* **212**, 1954.
Watson, D. H.. Russell, W. C., and Wildy, P. (1963). *Virology* **19**, 250.
Weinstein, L., and Meade, R. H. (1956). *AMA Arch. Intern. Med.* **98**, 91.
Weller, T. H. (1953). *Proc. Soc. Exp. Biol. Med.* **83**, 340.
Weller, T. H., and Witton, H. M. (1958). *J. Exp. Med.* **108**, 869.
Williams, B., and Capers, T. H. (1959). *Amer. J. Med.* **27**, 836.
Wright, E. T., and Winer, L. H. (1961). *Arch. Dermatol.* **84**, 242.
Young, R. C., Corder, M. P., Haynes, H. A., and DeVita, V. T. (1972). *Amer. J. Med.* **52**, 63.

Chapter 12

Cytomegaloviruses

Harry T. Wright, Jr.

I. Introduction

The cytomegaloviruses (CMV) are a group of species-specific agents capable of causing infection without symptoms or severe as well as fatal disease in man and in lower mammalian species. Infection with cytomegaloviruses, *in vivo* and *in vitro*, is characterized by distinctly enlarged cells (i.e., cytomegaly) containing intranuclear and cytoplasmic inclusions.

A. History

In 1904 Jesionek and Kiolemenoglou first described the presence of protozoonlike cells in the kidneys, lungs, and liver of a premature fetus, probably representing the first reported example of generalized cytomegalic inclusion disease (CMID). In the same year, Ribbert (1904) noted similar cells in the kidneys of a neonate and in the parotid glands of two older infants studied at postmortem. Goodpasture and Talbot (1921) described these cells in the kidneys, lungs, and liver of an infant dying with pneumonia at 6 weeks of age and believed that the giant cells were a result of chronic inflammation; they suggested the descriptive term "cytomegalia" to emphasize the size of the cells. Similar inclusions were observed by Tyzzer (1906) in biopsies of varicella skin lesions. Lipschütz (1921) recognized the similarity of the intranuclear inclusions to those seen in herpetic lesions and suggested this "inclusion body disease" was due to a virus. Von Glahn and Pappenheimer (1925) reported the first case of cytomegaly in an adult with ulcerative colitis and also noted the similarity of the inclusions to those seen in herpes simplex.

Cole and Kuttner (1926) inoculated infected salivary gland material from adult guinea pigs into young guinea pigs and subsequently saw typical inclusion-bearing cells develop.

Farber and Wolbach (1932) noted the characteristic cytomegalic inclusion-bearing cells in salivary glands in 12% of autopsy material from 183 infants and young children. Cappell and MacFarlane (1947) concluded that these infants demonstrated lesions as well as clinical signs and symptoms which were the result of dissemination of the human form of salivary gland virus. In 1950, Wyatt *et al.* emphasized the pantropic characteristics of disease with inclusion-bearing cells in many organs and suggested that the characteristic cells might be found in the urinary sediment in some cases and thus make possible the diagnosis during life. Fetterman (1952) reported two cases of salivary gland virus disease in whom the diagnosis was made antemortem by the discovery of the typical inclusion-bearing cells in the urinary sediment, thereby introducing exfoliative cytology as a diagnostic procedure. Smith (1954) succeeded in propagating the murine cytomegalovirus in explant cultures of embryonic mouse tissue. Finally, in 1956, the human salivary gland virus was successfully grown *in vitro* by Smith using tissue culture methods. Consequently, this virus was shown to be similar to two other human isolations from a liver biopsy by Weller and associates (1957) and from adenoidal tissue by Rowe *et al.* (1956). These agents could not be propagated in mouse tissue or produce disease in mice, indicating the high species specificity. Sever *et al.* (1963) and Hanshaw (1966a) have demonstrated that the complement-fixation test can be a useful tool in diagnostic and epidemiologic investigations. In 1964, Wright and associates examined human cytomegalovirus by high-resolution electron microscopy and characterized the morphology of the virus particles.

B. Physicochemical Properties

Early cytochemical procedures with infected cells indicated that the central core contained DNA, as demonstrated by acridine orange staining and also by the observation that virus replication was inhibited in the presence of 5-fluorodeoxyuridine (McAllister *et al.*, 1963; Goodheart *et al.*, 1963). The fluorescent antibody technique indicated the presence of viral antigen in the nuclear and cytoplasmic lesions, and infected cells stained with Sudan IV suggested that this was a lipid-containing virus, a fact confirmed by ether sensitivity and chloroform tests (McAllister *et al.*, 1963). Cytomegalovirus (CMV) is unstable at pH below 5; no hemagglutinin or hemadsorption activity has been demonstrated. Krugman and Goodheart (1964) have shown that this virus is heat-labile with a half-life of less than 1 hour at 37°C. It does not withstand storage at 5°C but is relatively stable at −60°C.

C. Methods of Diagnosis

1. Exfoliative Cytology

Inclusion-bearing cells may be detected in urine (Fig. 1), gastric washings, and cerebrospinal fluid, as well as in infected tissue such as liver, lung, or kidney. However, looking for infected cells in urine yields a high rate (up to 50%) of false negatives even in infants presenting with the classical manifestations of cytomegalic inclusion disease of infancy (Table I). The inclusion-bearing cells may be seen in unstained urine specimens but are better seen after staining with hematoxylin and eosin or Giemsa stain.

2. Virus Isolation

The best method of establishing CMV infection at any age is by the direct isolation of the virus. The agent may be propagated in a variety of human

TABLE I
SUMMARY OF USUAL CLINICAL MANIFESTATIONS AND LABORATORY RESULTS IN 26 INFANTS WITH CONGENITAL CMID[a]

Clinical Manifestations	Present	Not present	Not known
Sex (male/female)	15/11		
Low birth weight (< 2500 gm)	15	9	2
Jaundice	19	6	1
Microcephaly	11	14	1
Chorioretinitis	5	12	9
Petechiae	14	11	1
Hepatosplenomegaly	25	0	1
Laboratory results	**Present**	**Not present**	**Not known**
Anemia	9	12	5
Hyperbilirubinemia	15	4	6
Thrombocytopenia	11	10	5
Cerebral calcifications (skull X ray)	8	16	2
Urine—inclusion-bearing cells	7	13	6
Virus isolation			
Throat	10	4	12
Urine	25	0	1

[a]From H. T. Wright, Jr. (unpublished data).

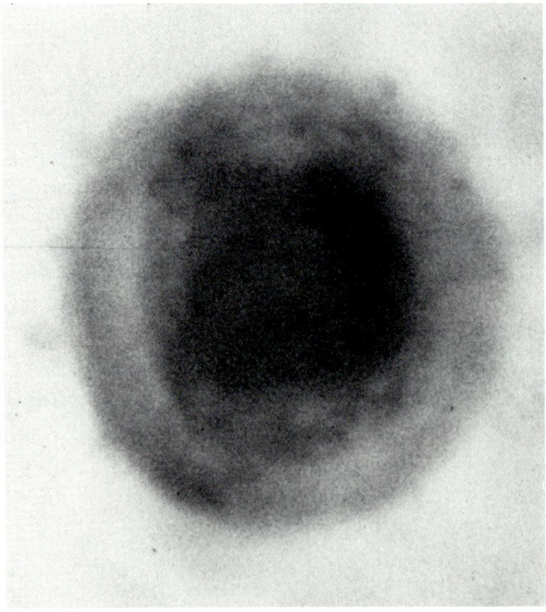

FIG. 1. Small epithelial cell from urine sediment with a diagnostic intranuclear inclusion body. Prepared from millipore filter stained by a modified Papanicolaou method.

embryonic fibroblastic cultures. Diploid cells derived from human embryonic lung (WI-38) are most frequently used as a tissue culture system. Virus cytopathic effect (CPE) may appear within 24 hours or may be delayed for as long as 6 weeks. The latter circumstance usually reflects a lower virus titer in the patient, but may also be due to a variety of technical factors related to the instability of the virus and the sensitivity of the tissue culture system.

For isolation purposes, urine specimens and throat swabbings are consistently the best source of CMV although leukocytes may harbor the virus. Virus has been isolated from patients as early as 1 day of age and some patients have continuously excreted virus up to 54 months of age (McAllister, 1966).

Specimens are collected and transported immediately to the laboratory for processing and inoculation into tissue cultures. If a delay in the transportation of specimens is anticipated, survival of the virus depends upon keeping the specimen cool but not frozen. Appropriately handled specimens have yielded live virus after 10 hours in transit and after 7 weeks if kept at refrigerator temperature. In the laboratory, specimens are treated with antibiotics and inoculated into tissue culture. Frequently, a cytopathic effect can be observed in tissue culture within 24 hours; however, characteristic intranuclear and intracytoplasmic inclusions cannot be demonstrated, by cytochemical methods, until about 48 hours after cytopathic effect first occurs.

The isolation of cytomegalovirus from the throat or urine establishes infection but does not establish the presence of disease due to this agent. This is especially true in isolations made after infancy.

3. Serologic Tests

Serum neutralization tests, complement-fixation tests, and indirect fluorescent antibody tests can be used to measure CMV antibody.

The serum neutralization test measures both IgG and IgM antibody. The 19 S antibody produced by the fetus is not distinguished from the 7 S antibody passively transferred from the mother (Hanshaw, 1969). Theoretically, pretreatment of the serum with 2-mercaptoethanol (ME) might be used to separate the two types of antibodies; however, at times it is difficult to obtain a significant reduction in ME-sensitive 19 S antibody. Except in special laboratories, the use of the neutralization test is unsuitable for the confirmation of the diagnosis of a suspected case.

It would appear that the complement-fixation (CF) test (Hanshaw, 1969) detects specific antibody against most strains of CMV using a single antigen. In this country, antigen made from AD 169 strain has been particularly useful; however, antigen made from other strains has been used. The CF test may be used in following antibody levels in infants suspected of having congenital infection. The persistence of CF antibody beyond 6 months of age suggests that a CMV infection occurred during intrauterine life or in early infancy. Passively acquired antibody with a half-life of approximately 3–4 weeks should show a progressive decline during the early months of life unless the infant is actively responding to CMV infection.

The indirect fluorescent antibody test for CMV is particularly useful in the serology of congenital infections, since the detection of specific CMV IgM antibody in cord serum is evidence of an active immune response by the fetus to CMV infection (Hanshaw *et al.*, 1968). Hanshaw (1969) has suggested that the detection of IgM antibody by immunofluorescence is the most valuable serologic test in the diagnosis of suspected congenital cytomegalic inclusion disease. With increasing age, production of IgG antibody may be enhanced while IgM antibody declines. Therefore, one cannot interpret the absence of CMV IgM antibody in the second year of life as negative evidence of congenital cytomegalic inclusion disease or even as evidence of inactive infection. Conversely, the diagnosis is improbable in the symptomatic infant under 1 year of age without detectable IgM in the serum. Although one usually thinks of IgM antibody as a transient, short-lived, and early response to infection, it is apparent that this is not the case in congenital CMV infection. Infected newborns usually continue to produce specific IgM antibody for weeks and months after birth (Hanshaw, 1969).

4. Assay by Counting Infected Cells

Goodheart and Jaross (1963) described an assay method for human cytomegalovirus based on counts of infected cells. Counts made 48 hours after infecting cell cultures, when preparations are fixed and stained, include all initially infected cells and are linearly proportional to the inoculum dilution.

5. Postmortem Specimens

Cytomegalic inclusion disease will continue to be diagnosed by pathologists, as the pathognomonic inclusions are noted in postmortem specimens.

6. Reference Antiserums

Early attempts to produce acceptable antibodies by immunization of various subhuman species failed. Investigations were restricted to studies of serum obtained from patients, their parents, or other humans (McAllister, 1966; Hanshaw, 1966b). More recently, albino rabbits have been immunized to produce specific neutralizing antibodies against human CMV (Martos *et al.*, 1970).

II. Disease States Associated with CMV (Essential Clinical Features)

A. Cytomegalic Inclusion Disease of Infancy

1. Classical

The effects of congenital infection with CMV have ranged from generalized damage to principal or multiple organs causing disease that is incompatible with life to an asymptomatic infection manifested by viruria. Infants infected with cytomegalovirus may be asymptomatic during the neonatal period and may be discovered to have extensive abnormalities, such as neurological findings, later in life. Although it may be difficult or impossible to determine if an infection detected later in the first year of life is congenital or acquired, characteristic signs and symptoms occurring in the first week of life in an infant, who is subsequently shown to be infected with CMV, are most likely due to congenital disease.

The important clinical features of CMID in the neonatal period as reported by a number of observers comprise a symptom complex which may include (1) jaundice; (2) petechiae; (3) chorioretinitis; (4) microcephaly (Fig. 2); (5) central nervous system disease, i.e., seizures, spastic diplegia, deafness, and microphthalmia; (6) pneumonia; (7) hepatosplenomegaly: (8) psychomotor retardation; (9) mental retardation; (10) diarrhea;

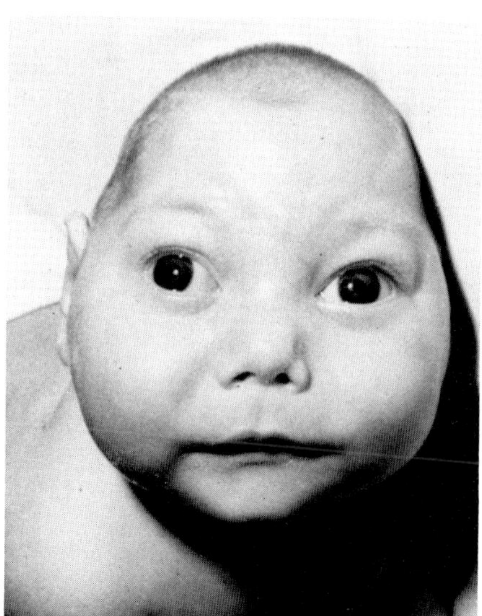

FIG. 2. A $7\frac{1}{2}$-month-old male infant with CMID of infancy showing remarkable microcephaly. (From Wright, 1971b).

(11) thrombocytopenia; (12) cerebral calcifications; (13) chronic gastroenteritis; and (14) prematurity (Mercer *et al.*, 1953; Nelson and Wyatt, 1959; Smith, 1959; Weller and Hanshaw, 1962; Medearis, 1964a; Emanual and Kenny, 1966; McAllister, 1966; Hanshaw, 1968; Osborn, 1970; Wright, 1971). Some of the symptoms attributable to congenital CMV infection suggest alteration in normal processes of morphogenesis and organogenesis (Sever and White, 1968).

The laboratory findings of anemia, thrombocytopenia, inclusion-bearing cells in the urine, and the presence of virus in throat swabbings and urine are also characteristic findings in these patients with congenital infection. The more common clinical manifestations and laboratory findings in one study are correlated in Table I.

2. Expanded Syndrome

Several years ago, Weller and Hanshaw (1962) suggested that nonfatal cases of CMID may have broad social significance, like rubella and toxoplasmosis, and they believed that it was important to accurately define clinical variants and sequellae of this disease. Since then, CMV has been considered by some to be equal to rubella virus as a potential fetal threat. It has been suggested that, since the hazard of CMV is largely in the risk to the fetus, expectant mothers should avoid contact with infants suspected of having CMID.

In a longitudinal study of 20 patients with CMID, McCracken and associates (1969) observed that patients with severe and prolonged illness due to CMV had growth retardation when compared with control patients. Several patients in this study had abnormal findings relative to the heart, although congenital heart disease has not been established as a part of this syndrome. Over one-third of the infants in this study had structural abnormalities of the derivatives of the first embryonic arch; these abnormalities included high arched palate, micrognathia, left facial weakness, cleft of the soft and hard palates, and deafness.

Radiographic changes in the long bone structure, similar to those seen in congenital rubella, have also been observed (Mercer *et al.*, 1953; Graham *et al.*, 1970).

In the classical article on developmental abnormalities associated with congenital CMV infection, Hanshaw (1970) has emphasized the possible teratogenic potential of CMV by summarizing all reported anomalies which have been observed in patients who were also infected with this virus. Unusual central nervous system abnormalities such as microcephaly, encephalomalacia, parietal lobe cyst, cerebellar aplasia, and dolichocephaly have been observed as well as unusual ocular abnormalities such as microphthalmia, cataracts, blindness, and malformation of the interior eye chamber. Certain extraneural abnormalities include the cardiovascular anomalies of atrial septal defect and anomalous venous return, gastrointestinal anomalies such as esophageal atresia and malformed pylorus, genitourinary anomalies such as hypospadias, pulmonary anomalies such as thymic hypoplasia, and musculoskeletal anomalies such as clubfeet and spastic diplegia. Other organs and systems were similarly involved.

Recently, Wright (1971) reported on the long-term follow-up of 15 patients with CMID of infancy and described an "expanded syndrome" (Table II). Some of these patients were followed from birth to 11 years of age (Fig. 3). Observations of these patients follow.

Most patients with abnormal electroencephalograms had nonspecific findings; however, three had specific findings: one patient had an EEG compatible with a paroxysmal disorder, another had an EEG characteristic of hypsarrhythmia, and another patient had a petit mal variant seizure disorder clinically manifested by staring spells.

Eye abnormalities included strabismus deformity, as well as bilateral optic atrophy with chorioretinal scars; one patient had microphthalmia and cataract in the left eye and anisocoria and posterior polar cataract in the right eye.

Examination of the dermatoglyphics in these patients indicated that they have (1) a higher frequency of complex pattern on the fourth and fifth fingers, (2) a high frequency of transitional transverse flexion creases, (3) transversely oriented palmar lines, (4) a high frequency of complex hypothenar patterns, (5) a high frequency of patterns in interdigital areas III and IV, and (6) a high

TABLE II
SUMMARY OF UNUSUAL CLINICAL MANIFESTATIONS IN LONG-TERM FOLLOW-UP OF 20 INFANTS WITH CONGENITAL CYTOMEGALIC INCLUSION DISEASE (14 MALES, 6 FEMALES)[a]

Abnormalities	Present	Not present	Not known
Eye defects	9	11	0
Hearing loss	4	13	3
Severe developmental retardation	9	11	0
Abnormal EEG	11	9	0
Congenital heart disease	2	18	0
Unusual dermatoglyphics	15	0	5
Retarded bone age	4	16	0
Hypoplastic lumbar spine	4	13	3
Unusual urine chromotography	8	9	3
Inguinal hernia	2	18	0

[a]From H. T. Wright, Jr. (1971 and unpublished data).

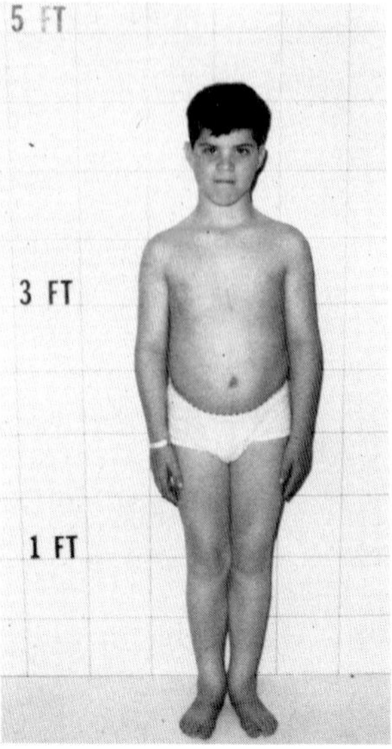

FIG. 3. A 10-year-old twin boy who had CMID disease of infancy manifested by jaundice, hepatosplenomegaly, and cytomegaloviruria. Abnormalities presently observed include congenital heart disease, scoliosis, defective visual acuity, abnormal electroencephalogram, and unusual dermatoglyphics. He functions well with a developmental quotient over 100 (the standard).

frequency of complex hallucal patterns on the soles (Wright *et al.*, 1972).

Defective hearing was manifest in four patients by partial or total deafness in one or both ears.

A retarded bone age was reported in four patients; the eldest was 8 years of age and his bone age was 6 years of age. The four patients with most severe developmental retardation had developmental quotients of 10, 11 and 20; the fourth patient had a developmental quotient so low it was unmeasurable.

Radiographs of the lumbar spine revealed two patients with scoliosis of the thoracolumbar spine, one of whom also had failure of fusion of neural arches L_3, L_4, and L_5. Another patient had hypoplasia of the left pedicles of L_1, L_2, L_3, and L_4 with some widening of the intrapedicular distances.

Two patients had congenital heart disease. One patient with pulmonary and mitral stenosis had successful surgical repair, and another patient had a murmur and abnormal EKG without a definite diagnosis.

Eight patients had unusual urine chromatography. Four patients had an increase in the normal range of the ten common amino acids, and three patients had unusual values of the phenolic acid metabolites. It is possible that these findings represent renal damage caused by the virus.

Prolonged follow-up observations of surviving infants with CMID have led to the recognition of an expanded syndrome. Certain abnormalities observed cannot be definitely attributed to the human cytomegalovirus; however, many of these anomalies have been seen in patients with other transplacental infections.

B. Syndromes Induced in Patients with Immunosuppressive States

1. Renal Homotransplant Recipients

> The transplant recipient has joined the growing legion of patients whose therapist treads a thin, barely observable line: too little therapy, and the patient succumbs to his biologic abnormality; and too much, and a new constellation of unrelated but equally ominous pathologic processes arises. To find and stay on the narrow middle road requires alert individualization of dose and a considerable delicacy of response to changes in the patient's condition. (Hill *et al.*, 1964).

Hill and associates (1964) reported that pulmonary infections were present terminally in 26 of 32 patients who died after receiving an organ transplant; many were infected with CMV. Hedley-Whyte and Craighead (1965) first recovered CMV from the lung tissue of a patient dying with pneumonia 36 days after renal homotransplantation. These authors found typical cytomegalic inclusions in the macrophages of five of 19 other patients dying after renal homotransplantation and suggested that the infection may be a complication of immunosuppressive therapy. Kanich and Craighead (1966) confirmed this association at autopsy by finding CMV in 32% of the renal homotransplant recipients who had been given drugs to suppress immunologic rejection of the graft. Craighead and associates (1967), by virologic and serologic studies, established CMV infection in 30 of 41 renal allograft recipients who survived one or more months after transplantation. Since some of these patients had demonstrable antibody at the time of surgery and some did not, they suggested that active CMV infection in renal homograft recipients can result either from the activation of "latent" virus or from exposure to the virus after transplantation. A similar study was performed in Denmark by Andersen and Spencer (1969) on the incidence and clinical significance of cytomegalovirus infection among renal allograft recipients. Evidence of infection was found in 33 of 36 (91%) patients occurring primarily during the first 2 months after transplantation. Although most infections were clinically inapparent, in four patients a febrile illness associated with relative lymphocytosis was seen, and in seven of 17 patients who came to postmortem CMV pneumonia was discovered; three of these patients had overwhelming bacterial pneumonia as well.

Balakrishnan and associates (1969) observed CMV mononucleosis in a patient after renal transplantation. The virus was isolated from the patient's blood on two occasions, 1 month apart. During the period of atypical lymphocytosis, a high CF antibody titer developed, and CMV appeared in the urine and saliva. These authors suggested that the source of the infecting CMV could be (1) the transplanted kidney, (2) transfused blood, or (3) an exacerbation of a latent infection. Other investigators in this country and abroad have observed CMV infection in patients following renal transplantation and have made speculations as to the clinical significance of this finding (Rifkind *et al.*, 1967; Armstrong *et al.*, 1971a; Nakao *et al.*, 1971).

In 1970, Fine and associates reported the isolation of CMV from specimens from 8 of 21 (38%) pediatric renal allograft recipients. This agent was associated with clinical symptomatology in 4 of the 8 patients; 3 had fever and 1 had anicteric hepatitis. In addition to fever, 1 patient had pneumonitis. All 8 patients had multiple positive urine cultures for up to 14 months.

2. Leukemia, Lymphoma, and Other Malignancies

In 1961, Hanshaw and Weller tested 50 children with leukemia, lymphoma, or Hodgkin's disease to explore the role of latent viruses as possible causes of complicating infections in the terminal stages of illness due to neoplastic disease. Cytomegalovirus was isolated two or more times from the urine of three patients with leukemia and from one with Hodgkin's disease. One of these patients had recurring respiratory symptoms and at postmortem CMV was identified in the lungs. In 1962, Gottmann and Beatty reported on 4 children in whom CMID was the terminal complication of leukemia and lymphosarcoma. In 1966, Cangir and Sullivan recognized a syndrome caused by CMV in 3 children who had received chemotherapy with agents known to have immunosuppressive properties. Cytomegalic inclusion disease presented in these children with acute leukemia as persistent fever, cough and rales, vomiting and diarrhea, and hepatosplenomegaly. Pancytopenia was present, and roentgenographic evidence of pneumonia appeared 3 weeks after the onset of symptoms. Abnormal liver function studies were late findings.

Duvall and associates (1966) recovered CMV from 11 of 32 adult patients with neoplastic disease, but from none of 17 control patients. In most instances, CMV infection did not seem to be solely responsible for causing clinical disease.

Rinker and McGraw (1967) reported the occurrence of disseminated CMID in patients with leukemia presenting as viral pneumonitis prior to death. Dyment and associates (1968) found cytomegaloviruria in 2% of children with acute leukemia tested for human cytomegalovirus, whereas none of the control patients yielded cytomegalovirus. Review of autopsy material in this same study revealed 3% of leukemic children with disseminated cytomegalic inclusions. These studies demonstrate the infrequent occurrence of CMV infection in children with leukemia in the population studied. A study from the Houston area suggested similar data (Benyesh-Melnick *et al.*, 1964). However, Bodey and his colleagues (1965) suggested that patients suffering from leukemia, lymphoma, and other malignancies or diseases treated with high doses of steroids exhibit increased susceptibility to CMV infection. In another report from Houston, Sullivan and associates (1968) performed longitudinal complement-fixation antibody titer determinations on 16 leukemic children and demonstrated nine seroconversions, with the median time for seroconversion being 2 months. A more recent study from the Memorial Hospital for Cancer and Allied Diseases and Sloan-Kettering Institute in New York suggests the incidence of infection with CMV did not differ from that found in other studies in non-leukemic and leukemic children (Armstrong *et al.*, 1971b). However, infection was asymptomatic without clinical manifestions of disease.

3. Combined Infections

When Hanshaw and Weller (1961) were exploring the role of latent viruses as possible causes of complicating infections in the terminal phases of illness due to neoplastic disease, one leukemic patient over a period of several weeks concurrently excreted two viruses in the urine: an adenovirus and a cytomegalovirus. The significance of this dual infection was obscure. When Hill and associates (1964) recognized pneumonitis in patients receiving immunosuppressive therapy for organ transplantation, multiple infections were common and consisted of a combination of such organisms as *Candida*, *Aspergillus*, *Nocardia*, *Pneumocystis carinii*, *Mycobacterium tuberculosis*, *Pseudomonas aeruginosa*, as well as other bacteria, and most frequently CMV. Buttrick and Roberts (1965) observed two infants with generalized CMID who had secondary fungal infections, one with aspergillosis and another with candidiasis.

Vietzke and associates (1968) have reported on a series of patients with simultaneous infections by the obligate intracellular parasite, *Toxoplasma gondii*, and CMV occurring with unexpected frequency in patients with disseminated neoplastic disease.

Wong and Warner (1962) describe 41 adults with CMID. Many of these patients not only had malignancies or Hodgkin's disease but also had other infections, such as *Pneumocystis*, *Toxoplasma*, herpes simplex, syphilis, and pneumonia.

C. *Infections and Syndromes Induced in Patients with Intact Immune Mechanisms*

1. Pregnancy

Mothers of infected neonates do not remember a particularly characteristic illness during their confinement, and prospective studies of large groups of pregnant women support the fact that CMV infection in healthy adults is usually asymptomatic. Mothers with asymptomatic disease but serologic evidence of infection with CMV may deliver infected infants; the clinical manifestations of congenital cytomegalovirus infection appear to be primarily a reflection of the duration of infection *in utero* (Monif *et al.*, 1972). About 3% of pregnant women infected with CMV may give birth to infants demonstrating no clinical involvement (Feldman 1969). On the other hand, infants may be born with no symptoms but may develop symptoms during the first 8 months of life (Starr *et al.*, 1970).

Primary maternal infection with CMV has occurred during the second trimester of pregnancy, with infection of the placenta but no fetal infection, resulting in a healthy baby from whom CMV was not isolated during the first year of life (Hayes and Gibas, 1971). In one study, human CMV has been isolated from the cervix more frequently than from the urine in pregnant women, the virus was recovered more often in the third trimester than in the second or first, and the virus was recovered more often from younger and primiparous women than from those who were older than 25 years and those who had had more than three pregnancies (Montgomery *et al.*, 1972). Since more women would be expected to have antibody as they become older, this latter observation might be anticipated. The outcome of pregnancy was not affected by this cervical infection, and it is speculated that the CMV infection of the cervix in pregnancy represents activation of latent infection by hormonally induced local changes—changes to which older, multiparous women are resistant.

2. Hepatitis, Gastrointestinal Tract

In 1965, Hanshaw and colleagues associated a spectrum of liver abnormalities in 28 of 29 children with acquired CMV infection. Hepatomegaly and abnormal liver function tests occurred in these children who were asymptomatic excreters of CMV, and this raised the important question of a possible etiologic role of CMV in idiopathic liver disease.

Toghill and others (1967) described two patients with hepatitis associated with high fever, atypical mononuclear cells in the blood, negative heterophil reaction, and episodes of hemolysis. In each case evidence of CMV infection was obtained and was considered the cause of the hepatitis.

Levine *et al.* (1964) reported four cases of nonfatal CMID of the intestinal tract of adults. The lesions were located in ulcerations associated with afferent loop obstruction, idiopathic steatorrhea, and ulcerative colitis.

3. Cytomegalovirus-Mononucleosis

Between 1965 and 1967 Klemola and Kääriäinen (1965; Klemola *et al.*, 1967; Kääriäinen *et al.*, 1966a,b) wrote several papers describing a syndrome resembling infectious mononucleosis caused by CMV. The disease was characterized by sustained fever, atypical circulating mononuclear cells, and frequent hepatic involvement; however, there was no pharyngitis or lymphadenopathy, and the heterophil test was negative. The disorder occurred in healthy persons as well as in patients receiving large quantities of fresh or relatively fresh whole blood.

Rifkind (1968) modified the characteristics of this syndrome to include fever, myalgia, headache, and frequent cough as well as a transient rubellaform rash appearing on the trunk and the extremities with associated findings of bilateral bronchopneumonia, myocarditis, pericarditis, and cholestatic hepatitis.

Unexplained rise of cold agglutinins seems to be a common feature of CMV-mononucleosis, and involvement of the liver with jaundice as a presenting sign also occurs (Lamb and Stern, 1966). Japanese investigators have observed a disease in young children characterized by fever, lymphadenopathy, and hepatosplenomegaly from whom CMV was isolated from the urine and saliva (Nakao *et al.*, 1967).

The term "cytomegalovirus-mononucleosis," used to describe this syndrome, suggests the close similarity to the more common infectious mononucleosis. Human CMV has been identified as a herpesvirus as has the Epstein-Barr (EB) virus, originally isolated from the EB cell line of Burkitt's African lymphoma but now causally implicated in classical heterophil-positive infectious mononucleosis (Henle *et al.*, 1968). In the case of both of these agents it appears that long-sustained infections of circulating leukocytes is a prominent pathologic mechanism.

Kapsenberg and associates (1970) have observed a patient with post-transfusion CMV-mononucleosis who developed heterophil, EB virus, and CMV antibodies and from whom CMV was isolated from the urine, representing a simultaneous infection with cytomegalovirus and EB virus.

4. Postperfusion Syndrome

Henson (1967) has reported a case of generalized CMID in a debilitated adult who died after receiving multiple blood transfusions for trauma, suggesting that CMV could be acquired from transfused blood or that multiple transfusions could activate a latent cytomegalovirus infection. Other investigators have observed CMV infections in patients following blood transfusions (Stevens *et al.*, 1970; Prince *et al.*, 1971; Diosi *et al.*, 1969). Human CMV has been recovered from the peripheral blood which would support such an association (Harnden *et al.*, 1967).

The postperfusion syndrome consists of fever, splenomegaly, and atypical lymphocytes in the peripheral blood appearing after cardiopulmonary bypass and occasionally after other operative procedures in which large quantities of blood are transfused; these signs develop 3–6 weeks after use of extracorporeal circulation for open heart surgery (Embil *et al.*, 1968; Reyman, 1966; Riemenschneider and Moss, 1966; Lang *et al.*, 1968; Lang and Hanshaw, 1969; Paloheimo *et al.*, 1968; Foster and Jack, 1969; Kantor and Johnson, 1970). With mild disease, the course is self-limited with a duration of approximately 3 weeks. However, this syndrome must be differentiated from more serious complications of open heart surgery such as bacterial endocarditis, hepatitis, postpericardiotomy syndrome, and the hemolytic-uremic syndrome.

Lang and associates (1968) confirmed an association between the postperfusion syndrome and CMV by observing patients with this syndrome who yielded virus from their urine and leukocytes and who demonstrated a rise in CMV-CF antibodies in serum.

Disseminated CMID has been observed in a burned adult who received 72 units of blood (Nash *et al.*, 1970).

Kahn and colleagues (1967) have observed a group of patients with prolonged fever, tachycardia, and mucosal lesions of the mouth occurring within a few days after a cardiac operation. These patients subsequently acquired recurrent fever, chest pain, pericardial and pleural friction rubs, and hepatosplenomegaly; however, the course was benign and symptoms slowly disappeared. Specimens taken from the mucosal lesions, pharynx, and blood yielded parainfluenza virus strain 3. This study would suggest that other viruses might be associated with a postperfusion and/or an infectious mononucleosis-like syndrome.

D. Miscellaneous Reports

Observers have associated CMV with a number of clinical manifestations. Feldman and Schwartz (1968) have reported isolating CMV from 3 of 6 patients with infantile spasms tested under 1 year of age; two of 28 controls also yielded virus. Frank *et al.* (1966) have reported a case of fetal ascites thought to be secondary to generalized CMV infection; virus was recovered from the mother's urine and from throat swabbings from the infant. Coombs (1968) reported a case of CMID associated with an acquired autoimmune hemolytic anemia in an adult. Stern (1968) has associated certain respiratory illnesses such as bronchitis and pneumonitis with CMV infection. Lang (1966) observed 11 of 14 males with CMID to have inguinal hernias. Brough and co-workers (1967) observed an hemorrhagic purpuric skin eruption made up of islands of dermal erythropoesis in neonatal infants and related this to CMV or rubella in 5 of 6 infants. Hanshaw (1966a) demonstrated CMV antibody in the serum of 44% of 41 infants and children with head circumferences 2 standard deviations below the mean. Jacox and co-workers (1964) repeatedly isolated CMV from the urine and sputum of an adult male who had hypogammaglobulinemia 2 years after surgical removal of a large thymoma. Thorell and Nathorst-Windahl (1965) observed an infant with generalized CMID in association with an omphalocele. Hagmann and associates (1969) reported a case of congenital aganglionic megacolon with histological findings compatible with CMID; human CMV was isolated from the urine, and CMV-CF antibody was present in serum. Characteristic cytomegalic inclusions have been demonstrated by light microscopy in the epithelial lining cells of the cochlear duct and semicircular canals of an infant dying with pneumococcal meningitis (Davis, 1969).

An infant is described with clinical and biochemical evidence of hypoparathyroidism, which is possibly a residual of severe generalized CMID (Curtis *et al.*, 1962). A newborn infant was observed with a cystic horseshoe kidney and congenital CMV infection, possibly related (Plotkin and Pasquariello, 1969).

As noted above, a number of abnormalities and diseases have been associated with the presence of CMV; whether they are causally or coincidentally related is unresolved in most cases.

III. CMV in Animals

In attempts to gain information about "inclusion body disease" seen in humans, an experimental model was sought. Cole and Kuttner (1926) were able to cause inclusion body formation in young guinea pigs injected with infected salivary gland material obtained from older animals. The inoculum remained infective after passage through a Berkefeld N filter but was not infective after heating. In the years that followed other observers saw inclusion-bearing cells in mice, hamsters, moles, dogs, monkeys, and chimpanzees. Inclusion-bearing cells were associated with a transmissable, filterable virus, but in each instance the virus proved to be entirely species-specific.

Congenital defects similar to those observed in the infant have not been demonstrated in experimental animals (Hanshaw, 1968).

A. Mice

In deciding upon a model for subsequent attempts to isolate the human virus, Smith (1954) undertook the propagation of the murine salivary gland virus in explant cultures of mouse embryonic tissue. Intranuclear inclusions were present in histologic sections of the salivary glands of each mouse. The virus was maintained by serial passages at intervals of 2–3 weeks in young adult mice from a special colony known to be free of salivary gland virus infection. Many focal cytopathic lesions composed of large rounded refractile cells appeared in the cultures about 1 week after initial inoculation. By the ninth to the twelfth day cytopathology in the culture was diffuse, and infected cells began to degenerate within 2–3 days after the focal lesion appeared. After three serial passages of the virus in culture, salivary gland virus disease characterized by large intranuclear inclusions was produced in mice by intraperitoneal inoculation of culture fluids.

In sublethal doses, murine CMV can produce a focal acute hepatitis without residual cirrhosis or permanent liver damage (Henson *et al.*, 1966). On the other hand, lethal doses result in cell necrosis and spreading foci of infection (McCordock and Smith, 1936). Henson and associates (1966) have shown that when virus is injected intraperitoneally it enters the liver via the portal veins causing infection. Irradiation does not interfere with virus-induced interferon production in mice but does abolish the Kupffer and inflammatory cell response that would ordinarily occur. Subsequently, there occurs expanding foci of necrosis, many inclusions, and tissue death.

B. Guinea Pigs

The guinea pig salivary gland virus has been propagated in homologous tissue cultures by Hartley *et al.* (1957). Virus that had passed through tissue cultures produced characteristic findings in guinea pigs from an uninfected colony. After intracerebral inoculation, meningitis with intranuclear inclusions in cells was observed.

C. Monkeys

Cytomegaloviruses are widely distributed in Old World monkeys. Smith *et al.* (1969) recently demonstrated that CMV was present in almost half of the Cercopithecus monkey kidney cell cultures tested, each of which had been derived from a single animal; each isolate could be propagated in human fibroblastic cell lines when subcultured.

D. Horses

An equine virus isolated from spontaneously degenerating cultures of horse kidney cells after prolonged cultivation has morphological, physicochemical, and biological properties suggesting that it is a CMV of the equine herpesvirus group (Hsiung *et al.*, 1969).

E. Comparison of the Viruses of Man and Animals in Tissue Cultures

1. Cytopathic Changes

Enlarged, rounded, refractile cells occur in cell cultures infected with CMV of man and animals. In early passages of the mouse virus, the focal lesions are numerous and progress rapidly to involve the entire culture in 2 or 3 days; whereas in cases of the human virus, sometimes days or weeks may be required for generalized involvement of the cultures, although this is not the rule (Smith, 1959).

2. Adaptation of Viruses to Tissue Culture

Adaptation of the viruses to *in vitro* growth is manifested by (1) earlier appearance of cytopathic effect, (2) more extensive cytopathic effect, and (3) more virus in supernatant fluids in subsequent, serial passages of virus in tissue culture. The mouse virus adapts very quickly, whereas slower adaptation may occur with the human and guinea pig viruses (Smith, 1959). Specific CF antigen is present in both supernatant fluids and cell extracts of adapted cultures of all tissue culture-adapted viruses.

3. Range of Pathogenicity or Cytopathic Effect

All viruses induce cytopathic effects in embryonic fibroblasts of the homologous species; however, no effect is produced in cultures of heterologous tissue by any of the viruses, except for the exception of monkey viruses in human cells (Smith *et al.*, 1969). This affinity for fibroblastic cells *in vitro* is in contrast to the frequently observed involvement of epithelial tissue *in vivo*.

It has been shown that when beef embryonic fibroblasts are exposed to human CMV no destructive changes occur; however, the virus can be recovered weeks later on transfer of the "infected" beef cells to cultures of human embryonic fibroblasts (Weller, 1971).

There is a remarkable similarity between the subclinical infections in man and animals (Smith, 1959).

4. Physical Characteristic

The CMV's of man and animals are similar in certain physical properties such as sensitivity to ether, inactivation by heating, sensitivity to freezing and thawing, and marked inactivation at pH of 4. However, they appear to be immunologically distinct.

IV. Pathogenesis and Pathology

A. In Tissue Culture

1. Susceptibility to Infection

Infection of human embryonic fibroblasts *in vitro* with a human strain of CMV produces characteristic cytopathic changes and eventual cell death. The first change consists of the appearance of large, round, refractile cells that contrast sharply with the uninfected fusiform fibroblasts. Focal lesions consisting of a number of these cells appear in infected cultures after 5–24 days and occasionally may be seen in spontaneously degenerating cultures of human adenoid tissue after 22–120 days in culture. The lesions gradually increase in size and number and eventually involve the entire cell sheet. The terminal event as demonstrated by phase contrast, time-lapse cinematography for a single infected cell is a dramatic cellular explosion with the cessation of all cellular activity (Wright *et al.*, 1968).

McAllister and associates (1963) have made cytochemical observations of intracellular lesion development in cultured cells infected with human CMV and have correlated these studies with viral synthesis and release from cells (Table III). These studies resulted in a growth curve which indicated that no virus was detected in either the cells or in the supernatant medium for the first 48 hours; however, mature virus accumulated in the cells and was detected in the medium after 72 hours.

Included in these studies were microscopic examinations of infected cells stained by various techniques and at various times following infection. A cytoplasmic lesion appeared next to the nucleus 24 hours after infection. Small intranuclear bodies appeared that contained viral DNA and viral antigen 48 hours after infection; the cytoplasmic lesion also contained viral antigen at this time. The cytoplasmic lesions contained DNA (Fig. 4) 72 hours after infection. The DNA of the cytoplasmic and nuclear lesions was resistant to DNase unless pretreated with pepsin which suggests that the DNA of the intracellular lesion is viral DNA surrounded by protein (McAllister *et al.*, 1963). Goodheart and associates (1964) performed autoradiographic studies of CMV-infected cells. Infected cell cultures were exposed

TABLE III

CORRELATION OF VIRAL SYNTHESIS AND RELEASE WITH MORPHOLOGICAL AND CYTOCHEMICAL CHANGES[a]

Basis of study	Hours after infection			
	24	48	72	>72
Virus	None detectable	None detectable	Intra- and extracellular infective virus	Same as 72 hours
Electron microscopy	No particles detected	Particles in nucleus	Same as 48 hours	Particles in nucleus and cytoplasm
Cytochemistry				
Cytoplasmic lesion	RNA halo, PAS +, lipid +	RNA, viral antigen, PAS +, lipid +	DNA, viral antigen, PAS +, lipid +	Same as 72 hours
Nuclear lesion	None detectable	DNA, viral antigen	Same as 48 hours	Same as 48 hours
Cell measurements	Nucleus smaller than uninfected nucleus	Not done	Nucleus larger than uninfected nucleus	Not done

[a]From McAllister *et al*. (1963).

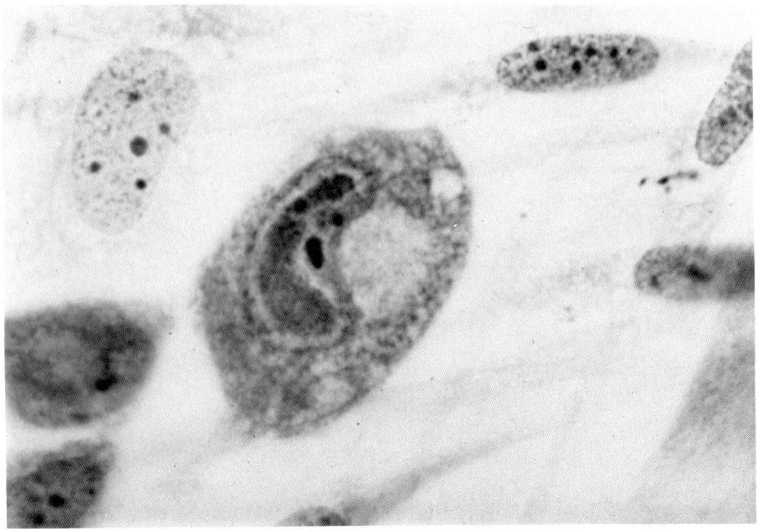

FIG. 4. Tissue culture of human embryo fibroblasts showing a cell infected with human CMV and demonstrating the intranuclear and intracytoplasmic lesions. × 1000. (From McAllister *et al.*, 1964).

to [H^3]thymidine and yielded information about the synthesis and migration of DNA found in the intranuclear and intracytoplasmic inclusions. The DNA of the intranuclear inclusion, presumably viral DNA, begins forming about 24 hours after infection and continues for at least 96 hours after infection. This DNA migrates to the intracytoplasmic inclusions by 72 hours after infection and is the only source of DNA found in the intracytoplasmic inclusion. These data suggest that virus particles are synthesized in the nucleus, migrate to the cytoplasm and are released into the medium (Goodheart *et al.*, 1964).

It is peculiar in the light of the extensive involvement of epithelial cells commonly observed *in vivo* that human fetal fibroblasts or myometrial cells are the only cultures which have proved suitable for cultivation of human CMV *in vitro*.

Interaction between CMV and *Pneumocystis carinii* has not been studied *in vitro*, since attempts to cultivate *Pneumocystis* have been unsuccessful.

2. Cellular Transformation

As recorded elsewhere in this book, certain members of the herpes group of viruses, such as EB virus and herpes simplex type 2, have been associated with cancer. At the moment there is no information indicating that the long-term persistence of CMV in the human host is similarly associated. Lang and Montagnier (1970) grew CMV-infected cells for several generations in agarose, and although transformation occurred in the form of altered clones of human fibroblasts, these eventually underwent lysis.

3. Morphology

The morphology of an infected cell, stained with May-Grünwald-Giemsa shows rounding of the cell, the intranuclear inclusion surrounded by a halo, and the juxtanuclear inclusion body in the cytoplasm (Fig. 4). The nuclear lesion is matured within 72 hours into a large patch of DNA occupying the center of a large nucleus and separated from the nuclear membrane by an unstained halo; the cytoplasmic lesion displays a prominent amount of DNA at this time (McAllister *et al.*, 1963). The morphology of mouse embryo cell cultures infected with murine CMV demonstrates similar lesions (Fig. 5).

B. In the Host

1. Transplacental Infection

The pathogenesis of congenital disease caused by human CMV is obscure; however, it is obvious that the virus must pass from the mother to the fetus because infants may be born with signs of generalized disease (Smith, 1959; Hanshaw, 1968; Wright, 1971). Transplacental infection probably occurs only when the mother is undergoing a primary infection, since it has been shown that usually the subsequent sibling of an infected infant does not excrete virus even though the mother may continue to excrete virus during the second pregnancy (Osborn, 1970). Whether the transplacental infection is caused by viremia and direct invasion of placenta and fetus, or whether the virus is transported by maternal leukocytes entering the placenta is unclear, although the former hypothesis is more consistent with the failure of second infection. Recently, Embil and associates (1970) reported on congenital CMV infection in two siblings from consecutive pregnancies. The first child had severe CMID and died at 30 days of age, and the second child born within 1 year, had hyperbilirubinemia, apnea, and viruria at birth. The second infant continued to excrete CMV, however; she did well during her postnatal period and was apparently a normal child at 4 months of age.

Although most infections of adults are subclinical, Davis and associates (1971) observed a 17-year-old pregnant female who developed CMV-mononucleosis during her first trimester. Cytomegalovirus was recovered from her urine and from amniotic fluid. Following a therapeutic abortion at

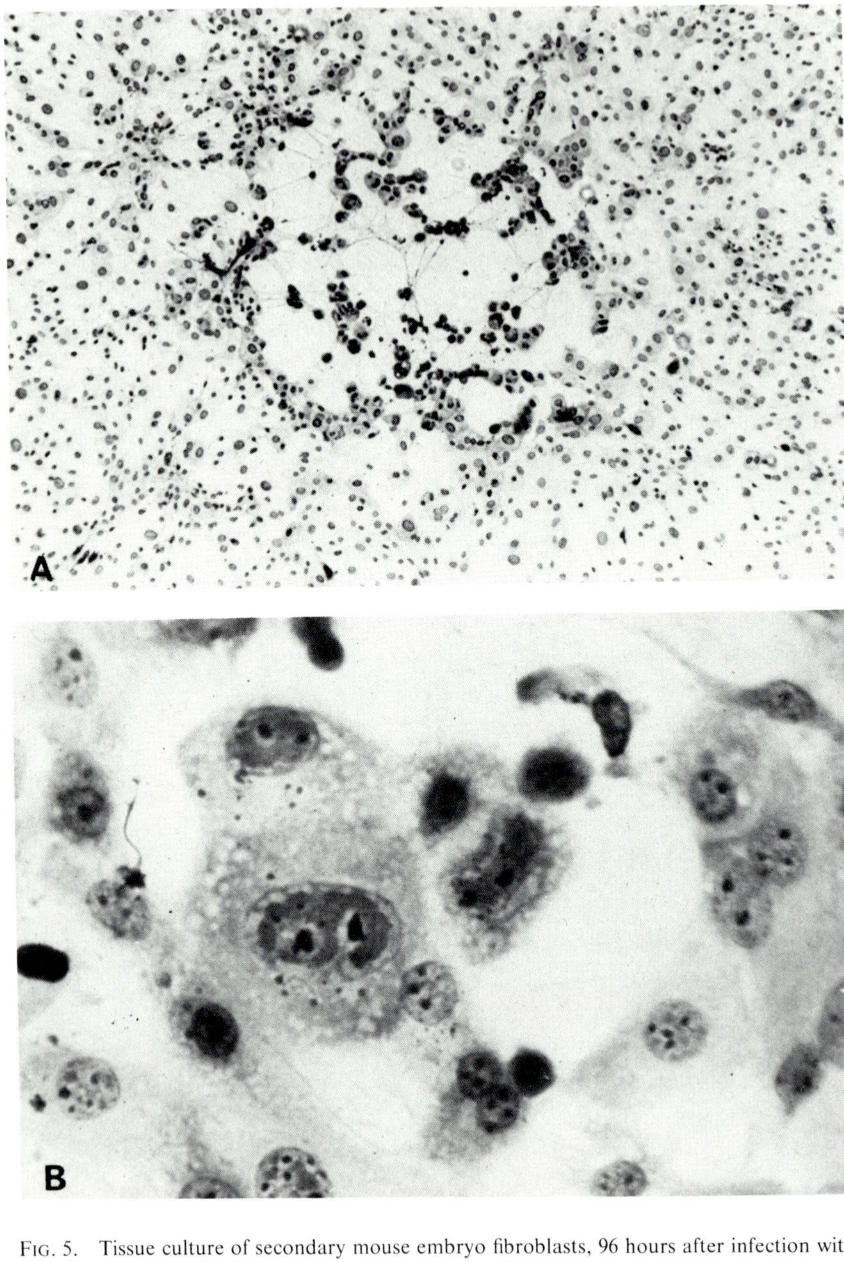

FIG. 5. Tissue culture of secondary mouse embryo fibroblasts, 96 hours after infection with murine cytomegalovirus. (A) Cytopathogenic effect showing representative plaques. × 40. (B) Cytopathogenic effect showing intranuclear lesions. × 400. (Figures kindly provided by Dr. June E. Osborn.)

22 weeks of gestation, CMV was recovered from a number of the organs of the fetus.

2. Prolonged Excretion of Virus

The marked difference in the response of the mother and the infant to infection with CMV is not fully explained. The infant tends to remain infected longer, to excrete higher titers of virus, even in the presence of significant neutralizing antibody, and to be more likely than the mother to have clinical symptoms related to his infection (Hanshaw, 1968). Medearis (1964b) has suggested that this difference in susceptibility is based on (1) the decreased integrity of the fetal blood–brain barrier, (2) the decreased phagocytic ability of fetal macrophages, (3) the delayed immunoglobulin response of the infant, (4) the greater number of viral receptor sites found on immature cells of the infant, and (5) the deficient interferon capacity of the immature infant.

3. Antibody

Antibody develops relatively early during CMV infection and is present throughout the long clinical course, seeming to correlate positively with the amount of virus excreted. It would appear that the more virus present, the more antibody present. This surprising finding probably reflects the capacity of this and many other herpesviruses to pass from cell to cell without sustained extracellular fluid contact (Osborn, 1970).

4. Disease versus Infection

When a developing fetus is infected with CMV, no disease may result, or there may be generalized, pantropic infection with inflammatory changes in many organs which may lead to eventual death or permanent sequellae. The factors determining variability in virulence are poorly understood.

Of the 26 infants born with congenital CMV infection reported by Starr *et al.* (1970), clinically apparent CMID was present in only one infected infant at birth.

Although some infected infants are born with a relatively benign disease, abnormalities in development may be observed later; therefore, once CMV infection has been diagnosed in early life, caution must be used in predicting subsequent development.

5. Latent State

Osborn (1970) has suggested that after the long period of demonstrable viruria in patients infected with CMV, the virus may be capable of entering a latent state. Should this prove to be the case, then perhaps other disease entities or abnormalities not presently recognized may prove to be etiologically related to CMV.

Viral replication with associated pathology, which is due either to activation of a latent process or to reinfection, is accepted as the by-product of iatrogenic modification of the host in the immunosuppressed organ transplant recipient. It has also been suggested that physiologic changes inherent in the state of pregnancy may reactivate a latent infection with CMV, explaining why isolation of CMV from cervical cultures of normal pregnant women were significantly greater during the third trimister than the first trimester (Montgomery *et al.*, 1972). Reactivation after a period of latency, with clinical manifestations quite different from those of the primary infection, is an established phenomenon with the herpes simplex and varicella–zoster agents; a reasonable assumption is that comparable late sequellae to infection with CMV may occur (Weller, 1971).

6. Characteristic Pathological Findings

The large inclusion-bearing cell, characteristic of CMV infections, attains a diameter of 25–40 μm with an intranuclear inclusion diameter of 8–10 μm (Hanshaw, 1970).

With the congenital infection, inclusion-bearing cells are found most frequently in the salivary glands, kidneys (Fig. 6), liver, and lungs, and less frequently in the retina, gastrointestinal tract, anterior pituitary gland, pancreas, adrenals, thyroid, parathyroid, bone marrow, spleen, thymus, lymph nodes, testes, ovary, heart, skin, blood vessels, and brain (Embil *et al.*, 1970). Pathological findings include chronic interstitial nephritis, pneumonitis, hepatitis with focal areas of necrosis, and meningoencephalitis with necrotizing granulomatous lesions and extensive calcifications. The pathologic basis for the hematopoietic changes of thrombocytopenia and hemolytic anemia are unknown, although Margileth (1955) has suggested that these are manifestations of the immune response of the host.

Typical inclusion-bearing cells have been described in the placenta, in urine, in gastric washings, and in most of the organs of the body. The ability of the pathologist to demonstrate inclusions is dependent upon the stage or severity of the infection at the time the tissues are examined (Hanshaw, 1968).

V. Immunity

A. Immunological Properties

Neutralizing and complement-fixing (CF) antibodies have been detected in the serum of infected infants and their mothers, and viral antigen has been

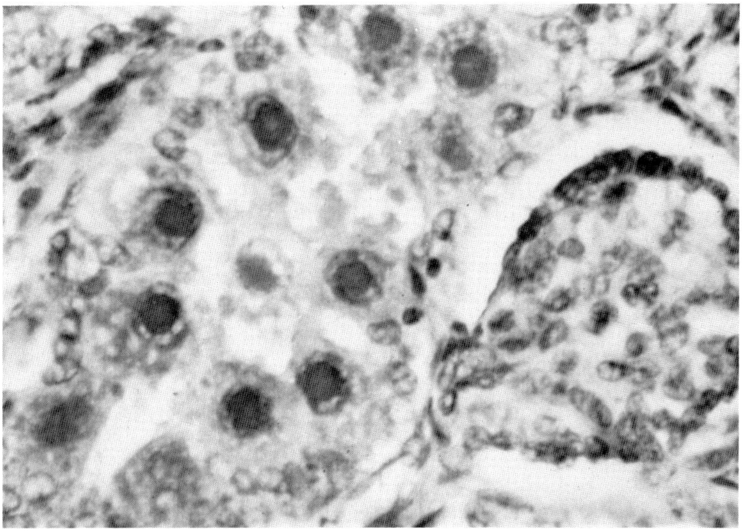

FIG. 6. Kidney tubule showing inclusion-bearing cells. This specimen is from infant who died at 3 days of age with overwhelming congenital CMID. He was the twin sibling of patient in Fig. 3.

detected in CMV-infected cells by means of fluorescein-labeled antibody (McAllister *et al.*, 1963; Weller, 1971). Recently, Krech and Jung (1969) inoculated rabbits, guinea pigs, and monkeys with human CMV and were able to detect the appearance of antibodies. The usual poor response of an experimental animal to immunization with the human CMV may in part reflect the past experience of that animal with its own CMV.

Congenital infections with human CMV result in the production of IgM and frequently IgA antibody, and these elevations are useful as screening tests in the detection of intrauterine infections due to CMV as well as rubella, toxoplasmosis, and syphilis (Steihm *et al.*, 1966).

Hanshaw *et al.* (1968) have demonstrated specific CMV macroglobulin in congenitally infected infants using an indirect immunofluorescent antibody method. This test is useful in distinguishing active antibody formation from passive immunity of maternal origin. Fluorescent antibody techniques are not only significant in congenital infections but have been applied to detect the early IgM antibody response in adults with CMV infections (Nordbring and Johansson, 1971).

Women giving birth to infected infants frequently have high CMV complement-fixing antibodies, and the infant receiving maternal IgG antibodies transplacentally will have low or undetectable levels by 5–6 months of age. Hanshaw (1966b) has suggested that a CF antibody titer greater than 1:8 in a 6-month-old infant usually results from active infection rather than passive transfer of maternal antibody. In older individuals acquiring infection for the first time, antibody usually rises over a 3-week period as in other viral infections. The durability of the antibody may be because of the persistence of CMV as an antigen in the host.

Black and associates (1963) as well as other investigators (Dreesman and Benyesh-Melnick, 1967) have noted a complement—fixation (CF) cross reaction between human and monkey viruses which was unexpected because of the usual strict species-specificities of members of the CMV. Cytomegalovirus-CF antibody in monkey serum was detected by both monkey and human antigens, but more efficiently by the monkey antigen; human sera reacted only with human CMV. In contrast, serum neutralization reactions with these two systems were species-specific.

The active CMV-CF antigen is cell-associated and is obtained by disruption and extraction of extensively infected cells either osmotically or mechanically by grinding or sonication.

Weller and associates (1960) have suggested that at least two serotypes of human CMV exist; these investigators felt that Davis and AD 169 strains were sufficiently different to warrant designations as type 1 and 2, respectively. Nothing is known concerning the relative pathogenicity of the two known serotypes; however, McAllister and associates (1964) reported that the Sec strain of CMV, serologically similar to Davis (type 1), was associated with the death of one twin and a nonfatal infection in the other twin.

Penttinen *et al.* (1970) have reported on a serological test based on the sedimentation patterns of washed platelets used as CMV antigen carrier; standardization was achieved by titration with antibody-positive human serum. There is some indication in patients with the postperfusion syndrome that the platelet agglutination test is more sensitive than the CF titer (Weller, 1971).

B. Immunological Distinctness

Hanshaw (1970) suggests there is evidence that CMV may be antigenically related to the Epstein-Barr (EB) virus seen in Burkitt's lymphoma and infectious mononucleosis and also to herpesvirus varicella. He suggests that CMV, EB virus, and varicella virus are more closely related to each other than they are to herpes simplex, and Plummer (1967) referred to these agents as the cell-associated herpesviruses or herpes B group.

VI. Epidemiology

A. Geographical Location

Cytomegalovirus is an ubiquitous agent having been reported from the United States, Canada, South America, Britain, Spain, France, Italy,

Germany, Scandinavia, Bulgaria, Lebanon, the East Indies, and China (Nelson and Wyatt, 1959). The incidence of CMID in infants is somewhat difficult to determine; however, in North America it ranged between 1 and 2% in unselected autopsies, but in view of the recent evidence of nonlethal forms of the disease, the true incidence is probably much higher (Nelson and Wyatt, 1959).

B. Age Incidence

Severe generalized infection is limited chiefly to newborn infants and to individuals with defense mechanism defects. In older children, asymptomatic infection is relatively common.

In adults, disease states are rare; however, infection must be a frequent occurrence, Rowe and associates (1956) demonstrated an increasing incidence of complement-fixing and neutralizing antibodies with age. Complement-fixing antibody was present in 14% of the serum specimens from infants 6–23 months of age, in 53% of serum specimens from young adults up to 25 years of age, and in 81% from individuals over 35 years of age. In newborn infants, 71% had antibody in their cord serum, and it was suggested that such antibody was passively acquired from the mother.

Hanshaw (1970) has reported that the prevalence of congenital infection, as determined by studies in Rochester and Cleveland, would approximate 1.3%. When these results are projected nationally, the birth of approximately 47,000 infants with congenital CMV infection would be expected in the United States annually.

C. Sex and Familial Incidence

The incidence of CMID is the same in the two sexes, and no obvious familial hereditary tendency has been observed. Li and Hanshaw (1967) have reported that 50% of 42 children of migrant workers from 1 to 13 years of age had serologic evidence of past or present infection with CMV, suggesting that CMV infection is more prevalent among migrant children than among other noninstitutionalized childhood populations studied to date.

D. Socioeconomic Factors

Cytomegalovirus appears to be endemic in all human societies. Statistics suggest that in the United States minimal infection rates at birth are approximately 1% as assayed by viruria (Hanshaw, 1970). The great majority of infected babies are asymptomatic; however, Hanshaw (1971) estimates that 10% of infected neonates are damaged. He further suggests that delayed recognition of certain sequellae, such as slow psychomotor development and impaired hearing, may make this figure conservative. Taking 1970 as an example, 3,700,000 live births occurred in the United States; therefore, the minimum estimate would indicate that 3,700 damaged infants secondary to CMV infection were born in this country in that year (Weller, 1971). An accurate assessment of the continuing responsibility imposed on society by this disease awaits completion of long-term prospective studies. Weller (1971) has suggested that in terms of personal tragedy, as well as economic loss, the accumulated toll attributable to congenitally acquired CMV infections exceeds that produced by congenital rubella. Wright (1971) has pointed out that these patients not only have severe brain damage but may have other long-term problems such as eye defects, hearing loss, and congenital heart disease.

Data on the importance of infection naturally acquired after birth are meager. Although it is known that CMV can produce hepatitis and can produce infectious mononucleosis-like disease, it is doubtful that these agents play a major etiologic role in these diseases.

Disease manifested in patients on immunosuppressive therapy is being recognized more frequently and presents as pneumonitis, hepatitis, gastroenteritis, and pancytopenia. In some studies, several agents were isolated at postmortem, and this would dilute the importance of CMV as compared to its being the only agent isolated.

E. Mechanisms of Transmission

1. Prenatal

Evidence that transplacental infection with CMV occurs consists of the finding of inclusion-bearing cells in stillborn infants and in newborns only a few hours old. Although there is usually no history of maternal illness that would yield information relative to the timing of the fetal infection, Davis *et al.*, (1971) described the occurrence of CMV-mononucleosis in a woman during her seventh week of pregnancy with the recovery of CMV not only from the mother but also from the placenta and fetus on interruption of pregnancy at the 22nd week. McAllister (1966) observed that mothers of infants with CMID are usually primigravida and from rural communities, suggesting that infection in the infant was due to an initial primary subclinical CMV infection in the mother coincidental with the pregnancy. McAllister's speculation is supported by the study of Starr *et al.* (1970) in which the mean age of mothers of infected newborns was 19 years, and 62% were primiparous.

It has also been suggested that intrauterine transfusions with fresh blood may be associated with fetal infection (King-Lewis and Gardner, 1969).

Berenberg and Nankervis (1970) observed that 7 of 12 mothers had pregnancies resulting in 14 live siblings and no miscarriages before birth of a baby infected with CMV, whereas after the birth of an infected child, 11 mothers experienced a total of 9 miscarriages during 24 pregnancies. This study suggests the possibility that the consequences of a congenital infection may extend to subsequent pregnancies and be expressed as fetal wastage.

2. Perinatal Transmission

As early as 1967, Diosi and colleagues isolated CMV from the cervix of pregnant or postpartum women. Recently, Montgomery *et al.* (1972) have isolated virus from the cervix more often in the third trimester than in the second or first.

Other evidence that would indicate that perinatal transmission is an important epidemiologic factor is the report by Levinsohn and colleagues (1969) which documents the appearance of viruria in certain infants between the first and third months of life. Correlation was established between infants with viruria and the CMV-CF antibody state of their mothers.

3. Postnatal Transmission

Since virus is present in the urine and saliva, it is likely that transmission is primarily through contact with these excretions. In view of the lability of the virus and sero-epidemiologic evidence now available, it is probable that transmission of the infection requires close physical contact. Patients, particularly infants with known or suspected active CMID, should be considered potentially hazardous to pregnant women as are infants with rubella infection.

Cytomegalovirus has been recovered from human breast milk, and it was suggested that the mother with protein–caloric malnutrition, under the additional stress of pregnancy and prolonged lactation, may disseminate virus in breast milk (Diosi *et al.*, 1967). Olson and associates (1970) have found CMV to be commonly present in the respiratory tract secretions of Thai children, suggesting the respiratory route may be a source of the extensive environmental contamination with this virus.

The use of fresh whole blood for transfusion entails risk of infection with CMV of the suspectible recipient, as does the use of organ transplantation.

VII. Treatment, Prevention, and Control

Infants congenitally infected with CMV have been treated with corticosteroids; however, there is no evidence that corticosteroids have improved or adversely affected the course of the infection (Osborn, 1970; Hanshaw, 1966b).

Passive immunization with hyperimmune serum would not be expected to help since CMV is capable of cell-to-cell spread without the necessity of an extracellular phase (Osborn, 1970). However, in one adult patient with hypergammaglobulinemia, pulmonary infection may have been improved with pooled gamma globulin injections given at frequent intervals (Jacox *et al.*, 1964).

In vitro studies show that poly IC, a synthetic double stranded RNA which is a potent interferon inducer, produces marked plaque reduction of human CMV in human fibroblasts which are sensitive to the antiviral action of interferon, while it is not active in other human fibroblasts which are relatively resistant to the action of interferon (Rabson *et al.*, 1969). Induction of high interferon blood levels by the administration of measles vaccine has not been found to diminish virus excretion.

Many reports relative to treating varicella–zoster and herpes simplex virus infections suggest that the viral infection responded favorably soon after cytosine arabinoside (ARA-C) was started, even when low doses were given for short periods (Hryniuk *et al.*, 1972).

In one patient with CMID of infancy, who has been treated with ARA-C intravenously on three occasions, virus has been eliminated from the urine on each occasion yet subsequently returned. After the third course of therapy which differed from the previous two in that the calculated drug was administered over a 12-hour period, it would appear that virus is remarkably reduced in titer but not completely eliminated (H. T. Wright, unpublished data).

Recently, Ch'ien and associates (1972) have treated three infants, who had severe, congenital CMV infections, with adenine arabinoside (ARA-A). Besides the decrease in virus excretion, patients appeared to have significant growth (height and weight) increase subsequent to therapy. Although drug dosages were high and prolonged, there was no evident toxicity or immunosuppression with this drug which suggests that it may be a better candidate drug for therapy than other drug considerations.

There are many problems associated with the development of a vaccine to control this infection. Of major concern is the fact that after live virus vaccination, the virus may persist for years as a latent infection, universal protection may not occur from vaccination with one strain, and the oncogenic potential of these agents is unknown (Hanshaw, 1971).

Therapeutic abortion may not be prudent as a control method, since it is not known whether the first 20 weeks is the vulnerable time for the fetus or not. It seems reasonable to presume that the infant with CMID of infancy is infectious, and hospitalized patients should be submitted to gown-type isolation and appropriate hand-washing procedures just as is required for the patient with the congenital rubella syndrome.

VIII. Summary

Cytomegalovirus is an ubiquitous agent, pantropic in character, found in many related and unrelated disease states, as well as in normal individuals with no symptoms of disease.

References

Andersen, H. K., and Spencer, E. S. (1969). *Acta Med. Scand.* **186**, 7.

Armstrong, D., Balakrishnan, S. L., Steger, L., Yu, B., and Stenzel, K. H. (1971a). *Arch. Intern. Med.* **127**, 111.

Armstrong, D., Haghbin, M., Balakrishnan, S. L., and Murphy, M. L. (1971b). *Amer. J. Dis. Child.* **122**, 404.

Balakrishnan, S. L., Armstrong, D., Rubin, A. L., and Stenzel, K. H. (1969). *J. Amer. Med. Ass.* **207**, 1712.

Benyesh-Melnick, M., Dessy, S. I., and Fernbach, D. J. (1964). *Proc. Soc. Exp. Biol. Med.* **117**, 624.

Berenberg, W., and Nankervis, G. (1970). *Pediatrics* **46**, 403.

Black, P. H., Hartley, J. W., and Rowe, W. P. (1963). *Proc. Soc. Exp. Biol. Med.* **112**, 601.

Bodey, G. P., Wertlake, P. T., Douglas, G., and Levin, R. H. (1965). *Ann. Intern. Med.* **62**, 899.

Brough, A. J., Jones, D., Page, R. H., and Mizukami, I. (1967). *Pediatrics* **40**, 627.

Buttrick, D. D., and Roberts, L. (1965). *Amer. J. Dis. Child.* **110**, 319.

Cangir, A., and Sullivan, M. P. (1966). *J. Amer. Med. Ass.* **195**, 616.

Cappell, D. F., and MacFarlane, M. N. (1947). *J. Pathol. Bacteriol.* **59**, 385.

Ch'ien, L. T., Benton, J. W., Buchanan, R. A., and Alford, C. A. (1972). *Pediat. Res.* **6**, 124.

Cole, R., and Kuttner, A. G. (1926). *J. Exp. Med.* **44**, 855.

Coombs, R. R. H. (1968). *Brit. Med. J.* **2**, 743.

Craighead, J. E., Hanshaw, J. B., and Carpenter, C. B. (1967). *J. Amer. Med. Ass.* **201**, 725.

Curtis, J. C., Dodge, W. F., and Daeschner, C. W. (1962). *Pediatrics* **29**, 52.

Davis, G. L. (1969). *Ann. Otol. Rhinol. Laryngol.* **78**, 1179.

Davis, L. E., Tweed, G. V., Stewart, J. A., Bernstein, M. T., Miller, G. L., Gravelle, C. R., and Chin, T. D. Y. (1971). *Pediatrics* **48**, 200.

Diosi, P., Babusceac, L., Nevinglovschi, O., and Kun-Stoicu, G. (1967). *Lancet* **2**, 1063.

Diosi, P., Moldovan, E., and Tomescu, N. (1969). *Brit. Med. J.* **4**, 660.

Dressman, G. R., and Benyesh-Melnick, M. (1967). *J. Immunol.* **99**, 1106.

Duvall, C. P., Casazza, A. R., Grimley, P. M., Carbone, P. P., and Rowe, W. P. (1966). *Ann. Intern. Med.* **64**, 531.

Dyment, P. G., Orlando, S. J., Isaacs, H., Jr., and Wright, H. T., Jr. (1968). *J. Pediat.* **72**, 533.

Emanuel, I., and Kenny, G. E. (1966). *Pediatrics* **38**, 957.

Embil, J. A., Folkins, D. F., Haldane, E. V., and van Rooyen, C. E. (1968). *Lancet* **2**, 1151.

Embil, J. A., Ozere, R. L., and Haldane, E. V. (1970). *J. Pediat.* **77**, 417.

Farber, S., and Wolbach, S. B.(1932). *Amer. J. Pathol.* **8**, 123.

Feldman, R. A. (1969). *Amer. J. Dis. Child.* **117**, 517.

Feldman, R. A., and Schwartz, J. F. (1968). *Lancet* **1**, 180.

Fetterman, G. H. (1952). *Amer. J. Clin. Pathol.* **22**, 424.

Fine, R. N., Grushkin, C. M., Anand, S., Lieberman, E., and Wright, H. T., Jr. (1970). *Amer. J. Dis. Child.* **120**, 197.
Foster, K. M., and Jack, I. (1969). *N. Engl. J. Med.* **280**, 1311.
Frank, D. J., DeVaux, W. D., Perkins, J. R., and Perrin, E. V. (1966). *Amer. J. Dis. Child.* **112**, 604.
Goodheart, C. R., and Jaross, L. B. (1963). *Virology* **19**, 532.
Goodheart, C. R., Filbert, J. E., and McAllister, R. M. (1963). *Virology* **21**, 530.
Goodheart, C. R., McAllister, R. M., and Filbert, J. E. (1964). *Virology* **23**, 603.
Goodpasture, E. W., and Talbot, F. B. (1921). *Amer. J. Dis. Child.* **21**, 415.
Gottmann, A. W., and Beatty, E. C., Jr. (1962). *Amer. J. Dis. Child.* **104**, 180.
Graham, C. B., Thal, A., and Wassum, C. S. (1970). *Radiology* **94**, 39.
Hagmann, R., Kuffer, F., Moser, R., and Bettex, M. (1969). *Schweiz. Med. Wochenschr.* **99**, 17.
Hanshaw, J. B. (1966a). *N. Engl. J. Med.* **275**, 476.
Hanshaw, J. B. (1966b). *Pediat. Clin. N. Amer.* **13**, 279–293.
Hanshaw, J. B. (1968). *Virol. Monogr.* **3**, 1–23.
Hanshaw, J. B. (1969). *J. Pediat.* **75**, 1179.
Hanshaw, J. B. (1970). *Advan. Teratol.* **4**, 63.
Hanshaw, J. B. (1971). *J. Infec. Dis.* **123**, 555.
Hanshaw, J. B., and Weller, T. H. (1961). *J. Pediat.* **58**, 305.
Hanshaw, J. B., Betts, R. F., Simon, G., and Boynton, R. C. (1965). *N. Engl. J. Med.* **272**, 602.
Hanshaw, J. B., Steinfeld, H. J., and White, C. J. (1968). *N. Engl. J. Med.* **279**, 566.
Harnden, D. G., Elsdale, T. R., Young, D. E., and Ross, A. (1967). *Blood* **30**, 120.
Hartley, J. W., Rowe, W. P., and Huebner, R. J. (1957). *Proc. Soc. Exp. Biol. Med.* **96**, 281.
Hayes, K., and Gibas, H. (1971). *J. Pediat.* **79**, 401.
Hedley-Whyte, E. T., and Craighead, J. E. (1965). *N. Engl. J. Med.* **272**, 473.
Henle, G., Henle, W., and Diehl, V. (1968). *Proc. Nat. Acad. Sci. U.S.* **59**, 94.
Henson, D. (1967). *J. Amer. Med. Ass.* **199**, 278.
Henson, D., Smith, R. D., and Gehrke, J. (1966). *Amer. J. Pathol.* **49**, 871.
Hill, R. B., Jr., Rowlands, D. T., Jr., and Rifkind, D. (1964). *N. Engl. J. Med.* **271**, 1021.
Hryniuk, W., Foerster, J., Shojania, M., and Chow, A. (1972). *J. Amer. Med. Ass.* **219**, 715.
Hsiung, G. D., Fischman, H. R., Fong, C. K. Y., and Green, R. H. (1969). *Proc. Soc. Exp. Biol. Med.* **130**, 80.
Jacox, R. F., Mongan, E. S., Hanshaw, J. B., and Leddy, J. P. (1964). *N. Engl. J. Med.* **271**, 1091.
Jesionek, A., and Kiolemenoglou, B. (1904). *Muenchen. Med. Wochenschr.* **51**, 1905.
Kääriäinen, L., Klemola, E., and Paloheimo, J. (1966a). *Brit. Med. J.* **1**, 1270.
Kääriäinen, L., Paloheimo, J., Klemola, E., Mäkelä, T., and Koivuniemi, A. (1966b). *Ann. Med. Exp. Biol. Fenn.* **44**, 297.
Kahn, D. R., Ertel, P. Y., Murphy, W. H., Kirsch, M. M., Vathayanon, S., Stern, A. M., and Sloan, H. (1967). *J. Thorac. Cardiov. Surg.* **54**, 682.
Kanich, R. E., and Craighead, J. E. (1966). *Amer. J. Med.* **40**, 874.
Kantor, G. L., and Johnson, B. L., Jr. (1970). *Arch. Intern. Med.* **125**, 488.
Kapsenberg, J. G., Langenhuysen, M. M. A. C., Nieweg, H. O., and Deiss, H. (1970). *Acta Med. Scand.* **187**, 79.
King-Lewis, P. A., and Gardner, S. D. (1969). *Brit. Med. J.* **2**, 603.
Klemola, E., and Kääriäinen, L. (1965). *Brit. Med. J.* **2**, 1099.
Klemola, E., Kääriäinen, L., von Essen, R., Haltia, K., Koivuniemi, A., and von Bonsdorff, C.-H. (1967). *Acta Med. Scand.* **182**, 311.
Krech, U., and Jung, M. (1969). *Arch. Gesamte Virusforsch.* **28**, 248.

Krugman, R. D., and Goodheart, C. R. (1964). *Virology* **23**, 290.
Lamb, S. G., and Stern, H. (1966). *Lancet* **2**, 1003.
Lang, D. J. (1966). *Pediatrics* **38**, 913.
Lang, D. J., and Hanshaw, J. B. (1969). *N. Engl. J. Med.* **280**, 1145.
Lang, D. J., and Montagnier, L. (1970). *Pediat. Res.* **4**, 462.
Lang, D. J., Scolnick, E. M., and Willerson, J. T. (1968). *N. Engl. J. Med.* **278**, 1147.
Levine, R. S., Warner, N. E., and Johnson, C. F. (1964). *Ann. Surg.* **159**, 37.
Levinsohn, E. M., Foy, H. M., Kenny, G. E., Wentworth, B. B., and Grayston, J. T. (1969). *Proc. Soc. Exp. Biol. Med.* **132**, 957.
Li, F., and Hanshaw, J. B. (1967). *Amer. J. Epidemiol.* **86**, 137.
Lipschütz, B. (1921). *Arch. Dermatol. Syph.* **136**, 428.
McAllister, R. M. (1966). *Ergeb. Mikrobiol. Immunitatsforsch. Exp. Ther.* **39**, 1–13.
McAllister, R. M., Straw, R. M., Filbert, J. E., and Goodheart, C. R. (1963). *Virology* **19**, 521.
McAllister, R. M., Wright, H. T., Jr., and Tasem, W. M. (1964). *J. Pediat.* **64**, 278.
McCordock, H. A., and Smith, M. G. (1936). *J. Exp. Med.* **63**, 303.
McCracken, G. H., Jr., Shinefield, H. R., Cobb, K., Rausen, A. R., Dische, M. R., and Eichenwald, H. F. (1969). *Amer. J. Dis. Child.* **117**, 522.
Margileth, A. M. (1955). *Pediatrics* **15**, 270.
Martos, L. M., Ablashi, D. V., Gilden, R. V., Sigüenza, R. F., and Hampar, B. (1970). *J. Gen. Virol.* **7**, 169.
Medearis, D. N., Jr. (1964a). *Bull. Johns Hopkins Hosp.* **114**, 181.
Medearis, D. N., Jr. (1964b). *Amer. J. Obstet. Gynecol.* **90**, 1140.
Mercer, R. D., Luse, S., and Guyton, D. H. (1953). *J. Pediat.* **11**, 502.
Monif, G. R. G., Egan, E. A., II, Held, B., and Eitzman, D. V. (1972). *J. Pediat.* **80**, 17.
Montgomery, R., Youngblood, L., and Medearis, D. N., Jr. (1972). *Pediatrics* **49**, 524.
Nakao, T., Chiba, S., Ohsaki, M., and Hanazono, H. (1967). *Lancet* **2**, 1153.
Nakao, T., Ikeda, S., Shiono, H., and Suzuki, M. (1971). *J. Amer. Med. Ass.* **217**, 697.
Nash, G., Asch, M. J., Foley, F. D., and Pruitt, B. A., Jr. (1970). *J. Amer. Med. Ass.* **214**, 587.
Nelson, J. S., and Wyatt, J. P. (1959). *Medicine (Baltimore)* **38**, 223.
Nordbring, F., and Johansson, S. G. O. (1971). *Scand. J. Infec. Dis.* **3**, 87.
Olson, L. C., Ketusinha, R., Mansuwan, P., and Snitbhan, R. (1970). *J. Pediat.* **77**, 499.
Osborn, J. E. (1970). *In* "Brennemann's Practice of Pediatrics," Vol. II. Chapter 37C, pp. 1–8. Harper, New York.
Paloheimo, J., von Essen, R., Klemola, E., Kääriäinen, L., and Siltanen, P. (1968). *Amer. J. Cardiol.* **22**, 624.
Penttinen, K., Kääiräinen, L., and Myllylä, G. (1970). *Arch. Gesamte Virusforsch.* **29**, 189.
Plotkin, S. A., and Pasquariello, P. S. (1969). *Amer. J. Dis. Child.* **118**, 515.
Plummer, G. (1967). *Progr. Med. Virol.* **9**, 302.
Prince, A. M., Szmuness, W., Millian, S. J., and David, D. S. (1971). *N. Engl. J. Med.* **284**, 1125.
Rabson, A. S., Tyrrell, S. A., and Levy, H. (1969). *Proc. Soc. Exp. Biol. Med.* **131**, 495.
Reyman, T. A. (1966). *Amer. Heart J.* **72**, 116.
Ribbert, H. (1904). *Zentralbl. Allg. Pathol. Pathol. Anat.* **15**, 945.
Riemenschneider, T. A., and Moss. A. J. (1966). *J. Pediat.* **69**, 546.
Rifkind, D. (1968). *Ann. Intern. Med.* **69**, 842.
Rifkind, D., Goodman, N., and Hill, R. B., Jr. (1967). *Ann. Intern. Med.* **66**, 1116.
Rinker, C. T., and McGraw, J. P. (1967). *Cancer* **20**, 36.
Rowe, W. P., Hartley, J. W., Waterman, S., Turner, H. C., and Huebner, R. J. (1956). *Proc. Soc. Exp. Biol. Med.* **92**, 418.
Sever, J. L., and White, L. R. (1968). *Annu. Rev. Med.* **19**, 471.
Sever, J. L., Huebner, R. J., Castellano, G. A., and Bell, J. A. (1963). *Amer. Rev. Resp. Dis.* **88**, Suppl., 342.

Smith, K. O., Thiel, J. F., Newman, J. T., Harvey, E., Trousdale, M. D., Gehle, W. D., and Clark, G. (1969). *J. Nat. Cancer Inst.* **42**, 489.
Smith, M. G. (1954). *Proc. Soc. Exp. Biol. Med.* **86**, 435.
Smith, M. G. (1956). *Proc. Soc. Exp. Biol. Med.* **92**, 424.
Smith, M. G. (1959). *Progr. Med. Virol.* **2**, 171.
Starr, J. G., Bart, R. D., Jr., and Gold, E. (1970). *N. Engl. J. Med.* **282**, 1075.
Steihm, E. R., Ammann, A. J., and Cherry, J. D. (1966). *N. Engl. J. Med.* **275**, 971.
Stern, H. (1968). *Brit. Med. J.* **1**, 665.
Stevens, D. P., Barker, L. F., Ketcham, A. S., and Meyer, H. M., Jr. (1970). *J. Amer. Med. Ass.* **211**, 1341.
Sullivan, M. P., Hanshaw, J. B., Cangir, A., and Butler, J. J. (1968). *J. Amer. Med. Ass.* **206**, 569.
Thorell, J., and Nathorst-Windahl, G. (1965). *Acta Soc. Med. Upsal.* **70**, 130.
Toghill, P. J., Bailey, M. E., Williams, R., Zeegen, R., and Bown, R. (1967). *Lancet* **1**, 1351.
Tyzzer, E. E. (1906). *J. Med. Res.* **14**, 361.
Vietzke, W. M., Gelderman, A. H., Grimley, P. M., and Valsamis, M. P. (1968). *Cancer* **21**, 816.
von Glahn, W. C., and Pappenheimer, A. M. (1925). *Amer. J. Pathol.* **1**, 445.
Weller, T. H. (1971). *N. Engl. J. Med.* **285**, 203 and 267.
Weller, T. H., and Hanshaw, J. B. (1962). *N. Engl. J. Med.* **226**, 1233.
Weller, T. H., Macauley, J. E., Craig, J. M., and Wirth, P. (1957). *Proc. Soc. Exp. Biol. Med.* **94**, 4.
Weller, T. H., Hanshaw, J. B., and Scott, D. E. (1960). *Virology* **12**, 130.
Wong, T-W., and Warner, N. E. (1962). *Arch. Pathol.* **74**, 403.
Wright, H. T., Jr. (1971a). *Proc. Int. Congr. Pediat., 13th*, Vol. 6, p. 341.
Wright, H. T., Jr. (1971b). *In* "The Mentally Retailed Child and His Family" (R. Koch and J. C. Dobson, eds.), pp. 69–80. Brunner/Mazel, Inc., New York.
Wright, H. T., Jr., Goodheart, C. R., and Lielausis, A. (1964). *Virology* **23**, 419.
Wright, H. T., Jr., Kasten, F. H., and McAllister, R. M. (1968). *Proc. Soc. Exp. Biol. Med.* **127**, 1032.
Wright, H. T., Jr., Parker, C. E., and Mavalwala, J. (1972). *Calif. Med.* **116**, 14.
Wyatt, J. P., Saxton, J., Lee, R. S., and Pinkerton, H. (1950). *J. Pediat.* **36**, 271.

Chapter 13

The Simian Herpesviruses

Robert N. Hull

I. Introduction

Extensive investigation during the past two decades into the viral flora of Old and New World subhuman primates has led to the discovery and characterization of many new viral agents indigenous in these populations. These agents, generally, are referred to as "simian viruses." Although various systems have been proposed for the classification of these viruses, it has been recognized that most of them could be placed into recognized, viral families such as, adenoviruses, herpesviruses, paramyxoviruses, picornaviruses, etc. (Hull, 1968a). This chapter pertains to a portion of the family of simian herpesviruses.

II. Introduction to and Origin of the Simian Herpesviruses

A. Introduction

At least 18 different herpesviruses, and herpeslike viruses, from a variety of simian species have been described in the literature. This group of viruses can be subdivided as indicated in Table I. The "typical herpesviruses" include four, or possibly, five agents which satisfy all the chemical, physical, and biological criteria generally attributed to herpesviruses. The fifth agent, THV, recently isolated from a tree shrew (a primitive primate) also may belong to this group. *Herpesvirus hominis* (herpes simplex) is listed, since it produces natural infection in monkeys and must be considered in all differential diagnosis because of its serological relationship with other members of the simian herpesvirus family. The viruses grouped under the other three headings in Table I share some properties with the "typical herpesviruses," but

TABLE I
TYPES AND NUMBERS OF SIMIAN HERPESVIRUSES

Typical herpesviruses	Cytomegaloviruses	Cell-associated varicella-like	Oncogenic herpesviruses
H. simiae	SA[a]	LVV[b]	*H. saimiri*[a]
H. tamarinus	Others[d–f]	Patas virus[g]	*H. saguinus*[h]
SA_8			SMHI[i]
SMV			*H. aotus* type 1[i]
THV			*H. aotus* type 2[j]
(*H. hominis*)			*H. aotus* type 3[j]
			H. ateles[j]
			AT-46[j]
			Chimpanzee[k]

[a]Malherbe and Harwin (1957).
[b]Clarkson *et al.* (1967).
[c]Melendez *et al.* (1968).
[d]Black *et al.* (1963).
[e]Swack *et al.* (1971).
[f]K. O. Smith *et al.* (1969).
[g]McCarthy *et al.* (1968).
[h]Melendez and Daniel (1970).
[i]Melendez *et al.* (1970).
[j]Melendez *et al.* (1971).
[k]Landon *et al.* (1968).

will not be considered further here. References indicated in the table will acquaint the reader with these agents. The four herpesviruses to be described and discussed in greater detail are identified in Table II, along with a listing of their synonyms and natural hosts.

B. *History of Isolation*

1. *H. simiae*

The first recognized simian virus, isolated and described by Sabin and Wright (1934), proved to be a herpesvirus. This virus, although isolated from a fatal human infection, was transmitted by the bite of a rhesus monkey (*Macaca mulatta*). The agent was labeled "B virus" by these authors (B, being the initial of the patient), but in a second paper, Sabin (1934a) described its immunological similarity to herpes simplex (*H. hominis*) and pseudorabies (*H. suis*) viruses, and subsequently it has been named *Herpesvirus simiae*. B virus has since been isolated many times from rhesus, and other macaques, as well as from additional human infections.

2. SA_8

SA_8 virus was isolated by Malherbe and Harwin (1958) from the spinal cord of an African vervet monkey (*Cercopithecus aethiops pygerythrus*). This animal, as well as a second animal a year later, had been inoculated intra-

TABLE II
THE TYPICAL SIMIAN HERPESVIRUSES

Name	Synonyms	Natural host
H. simiae	B virus	*Macaca* sp.
H. tamarinus	Herpes T	*Saimiri* sp.
SA_8	None	Vervets-Papio
SMV	None	*Ateles* sp.

spinally with inactivated poliomyelitis vaccine (Malherbe and Strickland-Cholmey, 1970). These monkeys became paralyzed, and a virus was recovered from the spinal cords of both monkeys, which later was given the designation of SA_8 virus. The virus could not be detected in the blood of either animal nor in the vaccine inocula; thus, it was assumed that the virus was latent in the spinal cords and was activated by the trauma induced by the vaccine inoculation. Malherbe and Strickland-Cholmey (1969) also reported the isolation of SA_8 virus from a rectal swab taken from a baboon (*Papio ursinns*). No other isolations of SA_8 virus have been reported in the literature, although large numbers of African monkeys have been used in vaccine research, production and control laboratories, and there is a fairly high incidence of SA_8 antibody in these animals.

3. *H. tamarinus*

Herpesvirus tamarinus has been known by various names, including, MHV (marmoset herpesvirus), herpes T, and *Herpesvirus platyrrhinae*. It was originally isolated and reported by Holmes *et al.* (1963) who recovered the agent from autopsy materials from six South American marmosets (*Tamarinus nigricollis*). These animals died rather suddenly within 2 weeks of their arrival in the laboratory and without signs of prior illness. The virus, also, was isolated from a throat swab taken from a sick marmoset prior to death. Melnick *et al.* (1964) independently isolated and described this same agent. In their laboratory the virus was recovered from cultures of marmoset kidney cells which had been prepared from the kidneys taken following natural death of the animal. The virus was further isolated from a homogenate of lung tissue from another dead marmoset.

4. SMV

SMV was recovered from a zoo-born and -reared New World spider monkey (*Ateles geoffroyi*). The parents of this animal also were born and raised in the zoo. The infected animal was a $5\frac{1}{2}$-month-old female, which was observed to be listless and clinging to its mother. The animal died within 24 hours, and specimens of brain, liver, and lip lesion were obtained at autopsy for virus isolation. The virus was isolated from brain tissue by the inoculation of homogenates into human fibroblast diploid cell strains and into the rabbit kidney cell strain, LLC-RK_1. The isolation and characterization of this virus was reported by Hull *et al.* (1972). No other isolations of SMV have been reported to date.

5. THV

The tree shrew herpesvirus, THV, only recently has been described by McCombs *et al.* (1971). It was isolated on a number of occasions from cultures of tissues prepared from apparently normal animals. The virus also was recovered from mouth swabs of healthy animals. These indications suggested that this virus is a latent agent in this species, and that infection is rarely manifested by clinical disease or lesions.

III. Nature of Infections Produced

A. In the Natural Hosts

1. *H. simiae*

Herpesviruses rarely produce overt disease in their natural hosts, and this is essentially true of these simian herpesviruses. When disease, or lesions are observed, they most likely are seen in infants or in stressed animals. Most observations involving *H. simiae* have been made in rhesus, or other *Macaca* species after recent capture, crowding, and rapid transportation to research or vaccine production laboratories. Generally, infection with *H. simiae* in macaques is asymptomatic. When lesions are present they consist of small vesicles on the tongue, buccal cavity, and mucoepithelial border of the lips which rupture and become ulcerated, as described by Keeble (1960). The type and extent of lesions will vary considerably from one individual to another; however, *H. simiae* infection should be suspected when vesicular lesions are observed in, or about the oral cavity, or on the skin of rhesus and other macaques or in other species exposed to macaques. Conjunctivitis also may be observed. In one study, Hull (1969) found that approximately 50% of the cases of nonbacterial conjunctivitis in rhesus monkeys was of *H. simiae* etiology. *Hespervirus simiae* rarely, if ever, produces encephalitis or other central nervous system disorders in the host species under natural conditions, but evidence of such disease with virus isolations, have been made from monkeys suppressed with cortisone and traumatized by intraspinal, intracerebral, and intramuscular inoculation with inactivated poliomyelitis vaccine (Committee Report, 1956; Keeble, 1960; Kirschstein and Van Hoosier, 1961). These animals, in addition to central nervous system (CNS) histopathology, also may have lesions in the viscera, especially in the liver, kidney, and lungs. These lesions consist of necrotic foci, or infiltration by leukocytes and monocytes. The class A intranuclear inclusions may be observed in cells within or around these lesions, especially if the infection is recent and not too far advanced.

2. SA_8

Little is known about disease caused by SA_8 virus in the African vervet monkey presumed to be the natural host. As noted above, it has been isolated only twice from this species and both times following trauma to CNS tissues. This paucity of knowledge and observations suggests that it is less likely to produce clinical disease in its natural host than is *H. simiae.*

3. *H. tamarinus*

Although *H. tamarinus* was isolated originally from marmosets, it was determined later that the squirrel monkey (*Saimiri sciureus*) was the natural host for this virus. Holmes *et al.* (1966) provided information from serological surveys of various New World species that squirrel monkeys, and possibly Cebus and spider monkeys, were candidates for the host species for *H. tamarinus.* Further and more convincing proof of the squirrel monkey as a natural host for *H. tamarinus* was seen in the report of Melendez *et al.* (1966), who isolated the virus from throat and anal swabs of a healthy squirrel monkey. This animal was a member of a closed colony of 10 animals held in isolation for 1 year prior to testing. One year later, King *et al.* (1967) again isolated the virus from 2 of 4 ill squirrel monkeys. Overt disease is rarely seen in the squirrel monkey, but when it does occur it resembles that seen in rhesus monkeys infected with *H. simiae*. Oral, lingual, and labial ulcers are seen which yield virus on isolation attempts and which demonstrate class A intranuclear inclusions in histopathological preparations.

4. SMV

SMV infection has been observed but one time, and as noted above (Section II, B, 4), this was in an immature spider monkey. This animal presented the picture of a typical herpesvirus infection. There were lesions on the lips and nose and large, deep ulcerated areas on the tongue, palate, and gums. Data from serological studies provided evidence that the spider monkey is the most likely natural host for this virus. Present knowledge, however, suggests that this fatal infection in a juvenile animal was an unusual event. No other member of this closed zoo colony of spider monkeys showed evidence of infection or of disease for long periods either before or after this event. Furthermore most sera from adult animals trapped in the wild had high titers of antibody against SMV, indicating prior infection and survival.

B. In Foreign Hosts and Experimental Animals

1. *H. simiae*

a. SUBHUMAN PRIMATES. Although the simian herpesviruses produce but limited disease in their native host under natural conditions, most of them are virulent for some other species, and in some cases, produce a devastating infection. Within the primate family, *H.simiae* has been found to infect rhesus (*M.mulatta*), cynomolgus (*M.fascicularis*), Japanese macaque (*M.fuscata*), and the stumptail macaque (*M.arctoides*), as reviewed by Hunt and Melendez (1969), as well as *M.cyclopsis* and *M.iris*. The African green monkey (*Cercopithecus aethiops*), the patas monkey (*Erythrocebus patas*), and the cynomolgus monkey have been experimentally infected, but without the production of disease (R. L. Kirschstein, personal communication, 1967). Natural infection in New World subhuman primates with *H.simiae* has not been reported, nor is there any information available relating to experimental infection in these species. The latter represents a void in our present knowledge of the virulence and epidemiology of *H.simiae* which should be filled. The virulence of *H.simiae* for man is discussed, in detail, in Sections VIII–XIII.

The most detailed account of the experimental infection of rhesus monkeys with *H.simiae* appeared in one of Sabin's (1934c) early papers. Antibody-negative animals were susceptible by a variety of routes of inoculation. A fatal encephalitis generally followed intracerebral inoculation, but invasion of the CNS did not follow other routes of inoculation. Intravenous inoculation was especially marked by the development of exanthema about the forehead and eyes and by enanthema of the buccal mucous membranes, tongue, palate, and conjunctiva. When the virus was given intraperitoneally an acute peritonitis followed, but only an occasional invasion of the abdominal viscera occurred. Intracutaneous inoculation produced a local area of acute inflammation and necrosis. Studies such as these have been difficult to undertake because of the need for antibody-negative rhesus monkeys. Keeble (1960) reported one instance in which a typical vesicular lesion was produced on the tongue of an antibody-negative monkey by the direct inoculation of the virus into the tongue.

b. LABORATORY ANIMALS. Other than in primates, *H.simiae* has extreme virulence for rabbits. This was first reported by Sabin (1934b), and the rabbit has become the test animal of choice for isolation and study of *H.simiae*. As few as 3 $TCID_{50}$ will produce a fatal infection following intradermal inoculation, and the rabbit is susceptible by all routes of inoculation, including ingestion (Hull, 1972). The most typical pathology and histopathology, is seen in animals sacrified at the first sign of CNS disease following peripheral inoculation. This is generally 7–8 days postinoculation and usually is represented by weakness of the hind legs or paralysis. Rabbits inoculated intracerebrally develop a rapid encephalitis with death in 3–4 days. Typical eosinophilic class A intranuclear inclusions are difficult to find in postmortem CNS tissue of these animals. *Herpesvirus simiae* has little virulence for the guinea pig, although skin lesions do appear following intradermal inoculation, and serum antibody is produced. The virulence of *H.simiae* for mice appears to vary with the strain. Sabin's original isolate produced infection in an occasional mouse, but the virus could not be serially passed in mice. The same observation was made with the B virus vaccine strain (Strain E2490) (Hull, 1972). Several strains recovered from human infections, however, have possessed virulence for the mouse. Strain E2490 is avirulent for white rats and adult chickens by intraperitoneal or intramuscular inoculation, but does stimulate the production of serum antibody. Cotton rats inoculated intraperitoneally, subcutaneously, and intracerebrally succumbed to the infection. Typical hindleg paralysis observed 7–8 days postinoculation proceeded death in those animals inoculated by the intraperitoneal and subcutaneous routes. Death occurred quickly, within 3–4 days after intracerebral inoculation, and progressive paralysis was not seen. In a series of four papers, Reagan and co-workers (Reagan *et al.*, 1952a,b, 1954; Reagan and Brueckner, 1953), described the adaption of *H. simiae* to Swiss mice, hamsters, baby white leghorn chicks, and cave bats. In the latter, infection was possible only by the intracerebral route; while in the other species, infection followed various routes of inoculation. *Herpesviruses simiae* also can be propagated in embryonated chicken eggs in which it produces pocklike lesions on the chorioallantoic membrane.

2. SA_8

a. SUBHUMAN PRIMATES. The experimental host range and virulence of SA_8 virus has not been thoroughly studied. As noted previously, it did produce disease in its presumed natural host, the vervet monkey, following trauma which, apparently, aroused the virus from latency. Experimentally, in a single vervet monkey, SA_8 inoculation produced but minimal lesions and no clinical disease (Hull, 1972). At the time of inoculation the monkey was thought to be antibody negative, but a repeat assay of preinoculation serum with a minimal dose of challenge virus, revealed that antibody was present in undiluted serum. The animal received 18.6×10^6 $TCID_{50}$ intradermally, and

6.2×10^6 $TCID_{50}$ was rubbed into a scarification on the lip. A small vesicular lesion appeared on the lip 3 days postinoculation, and some edema, but no vesicle formation nor necrosis, was observed at the site of the intradermal injection. On the fourth day, a small amount of fluid was aspirated from the lip lesion, and the virus was readily recovered in tissue culture. Both lesions healed within 9 days. Viremia could not be detected on the third through fifth days. Serum antibody titer rose to 1:1024 in 10 days.

b. LABORATORY ANIMALS. SA_8 has little virulence for small animals. It may produce local lesions in rabbits and guinea pigs following intradermal inoculation, and an occasional rabbit may show some signs of paralysis. The virus, however, has not been recovered from these rabbits. Both species, however, respond with the production of serum antibody. Weanling and suckling mice and weanling hamsters are resistant to intracerebral inoculation with high titer SA_8 virus (Hull, 1972).

3. *H. tamarinus*

a. SUBHUMAN PRIMATES. It has been noted that *H.tamarinus* is highly virulent for the marmoset, and this is true both under natural and experimental conditions. Fatality rates in either case approximate 100%. Holmes *et al.* (1964) were able to produce fatal infections by intradermal and intranasal inoculation and by gavage. Local hemorrhagic and necrotizing lesions were seen at the point of intradermal inoculation, and the animals developed progressive weakness and died between the fourth and seventh day postinoculation. Intranasal inoculation resulted in rhinitis and pneumonitis, terminating in death on the fourth or fifth day. Those animals infected by gavage became lethargic and died between 10 and 13 days. The owl monkey (*Aotus trivirgatus*) also develops a fatal infection following natural exposure to *H.tamarinus*. This has generally occurred after exposure to squirrel monkeys. Hunt and Melendez (1966) reported the investigation of a series of deaths in a colony of owl monkeys, from five of these monkeys *H.tamarinus* virus was isolated and identified. Forty-five animals were involved in this episode, and at least 25 died over a period of 5 months. These authors were able to reproduce the disease by experimental inoculation of owl monkeys. Four monkeys were inoculated intramuscularly with 100 $TCID_{50}$ of virus. Three of the four had neutralizing antibody in undiluted preinoculation sera, but all succumbed to the infection with death ocurring between 7 and 9 days. Gross and histopathologic changes in these animals were similar to those observed in the natural infection. Virus was readily recovered from numerous tissues.

Natural *H.tamarinus* infection in owl monkeys again was reported by Emmons *et al.* (1968). In this instance, the virus was recovered from an owl monkey which became ill and died in a pet shop. Several other animals in this shop, which housed 300 monkeys of 8 different species of South American primates, also became ill and died at this same time. In the subject animal, the virus was recovered from brain, liver, and tongue tissue suspension inoculated into human fetal diploid cell cultures and into suckling mice.

b. Laboratory Animals. Among laboratory animals, rabbits, adult and suckling mice, guinea pigs, hamsters, and embryonated chicken eggs show varying degrees of susceptibility to *H.tamarinus*. Rabbits develop hemorrhagic ulcerated skin lesions at the site of intradermal inoculation which heal after about 1 week with no sequelae. A slowly progressing meningoencèphalitis follows intracerebral inoculation with death by 9–12 days. Rabbits do not appear to be susceptible to intraperitoneal inoculation (Holmes *et al.*, 1964). Inoculation of the scarified cornea of the rabbit results in a purulent conjunctivitis which heals after 3–4 weeks without involvement of the central nervous system (Daniel *et al.*, 1967). Adult mice are susceptible by the intracerebral route, but not by intraperitoneal injection, while suckling mice are susceptible by either route. Death generally occurs within 3–5 days. *Herpesvirus tamarinus* behaves in the guinea pig much as *H.simiae* and SA_8 in that local lesions are produced by intradermal inoculation and that no other signs or symptoms are seen. Newborn and weanling hamsters are susceptible to intracerebral inoculation but are refractory to intraperitoneal, intramuscular, and subcutaneous inoculation. Herpes-like pocks are produced on the chorioallantoic membrane of the chicken embryo.

4. SMV

a. Subhuman Primates. SMV may be a cause of natural infection in several New World subhuman primates, but most likely does not produce a uniformly lethal disease. Serological studies revealed a high incidence of, and high titer of, antibody in adult spider monkeys (*Ateles geoffroyi* and *A. fusciceps*), and in occasional capuchin monkeys (*Cebus apella*, *C. albifrons*, and *C. capucinus*). Juvenile sera had a much lower incidence. Squirrel, marmoset, and woolly monkeys (*Lagothrix lagotricha*) were rarely antibody-positive. Experimentally, marmosets were shown to be equally as susceptible to lethal infection with SMV as they are to *H.tamarinus*. In a very limited study, one antibody-negative rhesus and one antibody-negative African green monkey proved to be refractory to inoculation with 7.6×10^6 $TCID_{50}$ of SMV. The dose was divided between subcutaneous and intradermal inoculations. Neither lesions nor disease developed in these animals, and serum antibody rose to only 1:4 in the African green monkey and to 1:32 in the rhesus by 1 month (Hull *et al.*, 1972).

b. LABORATORY ANIMALS. Rabbits inoculated subcutaneously with SMV do not uniformly develop clinical disease, but some may show evidence of a lesion at the site of inoculation and/or eventually develop CNS infection and die. Virus can be recovered from the brain, where a mild meningoencephalitis is seen. No infection results from intraperitoneal inoculation. The virulence of SMV for rabbits is similar to that of *H.tamarinus*, but is less so than that of *H.simiae*. In guinea pigs, following intradermal inoculation with SMV, local lesions develop but no other evidence of disease is seen. Serum antibody response follows such infections. Both suckling and weanling mice succumb to intracerebral inoculations within 5–9 days postinoculation. The LD_{50} (lethal dose) for weanling mice is about 1000 $TCID_{50}$ (Hull *et al.*, 1972).

C. *Natural* H. hominis *Infection in Simian Species*

Herpes simplex (*H.hominis*) is indigenous to man, but several species of subhuman primates are susceptible to this virus, and natural infections occur when these species are brought into association with man. Thus, in apparent herpesvirus infections in these species, and possibly others, the possibility of herpes simplex etiology must be considered. The disease in these species presents the typical herpetic syndrone which may include vesicular lesions, neurological disorders conjunctivitis, fever, and coryza. These infections are generally fatal. Species known to be susceptible and appropriate literature references are gibbons (*Hylobates lar*): P. C. Smith *et al.* (1969), Emmons and Lennette (1970), B. A. Kogan (personal communications, 1968), Hull (1972); owl monkeys (*Aotus trivirgatus*): Melendez *et al.* (1969), McClure and Keeling (1971); marmosets (*Tamarinus sp.*): M. R. Nilsson (personal communication, 1969), Hull (1972); tree shrews (*Tupaia glis*): McClure and Keeling (1971).

IV. Distribution and Prevalence

A. *H.simiae*

The distribution and prevalence of the simian herpesviruses in their natural hosts has been assessed by serological surveys, and in some instances the prevalence varies from animals bled in the wild, or soon after capture, to those held in laboratory colonies. More information of this type is available for *H. simiae* than for the other viruses. In one study (Hull and Nash, 1960), a 10% incidence of *H. simiae* antibody was observed in 99 rhesus monkeys at time of capture in India. Most of these animals were sexually immature. Shah and Southwick (1965) made a similar study in which they found no

H. simiae antibody in 39 juvenile rhesus monkeys, but 7 of 8 adult sera tested were antibody positive. A somewhat different population of rhesus monkeys was studied in the report of Shah and Morrison (1969) describing the incidence of antibody in monkeys on Cayo, Santiago Island. These animals constituted a free-roaming colony which had been established on the island nearly 30 years prior to the time of sampling. In 1- to 2-year-old animals, these authors found a 22% incidence of antibody to *H.simiae* which increased with age. All monkeys 5 years of age or older were antibody positive. This study demonstrated that *H.simiae* infection was perpetrated in the colony from its inception and that the incidence of infection was greater in this more compact population that it was in the free-ranging populations of India.

The incidence of *H.simiae* antibody in laboratory colonies will vary with the history of the animals and with the manner in which they have been housed. In situations which prevailed during the development and production of poliomyelitis vaccine when large shipments of rhesus monkeys were received and housed in gang cages, the incidence of *H.simiae* antibody was quite high, being 70% or greater (Keeble, 1960; Hull and Nash, 1960). Under better conditions of procurement and housing, the levels of infection with *H.simiae* can be reduced or controlled. Such a situation was described by DiGiacomo and Shah (1972) who also reviewed the literature on the prevalence of *H.simiae* antibody in rhesus monkeys. In their study only one of 39 laboratory-reared monkeys was found to possess neutralizing antibody. These monkeys were housed for a number of years in individual cages and at times were in the same room with other rhesus monkeys from India. In another instance, six immature male rhesus monkeys were trapped in India, placed in separate cages, and immediately flown to a laboratory in the United States. These animals were bled upon arrival, then placed in individual cages in separate rooms. One of the six monkeys was found to be positive for *H.simiae* antibody, and a rising titer was demonstrated in subsequent bleedings. The other five animals remained antibody-negative during nearly 1 year of residence in the laboratory (Hull, 1972). Thus, better care and isolation, or restricted contact between animals, can reduce the incidence of *H.simiae* infection in groups or colonies of rhesus monkeys.

The prevalence of *H.simiae* antibody in other *Macaca* species has been reported by Endo *et al.* (1960). Of 61 Japanese *Macaca fuscata*, 11% were antibody-positive, and 16% of 43 sera from the Formosan variety, *M.cyclopis*, were also antibody-positive. The incidence was as high as 35% in 86 *M.irus* monkeys from the Philippines, Indonesia, and Thailand. It is likely that these percentages would have been higher had these authors not heat-inactivated these sera prior to neutralization. The incidence of *H.simiae* antibody in a group of 46 recently captured Taiwan monkeys (*M.cyclopis*) was 24% as reported by Pryor *et al.* (1970).

The above serological data give indication of the incidence of past infection with *H.simiae*, but do not provide information as to the likely number of active infections within a colony of monkeys at any given time. Fewer studies have been done to acquire this type of information. Keeble *et al.* (1958) published one paper in which 2.3% of 1400 rhesus monkeys were found to have active *H.simiae* infections. These cases were seen shortly after arrival in the laboratory and were recognized mainly by vesicular or ulcerated lesions on the tongue and occasionally on the lip. The virus was recovered from these lesions and identified serologically. In an earlier group of 18 rhesus monkeys, they found as high as 33% to have active infections. Hartley (1964) found an incidence of 10% active infections in 300 recently imported cynomolgus monkeys (*M.irus*) that had not been exposed to rhesus monkeys at any time. The morbidity rates described in these papers determined from animals shortly after, or during, stress of capture, crowding, and shipment probably represent the extremes.

B. SA_8

There is but one report in the literature dealing with the prevalence of SA_8 antibody in simian populations. These authors, Kalter and Heberling (1971), found antibody-positive animals in various populations of African and Asiatic species, with the highest incidence being in African vervet and patas monkeys and in baboons. In one group of 40 vervet monkeys, 82% of the animals had neutralizing antibody, while 60% of a group of 37 patas monkeys were positive. An incidence of 100% was obtained from the assay of sera from 42 baboons. These figures represented the peak levels in their studies, while other groups of these same species, as well as of different species, had lower incidences. In most cases the same serum specimens were assayed also for antibody to herpes simplex and to *H.simiae*. A great deal of cross reacting occurred in their tests, and this will be dealt with subsequently. From a previously unpublished study (Hull, 1972) a total of 61 African green monkey sera from four different groups of animals were assayed for presence of SA_8 virus-neutralizing antibody and, in some instances, also for antibody to *H.simiae* and to herpes simplex. On the whole, 17 (or 28%) of these monkeys possessed antibody which neutralized SA_8 virus. Fourteen of the SA_8 antibody-positive sera, as well as others, were assayed also for *H.simiae* and herpes simplex antibody, and all but one neutralized both viruses. No serum neutralized either *H.simiae* or herpes simplex viruses which did not also neutralize SA_8 virus. A representation of the actual antibody titers, and the extent of crossreactions observed in this study are shown in Table III. This serological problem with this group of viruses will be considered in greater detail in Section VI,B,2. However, it seems reasonably safe to conclude that the antibody assayed in these African species was produced by

TABLE III
LEVELS OF SA_8. *H. simiae*, AND HERPES SIMPLEX ANTIBODY IN A GROUP OF AFRICAN GREEN MONKEYS

	Neutralizing antibody to		
Monkey No.	SA_8[a]	*H. simiae*[a]	Herpes simplex[a]
1	16*	32	16
10	256	32	64
18	64	64	128
38	128	64	64
99511	256	32	64
99526	256	< 16	< 16
99603	256	64	128
99901	128	32	64
60	< 256	32	32
15	256	512	256
28	128	> 2048	256
36	256	512	2048
100	256	64	64
380	128	64	64

[a] Reciprocal of serum dilution.

prior infection with SA_8 virus, rather than either of the other two viruses, so long as possible exposure to Asiatic species, or man, was eliminated. The findings of Kalter and Heberling (1971), however, created doubt as to which African species might be the true natural host for SA_8 virus. It may be that it is the baboon rather than the vervet monkey.

C. H. tamarinus

Holmes *et al.* (1966) found 73% of 121 adult squirrel monkey sera to contain neutralizing antibody against *H.tamarinus*, while only 8% of juvenile sera were antibody-positive. Similar percentages, based on small numbers of animals, were observed in Cebus and spider monkeys. In contrast, only 17% of the sera from 131 adult marmosets neutralized the virus. The antibody-positive data obtained from Cebus and spider monkey sera may have been misleading, since more recent observations (Hull *et al.*, 1972) have shown a strong one-way cross reaction between *H.tamarinus* virus and SMV, with the latter being the antigenic dominant. It is likely, therefore, that the antibody which they demonstrated in Cebus and spider monkeys was actually produced by prior infection with SMV. These, and other reports (Emmons *et al.*, 1968; Kalter and Heberling, 1971) have fairly well established that 70–90% of adult squirrel monkeys have experienced infection with *H.tamarinus* virus. In other than South American species, Kalter and Heberling

(1971) found only 1 of 302 sera from African subhuman primates and 6 of 101 specimens from Asiatic species that neutralized *H.tamarinus*. The significance of, or explanation for this, remained obscure, but it was evident that simians from either of the Old World geographical areas had had little, or no exposure, or susceptibility to *H.tamarinus* virus.

D. SMV

Studies on the prevalence of SMV have been limited to date. Such information as is available (Hull *et al.*, 1972) has been assembled in Table IV. The high incidence of 93% in adult spider monkeys, and the low of 18% in squirrel monkeys, are the most significant in respect to the number of sera examined. These data provided the evidence for the spider monkey to be the natural host for SMV, but also revealed that other South American species probably are susceptible, and occasionally become infected with SMV. Every serum which neutralized SMV, also neutralized *H.tamarinus*. Only a few of the squirrel monkey sera neutralized *H.tamarinus* alone.

V. Epidemiological Features

A. Effects of Stress and Latency

Some of the epidemiological features of these simian herpesviruses have been alluded to in the foregoing discussion. In some instances, active or clinical expression of infection in the native host has been induced by stress or trauma. Evidence for this in respect to *H.simiae* in rhesus monkeys, SA_8 in vervet monkeys, and *H.tamarinus* in squirrel monkeys has been cited. The stress of capture and crowding no doubt not only activates latent infections in some animals, but promotes the spread of the infection to others. The fact that some of these viruses (*H.simiae*, *H.tamarinus*, and THV) have been recovered from normal healthy animals, as well as from such animals' tissues cultivated *in vitro*, attests to the fact that they are carried as latent or silent

TABLE IV
PREVALENCE OF SMV NEUTRALIZING ANTIBODY IN SOUTH AMERICAN SUBHUMAN PRIMATES

Species	No. tested	No. positive	% positive
Adult spider monkeys	14	13	93
Juvenile spider monkeys	5	2	40
Squirrel monkeys	27	5	18
Capuchin monkeys	12	5	42

infections in their natural hosts. It is assumed, but not yet demonstrated experimentally, that these latent infections, in some animals, may result in a recurrent type disease such as is seen in man with herpes simplex virus infection.

B. Modes of Transmission

The mode of transmission of these viruses, whether within the species, or to foreign species, must be through direct contact with infected (active or silent) animals, or by virus contaminated fomites. Virus is present in saliva, vesicular fluids, conjunctival exudates, and possibly the stool of clinically infected animals. It also may be present in the saliva or stools of animals showing no overt disease. Evidence for the necessity of direct, or fairly close contact, between rhesus monkeys for the spread of *H.simiae* was provided in the report of DiGiacomo and Shah (1972). These investigators emphasized the housing of monkeys in individual cages as a means of controlling the spread of *H.simiae* in their colony. They noted, however, that this practice did not reduce incidence of antibody to respiratory viruses. Keeble (1960) and Hull (1968b) have made similar observations on the reduced incidence of *H.simiae* in animals held in separate cages.

VI. Diagnosis of Simian Infections

A. Clinical Features and Species Specificity

Diagnosis of herpetic infections in simian populations are based, first, on the clinical features which tend to distinguish these infections from those with other etiology. Principally, these include vesicular and ulcerated lesions, CNS system involvement, and keratoconjunctivitis. The latter is not necessarily indicative of a herpesvirus infection nor are certain respiratory symptoms, but both can occur. The species involved and history of possible exposure to other species should give the first indication as to the type of herpesvirus which might be responsible for the infection. Among South American species there is little reason to suspect *H.simiae* or SA_8 involvement although to date, the susceptibility of these species to these viruses has not been determined. *Herpesvirus tamarinus*, SMV, and herpes simplex viruses, however, must be considered. No herpesvirus other than *H.simiae* has been isolated from the Asiatic *Macaca* monkeys; thus, it should be the prime suspect in infections in these species. No information is available regarding the susceptibility of or of natural disease in Asiatic gibbons to *H.simiae*, but the susceptibility of this species to herpes simplex virus has been noted. Because of their geographic area of origin, however, possible *H.simiae* infection should be considered along with that of herpes simplex. Naturally occurring overt herpetic infections in African subhuman primates has not been reported except for the cell-associated varicella-like herpesvirus, LVV, (Table I). If such an infection should occur, SA_8 virus must be considered first, but the possibility of other etiological agents cannot be ignored.

B. Laboratory

1. Virus Isolation and Identification

The most certain diagnosis, in any case, can be made only by isolation and identification of the infecting virus. This can best be accomplished by the inoculation of vesicular fluids or tissue homogenates into appropriate tissue cultures. Cultures of choice, due to their uniformly high susceptibility to all of the simian herpesviruses, are primary vervet monkey, or rabbit kidney cells, or established strains of these cells such as BS-C-1 (Hopps *et al.*, 1963) and LLC-RK_1 (Hull *et al.*, 1965). Animal inoculation is less certain. It is more expensive and dangerous than the use of tissue culture, and a variety of animals would need to be inoculated because of differences in susceptibility to these viruses. Some indication of the possible identity of the virus may be gained at the time of virus isolation if cell cultures of various types are employed (Hull *et al.*, 1972). *Herpesvirus tamarinus*, SMV, and herpes simplex viruses, for example, will not grow in rhesus monkey kidney cells, and SA_8 virus does not grow in human amnion cells. All of the viruses, as noted above, proliferated in vervet monkey and rabbit kidney cells, but *H. simiae* is the only member of the group which can be cultivated in all the cell types mentioned. The cytopathic effects produced by these viruses are typical of herpesviruses, i.e., enlarged, giant cells with multinucleation are seen, generally in clusters or as foci of infection which enlarge to involve the entire cell sheet. In fixed and stained preparations the class A eosinophilic intranuclear inclusions are prominent.

Once the isolation has been made and a virus pool of known titer prepared, the virus is best identified by quantitative serum neutralization tests employing antisera for all the simian herpesviruses and for herpes simplex. The extent of this testing may be reduced when it is certain that no cross infection between Old and New World species might have occurred. If only New World species are involved, then it is necessary to test the isolate against *H. tamarinus*, SMV, and herpes simplex antisera. An Old World monkey isolate should be assayed against *H. simiae*, SA_8, and herpes simplex antisera. The antigenic similarity of these viruses has been pointed out on numerous occasions (Hull, 1968a; Hull *et al.*, 1972). The most specific antisera are produced in guinea pigs inoculated with formalin-inactivated viruses. Guinea pigs respond better to these antigens than do rabbits, and the degree of cross reaction appears to be lower when inactivated antigens are employed. *Herpesvirus simiae*, SA_8, and herpes simplex virus form one antigenic group; while *H. tamarinus* and SMV, constitute a second group. There is little difficulty with cross reactions between members of the two groups. Perhaps the least degree of cross reactions which might be anticipated among the viruses of a given group was seen in the sera employed in the cross neutralization test data presented in Table V. These data show why it is imperative that more than one serum be used and why the sera must be titered to extinction. When, or if, the results of cross neutralization tests leave the identity of an isolate in doubt it may be necessary to perform animal infectivity tests and to pool the information gained from growth in tissue culture, neutralization tests, and animal infectivity in order to arrive at the final identification.

2. Serological Diagnosis

Diagnosis by serological methods alone is extremely difficult, in many cases, even if paired sera are available. The extensive cross reactions in simian sera (presumably following natural infection) reported by Kalter and Heberling (1971) and by Hull *et al.*, (1972) attests to this fact. An attempt to experimentally infect a vervet monkey with SA_8 virus was described above (Section III, B,2,a), and it was noted that specific antibody rose from a level of positive in undiluted preinoculation serum, to 1 : 1024 in the postinfection specimen. The preinoculation serum from this same animal also neutralized *H. simiae* and herpes simplex when undiluted, but the postinoculation serum

TABLE V
Cross-Neutralization within Two Antigenic Groups of Simian Herpesviruses

Viruses	Sera: *H. simiae*[a]	Sera: SA_8[a]	Sera: *H. simplex*[a]
H. simiae	64	32	< 8
SA_8	16	256	8
H. simplex	32	64	< 1024
	H. tamarinus		SMV
H. tamarinus	2048		16
SMV	32		128

[a] Reciprocal of serum dilution.

had titers of greater than 1:2048 for *H. simiae*, and for herpes simplex. Thus, with these data, alone, it would be impossible to deduce that the infecting agent was SA_8 virus. In further pursuit of this problem two additional vervet monkeys were inoculated intramuscularly with 10^6 $TCID_{50}$ of herpes simplex virus (Hull, 1972). Preinoculation sera were antibody negative for herpes simplex, *H. simiae*, and SA_8 viruses at the 1:2 level. No evidence of disease was observed in these animals, but both developed a herpes simplex antibody titer in postinoculation sera of 1:64. The postinoculation sera had a 1:4 SA_8 neutralization titer, but failed to neutralize *H. simiae*. Thus, animals whose sera have high neutralizing antibody titers to all three of these viruses probably have not experienced infection with herpes simplex, but more likely, with SA_8 or *H. simiae*.

A similar problem exists with *H. tamarinus* and SMV in that animals infected either experimentally or naturally, with SMV develop antibody against both viruses. Only an occasional high-titered *H. tamarinus* antiserum will show a low level of cross reaction with SMV. Thus, one must proceed cautiously with this knowledge in attempting to diagnose herpesvirus infections in simians by serological methods. These same precautions apply to diagnosis of herpesvirus infections in man, as will be seen in Sections VIII–XIII.

VII. Prevention and Control

A. Procurement and Husbandry

The prevention and control of herpesvirus infections in laboratory simian populations can best be effected by good procurement and husbandry practices. This has been amply demonstrated in the foregoing discussions of the effects of stress, caging, and isolation of species on morbidity and transmission rates. Natural immunity exists in some cases due to nonspecific species immunity and to specific immunity induced by prior infection, either with the specific virus or with an antigenically similar virus. Latency, or even recurrent infection, may exist in these naturally immune animals, and, as such, they may constitute a threat to other nonimmune members of the group. If the facilities are available to do so, it would be wise to identify these immune (antibody-positive) animals and to house them in isolated quarters.

B. Active Immunization

Active immunization against infections by herpesviruses in laboratory primates has not been practiced. An experimental, inactivated vaccine, for use against *H. simiae* in man has been developed, but has been tested only once in rhesus monkeys (Hull and Nash, 1960). Well-conditioned, antibody-negative monkeys responded to this vaccine, but an attempt to evaluate its use in newly trapped animals in India failed, due to the poor condition of the animals and to a high death rate during their transportation to the United States. Daniel and Melendez (1970) have experimented with a live virus vaccine for *H. tamarinus* virus. A small-plaque variant was isolated which was avirulent for mice, hamsters, owl monkeys, and marmosets. Inoculation with this avirulent virus was reported to protect these species against direct challenge with the virulent parent strain. A live-virus vaccine would have one draw back, in that, if immunized animals were to be used as a source of tissue cultures, it is likely that the virus would appear as a latent agent in the cell cultures. If good vaccines were developed, they would be especially useful in the Primate Centers, or similar institutions, where laboratory rearing of subhuman primates is being practiced. In general, to attempt to carry out an effective immunization program in animals trapped in the wild against viruses indigenous to these species seems to be less likely to succeed because of the high incidences of infection prior to capture. Immunization of marmosets, or owl monkeys, however, against *H. Tamarinus* infection before possible exposure to squirrel monkeys, and hence exposure to the virus, in laboratories which employ both species would seem justified. One might include immunization against SMV and herpes simplex in these species if suitable antigens were available.

VIII. Simian Herpesviruses as Zoonotic Agents

A. Known Human Pathogens

The pathogenicity of B virus, or *H. simiae*, for man is well known, and this section deals almost exclusively with this virus. With but one possible exception, there are no recorded human infections with any of the other simian herpesviruses. Brief mention was made in an editorial (Schrier, 1966) that a research worker, who had been in contact with squirrel monkeys, developed an encephalitis, but was recovering. Reportedly, a rising titer to *H. tamarinus* virus was demonstrated in his serum. No attempt was made to isolate a virus. There was a suggestion, therefore, that *H. tamarinus* virus might have been involved. If this case truly represented a human infection with *H. tamarinus* virus, then one might speculate that this virus is somewhat less virulent for man than is *H. simiae*, and that the possibility of overt infection is rather remote in respect to the high frequency of infection in squirrel monkeys and to the numbers of these animals which have been used in research laboratories in recent years, enhancing the possible exposure of man to this virus. The number of cases of human infection with *H. simiae*, is also low in respect to the possibilities of exposure; however, a high percentage of humans have naturally occurring antibodies to *H. simiae*, which, in part, may explain this. There are no reports of serological surveys of human populations for *H. tamarinus* antibody.

B. *Speculation*

If *H. tamarinus* virus does possess some degree of virulence for man, then SMV should equally be regarded as a possible human pathogen, in view of the common virulence of these two viruses for laboratory primates and small animals. It is risky to speculate about the possible susceptibility, or resistance, of a species to a given virus based on the ability of the virus to propagate in cells of the species grown in tissue culture. *Herpesvirus tamarinus* and SMV, as well as *H. simiae*, grow and produce lethal cytopathology in several types of cultured human cells. SA_8 virus, however, does not do so in a human amnion cell strain, but the susceptibility of other cell types, such as human diploid fibroblasts or kidney cells, has not been investigated. SA_8 virus, also, has less virulence for laboratory animals than do the other members of this group. With the present limited knowledge, however, it is wise to consider all of these viruses as potentially dangerous to man.

IX. Epidemiologic Features of *H. simiae* Infection in Man

A. *Case Incidence*

At least 20 possible human infections with *H. simiae* have been recognized to date; however, only 10 of these have been confirmed by virus isolation and identification. Two other cases received partial confirmation by serological methods. Soper (1959) reviewed 15 cases, and mentioned a possible sixteenth case. Seven of these were confirmed by virus isolation, but only 7 of these possible 16 cases have been described in the literature, 3 of which were reported subsequent to Soper's review. The seventeenth case was reported by Love and Jungherr (1962). The eighteenth case is described below for the first time. Sumner-Smith (1966) described the nineteenth case which involved an African green monkey, but which had been exposed to rhesus monkeys. The twentieth, and most recent case, is reported below. Seventeen of these possible 20 cases resulted in fatalities.

B. *Descriptions of Two Previously Unreported Cases*

1. Case No. 18

A 53-year-old white male was caring for both rhesus and African green monkeys, but predominantly the latter. Fifty months prior to onset of symptoms, and before any association with either species of monkey, this individual was antibody-negative for *H. simiae*, SA_8, and herpes simplex viruses (Table VII). On approximately March 15 he complained of a respiratory infection. The infection persisted, and on March 30, he visited an Industrial Medicine Department because of this "cold-like" disease. The condition continued, increasing in severity, until April 6, when he showed signs of incoherence and was absent from work until April 13. On this latter date, he developed paralysis and was hospitalized. On April 14, while in the hospital, vesicular lesions were noted on the shoulder and on the thigh. The patient was comatose at this time, and he remained essentially in this state until his death, 3 years and 4 months from date of onset (J. H. Brown, personal communication, 1963).

Fluids aspirated from a vesicle on the shoulder yielded a herpeslike virus when inoculated into primary rabbit kidney, and LLC-RK_1 cells. No virus was recovered from spinal fluid collected on May 6. Attempts to identify the isolate by serum neutralization tests were somewhat inconclusive due to extensive cross reactions among the isolate, *H. simiae*, and SA_8 viruses. A one-way cross neutralization was obtained when the isolate was compared with herpes simplex virus, with the isolate being the dominant antigen. This is the type of cross neutralization which is generally seen when antiserum is prepared against live *H. simiae* virus. These serological data are presented in Table VI. As noted in the table, *H. simiae* antiserum failed to neutralize SA_8 virus in these tests. This, however, is not a common finding as can be seen by examination of data in Table V. These tests, therefore, failed to clearly identify the isolate as either *H. simiae* or SA_8 virus.

TABLE VI
CROSS-NEUTRALIZATION REACTIONS BETWEEN TWO SUSPECTED *H. simiae* ISOLATES AND OTHER RECOGNIZED HERPESVIRUSES

	Sera				
Viruses	Anti-18[a]	Anti-20	Anti-*H. simiae*[a]	Anti-SA_8[a]	Anti-herpes simplex[a]
Case 18	16	—[b]	16	16	<4
H. simiae	32	—	64	32	4
SA_8	16	—	<4	64	4
H. simplex	32	—	4	32	256
Case 20	—[b]	32	64	8	<4
H. simiae	—	64	128	64	<4
SA_8	—	16	8	256	4
Herpes simplex	—	8	4	32	256

[a]Reciprocal of serum dilution.
[b]Not tested.

Attempts to diagnose the cause of infection by serological methods proved equally as frustrating. As seen in Table VII, the patient had no neutralizing antibody to any of these viruses 50 months prior to onset of symptoms. The serum sample obtained after 2 months of infection neutralized all four viruses at essentially the same level. From previous experience (Hull *et al.*, 1962), it seemed very unlikely, however, that an individual with a natural herpes simplex antibody titer of only 1:32 would neutralize the two heterologous herpes viruses to levels comparable to the homologous virus. This, again, tended to minimize the possibility of a herpes simplex infection, but did not resolve the problem of distinguishing between *H. simiae* and SA_8 viruses.

The patient's virus was virulent for mice and rabbits, producing infection in the latter which was indistinguishable from that produced by *H. simiae*. As seen in Section III,B,2, SA_8 virus lacked virulence for these animals. Furtheremore, SA_8 virus never has been proved to be a human pathogen. Considering all data, this case was considered to represent an infection caused by *H. simiae* and is included among the confirmed cases in Table VIII (Hull, 1972).

2. Case No. 20

A complete clinical history of Case No. 20 has not been reported, nor is it the intent to do so at this time. A summary of the patient's history and of the onset of infection has been provided by Lennette and Emmons (1970). The patient, a 62-year-old, distinguished virologist, at the time of his illness, was engaged in research activities which did not involve the use of monkeys or monkey tissue cultures. The only primary monkey kidney cultures used in his institute during a period of 1 year and 5 months prior to his onset of infection had been purchased from a commercial supplier, who monitored such cultures for contaminating herpesviruses. All of eight lots purchased were found to be free of such agents. The patient, however, was not known to have used any of these cultures during an immediate period prior to his

TABLE VII
Neutralization Test Data Obtained from Two Different Serum Samples from a Suspected *H. simiae* Infection (Case No. 18)

Serum samples	Viruses			
	No. 18[a]	*H. simiae*[a]	SA_8[a]	*H. simplex*[a]
50 months before onset	<4	<4	<4	<4
2 months after onset	16	32	16	32

[a]Reciprocal of serum dilutions.

illness. The onset of illness was about March 1, and consisted of skin lesions (vesicles) and neuralgia of the face plus weeping eyes. At the time, it was thought to be typical of herpes zoster infection. During the next 2 weeks, however, additional lesions appeared on the chest, and bladder weakness, followed by urinary retention, and a slowly developing Landry-type paralysis was observed. A left-side paralysis progressed to a bilateral paralysis of the trunk and arms, and the patient became semicomatose. A tracheaotomy was necessary on March 26. By mid-April his condition was essentially stable, but with extensive paralysis, and respiration was assisted with a Bennett machine. The patient has been hospitalized and treated in various institutions, and, currently, 2 years after onset, he is alive and residing in a nursing home. The extent of the sequelae and the present condition of the patient is unknown to the author.

A virus was isolated from fluid aspirated from a vesicular lesion on the chest using human embryo kidney cell cultures (V. L. Bazeley, personal communication, 1970). Virus passed from these cultures to HeLa, BS-C-1, and additional human embryo kidney cells produced a herpetic-type cytopathology as early as 24 hours after inoculation. This was quite unlike the characteristics of herpes zoster virus in tissue culture. Fluorescence antibody studies performed on infected cell cultures indicated that the virus belonged in the herpesvirus group (Lennette and Emmons, 1970).

Attempts to identify the virus by cross neutralization tests met with some of the same cross reaction problems as described for the virus recovered from case No. 18; however, the patient's virus proved to be antigenically more closely related to *H. simiae* than to SA_8 virus. The results of one such test are seen in the lower portion of Table VI. These findings essentially eliminated a possible identification of the agent as herpes simplex virus. Cross neutralization between the isolate and *H. simiae* was reciprocal within the limits of a twofold serum dilution. Antiserum to the isolate neutralized twice as much homologous virus as SA_8, but SA_8 antiserum only neutralized the patient's virus to a 1:8 titer while it neutralized SA_8 to a 1:256 titer. Based on these results, the agent was tentatively identified as *H. simiae*.

TABLE VIII
POSSIBLE SOURCES OF INFECTION IN *H. simiae* CONFIRMED AND TOTAL CASES

Source	Confirmed cases	Total suspected cases
Bites (fairly certain)	1	4
Bites (possibly)	0	4
Laboratory accidents	3	3
Unknown	6	9

Serological diagnosis was aided by the availability of two preinfection serum samples and by multiple postinfection specimens. The results of neutralization tests performed on these sera are presented in Table IX. No antibody titer for *H. simiae* was detected in either of the preinfection sera, while very low levels (1:8 to 1:16) of herpes simplex antibody were present. The most significant finding was a rise in titer against *H. simiae* from 1:32 in onset serum, to 1:256 in a sample obtained 28 days later. Although antibody titers for SA_8 and herpes simplex were fairly high in the onset serum, no further significant increases occurred. Thus, these data tended further to confirm the *H. simiae* virus etiology in this case (Hull, 1972).

The virus was further characterized through animal virulence studies. Suckling mice inoculated intracerebrally became paralyzed on the third day, and died at 4–6 days. Brain tissues from these animals were positive for herpes-group antigen by fluorescence antibody staining. Adult mice were resistant. The virus behaved in rabbits much as *H. simiae*, although such studies were very limited.

The combined clinical and laboratory data strongly supported a diagnosis of *H. simiae* infection. This case, also, is included amongst the "confirmed" cases in Table VIII. Of greatest concern in this case, from an epidemiological point of view, was the failure to determine a possible source of infection. This was investigated more extensively by a committee of experts in this area, but no further suggestion of a source of infection was uncovered. Numerous biological reagents (cultures, sera, antigens, etc.) used in the patient's laboratory were tested for evidence of *H. simiae* contamination, but to no avail. The institute in which the patient was employed housed a colony of five rhesus monkeys. Sera from each of these animals neutralized *H. simiae*

TABLE IX

NEUTRALIZATION TEST DATA OBTAINED FROM SERIAL BLEEDINGS OF A SUSPECTED *H. simiae* INFECTION (CASE NO. 20)

	Viruses			
Serum Samples	No. 20	*H. simiae*	SA_8	*H. simplex*
50 months before onset	—[a]	<4	64[c]	16
13 months before onset	<4[b]	<4	<4	8
Onset	—	32	>128[c]	256
5 days after onset	—	8	>128[c]	256
20 days after onset	—	128	>512[c]	4096[d]
28 days after onset	64	256	128	256

[a] Not tested.
[b] Reciprocal of serum dilution.
[c] Very weak virus challenge dose employed.
[d] Human gamma globulin given prior to bleeding.

in titers ranging from 1:4 to greater than 1:64. These animals, therefore, constituted a possible local source of *H. simiae* virus, but there was no known contact between these animals and the patient. A group of thirteen squirrel monkeys also were housed in the institute, and all of these were antibody negative, except for one which neutralized *H. simiae* at 1:4 (Hull, 1972).

This patient had a long career in virus research, and had used monkeys and monkey cell cultures on many occasions in his research work over the years. This, plus the lack of an apparent source of recent infection, raises the very serious question of the possibility of *H. simiae* virus infection remaining dormant or latent, for long periods of time before clinical expression. The source of infection in approximately half of the suspected cases, (Section IX, C and Table VIII) was not determined; however, in these other cases the individuals did have known contact with monkeys.

C. Source of Infection

The first case reported by Sabin and Wright (1934) followed the bite of a rhesus monkey, and for a number of years this was considered to be the chief source of infection. A review of the total experience to date, however, does not substantiate this. Table VIII shows the available information relating to the source of infection, both for the cases confirmed by virus isolation and for the total number of cases. Four of the 20 suspected cases were associated with monkey bites, and four others possibly followed bites, but in nine, or nearly 50%, the source of infection remained unknown. Of the laboratory-confirmed cases, only Sabin's original case could be attributed to monkey bite. Of those eight cases possibly following monkey bites, four rhesus, three Asiatic cynomolgus, and one African green monkeys were involved. The nine cases with completely unknown sources of infection create the greatest concern to the laboratory investigator, since they create doubts as to the protective measures which should be taken to prevent such infections. All but one of these individuals, however, had known exposure to monkey populations, although no bites or other accidents could be immediately associated with their disease. The one exception is represented by the most recent case described above (No. 20).

The three cases listed in Table VIII associated with laboratory accidents include Sabin's (1949) second reported case, in which a minor cut on the finger of a physician was contaminated with saliva from a rhesus monkey, and the case of a laboratory technician who cut his finger on a broken culture flask containing primary monkey kidney cells (Hummeler *et al.*, 1959). The remaining case, according to Soper (1959) occurred in a postdoctoral student who was processing a monkey skull for study.

There has been no report of *H. simiae* tramsmission from man to man such as occurred in the "Marburg virus" cases (Martini, 1969), but there is every reason to believe that such transmission could occur. The infected human, or his tissues, probably presents the same degree of danger as does the infected monkey. Suspected cases, therefore, should be placed in strict isolation, and the greatest of care should be taken in handling potentially contaminated fomites, instruments, and other equipment coming in contact with the patient. Strict aseptic procedures should be employed during post-mortems performed on such patients, and adequate decontamination procedures should be used following completion of the examination.

D. Factors Relevant to Virus Transmission

Factors which influence the possible transmission of *H. simiae* infection to man are much like those associated with any infectious disease, i.e., source of infection, exposure, infecting dose, susceptibility of exposed host. The source of the virus must be infected monkeys or their tissues (active or latent), and, as indicated in Section VIII, these probably will be only Asiatic *Macaca* monkeys, or other species which have acquired the infection through prior contact with *Macaca* monkeys. The incidence of infection, or virus shedding in any group of monkeys, at the extreme, probably does not exceed 2–3% (Section IV,A). In established colonies, the incidence of infection at any point in time is likely to be much lower. Thus, the relative availability of the virus is important to the probability of human exposure. Based on rabbit experiments, the virus cannot penetrate the intact skin; thus, it must be introduced through wounds via the mouth, respiratory tract, or the eye. Virus is shed in the throat (saliva), vesicular fluids, conjunctival exudates, and, possibly, the urine and stool. It also may be present in blood, tissues, or tissue cultures of monkey cells. Exposure might be through direct contact with a virus-shedding animal (bites, scrathces, etc.), by contact with virus-contaminated fomites, or by contact with tissues containing virus. The virus is relatively unstable and does not persist for long periods (days), especially if drying occurs. Experimental animals have been infected by artificially prepared aerosols (Chappell, 1960), but it is doubtful that the virus is spread within a monkey colony by an airborne route as is the case with respiratory viruses (Section IV,A). Several of the human cases, however, had onset symptoms of respiratory disease; thus, the possibility of airborne infection must not be overlooked, however improbable it may seem.

The concentration of virus received may be a determinate of whether infection will follow, both in respect to nonspecific species' resistance and to naturally acquired active immunity. Human cells in tissue culture are less sensitive to *H. simiae* than are rabbit or monkey cells; thus, there exists the possibility that man, himself, might be less susceptible. A large proportion of adults have antibody to *H. simiae*, as will be discussed below; thus, the dose of virus necessary to produce an infection may be dependent upon these factors.

Several surveys for *H. simiae* antibody in human populations have been reported in the literature. Melnick and Banker (1954) tested 40 sera from Indians in the Bombay area, and found 11, or 27.5%, to possess *H. simiae* antibody; while 50% of the same group were antibody-positive for herpes simplex virus. Of the individuals in this group, however, 44% who were over 20 years of age were positive for *H. simiae* antibody. Two lots of USP human gamma globulin also were found to possess *H. simiae* antibody. In a group of 129 adult United States citizens, some of whom had been in contact with Asiatic monkeys, Hull *et al.* (1962) found 81.5% to be antibody-positive for herpes simplex, and 49.7%, for *H. simiae*. The percentage of sera containing both antibodies was highest when herpes simplex titers were 1:128 or greater. No herpes simplex antibody-negative sera contained *H. simiae* antibody. In a smaller sample of 13 human sera, Van Hoosier and Melnick (1961) found 8 containing *H. simiae* antibody, while all 13 neutralized herpes simplex. Cabasso *et al.* (1967) found 69% of 113 human sera to be positive for *H. simiae*, and 83% of the same samples contained herpes simplex antibody. These authors also found that the incidence of antibody to both viruses increased with age and that the presence, and levels, of *H. simiae* antibody were dependent upon the corresponding levels of herpes simplex antibody. There was no difference in the incidence of antibody to *H. simiae* in people who had, or had not, been in contact with monkeys. Four lots of human gamma globulin neutralized *H. simiae* and herpes simplex, and one lot had a higher titer for *H. simiae* than for herpes simplex. It is an established fact, therefore, that approximately 50% of the adult population have naturally acquired *H. simiae* antibody. This antibody was obtained as a heterologous response to infection with the antigenically related herpes simplex virus. There has been no evidence of subclinical infections in man with *H. simiae* virus.

If data obtained from rabbit experiments (Hull, 1971) can be extrapolated to man, then this naturally acquired antibody to *H. simiae* can be considered to be protective. Some rabbits infected with herpes simplex virus, or hyperimmunized with inactivated herpes simplex antigen (Hull and Peck, 1967), develop low levels of heterologous, *H. simiae* antibody comparable to those seen in man. These rabbits are solidly immune to direct challenge with *H. simiae* virus. Rabbits which do not develop *H. simiae* antibody, however, are susceptible to virus challenge, regardless of their levels of herpes simplex antibody. The low incidence of human infection with *H. simiae* lends credibility to this assumption.

X. Pathogenesis in Man

The tissues and organs involved in *H.simiae* infection, or the sequence of involvement, varies with the portal of entry of the virus. In infections incurred through breaks in skin (bites or wound contamination), the initial reaction was the development of vesicular lesions at the site of entry. The virus spread to regional lymph nodes producing a lymphadenopathy. Virus spreads to other organs and to the central nervous systems, but definitive information relating to the route(s) of this spread has not been elaborated. Viremia occurs in both rabbits and monkeys, and it probably occurs in man, but spread along nerve pathways must be considered and has been suggested in some cases. The fact that the abdominal viscera are involved and that virus has been isolated from these tissues procured at postmortem further suggests that virus may be disseminated via the blood or lymphatics. Hyperemia or congestion and focal necrosis of lymph nodes, heart and pericardium, spleen, liver, kidneys, adrenals, and lungs may occur, but has not been seen in every infection. The central nervous system, and especially the spinal cord and the medulla, has been the site of the most severe pathological changes; these changes include hyperemia, edema, inflammatory exudates (mostly mononuclear), perivascular round cell cuffing, and degeneration of motor neurons. The class A intranuclear inclusion bodies may be difficult to discern, especially if the infection has been of long duration.

The early symptoms in at least two cases were those of severe respiratory infection with evidence of pneumonitis. In one instance, the patient later developed a vesicle on his shoulder which yielded *H.simiae* on isolation attempts. Central nervous system disease of the general type described above follows the respiratory tract infection.

XI. Clinical Features

A. Symptomatology

Although a variety of clinical symptoms have been observed, the infection in man has followed two, or possibly three, general patterns. These are determined, at least, in part, by the portal of entry and the further dissemination of the virus. When infection was initiated through breaks in the skin (bites, scratches, cuts), local vesicular lesions appeared within 3–4 days at the site with regional lymphadenopathy. Additional vesicular lesions have occurred at other sites. A low-grade fever may be present at this stage of infection. Various signs and symptoms may be observed prior to, or along with, the onset of frank neurological symptoms. These include muscle pain, vomiting and intestinal cramps, stiff neck, difficulty in swallowing, photophobia, nystagmus, diplopia, and general malaise. Hyperesthesia or paresthesis of the limbs generally preceded weakness, loss of reflexes, and flaccid paralysis. Urinary retention was a marked feature at this stage of infection. Temperature elevation may be associated with the onset of neurological disorder. A transverse myelitis has been recognized at this point that ascended with an accompanying spread of paralysis. Mental competency has been fairly well retained in many of these cases, suggesting minimal cerebral involvement at this point of the infection. Depression of respiration occurred with the advancing paralysis. As brain involvement increased, the patients become comatose, some exhibiting convulsions, and cyanosis, with death occurring due to respiratory failure.

The clinical syndrome in at least two cases varied from the above-mentioned normal course since, the onset symptoms were those of a respiratory infection. It seems likely that the portal of entry in these cases was by this route. Symptoms included cough, sore throat, chest pains, and consolidation of the lungs, or a portion of the lungs. Chills, fever, and headache may be associated with these symptoms. One individual was said to have blisters in his throat. The interval between these onset symptoms, and the first evidence of neurological involvement was rather long, 3–4 weeks. In both instances, neurological disease and paralysis progressed very rapidly, and one patient died within 5 days. The other elapsed into a comma the following day and remained essentially in this state until he died 3 years later.

A third type of clinical onset was seen in the most recent case which has been described above (Section IX,B,2). Skin lesions and neuralgia of the face, plus weeping eyes, suggested a typical herpes zoster infection. The zosterlike vesicles spread to the chest, followed by bladder weakness and ascending spinal paralysis.

B. Incubation Periods

Due to the questionable source of infection in many of the suspected cases and to limited available case descriptions, it is difficult to assign finite incubation periods to *H.simiae* infection in man. The lack of such information in a number of cases, in fact, presents the alarming possibility that incubation periods might be quite long, or that the virus may have remained latent for periods of time before manifesting itself through overt disease. In Sabin's (Sabin and Wright, 1934) original case, local phenomena were observed 3 days after a monkey bite, the patient requiring hospitalization on the sixth day and death occurring 17 days following the monkey bite. No other case has been so well documented. In the case reported by Breen *et al.* (1958) the patient's first symptom occurred 13 days after bites from two monkeys, muscle weakness was reported on the nineteenth day, and the patient was hospitalized on the twentieth day. This patient recovered, however, and within 6–7 months was walking with aid of elbow crutches. One case, believed to have followed infection from a cut inflicted by a broken culture flask (Hummeler *et al.*, 1959) had an onset 2 days after the incident, although a prior episode of similar nature occurred 56 days before onset. This fatal infection terminated after a course of 22 days. In another case involving a monkey bite (Sumner-Smith, 1966), the onset of symptoms occurred 24 days later, and the case terminated in death on the thirty-fourth day after the presumed exposure. Thus, in these four cases in which the time of exposure was fairly well documented, the onset occurred between 3 and 24 days after exposure, while the first signs of neurological involvement were recognized between the fifteenth and about the twenty-fifth day of illnesses. Hummeler *et al.* (1959) described another case that probably followed monkey bites. This patient had a history of receiving bites 35, 80, and 158 days prior to the onset of his illness. Neurological symptoms developed 7 days after onset of the illness and death occurred on the twenty-fifth day.

As mentioned above, those cases for which the sources of infections were undetermined, and, therefore, the incubation periods undefinable, cause the greatest concern. One very rapidly progressing and fatal case occurred in a laboratory worker whose last recorded monkey bite, or accident, happened 4 months prior to the onset of his disease (Pierce *et al.*, 1958). In the case reported by Nagler and Klotz (1958), the patient had been engaged in rhesus monkey inoculation and autopsy, but had no history of bite or injury related to his work. Love and Jungherr (1962) describe a *H.simiae* infection in a man who had worked with monkeys for only 21 days prior to onset of illness, but who had no history of bites or accidents. This patient, however, did receive smallpox immunization 5 days before the onset of his illness. An immune reaction was noted on the first day of his illness, but there was no mention of vesicles or other evidence of infection at the site of his vaccination. In these, and other similar cases, the incubation period could not be determined, but all subjects were engaged in activities carrying the possibility of exposure. The most recent case, however, was seen in a research scientist who had had no known recent exposure to monkeys, or monkey tissue cultures (Section IX, B, 2).

C. Postmortem Findings

The most significant changes in the majority of the reported cases have been seen in the tissues of the central nervous system, the spinal cord and medulla showing the most extensive involvement. In the cord, the picture is that of a transverse meylitis which may also involve the regional ganglia. The lesions are a nonspecific type common to virus infections of the central nervous system. These include hemorrhagic foci, necrosis, inflammatory exudates, edema, and degeneration of motor neurons. Focal areas of demyelinization were reported in one case. Perivascular cuffing and infiltration with mononuclear and polymorphonuclear inflammatory cells may be seen in both brain and cord sections. The class A eosinophilic intranuclear inclusions, typical of herpesvirus infection, rarely have been seen in these cases. One case in which inclusions were reported (Pierce *et al.*, 1958) represented a very rapidly terminating case in which death occurred 3 days after onset. The disease has been represented as myelitis, encephalomyelitis, and encephalitis in individual cases.

As mentioned previously, the infection may involve a number of organs and tissues in addition to the central nervous system. These include most of the thoracic and abdominal viscera and lymph nodes. Changes in these tissues generally are represented by hyperemia and focal areas of hemorrhage and necrosis. The lungs may show a hemorrhagic pneumonic process.

XII. Clinical and Laboratory Diagnosis

A. Clinical

The possibility of *H. simiae* infection must be considered by the clinician when examining patients who have a history of exposure to, or association with, Asiatic *Macaca* monkeys, or other species if they have been housed or transported at any time with *Macaca* monkeys. This possibility becomes more probable if the patient has received bites or scratches, or has experienced a laboratory accident resulting in potential exposure to *H. simiae*. All further comment applies to patients with either of the above-mentioned histories. The obvious, or highly suspicious, case may be identified by the presence of herpetic-like vesicular lesions and regional lymphadenopathy. This is especially significant if the patient is not subject to recurrent herpes simplex infection, or if the lesions are anatomically located at sites other than those at which the recurrent herpes simplex lesions generally appeared. Neurological symptoms, other than actual paralysis, reflecting spinal cord or nerve injury such as paresthesis, muscle weakness or pain, nuchal rigidity, reduction in reflexes, abnormal gait, or impairment of coordination, either with or without accompanying vesicular lesions are suggestive of *H.simiae* infection in those patients with appropriate histories. Other neurological signs reflecting brain or cranial nerve involvement may be seen in the absence of myelic lesions. These may include facial neuralgia, delirium, temporary loss of consciousness, photophobia, nystagmus, and diplopia. Conjunctivitis alone has not been described as an initial symptom in any case to date; however, it would seem to be a possibility based upon animal studies. The onset of symptoms in some cases have been those of respiratory tract disease; and these cases, without other symptomatology, present a real problem to the diagnostician. The patient, however, with severe and persistent respiratory disease, and who does not respond to medication or other routine care, should be observed closely for the appearance of vesicular lesions and neurologic changes.

B. Aids to Laboratory Diagnosis

Serological diagnosis is difficult because of the antigenic similarity of certain of the simian herpesviruses and herpes simplex and because antibody to some members of this group are commonly found in the adult population. It is very helpful, therefore, to have preexposure, or preacute stage sera to compare with acute or convalescent samples. Thus, personnel working in areas where the threat of exposure exists, should be bled periodically and a bank of these frozen sterile serum samples maintained. Yearly serum samples from specific individuals would be satisfactory. Likewise, at the time of a known accident, such as monkey bite, a serum sample should be obtained and held for future reference. Sera should be collected aseptically and frozen immediately without heat inactivation.

C. Laboratory Diagnosis

1. VIRUS ISOLATION AND IDENTIFICATION

The recovery of a virus and its biologic and serologic identification as *H. simiae* provides the most convincing evidence of *H. simiae* infection. Procedures for virus isolation are essentially identical to those described for laboratory diagnosis of herpesvirus infections in simians (Section VI, B, 1). Appropriate specimens include vesicular fluids, tissue homogenates, and eye or throat swabs. Virus has been infrequently recovered from spinal fluids. An isolation was made from only 1 of 6 patients with confirmed infections (Pierce *et al.*, 1958). The methods for, and the problems associated with, the serologic identification of one of these herpesviruses isolated from man are the same as those outlined in (Section VI,B,1).

2. Serologic Diagnosis

The antigenic similarity of these viruses, as amply described in Section VI, B,2 presents the same problems to the serologic diagnosis of human infections as it does to those in monkeys. Most significant results can be obtained when preinfection serum and numerous post-onset specimens are available for assay. Examples of the value of such samples are seen in Tables VI and IX, and as described in Sections IX,B,1 and 2. The demonstration of a continuously rising titer to one of these viruses has diagnostic significance, while the finding of an approximately equal rise in titer to *H. simiae*, SA_8, and herpes simplex from preinfection to onset of infection, suggest that one of the two simian herpesviruses is involved rather than herpes simplex virus.

XIII. Preventive Measures

A. General Laboratory Techniques and Practices

Several authors have recommended laboratory practices which should be followed as precaution against *H. simiae* infection, both in monkeys and man (Perkins and Hartley 1966; Cole *et al.*, 1968; Hull, 1969). These consist mainly of adequate housing, isolation, and quarantine of new animals and the maintenance of barriers between animal and operator. Proper disinfection of cages before reuse, decontamination of all materials coming into contact with monkeys, and incineration of monkey carcasses has been stressed. All primary monkey cell cultures, as well as materials and equipment used in their preparation and maintenance, should be autoclaved before discarded. Strict aseptic technics, followed by proper disinfection, should be employed in all procedures such as inoculation, bleeding, physical examination, surgery, and postmortems. Immediate cleansing and routine care of wounds received has been emphasized, along with close follow-up of both the patient and monkey involved. In effect, the same procedures as normally employed when working with any known pathogen should be followed at all times, whether there is a suspicion of *H. simiae* infection or not. This suspicion, however, should always be in mind when dealing with Asiatic *Macaca* monkeys, and technicians and other personnel should be so advised. A further possible safeguard would be to employ only those people with natural *H. simiae* antibody in areas utilizing monkeys.

B. Passive Immunization

The use of hyperimmune serum, or gamma globulin, has not been shown to be effective in the treatment, or prevention, of human infection with *H. simiae* virus. Human gamma globulin has been administered to patients suspected of having *H. simiae* infection, and it has been demonstrated that most lots of human gamma globulin contain *H. simiae* antibody (Section IX, D). It is doubtful, however, that the levels of antibody in these preparations are adequate for protection or that the gamma globulin has been given soon enough after exposure to be beneficial. MacLeod *et al* (1960), demonstrated slight protection in rabbits by the administration of large doses of monkey gamma globulin concentrate within 1 hour of a minimal challenge with live virus. These authors also suggested that local infiltration of a wound with monkey gamma globulin within 10 minutes of infliction, might afford some protection against *H. simiae* infection. Buthala (1962b) prepared *H. simiae* hyperimmune horse and rabbit sera and employed these reagents in rabbit protection tests. Both sera showed evidence of protection against a challenge dose of 1000 PFU (plaque forming units) when infused immediately into the site of virus inoculation. Varying degrees of protection were seen when the antiserum treatment was delayed for periods of time and/or administered by different routes. The homologous serum was most effective, and serum titers were retained for 7 days. Serum antibody levels of the heterologous horse serum could not be detected by 36 hours after inoculation. Hull (1972) was unable to demonstrate any protection in rabbits treated with immune guinea pig serum by local infiltration of virus contaminated wounds, by intravenous inoculation, or by both, when serum treatment was initiated 15 minutes after exposure to virus. Levels of serum antibody, which were adequate to provide protection when actively acquired, were obtained following inoculation of guinea pig immune serum, but were ineffective. The duration of serum antibody levels was not determined, and it is likely that use of heterologous serum led to its rapid elimination from the circulation.

C. *Naturally Acquired Active Immunity*

As described in detail above (Section IX,D), approximately 50% of the adult population has naturally acquired *H. simiae* antibody, representing a heterologous response to prior infection with herpes simplex virus. The protective quality of this heterologous antibody in man has not been clearly demonstrated; however, in the few human cases where assays for pre-exposure antibody were reported none contained *H. simiae* antibody. It has been demonstrated, on the other hand, that *H. simiae* antibody produced in rabbits by hyperimmunization with herpes simplex virus is protective against direct challenge with *H. simiae* virus (Hull *et al.*, 1962). Thus, it is likely that naturally acquired antibody to *H. simiae* is protective. The very low incidence of infection in man further attests to this fact.

D. *Artificially Acquired Active Immunity*

Several reports have appeared in the literature describing attempts to prepare inactivated *H. simiae* vaccines (MacLeod *et al.*, 1960; Buthala,

1962a; Benda, 1965); however, only Hull and co-workers (Hull *et al.*, 1962, Hull and Peck, 1967; Hull and Nash, 1960; Hull, 1971) pursued the problem to the extent of clinical trials in man and, thus, to a possible licensed product for general use in persons at risk of exposure. Various degrees of success in the preparation of antigenic vaccines, through a variety of methods, were described in the other reports.

The vaccine most extensively studied has been referred to as B virus vaccine, and was prepared from virus propagated in primary rabbit kidney cell cultures. Serum-free culture supernatant fluids containing 10^6 to 10^8 $TCID_{50}/0.5$ ml of infectious virus, were clarified by filtration and inactivated with 1:400 (final dilution) formalin at 37°C. Extensive tests for residual live virus were negative. The vaccine stimulated antibody in a variety of experimental animals and was demonstrated to protect rabbits against severe challenge with live virus. Antibody levels equivalent to those found to be protective in rabbits have been produced in man; thus, if data obtained in rabbits can be extrapolated to man, it seems likely that immunization with this vaccine would provide protection to those persons who respond to the vaccine with antibody levels comparable to those seen in rabbits. In a group of approximately 300 persons immunized with this vaccine, and maintained on booster doses, the percentage of people without *H. simiae* antibody in prevaccination sera was reduced from about 50 to 20%, and the levels of antibody were generally enhanced. The 20% who failed to respond to immunization were essentially composed of the herpes simplex antibody-negative segment of this population. Many of these 300 subjects have been receiving this vaccine over a period of 12 years with no ill effects. Negotiations with the federal regulatory agency towards the eventual licensing of this vaccine have been instigated.

References

Benda, R. (1965). *J. Hyg., Epidemiol., Microbiol., Immunol.* **9**, 487.

Black, P. H., Hartley, J. W., and Rowe, W. P. (1963). *Proc. Soc. Exp. Biol. Med.* **112**, 601.

Breen, G. E., Lamb, S. G., and Otaki, A. T. (1958). *Brit. Med. J.* **2**, 22.

Buthala, D. A. (1962a). *J. Infec. Dis.* **111**, 95.

Buthala, D. A. (1962b). *J. Infec. Dis.* **111**, 101.

Cabasso, V. J., Chappell, W. A., Avampato, J. E., and Bittle, J. L. (1967). *J. Lab. Clin. Med.* **70**, 170.

Chappell, W. A. (1960). *Ann. N.Y. Acad. Sci.* **85**, 931.

Clarkson, M. J., Thorpe, E., and McCarthy, K. (1967). *Arch. Gesamte Virusforsch.* **22**, 219.

Cole, W. C., Bostrom, R. E., and Whitney, R. A., Jr. (1968). *J. Amer. Vet. Med. Ass.* **153**, 894.

Committee Report (1956). *Amer. J. Hyg.* **64**, 104.

Daniel, M. D., and Melendez, L. V. (1970). *Arch. Gesamte Virusforsch.* **32**, 45.

Daniel, M. D., Karpas, A., Melendez, L. V., King, N. W., and Hunt, R. D. (1967). *Arch. Gesamte Virusforsch.* **22**, 324.

DiGiacomo, R. F., and Shah, K. V. (1972). *Lab. Anim. Sci.* **22**, 61.
Emmons, R. W., and Lennette, E. H. (1970). *Arch. Gesamte Virusforsch.* **31**, 215.
Emmons, R. W., Gribble, D. H., and Lennette, E. H. (1968). *J. Infec. Dis.* **118**, 153.
Endo, M., Kamimura, T., Aoyama, Y., Hayashida, T., Kinjo, T., and Ono, Y. (1960). *Jap. J. Exp. Med.* **30**, 227.
Hartley, E. G. (1964). *Vet. Rec.* **76**, 555.
Holmes, A. W., Dedmon, R. E., and Deinhardt, F. (1963). *Fed. Proc., Fed. Amer. Soc. Exp. Biol.* **22**, 334.
Holmes, A. W., Caldwell, R. G., Dedmon, R. E., and Deinhardt, F. (1964). *J. Immunol.* **92**, 602.
Holmes, A. W., Devine, J. A., Nowakowski, E., and Deinhardt, F. (1966). *J. Immunol.* **96**, 668.
Hopps, H. E., Bernheim, B. C., Nisalak, A., Tjio, J. H., and Smadel, J. E. (1963). *J. Immunol.* **91**, 416.
Hull, R. N. (1968a). *Virol. Monogr.* **2**, 1.
Hull, R. N. (1968b). *Nat. Cancer Inst., Monogr.* **29**, 173.
Hull, R. N. (1969). *Ann. N.Y. Acad. Sci.* **162**, Art. 1, 472.
Hull, R. N. (1971). *Lab. Anim. Sci.* **21**, 1068.
Hull, R. N. (1972). Previously unpublished data.
Hull, R. N., and Nash, J. C. (1960). *Amer. J. Hyg.* **71**, 15.
Hull, R. N., and Peck, F. B., Jr. (1967). *Pan Amer. Health Organ. Sci. Publ.* **147**, 266.
Hull, R. N., Peck, F. B., Jr., Ward, T. G., and Nash, J. C. (1962). *Amer. J. Hyg.* **76**, 239.
Hull, R. N., Dwyer, A. C., Cherry, W. R., and Tritch, O. J. (1965). *Proc. Soc. Exp. Biol. Med.* **118**, 1054.
Hull, R. N., Dwyer, A. C., Holmes, A. W., Nowakowski, E., Deinhardt, F., Lennette, E. H., and Emmons, R. W., (1972). *J. Nat. Cancer Inst.* **49**, 225.
Hummeler, K, Davidson, W. L., Henle, W., LaBoccetta, A. C., and Ruch, H. G. (1959). *N. Engl. J. Med.* **261**, 64.
Hunt, R. D., and Melendez, L. V. (1966). *Pathol. Vet.* **3**, 1.
Hunt, R. D., and Melendez, L. V. (1969). *Lab. Anim. Care* **19**, 221.
Kalter, S. S., and Heberling, R. L. (1971). *Lab. Primate Newslett.* **10**, 25.
Keeble, S. A. (1960). *Ann. N.Y. Acad. Sci.* **85**, Art. 3, 960.
Keeble, S. A., Christofinis, G. J., and Wood, W. (1958). *J. Pathol. Bacteriol.* **76**, 189.
King, N. W., Hunt, R. D., Daniel, M. D., and Melendez, L. V. (1967). *Lab. Anim. Care* **17**, 413.
Kirschstein, R. L., and Van Hoosier, G. L. (1961). *Amer. J. Pathol.* **38**, 119.
Landon, J. C., Ellis, L. B., Zeve, V. H., and Fabrizio, D. P. A. (1968). *J. Nat. Cancer Inst.* **40**, 181.
Lennette, E. H., and Emmons, R. W. (1970). Information transmitted to author.
Love, F. M., and Jungherr, E. (1962). *J. Amer. Med. Ass.* **179**, 804.
MacLeod, D. R. E., Shimada, F. T., and Waloroft, M. J. (1960). *Ann. N.Y. Acad. Sci.* **85**, 980.
Malherbe, H., and Harwin, R. (1957). *Brit. J. Exp. Pathol.* **38**, 539.
Malherbe, H., and Harwin, R. (1958). *Lancet* **2**, 530.
Malherbe, H., and Strickland-Cholmley, M. (1969). *Lancet* **2**, 1427.
Malherbe, H., and Strickland-Cholmley, M. (1970). Document S38. Presented at a Symposium on the Production and Use of Laboratory Animals. South African Council for Scientific and Industrial Research, Pretoria, South Africa.
Martini, G. A. (1969). *Trans. Roy. Soc. Trop. Med. Hyg.* **63**, 295.
McCarthy, K., Thorpe, E., Laursen, A. C., Heyman, C. S., and Beatle, A. J. (1968). *Lancet* **2**, 856.
McClure, H. M., and Keeling, M. E. (1971). *Lab. Anim. Sci.* **21**, 1002.
McCombs, R. M., Brunschwig, J. P., Mirkovic, R., and Benyesh-Melnick, M. (1971). *Virology* **45**, 816.

Melendez, L. V., and Daniel, M. D. (1970). *In* "Medical Primatology" (E. I. Goldsmith and J. Moor-Jankowski, eds.), pp. 686–693. Albeit J. Phiebig, White Plains, N.Y.
Melendez, L. V., Hunt, R. D., Garcia, F. G., and Trum, B. F. (1966). *Symp. Zool. Soc. London* **17**, 393–397.
Melendez, L. V., Daniel, M. D., Hunt, R. D., and Garcia, F. G. (1968). *Lab. Anim. Care* **18**, 374.
Melendez, L. V., Espana, C., Hunt, R. D., Daniel, M. D., and Garcia, F. G. (1969). *Lab. Anim. Care* **19**, 38.
Melendez, L. V., Hunt, R. D., Daniel, M. D., and Trum, B. F. (1970). *In* "Infections and Immunosuppression in Subhuman Primates" (H. Balner and W. I. Beveridge, eds.), pp. 111–117. Williams & Wilkins, Baltimore, Maryland.
Melendez, L. V., Daniel, M. D., Barahona, H. H., Fraser, C. E. O., Hunt, R. D., and Carcia, F. G. (1971). *Lab. Anim. Sci.* **21**, 1050.
Melnick, J. L., and Banker, D. D. (1954). *J. Exp. Med.* **100**, 181.
Melnick, J. L., Midulla, M., Wimberly, I., Barrera-Ora, J. G., and Levy, B. M. (1964). *J. Immunol.* **92**, 596.
Nagler, F. P., and Klotz, M. (1958). *Can. Med. Ass. J.* **79**, 743.
Perkins, F. T., and Hartley, E. G. (1966). *Brit. Med. J.* **1**, 899.
Pierce, E. C., Peirce, J. D., and Hull, R. N. (1958). *Amer. J. Hyg.* **68**, 242.
Pryor, W. H., Jr., Chiang, H., Raulston, G. L., and Melendez, L. V. (1970). *Primates* **11**, 297.
Reagan, R. L., and Brueckner, A. L. (1953). *Amer. J. Trop. Med. Hyg.* **2**, 864.
Reagan, R. L., Day, W. C., Harmon, M. P., and Brueckner, A. L., (1952a). *J. Gen. Microbiol.* **7**, 327.
Reagan, R. L., Day, W. C., Harmon, M.P., and Brueckner, A. L. (1952b). *Amer. J. Trop. Med. Hyg.* **I**, 987.
Reagan, R. L., Delaha, E. C., and Brueckner, A. L. (1954). *Amer. J. Vet. Res.* **15**, 647.
Sabin, A. B. (1934a). *Brit. J. Exp. Pathol.* **15**, 248.
Sabin, A. B. (1934b). *Brit. J. Exp. Pathol.* **15**, 268.
Sabin, A. B. (1934c). *Brit. J. Exp. Pathol.* **15**, 321.
Sabin, A. B. (1949). *J. Clin. Invest.* **28**, 808.
Sabin, A. B., and Wright, A. M. (1934). *J. Exp. Med.* **59**, 115.
Schrier, A. M. (1966). *Lab. Primate Newslett.* **5** (No. 4), ii.
Shah, K. V., and Southwick, C. H. (1965). *Indian J. Med. Res.* **53**, 1.
Shah, K. V., and Morrisson, J. A. (1969). *Amer. J. Epidemiol.* **89**, 308.
Smith, K. O., Thiel, J. F., Newman, J. T., Harvey, E., Trousdale, M. D., Gehle, W. D., and Clark, G. (1969). *J. Nat. Cancer Inst.* **42**, 489.
Smith, P. C., Yuill, T. M., Buchanan, R. D., Stanton, J. S., and Chaicumpa, V. (1969). *J. Infec. Dis.* **120**, 292.
Soper, W. T. (1959). Technical Study 17. Biological Warfare Laboratories, Fort Detrick, Maryland.
Sumner-Smith, G. (1966). *Lab. Primate Newslett.* **5**, No. 1, 1.
Swack, N. S., Liu, O. C., and Hsiung, G. D. (1971). *Amer. J. Epidemiol.* **94**, 397.
Van Hoosier, G. L., and Melnick, J. L. (1961). *Tex. Rep. Biol. Med.* **19**, 376.

Chapter 14
Viruses of Other Vertebrates

Delbert G. McKercher

I. Introduction

Infections caused in man and the lower animals by viral agents now known as herpesviruses have been recognized for many years. Examples include "fever blisters," "shingles," and "pseudorabies."

Isolation of the causative agents of these diseases and characterization of their biologic properties were carried out largely by chicken embryo techniques. Additional viruses from infections in man and other mammals and birds were isolated, and, as in the past, each was named according to the disease which it produced. This system of nomenclature was satisfactory for viruses which caused distinctive clinical entities. However, it was of no value for those which apparently were not associated with disease, and which were isolated in great numbers after the introduction of cell culture procedures. Fortunately, by utilization of their physical and chemical properties, it was possible to separate most viruses into large groups. One such grouping, the herpesvirus group, was named after the herpes simplex virus, which was the first of its kind to be recognized.

With few exceptions, each species of domestic mammal and bird has its own specific herpesvirus or, in some instances, herpesviruses. The number continues to grow as these viruses are found in an ever-widening range of hosts. The list now includes free-living rodents and several cold-blooded species.

Herpesviruses cause a wide variety of clinical entities, ranging from such relatively mild conditions as conjunctivitis to highly fatal malignancies. The diverse nature of these syndromes, and the complex epidemiologic features associated with many, place them among the most interesting, as well as the most important, viral infections in the realms of human and veterinary medicine. In this chapter the most important herpesvirus infections of the domesticated animals are discussed.

II. Bovine Herpesvirus-1 Infections: Infectious Bovine Rhinotracheitis, Infectious Pustular Vulvovaginitis

A. Introduction

In the late 1940's and early 1950's a severe respiratory disease, clinically distinct from shipping fever and characterized by a severe laryngitis and tracheitis, swept through cattle in feedlots in Colorado (Miller, 1955). It then subsided for several years. A virus was suspected as the cause since the condition did not respond to antibiotic therapy. A similar although milder infection appeared several years later in large dairy herds in Los Angeles County maintained under the closely confined conditions peculiar to dairy operations in that part of the state (Schroeder and Moys, 1954). Later, the same infection, which was now believed to be identical with the one which had occurred earlier in Colorado feedlots, broke out among feeder cattle in California, (McKercher *et al.*, 1954) and was named "infectious bovine rhinotracheitis" (IBR) (McKercher *et al.*, 1955). Shortly thereafter the causative agent was isolated (Madin *et al.*, 1956) and identified subsequently as a herpesvirus (Huck, 1964).

In fairly rapid succession the virus was isolated from cattle affected with conjunctivitis (McKercher *et al.*, 1958), vulvovaginitis (Kendrick *et al.*, 1958), meningoencephalitis (French, 1962a,b; Barenfus *et al.*, 1963), and from aborted bovine fetuses (McKercher and Wada, 1964). The demonstration that this virus is the cause of *Bläschenausschlag*, a genital infection of cattle which was first described in central Europe almost a century earlier, established its origin, thus providing a working hypothesis of the probable manner in which it acquired the capacity to cause such a wide range of clinical syndromes in cattle (McKercher, 1963).

1. Classification and Properties of the Virus

Classification of bovine herpesviruses is in a state of flux at the moment, since several proposed schemes are under consideration. A provisional scheme in which these viruses are divided into subgroups according to host origin and subdivided on the basis of antigenic unrelatedness will be followed, where applicable, in this chapter. In the case of animal species in which only a single type of herpesvirus is known to cause disease, the virus will be referred to either by the name of the host species or the disease which it causes.

Bovine herpesvirus-1 (BHV-1) possesses morphologic features and physicochemical properties characteristic of members of the herpesvirus group. However, after prolonged culture of the virus in the presence of analogues of thymidine, mutants resistant to these analogues have been reported (Stevens and Groman, 1964).

The virus replicates readily in cell cultures prepared from a wide range of bovine tissues including kidney, embryonic skin, adrenal, thymus, thyroid gland, pancreas, testicle, lung, and lymph node, and it also replicates in lamb kidney and testicle and in goat, horse, pig, and rabbit kidney. It multiplies also in rabbit testicle and spleen cultures, as well as in human amnion and HeLa cells, but in the latter only after adaptation. Regardless of the type of cell culture employed, the cytopathic effects (CPE) produced are morphologically very similar. No replication occurs in monkey, mouse, guinea pig, or chicken embryo kidney; in chicken embryos, or in either KB or L cells. The above findings have been reported by numerous investigators and are summarized elsewhere (Gilbert and Saurat, 1970).

Plaques form readily under an overlay and increase in diameter from 1 to 2 mm on the third or fourth day to 5 mm by day 9 (Hahnefeld and Hahnefeld, 1962; Mondino *et al.*, 1964). Large and small plaques appear in the same culture, but it is not possible to select a mutant which yields plaques of uniform size (McKercher, 1964).

In coverslip cultures stained by Giemsa or hematoxylin and eosin, a few multinucleated giant cells are observed in the periphery of the foci, indicating limited syncytial formation, in contrast to other of the herpesviruses (Armstrong *et al.*, 1961). Cowdry type A inclusion bodies are present in infected cells *in vivo* and in cell cultures *in vitro*. Soon after CPE appear, small aggregates of finely granular, acidophilic material form among the nuclear chromatin and collect slowly into a mass which eventually occupies the major portion of the nucleus. The nucleolus either disappears or is displaced to the nuclear margin where it remains as a small basophilic body. The mature inclusion is round, oval, or irregular in contour, although it conforms generally to the shape of the nucleus. It is separated from the nuclear membrane by a clear zone or halo (Cheatham and Crandell, 1957).

Bovine herpesvirus-1 shares an antigenic component, or components, with equine herpesvirus-1 (EHV-1), which can be detected by complement fixation (CF) or immunodiffusion tests (Carmichael and Barnes, 1961).

2. Nature of the Infections

Bovine herpesvirus-1 undoubtedly possesses the broadest tissue tropism of any virus that infects domestic animals. It attacks the respiratory and the genital tracts causing, respectively, rhinotracheitis, vulvovaginitis, and balanoposthitis in the male. The genital infections are of a localized nature and are not characterized by sequelae. By contrast, infection of the respiratory tract results in concurrent conjunctivitis and secondarily in abortion, and it occasionally causes meningoencephalitis in calves. Experimental studies indicate that the virus may cause erosive lesions of the buccal cavity and occasionally of the digestive tract of newborn calves (Baker *et al.*, 1960). The etiologic role of the virus in keratoconjunctivitis has been suggested by a number of authors (Hughes *et al.*, 1964) but thus far conclusive evidence is lacking.

3. Natural and Experimental Host Range

Cattle are believed to be the only natural host of the virus. Recently, however, outbreaks of balanitis and vaginitis in swine in Sweden have been reported to be caused by a virus identical to BHV-1 (Onstad and Saxegaard, 1967). Also, recovery of BHV-1 from goats with severe respiratory illness accompanied by a marked keratitis, was reported recently (Mohanty *et al.*, 1972). Antibody to the virus has been detected in deer, and clinical disease, similar although milder than that occurring in cattle, was produced in this species by intratracheal inoculation of the virus (Chow and Davis, 1964). Neutralizing antibody to BHV-1 has been detected also in a high percentage of African buffalo and domestic cattle (76 and 85%, respectively), and in gnus in Tanzania (Rweyemamu, 1970). Also, precipitin antibody has been demonstrated in the serums of dogs, horses, and man (Afshar and Tadjbakhsh, 1970).

Cattle are readily infected by experimental means, but all other species tested, including sheep, swine, horses, guinea pigs, mice, dogs, and cats, are refractory. The response in goats is equivocal. Antibody is elicited in horses, goats, and sheep in response to inoculation, however (McKercher *et al.*, 1958). Infection cannot be reproduced in rabbits other than by intracerebral inoculation although antibody formation occurs (Persechino *et al.*, 1965).

3. Distribution, Prevalence, and Economic Importance

With the exception of South America, isolation of BHV-1 from cattle affected with at least one of the clinical syndromes which the virus causes has been reported from all continents. While the number of countries in which it has been recovered is relatively few, serologic surveys have disclosed the presence of BHV-1 antibody in cattle in practically all countries, including several in South America. A comprehensive serologic study conducted in the United States indicated that 35% of samples from 31 states were seropositive, whereas those from only 3 states were negative (Newberne *et al.*, 1961). In Italy, where vaccination against BHV-1 infections is not practiced, 30.4% of the mature cattle tested were seropositive (Castrucci *et al.*, 1966). Prevalence of the infection in England was found in limited studies to be only 2.0%, whereas in Chad and Nigeria the figures reported were 30 and 60%, respectively (Zwart, 1966).

Losses due to genital infection with BHV-1 in the female are minimal but are of more concern in the male. The respiratory disease, known commonly as IBR, causes heavy losses among feedlot cattle due to delayed weight gains, the cost of care and treatment of animals in which secondary bacterial infection develops, and, to some extent, death losses which occur mainly among such animals. While obviously heavy, the extent of the true economic impact of the disease on the feeder cattle industry in terms of dollars is not available. However, it has been estimated that losses due to outbreaks of IBR in dairy cattle amount to $51.00 per animal, chiefly from abortion (Pierson and Vair, 1965). Because of high mortality, the meningoencephalitis syndrome is costly insofar as individual outbreaks are concerned; however, it occurs so rarely that its overall economic importance is negligible.

B. Epidemiology

1. Influence of Ecologic Factors

For many years prior to its isolation, BHV-1 was confined to central Europe where it caused a relatively mild genital infection of cattle known commonly as *Bläschenausschlag*. or "coital vesicular exanthema." The nature of this infection was in keeping with the type of husbandry practiced during that particular period. Small village herds of cattle, isolated from each other, were the rule. The most common contact among such herds was the bull, which frequently serviced all herds in a village. As a consequence, veneral transmission of the virus was promoted, and the resultant immunity was adequate to protect cattle of breeding age against infection of the respiratory tract. While the virus undoubtedly reached the respiratory tract of young animals, adaptation to the point where it could produce clinical disease was not possible in the limited number of susceptible animals available in these small isolated herds.

It appears that the virus was introduced into the United States prior to 1930 when importation of cattle from Europe was permitted, since scattered outbreaks of a genital infection referred to variously as "vesicular vaginitis" and "vesicular veneral disease" were reported from different areas of the eastern United States (Jones and Little, 1927; Gibbons, 1944; Roberts, 1949). In retrospect it appears likely that the disease observed at that time was actually *Bläschenausschlag*, or infectious pustular vulvovaginitis (IPV) as it became known subsequently (Kendrick *et al.*, 1958). Evidence of this was the discovery that serum obtained from a calf in 1941 in New Jersey was found subsequently to contain neutralizing antibody to BHV-1, while seropositive cattle were detected in New York State in the absence of respiratory disease (Gillespie *et al.*, 1957). Thus, it is known that the virus was present in this country long before the appearance of the respiratory syndrome, which was first observed when it became established in large concentrations of cattle in Colorado feedlots.

The manner in which the virus became adapted to the respiratory tract of feeder cattle can only be surmised. Inasmuch as such cattle are reproductively inactive, the respiratory tract provided an alternate avenue of invasion. Possibly through a selective process, a mutant having a predilection for certain cell types of the upper respiratory tract emerged, or possibly by rapid serial passage through numerous cattle, the virus eventually became adapted to the upper respiratory tract acquiring, in the process, increased virulence for this system. Through extension via the lacrimal ducts, or by external contamination with infectious discharges, the virus reached the ocular tissue causing conjunctivitis. It was also carried into the blood stream in association with migrating macrophages as demonstrated subsequently, and then to the placenta where it multiplied profusely, invaded the fetus, and caused eventual abortion. It is conceivable that the virus reached the brain by hematogenous transport, thus accounting for the meningoencephalitis syndrome. An alternate route to the brain would be via the olfactory bulb and the major nerve trunks to which virus in the upper respiratory tract would have access.

2. Latency and Latent Infection

The manner in which BHV-1 is maintained between epidemics is still uncertain. Being a herpesvirus, however, its survival is attributed to the property of latency.

It has been reported that the virus was shed intermittently over a maximum period of 578 days by three cows and one bull inoculated via the intravenous, the vaginal, or the preputial route (Snowdon, 1965). However, according to the experimental design, these results could be interpreted also as evidence for an infection maintained in a small group of cattle by genital transmission, much as *Bläschenausschlag* is assumed to have been perpetuated in the past in the small, closed village herds of central Europe. Perhaps significantly, two uninoculated calves held in isolation with two nasally inoculated contact animals both became infected. However, neither these two calves nor the latter two shed virus beyond day 14. Also, one of two calves inoculated intracerebrally (the second calf was killed on the fourth day postinoculation) also shed virus only through day 13 postinoculation (Snowdon, 1965). The virus has been recovered from an experimentally infected bull on the 26th day after inoculation, preceded by an interval during which virus was not recovered (Studdert *et al.*, 1964).

Evidence that the virus is carried latently in the nasal passages of recovered cattle is less convincing, although frequent reports of IBR occurring in feeder cattle from 10 days to a few weeks after the introduction of new cattle would suggest such a possibility. In one study, cattle recovered from experimentally produced IBR were exposed alternately to the stress of extreme ambient temperatures for a period of several days. None showed clinical evidence of disease, and virus was not recovered from any during or immediately after the period of stress, or at intervals over the subsequent several months. In another study, however, virus was recovered from the nasal secretions of two cows in a group of 20 on the 68th day after experimental infection. Inasmuch as these cattle were not held under strict isolation, the results were considered to be equivocal (McKercher *et al.*, 1963).

3. Reservoir Hosts

To date, reservoir hosts of the virus, other than the possible exception of cattle, have not been demonstrated. However, the finding that swine, goats, and possibly deer undergo natural infection with the virus, although apparently very rarely, indicates that current epidemiologic concepts of BHV-1 infections in the bovine might have to be modified.

C. *Pathogenesis*

1. Transmission

Bovine herpesvirus-1 invades the body by way of either the respiratory or the genital tract. Infection of the latter results sometimes from venereal exposure. While the virus has been isolated from semen, its presence was believed due to contamination with prepucial discharges in which the virus attains quite high titers (Spradbrow, 1968). Infection can be produced also by transfer of infectious vaginal discharges to susceptible cattle in various ways including tail switching, the careless use of vaginal speculums, sponges and the like, and by viral contaminated bedding. Some investigators feel that the virus is carried latently by clinically recovered animals and that periodic exacerbations of disease occur as a consequence (Kendrick, 1971). The virus apparently does not reach the genital tract by hematogenous transport. The respiratory infection is contracted by droplet exposure and possibly from vaginally infected animals through the propensity of cattle to lick and nuzzle others of their kind. Meningoencephalitis and abortion result as sequelae to the respiratory infection, although abortion ensues also from the parenteral administration of BHV-1 vaccine. There is no evidence for vector transmission of the virus.

2. Clinical Features of the Infection

Bovine herpesvirus-1 causes two primary infections. The first is IBR, which is frequently accompanied by conjunctivitis, with abortion or meningoencephalitis occurring as sequelae. The second is a localized genital infection known as IPV in the female and as balanoposthitis in the male.

a. Respiratory Infection. The incubation period of experimentally produced IBR usually lasts 2–3 days, although that of the field infection is believed to be considerably longer, probably as long as 1 week.

The cells of the upper respiratory tract become infected within a short time after exposure, resulting in an acute catarrhal inflammation. Within 24–48 hours infected animals become febrile and depressed. Initially serous, the nasal exudate becomes increasingly mucoid as the disease progresses, and finally mucopurulent in nature. Coughing is not a constant sign, but dyspnea, ranging from mild to severe, invariably occurs. The appetite is usually diminished to some extent and consequent loss of weight may occur. Conjunctivitis frequently accompanies the respiratory syndrome. The course of the uncomplicated infection lasts 7–10 days, improvement beginning at this point, and most animals make a rapid recovery and weight losses are soon regained.

In animals that undergo severe disease, bronchopneumonia sometimes occurs because of secondary bacterial infection resulting from the inhalation of infectious tracheal exudates into the lungs. Death in these cases may be sudden or delayed if the condition becomes chronic. Animals that survive the pneumonia never regain their former condition.

Infectious bovine rhinotracheitis may have either of two sequels. The infection in calves 4–6 months of age has resulted occasionally in meningoencephalitis, and cows may abort, particularly if exposure occurs between $5\frac{1}{2}$ and $7\frac{1}{2}$ months of gestation.

Prior to the latter determination, abortion which occurred in cows that had been vaccinated against IBR while pregnant, made the virus suspect of being the cause. However, since viremia could not be demonstrated in experimentally inoculated cattle, it was not apparent how the virus could reach the fetus. Later, when it was found to be associated with leukocytes in the blood stream of either nasally or parenterally inoculated cattle, the probable manner in which fetal infection occurs became apparent. It is now believed that in response to nasal exposure, the macrophages which migrate into the infected areas to assimilate the cellular debris carry virus with them on their return to the blood stream. Presumably a similar response is elicited in the adjacent tissues by parenteral injection of the vaccine. As the virus cannot be isolated from the blood buffy coat fraction of cattle that have any detectable level of neutralizing antibody, it would appear that it is located on the surface of the leukocyte cells where it is exposed to the action of antibody. Moreover, failure to isolate the virus from whole blood of infected cattle indicates that viral multiplication does not occur in the blood vascular system. The virus apparently lodges in the caruncles and then invades the fetal portion of the placentome where it replicates. Damage is not marked, however, being limited to necrosis of an occasional trophoblast cell. The fetus invariably dies from 1 to several days before expulsion (Kendrick and Straub, 1967).

Meningoencephalitis infection in calves due to BHV-1 has occurred only rarely, although in widely separated parts of the world. The disease has usually appeared in 4–6-month-old calves. None of the reports mention signs of respiratory tract infection either preceding or during the infection, although it undoubtedly occurs in a mild form. Signs include incoordination, ataxia, and periods of depression alternating with intervals of hyperexcitability during which the animals undergo tetanic seizures. Some affected animals appear to be blind. The course of the infection lasts 4–5 days and almost without exception it terminates fatally. Studies indicate that the infection is not acquired *in utero*, and is believed to be associated with strains of the virus which are primarily neurotropic in nature (McKercher *et al.*, 1970). This would account for the mild or subclinical nature of the respiratory infection, which presumably precedes the signs of neurotropic disease. Also, the fact that most outbreaks have occurred in calves within a narrow age range indicates an age susceptibility.

The manner in which infection takes place under natural conditions is not apparent, although it seems logical that if the strains involved are neurotropic in nature, they would invade the brain by direct extension along branches of the cranial nerves located in the upper respiratory tract rather than by hematogenous transport.

b. Genital Infection. The incubation period of IPV is short, lasting 24–72 hours, and is followed by an undulating febrile response of several days duration. The vulva may be slightly swollen, with a small amount of tenacious discharge adhering to the vulvar hairs. Affected cattle usually stand with the tail slightly elevated and make frequent and obviously painful attempts to urinate. The appetite is not affected, however, and no significant decrease in milk production results. In mildly affected cattle, the vulvar mucosa is inflamed with few to numerous small, whitish pustules scattered over its surface, with some forming a linear pattern. The vaginal mucosa is also slightly congested but pustules are absent, although a variable amount of the yellowish exudate usually is present on the vaginal floor. In more severely affected cattle the vulvar pustules coalesce to form yellowish raised plaques or sheets, while hemorrhagic foci appear in the inflamed mucosa, accompanied by large accumulations of the vaginal exudate. After several days the hemorrhagic foci slough, exposing circular areas of denuded, underlying epithelium. Clinical recovery occurs in 10–14 days, although the vaginal exudate may persist for several weeks.

In the male, hyperemia of the genital mucosa occurs, after an incubation period of 2–3 days, preceded by a mild transitory febrile response. In such cases, the hyperemia regresses after a day or two, and recovery takes place within several days. More severe infection is characterized by a diphasic temperature rise, and pustules, similar to those occurring in the female, appear chiefly in the mucosa of the prepucial folds and to some extent in the area of the glans, while a few are scattered over the body of the penis. Swelling of the prepuce and penis usually occur. Within several days the pustules slough, leaving craterlike ulcers. Healing begins about 1 week after the appearance of lesions and is usually complete after an additional week. Occasionally adhesions form between the penis and the prepuce. The condition can be rectified by surgical intervention when the adhesions are not extensive.

3. Pathologic Findings

a. Respiratory Infection and its Sequelae. In mild, uncomplicated IBR, the changes consist essentially of a slight to moderate rhinitis, with slight serous exudation into the nasal cavity. In more severely affected animals, the inflammation involves also the pharynx and the trachea. The exudate, at first serous, becomes catarrhal and eventually fibrinous in nature as necrosis of the inflamed surfaces occurs. It adheres to the walls of the nasal passages, the larynx, and the trachea in which it forms a yellowish, fibrinous pseudomembrane. The underlying mucosa is intensely inflamed and contains petechiae in addition to the necrotic foci. Bronchopneumonia is sometimes found in advanced cases, particularly when marked secondary bacterial infection occurs.

On histopathologic examination, the mucosa is found to contain migrating neutrophils, while lymphocytes, macrophages, and plasma cells infiltrate the submucosa. The pseudomembrane is also infiltrated with neutrophils and contains colonies of bacteria. Cellular desquamation and diffuse necrosis occur at the point of attachment of the membrane to the underlying epithelium. Eventually the entire epithelial surface is destroyed, accompanied by congestion of the underlying blood vessels. In most fatal cases, histopathologic evidence of bronchopneumonia is observed. Inclusion bodies are present in the tracheal epithelium after 36 hours, and by 48–60 hours they are found also in the cells of the turbinates and the bronchi (Crandell *et al.*, 1959).

The gross pathologic changes which are observed in aborted fetuses are of a postmortem nature and, as such, are of no diagnostic significance. Histopathologically, the typical lesion is a diffuse focal necrosis, occurring most consistently in the liver but also present in the lungs, spleen, thymus, lymph nodes, and kidney. Necrosis, typical of that present in the fetal organs, has been reported to occur in the placenta. Inclusion bodies are difficult if not impossible to find, mainly because of the autolytic changes which occur. In contrast to the gross lesions, the histopathologic changes are considered to be specific for the infection (Kennedy and Richards, 1964).

Other than slight congestion of the meninges, gross lesions are not apparent in calves which die of meningoencephalitis. However, histologic lesions are present in all parts of the brain but are more severe in the cerebrum, thalamus, and basal ganglia. An extensive lymphocytic meningitis and perivascular cuffing with mononuclear cells are the principal lesions. Gliosis and glial foci are widespread, with an occasional polymorphonuclear cell present among the glial cells. Nuclear changes occur in a few of the neurons in affected areas, but inclusion bodies were not reported in a naturally occurring outbreak (Gardiner *et al.*, 1964). However, Cowdry type A inclusions were present in the brain and cord of an experimentally infected calf (French, 1962c).

b. Genital Infection. Infectious pustular vulvovaginitis is manifested clinically by a vulvitis and vaginitis. Histologically the basic lesion is necrotic in nature, with an accumulation of neutrophils in the necrotic foci and lymphoid cell infiltration of the surrounding connective tissue. A narrow zone of degenerating cells, in which inclusion bodies are present, separates the normal epithelium from the necrotic foci. Inclusion bodies are difficult to detect after the sixth day, when healing usually begins. The healing process is accompanied by the appearance of macrophages, and extensive lymphocytic infiltration of the tissues remains for some time.

D. *Morbidity and Mortality*

The morbidity associated with BHV-1 infections depends on the nature of the infection and the circumstances surrounding the outbreak. In feeder cattle, IBR occurs almost exclusively, usually accompanied by conjunctivitis. The morbidity on a clinical basis ranges from 20 to 30%, although by serologic testing the figure would be much higher, as many cattle undergo very mild and sometimes subclinical infection. Mild IBR is also quite common in large dairy herds and is frequently followed by abortion in as many as 50% of the cows infected after the fifth month of gestation. Infectious pustular vulvovaginitis is more common than IBR in small dairy herds where it occurs sporadically.

In contrast to the morbidity figures, the mortality rate is relatively low although it varies with the type of infection. It ranges from 2 to 10% for IBR among feeder cattle but is much lower for dairy type animals. Meningoencephalitis occurs very rarely, but the morbidity rate is high while the mortality rate is essentially 100%.

E. *Immunity*

1. Passively Acquired

Passive BHV-1 serum antibody titers, which reach levels almost as high as those of the dam, are acquired by the newborn calf within 15 minutes of nursing. The findings of various investigators differ, however, with respect to the duration of passive immunity, ranging from 7 to 21 days to 2½ to 3½ months or longer. The latter range is regarded as the more accurate.

2. Actively Acquired

The duration of immunity resulting from naturally occurring BHV-1 infection depends on the infection involved. The serum antibody level elicited by genital infection with BHV-1 develops more slowly and attains lower levels than after nasal infection (McKercher *et al.*, 1959). After recovery from IPV, animals are refractory to vaginal challenge for several weeks. Challenge inoculations after 1 month, however, cause a mild infection, characterized by the presence of a few pustules which disappear rapidly (Kendrick *et al.*, 1958).

To date, vaginal mucus has not been assayed for neutralizing antibody to the virus. However, because immunity to IPV appears to wane more rapidly than to IBR, and since local antibody affords relatively short term protection, indications are that the resistance to IPV might be due almost entirely to extravascular (IgA) antibody. Essentially nothing is known regarding the duration of immunity following balanoposthitis infection in bulls.

It is becoming more apparent that the immunity elicited to IBR either by experimental or natural infection is extremely durable. Two long-term studies demonstrated that resistance to experimental challenge lasts for at least $4\frac{1}{2}$–$5\frac{1}{2}$ years after one injection of virulent BHV-1, given either intranasally or intratracheally or by intramuscular injection (McKercher, 1962; Chow, 1972). Each experiment was terminated before an immunity endpoint was reached because of the condition of the cattle after $5\frac{1}{2}$ years in isolation quarters in one experiment, and because the number of animals (20) on trial in the other was insufficient to reach an immunity endpoint on the basis of the challenge schedule followed.

A serum antibody titer of 1:2 or 1:3 suffices to protect against experimental challenge via the nasal route. Recent studies have shown that nasal antibody (IgA) is secreted to a low level following either local or parenteral inoculation of vaccine virus (McKercher and Crenshaw, 1971) and that this antibody plays a protective role. However, IgA antibody could not account for a durable immunity because of its relative transitory presence in the nasal secretions.

It has been suggested that serum antibodies can prevent clinical evidence of reinfection in man with type 4 adenovirus. This is attributed to the fact that apparently this adenovirus multiplies in the subepithelial tissues of the respiratory tract, where it comes into contact with serum antibody (Chanock, 1969). Bovine herpesvirus-1 produces a quite severe respiratory infection, as compared with either parainfluenza-3 (PI-3) or bovine rhinovirus infection, so it might also multiply in the subepithelial tissues. In this event, the virus also would come under the influence of systemic antibody so that reinfection would be prevented for as long as an appreciable level of circulating antibody persisted. It is possible also that some cattle remain latently infected, as claimed by some (Snowdon, 1965) and that periodic exacerbations of disease in such animals boost their own immunity, and possibly that of contact cattle through viral reexposure.

Resistance to abortion and possibly to meningoencephalitis depends on the immune status of the respiratory tract, since virus must first multiply in these tissues before it can invade the blood stream. Moreover, should virus reach the blood vascular system of an immune animal, the presence of neutralizing antibody, even in low titer, would provide an effective barrier to further dissemination. It is possible that virus reaches the brain directly by way of the cranial nerves, and thus it escapes neutralization by serum antibody. However, the route or routes by which brain invasion occurs has not been elucidated to date.

F. Diagnosis

1. Clinical

With experience, a diagnosis of BHV-1 infection can usually be made on a clinical basis. Factors to consider are the nature of the operation involved, the circumstances surrounding the outbreak as, for example, the introduction of new animals, and the vaccination history of the herd.

2. Laboratory

The virus can be isolated most readily from nasal, conjunctival, vaginal, or prepucial swabbings during the acute stage of the infection. In the few reported outbreaks of meningoencephalitis, virus was recovered from the brain tissue (French, 1962a).

Aborted fetuses are invariably dead on expulsion and are highly autolyzed. Because of the autolysis, inclusion bodies are difficult to demonstrate, while the gross lesions are nonspecific. Confirmation of BHV-1 etiology can be made by viral isolation from the fetal tissues of the placentomes or the amniotic fluids or fetal heart blood, pericardial or pleural fluids, lungs, kidneys, or spleen (McKercher and Wada, 1964). Identity of BHV-1 isolates is determined either by the serum neutralization (SN) test or by direct immunofluorescence, using appropriate antiserums. A retrospective diagnosis also is possible by serologic means.

G. Prevention and Control

1. Vaccination

Prevention of IBR by means of a modified, live virus vaccine has been outstandingly successful, although vaccination is not practiced against IPV per se. Protection is afforded 10–14 days after vaccination, but the vaccine causes a high abortion rate, particularly in cattle from the fifth through the seventh month of gestation. Thus, its use is contraindicated in the face of an IBR outbreak or when abortion is occurring in a herd.

A recently marketed vaccine, given by intranasal administration, confers protection between 40 and 72 hours after administration, and it can be used without risk in pregnant cattle (Todd *et al.*, 1971). The early protection is attributed to viral-induced interferon in the nasal secretions. Between the eighth and tenth days, when the interferon effect has largely worn off, the locally produced nasal and the systemic antibody levels are sufficient to maintain the immune status. Failure of the vaccine to cause abortion is difficult to explain and must be attributed either to the strain of virus employed, or the manner in which it was attenuated, or both.

2. Other

Passive immunization is not practiced per se, although by vaccination of breeding cows, the offspring benefits from the prophylactic effects of colostral antibody.

Bovine herpesvirus-1 stimulates the production of (endogenous) interferon in cattle, with higher levels being attained after intravenous than after nasal inoculation (Rosenquist and Loan, 1969). The nasal secretions were not assayed for interferon in the above study, but a relatively high level was obtained in the nasal secretions of cattle following nasal administration of a BHV-1 vaccine (Todd *et al.*, 1971, 1972). Evidence is substantial that the protection afforded to challenge virus for the first 10 days was due to this interferon. However, while exogenous interferon therapy offers few prospects of success, there are indications that within the forseeable future endogenous interferon therapy against herpesvirus infections, stimulated either by viral agents or other biological materials or by synthetic inducers, will prove to be a feasible prophylactic measure for short-term protection in emergency situations.

III. Bovine Herpesvirus-2 Infection: Bovine Herpesvirus Mammillitis

A. *Introduction*

Bovine herpesvirus mammillitis (BHM) was first observed in Scotland in 1963 where the initial isolation of the virus was made (Martin *et al.*, 1964, 1966a). Subsequently the virus was isolated by investigators in several parts of the United Kingdom (Deas and Johnson, 1966; Pepper *et al.*, 1966; Rweyemamu *et al.*, 1966). In 1970 it was recovered in the United States from cattle affected with a condition resembling "lumpy skin" disease (Yedloutschnig *et al.*, 1970) but subsequently the mammillitis syndrome appeared to a limited extent in other parts of the country (Fox, 1972). The clinical disease has not been observed thus far in continental Europe, although a virus with characteristics of the one causing BHM, and closely related to it serologically, was isolated in Italy from oral lesions of a calf which died of an apparent alimentary tract infection (Castrucci *et al.*, 1972).

1. Classification and Properties of the Virus

The causative virus of BHM is provisionally classified as bovine herpesvirus-2 (BHV-2). Its morphologic and physicochemical properties are similar to those of other herpesviruses, but it is unrelated to those of other species with which it has been compared serologically. However, it cannot be distinguished from the Allerton virus, the prototype strain of BHV-2, by conventional serum neutralization (SN) or agar gel precipitin tests (Martin *et al.*, 1966b; Castrucci *et al.*, 1972).

The virus was isolated originally in monolayer cultures of calf lymph node cells but it has since been propagated in calf, lamb, baby pig, kitten, and hamster kidney (BHK21/C 13) cells, in calf thyroid and conjunctival cells, and in cells of lamb testes and kitten lung. Replication does not occur in HeLa, porcine, or rabbit cell line cultures or in chicken embryos or birds (Rweyemamu and Johnson, 1967; Castrucci *et al.*, 1972). In cell culture the virus produces marked cytopathic effects (CPE). Discrete circular plaques with irregular borders, measuring 1–3 mm in diameter, are formed in monolayer cultures under agar (Castrucci *et al.*, 1972).

2. Nature of the Infection

Naturally occurring BHM is an ulcerative condition of the skin of the teats and sometimes of the udder which, insofar as is known, affects only lactating and recently "dried off" cows. Despite the close relationship of BHV-2 and the Allerton virus, each causes a clinically distinctive disease entity. One is the ulcerative condition referred to above which occurs in cattle mainly in the United Kingdom, and the other, caused by the Allerton virus, is a nodular infection of the skin of cattle which occurs in parts of Africa and which resembles lumpy skin disease. The latter is a severe infection caused by a poxvirus (Alexander *et al.*, 1957). By contrast, infection caused by Allerton virus is mild, and its chief importance is the fact that it is sometimes mistaken for true lumpy skin disease (Weiss, 1963). Some investigators consider that Allerton viral infection should not be regarded as a specific disease entity.

3. Natural and Experimental Host Range

The domestic bovine is the only known natural host of BHV-2, although a fairly wide range of heterologous host cell types supports replication of the virus *in vitro*. Teat lesions can be induced in lactating cows by intradermal (id) inoculation or by the application of virus to lesions induced in the skin of the teat by chemical irritants. Following id inoculation, nodules develop at the inoculation sites. Disseminated skin lesions occur, although limited, after intravenous (iv) inoculation of virus (Haig, 1967; Martin *et al.*, 1969).

Mature and immature rabbits are susceptible to infection by the id route but not by intraperitoneal (ip) injection, and erythematous lesions develop which later exfoliate. Stunting occurs in immature rabbits, accompanied by loss of hair around the inoculation sites. Stunting is noted also in adult guinea pigs, with relatively severe lesions in the skin which become confluent. Following intramuscular (im) or ip inoculation, nodular lesions develop at the inoculation sites. Mice 7 days of age or older are refractory to infection, but skin lesions are produced in baby mice. Newborn mice can be fatally infected, but the virus cannot be maintained by serial passage in this host (Martin *et al.*, 1966b; Rweyemamu *et al.*, 1968a; Castrucci *et al.*, 1972).

4. Distribution, Prevalence, and Economic Importance

Insofar as is known, BHM occurs only in the United Kingdom and to a limited extent in parts of the United States. A condition reported from Ruanda-Urandi, which affected the teats of cattle, possibly was BHM (Huygelen, 1960). As the virus was isolated in Italy, although from a calf which died of an enteric infection, it is possible that BHM exists in that country and is not recognized as such.

There are no data available regarding the prevalence of the disease by serologic testing, other than in west England where 19.5% of the cattle tested were found to have had previous exposure to the virus (Rweyemamu *et al.*, 1969).

In severely affected herds, the marketable milk yield is reduced by as much as 20% through contamination by blood, difficult milking, and intercurrent mastitis. In some instances severely affected animals have to be slaughtered because of problem milking.

B. *Epidemiology*

1. Influence of Ecologic Factors

Little is known about the epidemiology of BHM, but in view of the close relationship, if not identity, of BHV-2 with the Allerton virus, some link must have existed between these two viral strains in the past.

As BHM is the more recently recognized infection it seems reasonable that the virus was introduced into the United Kingdom from Africa. In view of the high natural host specificity of the virus, the carrier must have been a latently infected cattle beast. In Africa, where climatic conditions maintain diverse and abundant insect populations, the Allerton virus is believed to be vector transmitted. However, climate and the density of the insect populations in the United Kingdom differ drastically to those in Africa. Were some specific vector involved in transmission of the virus in its African habitat, the likelihood of the same vector existing in the United Kingdom obviously would be slight. In this respect, the virus was in much the same situation as was bovine herpesvirus-1, when introduced into feedlot cattle in the western United States. In that particular situation the virus adapted to the respiratory tract, with the emergence of a new disease which became known as infectious bovine rhinotracheitis (IBR). In the United Kingdom, the Allerton virus apparently found its way into abrasions in the teats of cattle and thus was able once again to replicate in the natural host. Transmission by indirect contact then ensued, with gradual adaptation of the virus to the skin of the mammary gland, and the eventual appearance of the mammillitis syndrome.

Although proof is lacking that such a series of events occurred, certain facts nevertheless support this concept, at least in part. Possibly the most significant is the fact that when BHV-2 is inoculated id, a route simulating vector transmission, skin nodules similar to those associated with Allerton viral infection are produced (Haig, 1967; Castrucci *et al.*, 1972). Although disseminated skin lesions occur only after iv inoculation, the reason might be that in adapting to a localized existence in the mammary gland skin, the virus lost much of its original invasiveness. It thus became incapable of invading the blood stream from the dermal location, thus precluding the development of disseminated skin lesions.

The fact that BHV-2 was first recovered in the United States from cattle with disseminated skin nodules (Yedloutschnig *et al.*, 1970) suggests that the strain of virus was invasive and that transmission occurred by biting insects. The latter possibility is in keeping with the fact that the disease outbreak occurred during early August when the insect population is high throughout the country. Subsequently, however, the typical mammillitis syndrome appeared among dairy cattle in New York State, and the virus was isolated subsequently (Fox, 1972).

2. Latency and Latent Infection

There is no direct evidence that BHV-2 causes latent infection, or that a reservoir host or hosts of the virus exists. It is speculated, however, that it might behave in cattle as herpes simplex virus does in man (Martin *et al.*, 1966a). Because of the long association between man and the latter virus, clinical infection occurs only rarely and then only under unusual environmental circumstances. Such a pattern might exist in cattle, particularly if the immune response to BHV-2 is insufficient to eliminate it from the body. It could, therefore, be carried latently and cause overt disease when favorable conditions arose. The finding of BHV-2 neutralizing antibody in nonlactating cattle in the absence of clinical disease is in keeping with this possibility (Rweyemamu *et al.*, 1969).

C. Pathogenesis

1. Transmission

The manner in which BHM viral infection is introduced into a herd is unknown. Most outbreaks occur in herds in a particular area although isolated outbreaks have also been reported. It is suggested that transmission of the virus among nonlactating cattle is due to vectors (Rweyemamu *et al.*, 1969), but this would not account for its introduction into milking herds. Spread of the infection within a herd appears to occur by mechanical transfer of the virus, particularly by the hands of the milker and the milking equipment. Inasmuch as preexisting lesions are necessary for infection to occur, the fact that the disease occurs during the fall months when the cold, damp conditions predispose the teats to chapping and cracking, is consistent with mechanical spread of the virus. During the winter months when cattle are housed, incidence of the infection decreases markedly (Martin *et al.*, 1966a).

2. Clinical Features of the Infection

After an incubation period of 5–10 days, lesions appear on the teats and occasionally on the skin of the udder. Infected animals show no evidence of systemic illness and remain afebrile. Severe lesions are preceded by swelling and rigidity of the teat. Serous exudation occurs, followed by sloughing of the skin. In these cases, the ulceration becomes extensive and involves most of the teat. In less severe cases, plaques develop within the teat wall, and the overlying skin becomes dry and dark in color. In other cases, soft circular plaques are observed which ulcerate. These ulcers sometimes coalesce and cover much of the teat surface. They frequently have sharply demarcated borders and many remain edematous throughout the course of the disease. Thick dark scabs form over others, resulting in bleeding when they are removed although some survive machine milking. Vesicles are rarely seen. On healing, scars remain and loss of pigment occurs.

About 10% of affected cows develop concurrent cutaneous udder infection which, in severely affected animals, involves much of the skin. The lesions exude as serous fluid and scabs eventually form. In less severe cases a dry crust results rather than scab formation.

The course of the disease in individual animals ranges from 10 days in mild cases to 12 weeks in those severely affected. The duration of herd outbreaks is 6–15 weeks, with the more severe and prolonged infections occurring during the early part of the winter (Martin *et al.*, 1966a). Mastitis is a common sequel, occurring most frequently when the lesions render milking difficult or when the sphincter of the teat is involved.

3. Pathologic Findings

The skin lesions are characterized by vesiculation and syncytial cell formation, and by the presence of intranuclear inclusion bodies. Early changes following either id or iv inoculation of virus include intercellular edema and the accumulation of small groups of polymorphonuclear cells scattered throughout the epidermis, followed by congestion and perivascular edema of capillary vessels in the dermal layer. Replicating virus can be detected by electron microscopy although it cannot be isolated until approximately 48 hours later. Extracellular fluid accumulates in the epidermis, accompanied by hydropic degeneration of the cells of the Malpighian layer, resulting in vesiculation. The epidermis becomes increasingly infiltrated with polymorphonuclear and mononuclear cells, and inclusion bodies appear in the syncytia present in the vesicles. The cells of the stratum corneum disintegrate with an outpouring of exudate, and cellular infiltration of the sebaceous glands occurs, accompanied by the appearance of inclusion bodies in some differentiated sebaceous cells. By the eighth day, the lesions reach their maximum. The epidermal vesicles begin to coalesce and eventually rupture. A serosanguinous exudate accumulates on the vesicle floor, with subsequent scab formation. At this time replication and release of virus are at their peak. Shortly thereafter new epithelium commences to form under the scabs and regeneration occurs quite rapidly. Within a few days inclusion bodies are no longer discernible in the dermal layer by electron microscopy examination. However, virus can be recovered from scab material through the 17th day postinoculation. In essence the ultrastructural aspects of BHM viral lesions are basically similar to those of herpes zoster infection in man (Lepper *et al.*, 1969).

D. *Immunity*

Neutralizing antibody appears in the serum 7–9 days after lesions appear and peak levels are attained 2–3 weeks later. The titers are relatively low and vary greatly from animal to animal. They decline quite rapidly, and in most cases antibody cannot be detected 4 months after infection (Martin *et al.*, 1969). Other studies, however, indicate that the titers persist for as long as 2 years (Rweyemamu *et al.*, 1969). Little is known about the duration of immunity but reinfection has been reported to occur 13 months after a previous episode (Martin *et al.*, 1966a). Again, others believe that the immunity is of longer duration (Rweyemamu *et al.*, 1969). Passive antibody is believed to persist in calves for 6 months (Rweyemamu *et al.*, 1969).

E. *Diagnosis*

With experience, BHM can be differentiated on a clinical basis from cowpox (vaccinia) and pseudocowpox (paravaccinia) or milker's nodule (the lesion in man). A diagnosis of BHM can be confirmed by isolation of the virus from teat or udder lesions. Because of the early appearance of neutralizing antibody, a diagnosis can be made serologically while the infection is still in progress.

F. Prevention and Control

A vaccine consisting of viable, unmodified virus, which is administered by im injection, was developed when it was found that inactivated or modified, live virus vaccines were ineffective. The vaccine can be used in pregnant cows without risk, and the virus does not spread by direct contact. However, since it consists of unmodified virus, its recommended use is limited to infected premises. Protection develops 1–2 weeks after vaccination and lasts for approximately 3 months. Over the next 5-month period, vaccinated cattle may become infected but the lesions are much less severe than in unvaccinated animals, and the healing time is greatly reduced (Rweyemamu *et al.*, 1968b; Rweyemamu and Johnson, 1969).

IV. Equine Herpesvirus Infections: Equine Rhinopneumonitis, Equine Coital Exanthema

A. Introduction

During the early 1930's an abortion syndrome, which was first observed in horses in Kentucky, was shown by filtration studies to be caused by a virus (Dimock and Edwards, 1932). This virus became known subsequently as the "equine abortion virus." Later, similar findings were reported from Europe (Meissner and Harms, 1937; Hupbauer, 1938; Sedlmeier, 1938). It was observed, however, that pregnant mares inoculated with the European isolates developed clinical signs of influenza and subsequently many aborted. However, the gross and histopathologic changes in these fetuses closely resembled those described by Dimock and Edwards in aborted fetuses of mares with equine abortion infection. In view of this, it was concluded by the European investigators that abortion was a sequel to equine influenza (Manninger and Csontos, 1941). Subsequently, the equine abortion virus was compared serologically with a virus isolated from horses suffering from a condition clinically diagnosed as influenza (Doll and Kintner, 1954). Surprisingly, both viruses were found to be identical. Since abortion was a sequel to infection of the respiratory tract with this hitherto unrecognized virus, and inasmuch as this virus caused abortion secondarily, it was named the "rhinopneumonitis" virus (Doll *et al.*, 1957). The virus was isolated in cell culture (Randall *et al.*, 1953; Shimizu *et al.*, 1959) and identified subsequently as a herpesvirus (Tajima *et al.*, 1961).

1. Classification and Properties of the Viruses

Three main groups of herpesviruses have been isolated from horses. These are (1) equine herpesvirus-1 (EHV-1) (equine rhinopneumonitis virus), (2) equine coital exanthema (ECE) virus, and (3) equine cytomegaloviruses (ECM). Only the first two are associated etiologically with disease. Two subtypes of EHV-1 are recognized, subtype 1 being represented by the Kentucky D strain and subtype 2 by Army 183 and several European strains (Mayr *et al.*, 1965). The three groups of equine herpesviruses are immunologically distinct, but they probably share common complement fixing (CF) antigens (Plummer, 1964). Equine herpesvirus-1 cross reacts in CF and gel diffusion tests with infectious bovine rhinotracheitis (IBR) virus (Carmichael and Barnes, 1961), and it shares a CF antigen with herpes simplex virus (Plummer, 1964).

The equine herpesviruses are morphologically indistinguishable from each other and from other herpesviruses, and their physicochemical properties are the same as those of other members of the herpesvirus group.

Equine herpesvirus-1 can be cultivated in the chorioallantois of chicken embryos (Doll and Wallace, 1954), but other methods give inconsistent results (Randall, 1955; Doll *et al.*, 1956b). It replicates in Maitland type cultures of fetal equine, cat, and hamster tissues (Randall *et al.*, 1953), and also in monolayer cultures of equine, porcine, and ovine cells but less rapidly in bovine cells (McCollum *et al.*, 1962; Kawakami *et al.*, 1962). Inconsistent results were reported for monkey kidney, while no replication occurred in either rabbit kidney or mouse fibroblast (L) cells (Woyciechowska, 1962). However, others report that the virus multiplies readily in rabbit kidney cells (Plummer and Waterson, 1963; Girard *et al.*, 1963). Conflicting results were obtained in attempts to propagate the virus in HeLa cells (Pleva and Gois, 1964; Randall and Lawson, 1962).

Equine cytomegalovirus strains have a more restricted host cell range (Plummer and Waterson, 1963) while the ECE virus replicates only in cells of equine origin (Pascoe *et al.*, 1969).

The CPE associated with the replication of EHV-1 and the ECE virus develop more rapidly than those produced by ECM viruses. Both the ECE virus and ECM viruses form large syncytia, while syncytial formation by EHV-1 is limited (Pascoe *et al.*, 1969). All three form plaques under overlays. Those produced by EHV-1 and the ECE virus form within 24–48 hours, whereas plaques of ECM viruses develop much more slowly.

Intranuclear inclusion bodies are formed by EHV-1 although in small numbers, but in cultures of either the ECE virus or ECM viruses the inclusions are quite numerous (Plummer *et al.*, 1969; Pascoe *et al.*, 1969).

2. Nature of the Infections

Equine herpesvirus-1 causes primarily rhinopneumonitis and secondarily abortion (Doll, 1952) and occasionally a form of nervous paralysis (Saxegaard, 1966; Bitsch and Dam, 1971). A relatively rare vesicular infection of the mucosa of the genital tract of male and female animals, known as equine coital exanthema, is caused by the ECE virus. Equine cytomegaloviruses have been isolated from clinically normal horses but thus far they have not been associated with any disease condition in this species (Bryans, 1968).

3. Natural and Experimental Host Range

The horse and the mule are the only species susceptible to naturally occurring infection with equine herpesviruses (Henning, 1946; Matumoto *et al.*, 1965). However, EHV-1 has a relatively wide host range by experimental inoculation although adaptation is required in the case of several of these hosts. Experimental hosts include unweaned and 4–6-week-old Syrian hamsters (Doll *et al.*, 1953, 1956a; Randall *et al.*, 1954), baby mice (Kaschula *et al.*, 1957), kittens (Hatzolios and Reagan, 1960), and unweaned guinea pigs after treatment with immunosuppressive drugs (Semerdijiev and Christov, 1958). Infection of rabbits is questionable (Plummer and Waterson, 1963), while adult mice, rats, cats, and calves are refractory (Jones *et al.*, 1948), as is man (Bracken, 1960). The hamster is the most satisfactory laboratory host as titers of 10^9–10^{10} LD_{50} per gram of tissue may be obtained 6–9 hours after infection.

4. Distribution, Prevalence, and Economic Importance

Viral isolation and serologic surveys indicate that EHV-1 infection occurs throughout the world, with the prevalence being high in many countries. Equine cytomegaloviruses are of much narrower distribution although, with the exception of South America, their isolation has been reported from all continents. Thus far isolation of ECE virus has been reported only from Germany (Petzoldt, 1967b), the United States (Bryans, 1968), Canada (Girard *et al.*, 1968), and Australia (Pascoe *et al.*, 1968). The prevalence of equine herpesvirus infections in these countries apparently has not been established to date.

Figures indicating the losses due to EHV-1 infection in the United States are not available, but it is apparent that they are considerable. Estimates for single breeding farms have been placed as high as 1 million dollars per year as a consequence of abortion among highly valuable racing stock (Bittle, 1969). Respiratory infection among young horses in training and on the track results in indirect financial losses in terms of training costs and decreased revenue to the racetracks. The mortality losses from the uncomplicated infection are negligible but secondary infections are costly due to debilitation, delayed recovery, and the costs of treatment.

B. Epidemiology

There is no evidence that ecologic factors or husbandry practices played any role in the evolution of the pathogenic scope of EHV-1 or, in fact, that the virus ever produced primary infection in any system of the body other than the respiratory tract. The etiologic agent of ECE is antigenically different from the herpesvirus causing rhinopneumonitis, hence there is no etiologic relationship between the two syndromes such as that which exists between the corresponding conditions, i. e., IBR and IPV, in cattle.

Epidemics of rhinopneumonitis, which begin around mid-October and last through December, occur annually in young stock after weaning, accompanied by reinfection of older animals (Doll *et al.*, 1954). Abortions begin in December and continue through March, with the majority occurring in January and February. This sequence of events is in keeping with the reinfection of pregnant mares, the length of the incubation period associated with the abortion syndrome (from 3 weeks to 3 months) (Doll and Bryans, 1962b) and the increased susceptibility of the fetus to the infection during the ninth and tenth month of gestation (Doll and Bryans, 1963c). Some consider that abortion at this stage of gestation is related to the time of exposure of mares to infected foals rather than to an increased susceptibility on the part of the fetus during the latter stages of the gestation period (Kendrick, 1972).

The source of virus initiating abortion epidemics is not known, although in some instances it can be traced to infected stock, such as horses returning from training, or by the addition of infected mares which later abort with consequent dissemination of virus from the placental and fetal tissues (Petzoldt, 1967a). The existence of immune carriers or a natural reservoir of the virus has been postulated but not demonstrated thus far (Doll, 1963; Turner *et al.*, 1970; Burrows, 1970). Indications are, however, that repeated infection occurs as a consequence of reinfection rather than by reactivation of latent infection.

C. Pathogenesis

1. TRANSMISSION

Equine rhinopneumonitis (ERP), the name commonly used for EHV-1 respiratory infection, is a highly contagious disease, and the virus is transmitted readily by aerosol or droplet exposure once the infection has been introduced into a stable. There is some evidence that infection may result also from the ingestion of infectious material.

2. Clinical Features of the Infections

a. Respiratory Infection. The incubation period of naturally occurring ERP in young stock is short, probably not exceeding 2–3 days. The disease is characterized by sudden onset with temperatures which reach 105.0° F and last for 2–5 days, and by an intermittent nasal discharge which is accompanied by hyperemia and congestion of the nasal and conjunctival mucosa. The appetite is sometimes decreased temporarily. Enlargement of the submaxillary lymph nodes and edematous swelling of the subcutis occur, while tendonitis of the limbs also has been reported. Ordinarily recovery takes place within 1 week to 10 days.

Rhinopneumonitis in adult horses is essentially subclinical although infected animals become febrile for a short period. Secondary bacterial infection results in rhinitis, pharyngitis, and laryngitis, accompanied by a mucopurulent nasal discharge. A harsh, dry cough sometimes develops which persists for 1–3 weeks. Pneumonia or pleurisy may also develop secondarily (Mahaffey, 1962).

A common sequel of ERP is abortion. As in the case of IBR in cattle, macrophages are believed to pick up virus from the infected nasal mucosa and carry it via the blood stream to the placenta. Multiplication occurs in the placental tissues, followed by invasion of the fetus. Abortion occurs spontaneously and without impending signs from 3 weeks to 3 months after infection of the respiratory tract. Some fetuses nearing term are alive when aborted but rarely survive beyond 36 hours. The health of the mare is rarely affected and neither sterility nor other sequelae occur.

Involvement of the CNS is a rare sequel, presumably of the respiratory infection. The condition has been reported from Europe (Saxegaard, 1966; Bitsch and Dam, 1971) and has recently been recognized in the United States (Kendrick, 1972). Clinical and serologic studies suggest that it results from reinfection which occurs about 1 week prior to the appearance of CNS signs of illness. It varies in severity from mild ataxia to extensive paralysis. Thus far, however, the virus has not been recovered from affected horses.

b. Genital Infection. Equine coital exanthema is contracted by venereal means only. The incubation period usually lasts about 1 week and is followed by the appearance of vesicular lesions, which later become pustular, on the penile and vulvar mucosa. Ordinarily, healing takes place within 2 weeks, accompanied by depigmentation of the skin of the affected areas.

3. Pathologic Findings

In young horses, the inflammatory and erosive changes in the upper respiratory tract are followed by lung involvement characterized by edema and fibrinous infiltration of the interstitial tissues, and subsequent organization and fibrosis (Jones and Maurer, 1943). Small atelectic areas are present in the apical lobes of the lungs. Necrosis of the bronchial epithelium and the germinal centers of the lymph nodes, with the presence of intranuclear inclusion bodies, have been reported. Seropositive horses show little change other than hyperplasia of the regional lymph nodes (Prickett, 1970).

Lesions in fetuses aborted prior to the seventh month of gestation are rather nonspecific. They include widespread autolysis but with little evidence of local tissue reaction. Classical lesions are present in fetuses which are aborted subsequent to the seventh month. Such fetuses are frequently jaundiced, and petechiation is present throughout the visible mucous membranes and on the surface of the heart, spleen, and lungs. Subcutaneous and pulmonary edema occur, with the accumulation of fluid in the pleural and peritoneal cavities. Occasionally small necrotic foci are found in the liver and lungs.

Microscopic examination discloses necrotic lesions in the liver, lungs, and spleen but without cellular infiltration of the tissues. The bronchial and alveolar epithelium is also necrotic. Typical intranuclear inclusions are found most readily in the periphery of the lung and liver lesions (Dimock, 1940).

The marked differences in the nature of the lesions found in fetuses aborted prior to the seventh month and in those aborted subsequently are ascribed to maturation of the immune mechanism, which becomes operative at approximately the seventh month of gestation (Prickett, 1970).

D. Morbidity and Mortality

Because ERP is a highly contagious disease, the morbidity rate is high while the abortion rate ranges from 10 to 90% of mares on the same premises. With the exception of stillbirths, and congenitally infected foals which die subsequent to birth, death losses are negligible. Although deaths result from the CNS syndrome the condition is of little economic significance because of its extremely low prevalence.

E. Immunity

The development of a serologic response to ERP resembles in some respects that to IBR in cattle. Neutralizing antibody appears 1 week to 10 days after evidence of clinical disease. Peak titers are attained between weeks 3 and 5, and persist for 4–5 months before beginning to decline gradually. Complement-fixing titers rise rapidly between the 10th and 14th days after infection but disappear from most animals 3–6 months later. Foals become seronegative even sooner (Doll and Bryans, 1962a), as the colostral antibody disappears quite rapidly.

Immunity to ERP lasts for approximately 4 months, since the local immunity is of relatively short duration. However, resistance to the abortion syndrome is more durable, probably because of the relatively longer persistence of systemic antibody which affords the fetus at least some protection.

On the basis of studies conducted on foals and pregnant mares, there appears to be a correlation between serum antibody titers and resistance to infection via nasal exposure to virus. Pregnant mares with EHV-1 serum neutralizing indices (NI's) of 2.0 or greater rarely undergo infection of the respiratory tract, they fail to become viremic or to abort or develop a secondary antibody response following nasopharyngeal exposure to virus. However, in animals having an NI of less than 2.0, respiratory exposure results in viremia and a secondary serologic response, and abortion may occur. The situation in foals is similar (Bryans, 1969).

Although assays of nasal secretions for EHV-1 neutralizing antibody have not been reported, equine influenza virus administered via the nasal route stimulates locally produced IgA nasal antibody (Todd, 1969). It is possible, therefore, that an NI of 2.0 or greater indicates the presence of nasal antibody in sufficient concentration to prevent spread of EHV-1 from the nasopharynx, thus precluding viremia. Conversely, one could postulate that in animals with an index of less than 2.0, the interval following the previous infection is sufficiently long for disappearance of the local antibody to occur. As a consequence, the virus replicates in the nasopharynx and is carried into the blood stream, probably in association with macrophages, and a leukocyte-associated viremia results.

Correlation between serum antibody levels and resistance to abortion differ in bovine and equine herpesvirus infections. A very low serum antibody titer will prevent BHV-1 viremia, and hence abortion, following parenteral inoculation, whereas EHV-1 can exist in the presence of homologous circulating antibody. This finding suggests that the latter virus is located within the macrophages, or other cells of the leukocytic series which are associated with viral transport, where it is protected against the action of antibody (Bryans, 1969). Nevertheless, seropositive mares which become viremic after parenteral inoculation of virus may abort. However, the neutralizing antibody appears to exert some degree of protection inasmuch as mares with NI's of 2.0 or greater abort less frequently than do those having indices of less than 2.0.

The explanation for this situation is not clear, but it must relate in some manner to the release of virus from macrophages or other cells with which the virus is associated in the blood stream. Virus has been isolated from the buffy coat of seropositive mares over a period of 24 days (Bryans, 1969). This virus must have been released either when the virus-containing cells disintegrated or from viable cells in which viral replication was occurring. Regardless of the source of virus, antigen–antibody complexes would be formed in the presence of homologous antibody. Theoretically at least the virus would now be neutralized and incapable of causing infection. Obviously this is not the case, since fetal infection, with ensuing abortion occurs, indicates that free virus must have had access to the fetus. In view of this it may be postulated that the stability of the antigen–antibody complexes is dependent on the ratio of available antibody molecules to viral particles in the complex. As mares with high serum titers rarely abort, it would appear that EHV-1 antigen–antibody complexes are more stable when the ratio of antibody to virus is high. Conversely, mares in which this ratio is low frequently abort, suggesting that the complexes dissociate, with release of free virus which brings about infection of the fetus and its eventual expulsion.

The paradox of a virus capable of existing *in vivo* in the presence of relatively high levels of homologous antibody poses an extremely interesting situation. Its elucidation would contribute much to a better understanding of the nature of the immunity associated with EHV-1 infection and possibly of the dynamics of antigen–antibody reactions in general.

F. Diagnosis

A clinical diagnosis of ERP usually can be made quite readily. The disease is more severe in young than in mature animals. However, it is less severe than equine influenza which affects both young and old alike. A clinical diagnosis can be confirmed by isolation and identification of the virus or by the demonstration of typical inclusion bodies in cell cultures. A retrospective diagnosis is possible by serologic means.

Spontaneous expulsion of the fetus and the placental membranes during late gestation is presumptive evidence of EHV-1 abortion, especially if accompanied by the typical gross lesions (see Section IV, C, 3). Confirmation can be made by virus isolation or demonstration of intranuclear inclusion bodies in the liver or lungs.

G. Prevention and Control

Since indications were that loss of antigenicity occurred concurrently with attenuation of EHV-1 (Doll, 1961), a program based on controlled infection was instituted (Doll and Bryans, 1963a,b). The vaccine is only slightly modified and consists of an emulsified preparation of infected hamster liver (Doll *et al.*, 1955; Doll, 1961). It is given by nasal instillation on a biannual basis. The first vaccination coincides with the end of the foaling season in early June or July. The second is given in October when the mares are in early gestation and still possess residual immunity from the previous vaccination, and when the fetus is considered to be relatively resistant to infection. The foals are weaned by this time but possess some passive immunity. The object of revaccination is to maintain the existing immunity in anticipation of the respiratory disease which usually occurs during the late fall months. In this way a relatively strong immunity is assured in both the young and adult animals if an epidemic should occur, thus protecting the young against the respiratory disease and the mares against subsequent abortion. In general, the program has been quite effective. However, since the virus vaccine is capable of producing disease and abortion in susceptible horses, the program can be utilized only on farms where a seasonal breeding schedule is followed.

A vaccine used in Europe is prepared from a strain of EHV-1 serotype 2 virus, isolated in golden hamsters from an aborted equine fetus and modified by prolonged serial passage in primary cultures of piglet kidney cells. It is a lyophilized product and given intramuscularly in a dose of 5.0 ml per animal on a biannual basis. The vaccination schedule follows closely that adopted in the United States. This vaccine apparently does not cause untoward vaccinal reactions such as have been reported for parenteral EHV-1 vaccines in this country (Mayr, 1970).

V. Porcine Herpesvirus Infection: Pseudorabies

A. Introduction

Pseudorabies (PR) was among the earliest of the viral diseases to be recognized, and reports dealing with it have appeared in the scientific literature since 1902. At that time, Aujeszky described the condition in cattle, dogs, and cats and demonstrated that it is transmissible to rabbits in which it causes signs typical of the naturally occurring infection (Aujeszky, 1902). The disease then became known as "Aujeszky's disease" and subsequently also as "pseudorabies" because of its clinical similarity to rabies.

A disease of cattle which was referred to by farmers as "mad itch," because of the intense itching associated with it, was described in a number of farm journals during the early and midpart of the last century. These early references are reviewed by Hanson (1954). On the basis of Aujeszky's studies the belief that mad itch and Aujeszky's disease were one and the same entity gained increasing acceptance. This relationship was confirmed subsequently by Shope whose studies did much to elucidate the nature of the disease and particularly its epidemiologic features (Shope, 1931).

1. Classification and Properties of the Virus

The pseudorabies virus (PRV) is the only known herpesvirus to cause natural infection of swine; accordingly it was assigned the binomial of Herpesvirus suis (Andrewes, 1962). The properties of this virus are reviewed in detail elsewhere (Kaplan, 1969).

Antigenic differences have not been detected among strains of PRV examined thus far (Kaplan, 1969). The virus is unrelated to other herpesviruses with the exception of minor crossing between it and B (simian herpes) virus (Sabin, 1934; Burnet *et al.*, 1939), and Marek's disease virus (MDV) (Sharma *et al.*, 1972). Demonstration of the latter relationship was limited to direct fluorescent antibody (FA) staining. A relationship was not detected by means of gel diffusion, viral neutralization, or cross immunity tests. No relationship between PRV and herpesvirus of turkeys could be demonstrated by any of these procedures.

The virus has a wide cell culture host range, replicating in rabbit, swine, lamb, dog, and monkey kidney; in HeLa cells; mouse fibroblasts; and in chicken embryos (Kaplan, 1969). The virus produces pocklike foci or massive ulceration in the chorioallantois, depending on the dilution of the inoculum. It also invades the embryo causing hemorrhagic bulging of the cranium and destruction of the nerve tissue. Inclusion bodies are numerous in nerve cells and the cells of the chorioallantois (Bang, 1942).

In cell monolayers the virus produces either syncytial formation or granulation and clumping of cells with eventual lysis. The nature of the cytopathic effect (CPE) produced is governed by several factors, including the strain of virus and the type of cell culture. Usually both types of CPE's are observed in the same monolayer but one will predominate.

2. Nature of the Infection

Pseudorabies causes two types of infection. In the pig, which is the natural host, the infection is latent in the adult but severe in the newborn. In cattle and most other susceptible species, it is manifested as a rapidly fatal systemic disease characterized by signs referable to the central nervous system (CNS).

3. Natural and Experimental Host Range

Pseudorabies occurs most frequently in swine, cattle, sheep, dogs, and cats and to a limited extent in rats and mice (Gustafson, 1970). It has been reported also in mink, polar bear, silver foxes (Ljubashenko *et al.*, 1958), blue foxes (von Hartung and Fritsch, 1964), and field mice (Lukashev and Rotof, 1939). With the exception of man and apes, infection has been reproduced experimentally in all species of mammals and many birds.

4. Distribution, Prevalence, and Economic Importance

The disease occurs throughout central and eastern Europe where it causes significant losses among cattle and swine, particularly in the Balkan countries. It is present also in China (Lin, 1947), Iran, and possibly parts of North Africa but not in either Japan or Australia (Gustafson, 1970).

During the first part of the present century, the disease was reported from the midwestern part of the United States to the Atlantic coast. At the present time it occurs mainly in the hog-raising areas of the midwest, although sporadic outbreaks have occurred throughout the country, including the west coast (Howarth, 1969).

The prevalence of the disease is not known. However, a serologic survey conducted in Indiana indicated that the swine population of that state had a high susceptibility rate. This finding and the occurrence of only 13 epidemics of the disease over a 21-month period, 10 of which were in pigs and 3 in cattle, in an area where hog raising is a major agricultural pursuit, suggest that the prevalence of PR on a national scale is relatively low (Saunders and Gustafson, 1964). Losses incurred by the swine industry in the United States due to the disease are considered to be relatively minor.

B. Epidemiology

1. Influence of Ecologic Factors

While PR is a more severe disease of swine in Europe than in the United States, the American strains of virus appear to have acquired enhanced virulence over the past 10–12 years. This is reflected in the occurrence of mortality in pigs of all age groups, in contrast to the past when only suckling pigs died of the disease. This more severe infection is attributed to the emergence of strains or variants of high virulence (Saunders *et al.*, 1963; Gustafson, 1967). Several such strains were shown to be antigenically similar to earlier PRV isolates, but they attained much higher titers in cell culture (Saunders *et al.*, 1963). The circumstances which brought about this increased pathogenicity in the virus are not known. However, in keeping with the behavior of certain other herpesviruses, it probably resulted from a combination of management practices and ecologic factors.

This situation would seem to apply particularly to large garbage-feeding operations where severe outbreaks of PR occur sporadically. Large numbers of weaned, seronegative pigs are introduced periodically into these establishments, resulting in a dense population of susceptible animals under conditions which are ideal for the spread of disease. Subclinical PRV infection occurs, as indicated by the fact that about 50% of these pigs are found eventually to have become seropositive (Howarth, 1969). Rapid passage of virus through a large susceptible population such as this provides circumstances which frequently lead to the emergence of virus mutants or to the enhancement of viral virulence. It is apparent that the virus does acquire increased pathogenicity under these conditions, since severe outbreaks of disease occur, characterized by a high death rate and, in most cases, by marked signs of CNS involvement, including blindness (Howarth and De-Paoli, 1968). These outbreaks usually take place during the winter and summer months when the stressful effects of temperature extremes come into play.

2. Latency and Latent Infection

In a series of brilliant experiments, Shope demonstrated that Aujeszky's disease and "mad itch" were the same disease entity (1931, 1932). He found that it occurred in swine as a latent although contagious infection and that the virus was present in the nasal secretions (Shope, 1935a). Cattle became infected when the secretions from infected pigs were introduced through existing abrasions in the skin or slight wounds inflicted by hogs, particularly in the rear limbs of cattle, since the two species comingled while feeding. The disease in cattle was not contagious, hence swine served as a reservoir of the virus for the bovine species. Shope also demonstrated that rats were moderately susceptible to the infection and that many died from it (Shope, 1935b). He concluded that swine contracted the disease through the eating of infected rats and then infected other swine by contact. Rats, in turn, became infected, presumably from cannibalism or while fighting, or by feeding on tissues of cattle or other animals, such as dogs or cats, that died of the disease (Shope, 1935a). Because of their migratory habits, Shope suspected that rats are responsible for the spread of the infection from farm to farm (Shope, 1935b).

3. Reservoir Hosts

In view of the ubiquity of both rats and swine, these two species alone could account for perpetuation of the disease in nature. The survival of gray rats infected with the virus is relatively high (20%), and such rats have been found to shed the virus for as long as 131 days (Nikitin, 1960). The possible existence of other reservoir hosts of the virus cannot be ignored, however, in view of the occasional occurrence of PR in closed swine herds and in sheep and cattle not associated with swine.

Virus initiating the infection in garbage-feeding operations is probably introduced in subclinically infected pigs. Such animals shed the virus over prolonged periods, and, with the constant introduction of replacement pigs, a susceptible population is always present. This situation would subscribe to the view that once the infection is established on a premises, it is perpetuated entirely in the swine themselves as a subclinical infection. It is highly unlikely that rats or other reservoir hosts of the virus play any role in the epidemiology of the disease in these situations.

C. Pathogenesis

1. Transmission

Naturally occurring PRV infection apparently is acquired by droplet infection or by ingestion, since nasal exposure to the virus by experimental means causes signs characteristic of the natural disease, whereas inoculation via other routes, including intramuscular (im), intratracheal (it), or intragastric results in atypical infection (Gustafson, 1970).

Viral multiplication occurs in the tonsillar and pharyngeal tissues and in the olfactory epithelium. From these sites, virus reaches the medulla by way of the olfactory nerve system and the epineural lymph of the trigeminal and glossopharyngeal nerves and, on further multiplication, spreads throughout the brain (McFerran and Dow, 1965; Gustafson, 1970). Evidence for transmission of the virus along, or in, nerve trunks is shown in rabbits inoculated subcutaneously in an area deprived of its nerve supply. Clinical signs are delayed since the virus must be carried in the blood to visceral areas where foci of infection are established. From these foci, infection of the CNS occurs secondarily (Hurst, 1934).

Multiplication of the virus in the upper respiratory tract of swine facilitates its spread within the body, since leukocytes, attracted to the infected area, pick up virus and carry it to various body organs, particularly to the placenta in which it multiplies with the subsequent invasion of the fetus followed by abortion. The fact that the virus can be isolated from the buffy coat cells, although with difficulty, but not from whole blood indicates that it is carried passively, either within or adsorbed to the leukocytes.

2. Clinical Features of the Infection

The incubation period of PR varies from 36 to 72 hours, the course may be short or prolonged, with the mortality ranging from 100% in the newborn to essentially nil in adult swine. The most acute and fatal form of the disease occurs in newborn pigs, in which the course does not exceed 72 hours. One-month-old pigs are less severely affected, but the duration of the disease is slightly longer than in the newborn and the mortality is considerably less. In 5–6-month-old pigs the course lasts as long as 8 days. Adult pigs undergo subclinical or very mild infection, and rarely, if ever, will an adult animal die from the disease. However, the abortion rate may reach 50% of affected sows (Gustafson, 1970).

The signs of PR, all or several of which only may be observed, depending on the age of the pigs, include fever, with temperatures which sometimes reach 107.0°F, anorexia, depression, slight coughing, and vomiting, with diarrhea in some and constipation in others. Pigs which recover begin to show improvement at this point. Sows in early gestation may abort, whereas in later gestation the fetuses die *in utero*. Pigs which eventually succumb become reluctant to move and are oblivious to all but extreme stimuli. Tremors appear in the tail and muscles of the flank followed by incoordinated movements, particularly of the rear limbs. Some pigs have epileptiform seizures and fall as tonic spasms cause the limbs to stiffen. While recumbent the animal may make paddling movements. Within 1–2 minutes, it will regain its feet but the seizure is usually repeated a number of times before the animal becomes comatose. Death usually occurs within the next 12-hour period. Blindness has been reported in hogs in garbage-feeding establishments (Howarth and DePaoli, 1968). Only rarely is pruritis observed (Gustafson, 1970), although it may occur in pigs inoculated nasally with virulent virus (Howarth, 1970).

Pseudorabies in cattle assumes a rapid and fatal course. The first sign is a decrease in milk yield, followed by violent licking of any part of the body, but particularly the nostrils, the skin between the udder and the rear limbs, or the rear limb itself. The area becomes denuded of hair and hyperemic. As the pruritis increases in intensity, the animal becomes frenzied and bellows, bites and gnaws at the skin, and rubs the head and neck violently against hard objects. Within 24 hours the buttocks and thighs become swollen and discolored, and ooze a serosanguinous fluid. The latter stages of the disease are characterized by progressive weakness, profuse salivation, bruxism, and the inability to stand. However, the urge to lick continues until the animal is exhausted. Death usually occurs 36–48 hours after the first signs of illness appear (Galloway, 1938).

Cats are more susceptible to PR than are dogs, and the infection sometimes progresses so rapidly that death occurs before signs of pruritis appear. Ordinarily, signs of PR in these animals are very similar to those observed in cattle. They remain afebrile and the pruritis is intense, as indicated by frenzied attempts to alleviate the itching by scratching and tearing at the skin. A bulbar paralysis develops soon after infection, followed by paralysis of the mandibular and pharyngeal muscles. The animals may whimper and cry and salivate excessively. They remain conscious until death, which usually intervenes from 24 to 36 hours after the appearance of clinical signs (Galloway, 1938).

Rabbits are highly susceptible to the virus by inoculation, whereas guinea pigs are about 1000-fold more resistant. Rabbits were, therefore, used extensively for diagnosis of the disease in the past.

3. Pathologic Findings

Gross pathologic lesions of PR are absent except in those species in which pruritis occurs. In addition to extensive skin damage, a hemorrhagic subcutaneous edema is present. The lungs are sometimes congested and edematous, a finding which is associated with severe congestion of the nasal mucosa. In the early stages of CNS involvement, the meninges are congested and excessive amounts of cerebral spinal fluid are present. In swine, petechiation of the renal cortex may also occur.

The main histopathologic lesions consist of a diffuse nonsuppurative meningoencephalitis and a ganglioneuritis, perivascular cuffing with small mononuclear cells, and diffuse and focal gliosis with extensive neuronal and glial necrosis. The cerebrum is invariably involved, with the white and gray matter about equally affected. Intranuclear inclusions are present in the neurons and astrocytes of the cerebral cortex and the subcortical white matter but in limited numbers. Inclusions are present also in the large reticular cells adjacent to the hyperplastic germinal centers or in the sinusoids of the affected lymph nodes (Olander *et al.*, 1966).

D. Morbidity and Mortality

The morbidity and mortality for PR in swine ranges from essentially 0–100%, since the disease is almost uniformly fatal in the newborn but rarely, if ever, for adults. Figures for intermediate-aged pigs range between these values. The mortality rate in cattle, dogs, and cats approximates 100%.

E. Immunity

Passive immunity acquired through the ingestion of colostrum provides a relatively low degree of protection against PR. Pigs from immune dams can be infected by intranasal inoculation, although the severity of the infection is modified. However, such pigs may sicken and die in a contaminated environment. Some sows do not produce antibody in response to natural infection, thus leaving the offspring fully susceptible (Gustafson, 1970).

Recovery from naturally occurring PR confers a high degree of immunity. Antibody titers attain maximal levels by 3 weeks after recovery and are maintained for at least 18 months (Gustafson, 1970).

It is possible that periodic exacerbations of PR in latently infected pigs may be due to the limited duration of local immunity. Determination of the presence of neutralizing antibody in the nasal secretions of pigs apparently has not been made. However, it would be unusual if local antibody were not present, since it has been demonstrated to be present in man, cattle, and horses following recovery from herpes and other viral infections.

F. Diagnosis

The clinical signs of PR are sufficiently characteristic to enable a provisional diagnosis to be made on this basis. The gross lesions are not pathognomonic of the disease, and, apart from the presence of marked inflammation of the meninges, they are of little diagnostic value. The demonstration of inclusion bodies in the CNS, the nasopharyngeal mucosa, or the lymph nodes is of significance. However, the infrequency with which inclusions can be demonstrated in cadavers renders this feature of little value in diagnosis.

A definitive diagnosis can be made most readily by isolation of the virus in cultures of rabbit or swine kidney cells or in chicken embryos by chorioallantoic inoculation. The material of choice for isolation is tonsillar tissue. The presence of virus is indicated by syncytial formation in the cell monolayer, accompanied by the presence of eosinophilic intranuclear inclusion bodies. Pocklike lesions or ulcer formation occur in the chorioallantois, with the presence of typical inclusion bodies in the cells. Virus is recoverable from the brain for only several days after clinical signs appear (McFerran and Dow, 1965).

A diagnosis can be made retrospectively by serologic means, providing acute and convalescent serum samples are available.

G. Prevention and Control

1. Vaccination

It is generally conceded that inactivated vaccines are inferior to those consisting of modified, live virus for protecting swine, cattle, and sheep against PR. Moreover, the inactivated vaccines must be given in multiple injections, and the antibody response develops slowly. For these reasons some investigators consider the inactivated products to be of little or no value (Kretzschmar, 1964; Zuffa, 1963).

In areas such as central and eastern Europe where PR poses a constant threat to the swine industry, the use of modified, live virus vaccines has materially reduced the incidence of epidemics of the disease. However, all pigs must be vaccinated, although the vaccine may cause infection in the newborn (Skoda *et al.*, 1970). The latter can be protected by the use of antiserum until such time as the vaccine can be administered safely. A variable proportion of pigs shed virus for almost 1 year after vaccination, although neutralizing antibody is present in the serum of many (Sabo and Grunert, 1971). Nevertheless, shedding plays an important role in protection, since it maintains the immunity of vaccinated animals, and limits the occurrence of natural infection on a premises to the occasional pig in which the vaccine failed to elicit an immune response.

2. OTHER

Since the onset of epidemics of PR is invariably sudden, and since these outbreaks do not usually last for more than 2 weeks, prophylactic serum therapy is recommended for short-term protection of newborn and suckling pigs. Serum from "hyperimmunized" swine and horses is less satisfactory than gamma globulin from the whole serum (Mermerski *et al.*, 1968; Popescu, 1962), while swine gamma globulin is more effective than that derived from heterologous species.

Passive immunization is relatively ineffective after the animal has been exposed to the infection. Pseudorabies is, to a large extent, neurotropic in nature and is characterized by a very mild viremia. The virus multiplies in the cells of the upper respiratory tract and invades the brain by way of certain cranial nerves, followed by further multiplication in the CNS. Moreover, since virus that reaches the viscera is believed to be transported mainly by the lymphatics, and to a limited extent by the blood, there is little opportunity for serum or colostral antibody to interact with it. However, such antibody probably can modify the severity of the disease in exposed animals by neutralizing virus that might be present in the blood and the body fluids (Gustafson, 1970).

While an interferon inducer (statalon) protected a high percentage of newborn mice against PR virus, induction of interferon in the serum of swine by poly I: poly C or statalon, or by infection with Newcastle disease virus, hog cholera virus, or PRV was unsuccessful (Mitchell and Gustafson, 1971).

VI. Canine Herpesvirus Infection

A. Introduction

Death losses, particularly among puppies in large kennels, are a relatively common occurrence. A study of 11 kennels involving 103 dams from $1\frac{1}{2}$–6 years of age revealed that the overall mortality from birth to weaning was 21.9%. The great majority (19.6%) of the deaths occurred at birth or shortly thereafter (Andersen, 1970).

A number of factors are involved. They include trauma, diet, rejection by the dam, environmental conditions, and infection. Nevertheless, the microbial agents believed to be implicated etiologically are poorly defined, although infectious canine hepatitis (ICH) virus is considered to be a common one.

A significant advance in the clarification of the cause of these deaths was made with the isolation of a herpesvirus from sick and dead neonatal puppies and subsequently from spontaneously degenerating cell cultures prepared from puppy kidney tissues (Carmichael *et al.*, 1964, 1965a). Similar findings were made shortly afterwards in several other laboratories in the United States (Stewart *et al.*, 1965; Spertzel *et al.*, 1965; Schwartz and Martin, 1966; Prydie *et al.*, 1966).

A prominent pathologic finding in puppies from which these viral isolations were made was extensive hemorrhage and the presence of necrotic foci throughout the liver, kidney, and spleen. However, fetal or neonatal puppies whose kidney cells yielded the virus on *in vitro* cultivation appeared normal.

Isolation of the virus has been reported also from adult dogs with respiratory disease in Japan (Motohashi and Tajima, 1966) and in the United States (Binn *et al.*, 1967) from clinically normal dogs (Motohashi and Tajima, 1966; Karpas *et al.*, 1968), and from dogs with tracheobronchitis ("kennel cough") (Karpas *et al.*, 1968).

1. Classification and Properties of the Virus

Canine herpesvirus (CHV) possesses morphologic and biologic properties compatible with those of members of the herpesvirus group. It is unrelated antigenically to all herpesviruses thus far tested (Carmichael *et al.*, 1965b), with the exception of herpes simplex, with which it shares some neutralizing activity (Aurelian, 1968).

Thus far CHV has been propagated only in primary or line cultures of dog kidney (DK) cells although "limited" multiplication has been reported to occur in cell cultures of cynomolgus monkey, calf, pig, and rabbit kidney (Prydie *et al.*, 1966). Cell cultures prepared from fetal or neonatal puppy kidney appear to be more susceptible to infection than are cultures derived from tissues of dogs over 3 months of age (Carmichael *et al.*, 1965a). No evidence of multiplication has been obtained in cells of the chorioallantois of chicken embryos (Cornwell *et al.*, 1966). The virus in cell culture is largely cell-associated (Carmichael *et al.*, 1965b).

The cytopathic effects (CPE's) are typical of those caused by members of the herpesvirus group. When cultured under agar or methylcellulose, the virus produces small plaques with sharply defined, irregular borders (Prydie *et al.*, 1966). Typical herpetic inclusion bodies are found only rarely, probably due to the rapidity by which the CPE occur.

The temperature range for viral multiplication is 33.5°–37° C (Cornwell *et al.*, 1966) with an optimal temperature of 35°–36° C (Huxsoll and Hemelt, 1970; Carmichael, 1970). At 39° C, which is the normal body temperature of dogs after age 2 weeks, viral multiplication is minimal. It has been suggested that the failure of the virus to produce lesions in dogs after weaning is due to the development of an efficient thermoregulatory system in the body (Carmichael *et al.*, 1970). Body temperatures of newborn puppies are frequently lower, falling into the range that is optimal for multiplication of CHV.

2. Nature of the Infection

Canine herpesvirus causes primarily an infection of the upper respiratory tract. In puppies less than 1 week of age the infection becomes generalized, terminating almost invariably in death. In 1–2-week-old puppies it may become generalized, in which case it usually terminates fatally, or it may remain localized in the upper respiratory tract with mild signs of disease followed by recovery. The disease in older dogs is asymptomatic, with viral multiplication being limited to the mucosa of the upper respiratory or the genital tracts (Carmichael, 1970).

3. Natural and Experimental Host Range

The dog is the only known host, either natural or experimental, of CHV. There is no evidence of breed susceptibility. While antibody to the virus has been detected on rare occasions in man (Lundgren and Clapper, 1969), it has been found by means of a highly sensitive plaque reduction test that CHV cross reacts with herpes simplex antiserum (Aurelian, 1968). It is possible, therefore, that the presence of antibody in man to CHV indicates the existence of latent herpesvirus infection rather than previous infection with the canine virus.

4. Distribution, Prevalence, and Economic Importance

Thus far CHV infection has been reported from the United States, England, Scotland, France, Japan, and, recently, Australia (Geldard *et al.*, 1971). Although only limited serologic surveys have been conducted, the disease is believed to be widespread in the United States, since virus has been recovered from dogs originating in widely separated areas (Carmichael *et al.*, 1964). Also, CHV antibody has been detected in commercially prepared canine globulin, also suggesting that the disease is of wide distribution. Nevertheless, it is believed that only a small proportion of the deaths that occur in puppies is due to this infection (Carmichael *et al.*, 1965a). Epidemiologic data acquired in European countries give little indication of the distribution and prevalence of the disease in those areas.

The economic importance of CHV infection is not known because of the uncertainty of its distribution in this and other countries. However, losses sustained in individual kennels could be substantial when highly valuable breeding stock is involved.

B. Epidemiology

1. Influence of Ecologic Factors

Until recently there was no evidence that the pathogenic potential of CHV had been enhanced through management practices or ecologic factors. However, a virus isolated from dogs in England with associated infertility, abortion, and stillbirth (Poste and King, 1971) was believed to be a new canine herpesvirus because of the severity and diverse nature of the infection produced (Poste, 1972). This isolate was shown later to be antigenically identical with strains of CHV isolated earlier in the United States. Thus, it may be more properly regarded as a variant (Carmichael, 1972). Its marked virulence, nevertheless, is in keeping with a trend towards more severe clinical disease associated with CHV infection. This trend is reflected in the finding that dogs as old as $3\frac{1}{2}$ months have died of generalized herpesvirus infection, an occurrence which hitherto had been limited to puppies under 1 week of age. Although concurrent infection with adenovirus was involved in this particular instance, and the circumstances under which death occurred reflected a stressful environmental situation, the clinical infection was nonetheless that of generalized herpesvirus disease. The picture that is emerging appears to be one of increasing virulence on the part of the virus, complemented by stressful environmental situations and possibly psychologic factors, combining to cause a clinically more severe infection. Undoubtedly this situation is more prevalent than realized, but its extent will not be known until extensive diagnostically oriented laboratory studies have been conducted.

2. Latency and Latent Infection

Initially it was felt that latency was not a feature of CHV infection. This was based mainly on the observation that bitches which had delivered an infected litter earlier, subsequently gave birth to normal litters. It was demonstrated recently by the administration of steroids to dogs, which had been infected experimentally 6 months earlier and which did not shed virus in the meantime, that most remained latently infected (Carmichael, 1972). The reactivated infection was not associated with overt disease other than a slight nasal discharge which lasted for several days, but viral shedding occurred. Such minor signs would usually be overlooked, even by a veterinarian much less the owner, or be attributed to other factors. While the stressing agent employed was highly artificial, the fact remains that the virus can persist latently in the body, and the infection can be reactivated. It is entirely possible that commonplace stress factors would be equally as effective as steroids in precipitating active disease. Hitherto some recovered dogs were believed to remain carriers of the virus, but in view of this more recent finding, latency and latent infection must also be included as a feature of the CHV syndrome.

3. Reservoir Hosts

There are no indications that hosts other than the dog harbor CHV or that other species play a role in the epidemiology of the disease.

C. Pathogenesis

1. Transmission

Naturally occurring CHV infection is believed to be transmitted in several ways. The most common is by ingestion or inhalation of infectious secretions during birth as the pup passes through the vaginal canal of the infected dam (Carmichael *et al.*, 1965a). The virus is transmitted also by droplet exposure from an inapparently infected bitch to her puppies and also between littermates, with establishment of the infection in the upper respiratory tract (Carmichael, 1970). Isolation of the virus from stunted puppies removed by cesarean section from healthy bitches approaching term (Stewart *et al.*, 1965) and from primary cultures of fetal DK which underwent spontaneous degeneration (Carmichael *et al.*, 1964); deRatuld and Werner, 1965; Spertzel *et al.*, 1965) can be accounted for only on the basis of transplacental infection. Presence of virus in the kidneys of neonatal puppies probably results from infection of the upper respiratory tract, with transport of the virus from the primary focus to the kidney and possibly other organs. While viral persistence in the upper respiratory tract has not been demonstrated beyond 3 weeks, it is believed that it can persist at low levels in various body organs for relatively long periods of time (Carmichael, 1970).

Puppies 1 week of age or less can be readily infected by oronasal exposure to virus or by intraperitoneal (ip) injection (Carmichael *et al.*, 1965a). Oral, oronasal, or aerosol exposure of weaned puppies to the virus produces either signs of mild rhinitis and pharyngitis or inapparent infection, whereas virus administered by intracerebral (ic), intraocular, subcutaneous (sc), intravenous (iv), or ip injection fails to elicit observable signs of disease (Cornwell *et al.*, 1966). Dogs exposed via the vaginal route develop a mild vaginitis only (Carmichael, 1965; Poste and King, 1971).

2. Clinical Features of the Infection

Canine herpesvirus infection in dogs from the age of 5 weeks through adulthood is essentially asymptomatic, although recently death in $3\frac{1}{2}$-month-old animals has occurred (Carmichael, 1972). Dogs 2–5 weeks of age display mild signs of rhinitis and pharyngitis, but, on occasions, generalized infection occurs which sometimes ends fatally. However, puppies under 1–2 weeks of age undergo generalized infection which terminates almost invariably in death.

The naturally acquired infection usually appears within a few days of birth. Infected puppies do not become febrile; they are usually dull and listless and have little or no inclination to nurse. They may cry persistently and evince abdominal pain when handled. In other cases, the puppies appear quite healthy and active but frequently vomit or retch after feeding. Death ensues 6–12 hours later. Survivors of the initial infection frequency exhibit evidence of CNS involvement manifested by ataxia, circling in one direction, and blindness (Percy *et al.*, 1971). Similar signs are observed in some puppies following experimental inoculation (Carmichael *et al.*, 1965a). The virus localizes in the mucosal cells of the turbinate bones, the tonsils, and the pharynx (Carmichael, 1970). Foci of epithelial cells and macrophages containing virus are detected in the lamina propria within 24 hours of experimental infection by fluorescent antibody (FA) staining. In the case of dogs 2 or more weeks of age, the infection usually remains limited to the upper respiratory tract and the lymph nodes draining the area. Virus can be isolated over a period of 2–3 weeks from nasal and pharyngeal swabbings, from the nasal and tonsillar mucosa, and occasionally from the lungs. Dissemination of virus occurs apparently by way of the secretions bathing the mucosal surfaces. On occasions, virus is recovered from the bronchial lymph nodes also. In young puppies, the infection becomes generalized 3–4 days after exposure, and virus can be detected in the reticuloendothelial (RE) cells of the lymph nodes and spleen. The appearance of virus in these locations following its presence in the macrophages in the lamina propria provides rather convincing evidence that it is carried into the blood stream within the RE cells from the foci in the lamina propria. Further evidence of leukocytic transport is the fact that the virus can be recovered from buffy coat but not from the serum plasma. It appears also that its dissemination to the various internal organs takes place by hematogenous transport, while the distribution of lesions in the CNS of experimentally infected puppies is also compatible with this mode of dissemination. There is some evidence also of brain invasion via the cranial nerve trunks, however (Percy *et al.*, 1968).

3. Pathologic Findings

Lesions associated with either naturally acquired or experimentally produced CHV infection are essentially similar. The main gross changes include the presence of serosanginous fluid in body cavities, and sharply demarcated foci of renal necrosis and focal subcapsular hemorrhage which give the organ a mottled appearance. The necrotic foci frequently extend into the cortex. Pethechial hemorrhages are noted in the mucosa of the intestinal tract. Lungs of affected puppies are edematous and contain a frothy exudate, with very small hemorrhagic or grayish foci scattered throughout the lobes. The spleen is enlarged and a generalized lymphadenitis is present. Histopathologic examination reveals focal necrosis and hemorrhage in all major organs of the body, including the kidney, liver, spleen, adrenal glands, lung, and brain. The most severely affected organ is the kidney (Carmichael *et al.*, 1965a).

Typical herpetic type A inclusion bodies are few in number and are difficult to demonstrate in smear preparations. When present they are confined to the necrotic lesions. However, FA staining readily reveals CHV antigen in these foci. The gross and microscopic brain lesions resemble those caused in other species by herpesviruses. They vary from discrete neuronal degenerative foci, with perivascular cuffing, to a diffuse meningoencephalitis characterized by necrosis, cavitation, and hemorrhage. The presence of inclusion bodies in the brain is doubtful (Percy *et al.*, 1968).

D. Immunity

It is difficult to determine the duration of immunity to CHV infection, since dogs over 4 weeks of age do not become febrile or show clinical signs of disease in response to either natural or experimental exposure to the virus. Therefore, in the absence of any parameters of infection, immunity challenge is of no value in determining either the presence of immunity or its duration. It is also doubtful whether a direct correlation exists between antibody and the degree of immunity, so that serologic testing would not necessarily indicate the immune status of an animal. However, newborn puppies which nurse bitches having a serum antibody titer of 1:4 or greater do not develop clinical signs of disease or die from experimental inoculation. Nevertheless, they apparently become infected, as shown by the presence of presumably replicating virus in the nasal secretions for several days after exposure to the virus. Also, ip injection of newborn puppies with serum from bitches that had given birth to an infected litter, prevented death losses (Carmichael, 1970). Antiserum, therefore, is of value in protecting puppies during the period when they suffer severe CHV infection. However, it is difficult and costly to prepare (Carmichael, 1970).

Possibly a more practical approach is the vaccination of breeding bitches in order to provide the puppies with maternal antibody. Unfortunately, CHV is a relatively poor antigen, and little success has been experienced thus far in its attenuation. Limited study has indicated that multiple injections of inactivated virus, with added adjuvant, are required in order to induce appreciable antibody levels (Carmichael, 1970).

E. Diagnosis

A clinical diagnosis of CHV infection is not reliable because of the variability of the signs. Also, the signs somewhat resemble those of other infections, including streptococcal septicemia and ICH, which occur frequently in neonatal puppies (Carmichael *et al.*, 1965a). However, the gross lesions, and particularly the renal necrosis, focal hemorrhage, and splenomeglia are of diagnostic significance, as are the histopathologic changes. Inclusion bodies are atypical and appear too inconsistently and in too small numbers to be relied upon for diagnostic purposes. Fluorescent antibody staining, however, reveals large amounts of viral antigen in the necrotic foci and can be used successfully for rapid diagnosis (Cornwell *et al.*, 1966). Isolation and identification of the virus also is a reliable diagnostic procedure.

Neutralizing antibody to CHV is difficult to detect by conventional serologic procedures. However, by the addition of fresh guinea pig complement to the virus prior to its addition to the diluted serum samples, antibody titers are enhanced several fold (Carmichael, 1970).

F. Prevention and Control

Canine herpesvirus vaccines are not available, although vaccination of bitches prior to conception, in order to provide the newborn with passive protection, appears feasible. An alternative approach is the use of antibody globulin to protect the newborn during epidemics in kennels (Carmichael, 1970). Vaccination of puppies is not indicated.

Routine sanitary measures such as the disinfection of cages and pens occupied by infected dogs, and the separation of bitches that had infected litters from those with normal litters is recommended.

Reports that induced hyperthermia (38.4°–39.5° C) prolongs the survival of CHV-infected puppies indefinitely suggest that this measure may be applied to advantage in inducing resistance to the infection until the puppies attain 3 weeks of age. At this age the pup can maintain a stable body temperature. It is apparent, however, that factors other than body temperature regulation are involved in age-associated resistance (Carmichael *et al.*, 1970).

VII. Feline Herpesvirus Infection: Feline Viral Rhinotracheitis

A. Introduction

Cats suffer from a number of respiratory tract infections caused by several agents acting singly or in concert with others. Clinically these conditions resemble each other so closely that they may be referred to collectively as a respiratory disease complex.

The first pathogen of the respiratory tract of cats to be recognized was a chlamydial agent which was isolated in 1942, and the condition named feline pneumonitis (FP) (Baker, 1942). Although characterized clinically by rhinitis and conjunctivitis, pneumonitis is apparent at necropsy. The initial feline viral respiratory pathogen was recovered from kittens with an acute upper respiratory tract infection resembling FP. The isolate was identified as a herpesvirus, and the condition designated as feline viral rhinotracheitis (FVR) (Crandell and Maurer, 1958). Subsequently, picornaviruses (Bittle *et al.*, 1960) and a feline reovirus (Scott *et al.*, 1970), both of which are associated with respiratory illness, have been recovered. Recently, syncytial viruses have also been isolated from clinically normal cats and from cats affected with a variety of conditions, including respiratory disease (Gaskin, 1970; Scott, 1971).

After isolation of the feline herpesvirus in several geographic locations in the United States (Bittle *et al.*, 1960; Crandell *et al.*, 1960), the same virus was recovered in Switzerland (Bürki, 1963), Canada (Ditchfield and Grinyer, 1965), Hungary (Horvath *et al.*, 1965), and England (Johnson and Thomas, 1966).

1. Classification and Properties of the Virus

The causative agent of FVR is the only feline herpesvirus described thus far. Its physical and biological properties are consistent with those of herpesviruses of other species.

The virus is highly host specific and thus far has been cultivated readily in feline kidney cell cultures only. Evidence for its replication in monkey and dog kidney cells has been reported (Piercy and Prydie, 1963), as has its replication in cell cultures of rabbit kidney (Ditchfield and Grinyer, 1965).

Foci of opaque, rounded cells appear in monolayer cultures 24–30 hours after inoculation, followed by the formation of multinucleated giant cells (Crandell and Maurer, 1958). All isolates of the virus tested to date have been found to be closely related antigenically, if not identical.

2. Nature of the Infection

Naturally occurring FVR is manifested primarily as an acute rhinotracheitis (or coryza), accompanied by fever, conjunctivitis, and occasionally by glossitis. Abortion has been reported as a sequel to intranasal (in) or intravenous (iv) inoculation of germ-free cats (Hoover, 1970) but is not well documented for the natural disease. Vaginal exposure of conventionally reared cats results in vaginitis and congenital infection (Bittle and Peckham, 1971). However, these sequelae have not been reported thus far to be associated with naturally occurring FVR.

3. Distribution, Prevalence, and Economic Importance

The fact that the feline herpesvirus was isolated over a short period from cats in different areas of the United States as well as in several European countries indicates that the disease was of wide distribution prior to the initial isolation of the virus. However, since cats are normally territorial animals tending to commingle with their kind only in the immediate vicinity, it is possible that the disease, although widespread, might be focally distributed.

The prevalence of FVR has not been determined, mainly because of the transient nature of the antibody response of convalescent animals. In view of this and the possible focal distribution of the disease, a true indication of its prevalence would require repeated wide-scale serologic testing.

The economic importance of the disease can be assessed only on the basis of the debilitation incurred due to the respiratory syndrome in adult cats and death losses which occur among young kittens. Again, since the prevalence of the disease has not been established and since the full pathogenic potential of the virus still might not be fully delineated, the true economic importance of the disease is not known. The infection is of considerable nuisance value, however, in animal hospitals and catteries because of its highly contagious nature and the fact that it is transmitted by asymptomatic carrier animals.

B. Epidemiology

1. Influence of Ecologic Factors

The increased popularity of cats as pet animals over the past 10–15 years, together with a growing demand for this species in research studies, has resulted in a great proliferation of breeding and reasearch colonies, commercial pet shops, and other establishments where large numbers of cats of different ages and from diverse sources are housed under closely confined conditions. Such a situation favors the spread of disease and probably contributes to increased virulence of the viruses involved, as a result of rapid passage through large numbers of the host species. Nevertheless, these factors do not appear to have caused altered or new trends in the epidemiologic pattern of FVR similar to that which occurred in the case of herpesvirus infections of cattle.

This situation might be more apparent than real, however. It would appear that once a virus has established itself as a respiratory tract pathogen, it is in a highly favored location to exert its full pathogenic potential on the host, since it has essentially direct access to all important organs and systems of the body. For example, until bovine herpesvirus-1 became a respiratory pathogen, it caused only a relatively mild, localized, genital infection. The increased pathogenic scope of the virus was acquired within a relatively short time after it became capable of causing respiratory disease. Inasmuch as FVR has been recognized for at least 15 years and possibly longer, it is conceivable that the virus has already attained its full pathogenic capability and that outbreaks of undiagnosed abortion and the occasional case of encephalitis in cats is evidence of this. Proof, however, can be obtained only by more intensive diagnostic study and continued research. On the other hand, if highly invasive and neurotropic mutants of the virus, capable of invading the blood stream and replicating in the central nervous system still have not emerged, it is highly doubtful whether they ever will.

It would not necessarily follow, however, that new infectious syndromes due to this virus will not appear, since enhanced invasive capabilities or altered tropisms are not necessary in situations where the virus can be mechanically transferred from an infected to a noninfected site of the body. An example of such is the vaginal infection which, thus far, has been induced only by experimental means. However, in view of the grooming habits of cats, it is possible for the virus in the respiratory passages to be introduced into the genital tract, with vaginitis resulting. Also, as in the case of infections pustular vulvovaginitis (IPV) in cattle, the virus plausibly could be transmitted by venereal contact. However, the seasonal nature of the estrus cycle in the cat would preclude the occurrence of such infection, except during the relatively short biannual breeding period.

2. Latency and Latent Infection

True latent feline herpesvirus infection has not been demonstrated thus far. However, it is well established that at least some recovered animals shed the virus for a considerable time (Crandell *et al.*, 1961; Johnson and Thomas, 1966; Povey and Johnson, 1967). Thus, the presence of convalescent carrier animals among the cat population suffices to perpetuate the disease in the absence of known reservoir hosts of the virus.

C. *Pathogenesis*

1. Transmission

Naturally occurring FVR is acquired through contact exposure. The infection can be induced experimentally by nasal exposure to the virus, while vaginal inoculation causes vaginitis and, in the case of pregnant queens, prenatal infection in at least some cases (Bittle and Peckham, 1971). Parenteral exposure of germ-free cats to the virus also causes abortion or stillbirths and placental lesions. Evidence that intranasal inoculation of germ-free cats also results in abortion is less convincing (Hoover, 1970).

2. Clinical Features of the Infections Produced

The development of FVR infection corresponds closely to that of herpesvirus respiratory syndromes in other species. The virus enters the respiratory system in association with droplets of saliva or ocular and nasal secretions. It localizes in the cells of the upper respiratory tract and replicates rapidly, causing clinical signs of infection characterized by excessive salivation and sneezing approximately 48 hours after exposure. Rhinitis and conjunctivitis then develop, accompanied by mild fever, depression, and inappetence. The nasal and lacrimal discharges are clear at first but become mucopurulent as the infection increases in severity. Clinical signs usually subside after 1 week but persist in those animals that become chronically infected. Coughing and labored breathing, accompanied by the development of sinusitis, are characteristic signs of the chronic form of the disease (Bittle, 1972).

The mortality rate may reach 50% in young kittens but death is rare in adult animals. The morbidity, however, approaches 100% of susceptibles in the case of either immature or mature cats.

3. Pathologic Findings

The lesions are confined to the respiratory tract. The mucosa of the nasal passages and the turbinate bones becomes diffusely congested, followed by inflammatory changes in the larynx and the trachea. Several days after the initial signs of disease, focal areas of necrosis develop but remain confined to the mucosa of the nasal passages and the turbinate bones. The tonsils and cervical lymph nodes become enlarged, accompanied usually by slight to moderate petechiation, while the mediastinal and bronchial nodes sometimes are congested and slightly larger than normal. A mild to severe glossitis occasionally occurs. In chronically infected cats, a sinusitis is sometimes disclosed at necropsy (Crandell *et al.*, 1961).

Typical type A intranuclear inclusion bodies and associated cell changes are present in all tissues of the upper respiratory tract from days 2 through 5 postinfection. The inclusions are most numerous in the mucosal cells of the nasal septum, the turbinate bones, the tonsils, and the nictitating membrane. Fewer are present in the epiglottis and trachea (Crandell *et al.*, 1961).

A rather unusual pathologic change is resorption of the turbinate bones (Crandell *et al.*, 1961). Studies conducted in germ-free cats indicate that this process is due most likely to the characteristic vascularization of these bones that permits extravascular localization and proliferation of the virus (Hoover and Griesemer, 1971).

D. Immunity

Most investigators regard immunity to FVR as relatively weak and transient, since many recovered cats become asymptomatic carriers of the virus (Johnson and Thomas, 1966; Povey and Johnson, 1967). Recent studies revealed that kittens infected by aerosol exposure were refractory to immunity challenge 21 days later, and they did not shed virus. However, the third exposure to virus in the same manner 5 months later resulted in moderate clinical disease with viral shedding (Walton and Gillespie, 1970). Thus it appears that immunity to FVR is of longer duration than originally suspected.

Antibody levels are detected 14–21 days after exposure although some cats do not respond serologically. On reexposure, however, the titers of seropositive animals increase, although not as markedly as when reexposure occurs after a long interval (Walton and Gillespie, 1970). Antibody levels drop fairly rapidly in the absence of reexposure. There is usually a correlation between immunity and antibody levels, although some adult cats, with or without detectable antibody, have been found to be refractory to infection (Povey and Johnson, 1967). Resistance to challenge has been associated in younger cats with antibody titers as low as 1 : 4 (Walton and Gillespie, 1970).

There is little or no information relative to naturally acquired passive immunity to FVR or the response of newborn kittens from seropositive mothers to experimental or naturally acquired infection. Apparently assays of nasal secretions for extravascular antibody or interferon have not been made.

E. Diagnosis

Clinically, FVR, feline picornavirus (FPV) infection, and FP resemble each other closely. However, the presence of intracytoplasmic chlamydial inclusions in smears of conjunctival swabbings stained by Giemsa is indicative of FP. Although FPV infection is said to be milder than FVR (O'Reilly,

1971), isolation and identification of virus provides the most reliable method of differentiating the two. Occasionally FVR is characterized by a mild to severe glossitis, but the inconstancy of this sign limits its value as a differential feature. In cadavers, the presence of intranuclear eosinophilic inclusion bodies, particularly in cells of the upper respiratory tract tissues, is of diagnostic significance.

A retrospective diagnosis usually can be made serologically, although, as already mentioned, some cats do not develop neutralizing antibody while antibody titers of others are low. Nevertheless, low titers to FVR are significant. Many cats still have appreciable titers 3 weeks after exposure, although these titers decline quite rapidly thereafter.

A hemagglutination inhibition test specific for feline herpesvirus antibody has been reported but thus far it has not been used to any extent (Gillespie *et al.*, 1971).

F. Prevention and Control

Despite the relatively transient immunity to FVR, indications are that a vaccine would be useful in minimizing the severity of recurring infection. One report indicates that a vaccine has been used in Switzerland but specific details are lacking (Lindt *et al.*, 1965). It was found, however, that the original feline herpesvirus isolate still retained the capacity to cause marked clinical disease in kittens after 100 serial transfers in cell culture (Crandell, 1971). The same investigator found that β-propiolactone-inactivated virus failed to protect kittens against challenge with virulent virus.

The removal of diseased cats, followed by disinfection of the cages and pens, is recommended as a means of controlling spread of the disease in a colony. There are no data regarding the availability or efficacy of antiserum, used either prophylactically or therapeutically, in the prevention or control of the disease.

VIII. Cottontail Herpesvirus Infection

A. Introduction

With the exception of sheep, naturally occurring herpesvirus infections are found among all of the common domestic animal species including chickens, ducks, and turkeys. Thus far, however, the number of wildlife species examined for the presence of these and other viruses, especially mammalian species, has been limited. Nonetheless, the recent isolation of a herpesvirus from the cottontail rabbit (*Sylvilagus floridanus*)—probably among the first of the wild mammals to be examined—indicates that the host range of herpesviruses among wildlife might well be as broad as it is among the domestic species.

1. Classification and Characteristics of the Virus

The virus was isolated from clinically normal, mature cottontail rabbits that had been trapped in different areas of southern and central Wisconsin (Hinze, 1968). It possesses the physical and chemical properties common to all herpesviruses but much of the virus appears to be cell-associated (Ley and Burger, 1970). It is antigenically distinct from herpesviruses of a wide range of animal host species and also from virus III, the only other known herpesvirus of rabbits (Hinze, 1968). The name Herpesvirus sylvilagus has been proposed for it (Hinze, 1971a).

2. Nature of the Infection

The naturally occurring infection is inapparent, but a generalized proliferative disease that is frequently benign but which, in its most severe form, histologically resembles a malignant lymphoma is produced by experimental inoculation of the virus (Hinze, 1969).

3. Natural and Experimental Host Range

Studies to date indicate that the cottontail is the only host of the virus. Experimental species, including young and mature New Zealand white rabbits, newborn and adult white Swiss mice, Syrian hamsters, and adult guinea pigs are refractory. However, the virus has been propagated in kidney cell cultures of New Zealand white rabbits and the natural host. Multiplication did not occur in a wide range of other cell types or in chicken embryos inoculated via the chorioallantois.

4. Distribution, Prevalence, and Economic Importance

Beyond the fact that this infection exists in certain areas of Wisconsin in apparently normal cottontail rabbits, nothing is known of its distribution or prevalence. The infection is of no known importance, economically or otherwise, other than as a possible model for studies of herpesviral neoplasias.

B. Epidemiology

Inferences only can be drawn from the limited observations and studies published to date. Seemingly, the infection is not contagious. The fact that it can be reproduced only by parenteral inoculation suggests that the virus might be transmitted by a vector or by wound infection incurred in fighting. The disease is apparently latent in nature, with the host species serving as the reservoir of the virus.

C. Pathogenesis

The pathogenesis of the infection has been studied only in experimentally infected cottontail rabbits (Hinze, 1971b). Generalized lymph node enlargement occurs 1–2 weeks after inoculation, with a 20-fold increase occurring in the size of some nodes. A low grade viremia, which appears to be cell-associated, is detected at this time and persists for the remaining life of the host. A lymphocytosis, consisting in part of large numbers of immature and abnormal lymphoid cells, occurs 2–3 weeks after infection. It reaches maximal intensity between 4 and 8 weeks, when the cell count attains double its normal value, and the lymphocyte fraction increases from 55% to over 90%. The total and the differential counts return to essentially normal 6–8 weeks later. By the fourth week, virus is present in the lymph nodes, spleen, and kidneys but only in those animals which develop the lymphoma-like disease. In such animals there is massive infiltration of most organs by immature, mitotically active lymphocytes by the sixth week. This cellular invasion, in conjunction with loss of normal architecture, is suggestive of malignant lymphoma. However, the disease has not been shown to be irreversible, and lymphocytes do not appear to be arrested at one stage of maturation. These features would mitigate against the likelihood of the disease being a true neoplasia. It appears that the virus causes lymphocytic proliferation by direct stimulation rather than inducing lymphoid hyperplasia by means of antigenic stimulation. This is in keeping with the probability that it is cell-associated in the blood stream and the fact that it cannot be isolated from nonlymphoid cells of infected organs. The virus behaves somewhat like the Epstein-Barr virus in that it produces a benign disease in some members of the host species and a seemingly malignant process in others (Hinze, 1971b).

Histopathologic Changes

The histopathologic changes are compatible with those of a marked stimulation of the lymphoid organs (Hinze, 1971b). These changes include spleen and lymphoid hyperplasia, with architectural changes in the lymph nodes occurring after 4 weeks as a consequence of proliferating blast cells. Similar changes occur in the spleen, with large germinal centers containing masses of immature lymphocytes. Cellular infiltration of other organs takes place, particularly of the kidneys, liver, and myocardium in most infected animals although the infiltration is limited to small foci in these cases. It is more marked, however, and involves, in addition, the lungs, pancreas, submaxillary gland, and intestinal wall of animals in which the normal structure of the lymph nodes is lost. Inclusion bodies have not been demonstrated at any time in either the invading lymphocytes or the tissue cells of any of the involved organs.

D. Immunity

No information is available regarding the immunity associated with either the naturally occurring or the experimentally induced disease. Neutralizing antibody has been produced by inoculation of the natural host but attempts to produce antibody in New Zealand white rabbits were unsuccessful. Apparently the only diagnostic procedure is recovery of the virus from the blood by cell culture procedures.

IX. Herpesvirus Infection of Chickens: Infectious Laryngotracheitis

A. Introduction

Laryngotracheitis (LT) was first described in 1925 in the United States under the name of "tracheolaryngitis" (May and Tittsler, 1925). Although the disease had been observed earlier, it was known by a number of names including "infectious bronchitis" and "bronchopneumonia" (Beaudette, 1949). Later it was assigned the name by which it is currently known (Graham *et al.*, 1931). The disease has been diagnosed in Canada (Gwatkin, 1925), Holland (Van Heelsbergen, 1929), the United Kingdom (Dobson, 1935), Australia (Seddon and Hart, 1935), Sweden (Magnusson, 1940), Poland (Marek, 1948), Germany (Fritzsche and Gerriers, 1959), and Finland (Rislakki, 1965).

1. Classification and Properties of the Virus

The causative agent of LT was demonstrated by filtration studies to be a virus (Beaudette, 1930; Beach, 1930). More definitive studies by means of negative staining revealed that its structure was essentially identical to that of herpes simplex (Cruickshank *et al.*, 1963).

The LT virus is highly host specific, being propagated readily only in tissue cells of chickens, pheasants, and their hybrids. It was cultivated initially in Maitland type tissue culture (Beach, 1932) but fertile eggs proved subsequently to be a much more suitable culture system. Inoculation of diluted virus to the chorioallantois results in the formation of foci from 4–5 mm in diameter with opaque, raised edges and a centrally depressed grayish area consisting of necrotic cells (Beveridge and Burnet, 1946). With less dilute inoculum the membrane becomes thickened and edematous without the formation of characteristic pocklike foci. Acidophilic inclusion bodies appear 24 hours after inoculation and eventually occupy the greater portion of the nuclear area (Beveridge and Burnet, 1946). Embryos die from 2 to 12 days after inoculation. Virus inoculated into the allantoic sac produces lesions on the endothelial surface of the chorioallantois which are characterized by inflammation and hyperplasia, but virus yields are inconsistent (Beveridge and Burnet, 1946). The yields are likewise poor following amniotic sac inoculation, while the virus cannot be propagated in the yolk sac of embryos (Brandly, 1934).

It was almost 30 years after Beach demonstrated that the virus can replicate in Maitland type tissue culture that its multiplication in monolayer cultures of chicken embryo fibroblasts and chick respiratory epithelium was reported (Atherton and Anderson, 1957; Pulsford, 1957, 1960; Chomiac *et al.*, 1960). Eventually a wide range of chicken embryonic tissues was found suitable, with best results being obtained with cell monolayers initiated by numerous minute cell explants or partially trypsinized cell clumps (Buthala and Mathews, 1957; Pulsford, 1958). Since the virus is cytopathic it was possible to develop a serum neutralization (SN) test (Atherton and Anderson, 1957). A reproducible plaque system for assay of the virus has also been developed (Sharma and Raggi, 1969). Nevertheless, the chicken embryo is still the most widely used indicator host for the SN test in identifying virus or detecting the presence of LT neutralizing antibody.

In cell culture, virus of virulent strains is released into the extracellular fluid soon after its appearance in the cells, but with strains of low virulence the release is delayed or minimal (Pulsford, 1960). It thus appears likely that the virus is cell-associated and, hence, passes directly from cell to cell, a form of spread which might account for its ability to form pocks on the chorioallantois (Atherton and Anderson, 1957).

2. Nature of the Infection

The virus produces a respiratory disease syndrome of variable intensity in chickens. It is not followed by sequelae which frequently characterize herpesvirus infections of other species.

3. Natural and Experimental Host Range

Laryngotracheitis is a highly host-specific disease with chickens, pheasants, and their hybrids only being susceptible. However, the infection is not transmitted between chickens and pheasants (Kernohan, 1931). Propagation of the virus on the chorioallantois of turkey eggs has been reported (Brandly, 1936), and recently turkey poults were found to be susceptible to inoculation (Winterfield and So, 1968).

4. Distribution, Prevalence, and Economic Importance

The widespread distribution and the high mortality associated with LT make it a disease of considerable economic importance. Additional losses are incurred through lowered egg production and general unthriftiness of affected birds (Raggi *et al.*, 1961).

B. Epidemiology

Influence of Ecologic Factors

It is postulated that the epidemic or peracute form of LT, which first appeared during the early 1920's, developed over a period of time during which the virus evolved from an orphan virus, or one of low virulence, to a virus of high virulence. There is evidence that this change was brought about by mass production methods which, by inducing stress on the birds, promoted the spread of disease with consequent increase in the virulence of the virus (Pulsford, 1953, 1954, 1961).

The LT virus of low virulence and the highly virulent virus differ in properties which are of epidemiologic significance. Strains of low virulence are only weakly neutralized by antibody, and the virus apparently is largely cell-associated (Atherton and Anderson, 1957). Transmission from infected hens to their offspring is, therefore, by contact (Pulsford, 1954, 1961). Such infection is frequently subacute or chronic, with only slight damage resulting to the host. Clinical infection appears in many cases only after the intervention of some predisposing factor such as concurrent viral infection or adverse environmental conditions. As the antibody has only a low avidity for the virus, the latter is able to persist in an immune environment, despite high antibody levels in the bird population.

By contrast, the highly virulent epidemic viral strains are tracheal pathogens. The virus is released from infected cells and is thus spread by droplet infection (Pulsford, 1958). Since the virus is readily neutralized by homologous antibody, it attacks only highly susceptible birds, causing severe disease terminating in death in a high percentage of cases.

Laryngotracheitis is not characterized either by latency or the existence of reservoir hosts. However, carrier birds appear to play an important role in perpetuating the infection on a premises (Gibbs, 1932; Beaudette, 1937). Virus has been isolated from the tracheas of birds from 6 days to 16 months after recovery from the disease (Komarov and Beaudette, 1932).

C. *Pathogenesis*

1. Transmission

The LT virus is transmitted mainly by droplet infection, with birds in the preclinical incubative stage of the disease transmitting the virus more readily than those with clinical signs of infection (Hinshaw *et al.*, 1931). Experimental study has largely discounted the likelihood that transmission occurs through the egg (Brandly, 1934). Experimentally, the infection can be reproduced consistently by intratracheal (it) or intraocular exposure to infectious material, frequently by intraperitoneal (ip) inoculation, and inconsistently by the intravenous (iv) route. Spread of the virus by fomites such as contaminated cages has been reported (Dobson, 1935). Indirect spread of the infection has been attributed to poultry dealers, rats, crows, and dogs (Kingsbury and Jungherr, 1957).

2. Clinical Features of the Infection

The incubation period of naturally occurring LT varies from 6 to 12 days and from 2 to 3 days following intratracheal exposure (Seddon and Hart, 1935; Raggi *et al.*, 1961). Most investigators consider that birds of all ages are equally susceptible. However, the infection occurs in most flocks when the birds are under 12 months of age but older than 10–12 days (Hinshaw, 1931; Hinshaw *et al.*, 1931).

The acute or epidemic form of the disease is characterized by a number of clinical signs of varying degrees of intensity, several or all of which may occur in the same bird. The onset is sudden, with the first indication of disease often being the death of a few birds. Dyspnea is probably the most characteristic clinical sign. It is usually preceded by lacrimation, or by the appearance of a frothy, ocular exudate which is followed by conjunctivitis. The ocular exudate becomes mucoid and may seal the eyelids together. A nasal discharge is often present. Spasmodic coughing occurs, during which blood or mucus is expelled, and moist rales are detected in many birds. The dyspnea is severe, with the birds extending and raising the head as they gasp for breath. Inspiration is usually labored and accompanied by a high-pitched wheezing sound. Convulsions and choking often occur immediately prior to death (Beach, 1926; Kernohan, 1931; Hinshaw *et al.*, 1931).

Signs of the mild or endemic form of the infection include conjunctivitis, with swelling of the infraorbital sinuses, and a persistent nasal discharge. In some cases the signs are limited to mild coryza.

The average duration of the acute disease ranges from 12–15 days while that of the mild or endemic form is approximately 3 weeks.

The productivity of laying hens drops materially during an outbreak, and significant deterioration in shell thickness occurs which lasts for 1–2 days only after affected egg layers return to production (Raggi *et al.*, 1961). In the case of infectious bronchitis the inferior shell quality may persist for several months.

3. Pathologic Findings

Gross lesions are confined to the respiratory tract and the conjunctiva. The initial changes occur 36–42 hours after infection and consist of inflammation of the larynx, trachea, and bronchi accompanied in some cases by congestion of the lungs. In severely affected birds, the most prominent lesion is a hemorrhagic tracheitis. Diphtheritic inflammation and a mucoid exudate are commonly present in both acutely and mildly affected birds (Graham *et al.*, 1930). Occlusion of the larynx and occasionally the trachea with caseous or diphtheritic material is a frequent cause of death (Seifried, 1931).

Histologic changes resulting from either the naturally occurring or the experimentally induced disease are very similar. Early in the infection the surface epithelial cells become edematous, swell, and lose their cilia. The edema increases, accompanied by cellular infiltration of the mucosa and the submucosa, and hemorrhage from small vessels sometimes causes separation of the two layers. The structural identity of the cells and mucous glands is gradually lost and by the fifth day marked degenerative changes are apparent, with sloughing of entire sections of mucosa occurring. In addition, microscopic lesions occur in the lungs, kidneys, epicardium, and liver of naturally infected birds. They were attributed by some workers to systemic viral invasion (Thorp and Graham, 1934; Beach, 1931). Others, however, were unsuccessful in attempts to isolate virus from the blood and internal organs (Komarov and Beaudette, 1931; Burnet, 1936; Kernohan, 1931; Seddon and Hart, 1936; Jordan, 1963). It appears that should viremia occur, it is of a very transitory nature.

Intranuclear inclusion bodies are present by 12 hours postinfection but are most numerous approximately 48 hours after clinical signs of disease appear. By the fourth day, however, few can be found (Seifried, 1931).

D. Morbidity and Mortality

In epidemics of LT the morbidity may reach 90–100% and the mortality from 5 to 80%, the average being 20%. The majority of deaths occurs between the tenth and twelfth days of infection. The morbidity associated with the milder chronic disease does not exceed 5%, and deaths are rare (Raggi *et al.*, 1961).

E. Immunity

There is substantial evidence that neutralizing antibody is present in the yolk from eggs of vaccinated hens, from hens in endemic areas (Pulsford and

Watts, 1961), and in the serum of the progeny of such hens for at least several weeks after hatching (Benton *et al.*, 1960). However, opinion is divided regarding the significance of passive antibody in disease protection, or in the development of immunity to vaccination (Hitchner and Winterfield, 1960; Satriano *et al.*, 1957; Pulsford and Watts, 1961). Available evidence, however, tends to support the view that the presence of passive antibody affords protection for the first few weeks after hatching but adversely affects the response to vaccination.

The immunity following natural infection lasts for 1 year or longer, whereas vaccination affords protection over a period of 6 weeks to 1 year (Beaudette, 1949; Shibley *et al.*, 1962; Raggi and Lee, 1965). Evidence of a correlation between neutralizing antibody and immunity is conflicting. Some workers (Hitchner *et al.*, 1958) report that neutralizing antibody provides a valid indication of the immune status of vaccinated birds, whereas others report the opposite finding (Shibley *et al.*, 1962).

F. Diagnosis

Signs such as expectoration of blood-tinged mucus, hemorrhagic tracheitis and associated blood clots, and high mortality are pathognomonic of the peracute disease (Delaplane, 1945; Van Roekel, 1955). Because of its clinical similarity to a number of respiratory infections of birds, the mild form of LT, however, cannot be diagnosed with certainty on a clinical basis. The most common laboratory procedure for diagnosis of the latter form is the demonstration of typical intranuclear inclusion bodies in lesions which develop in the chorioallantois following the inoculation of suspect material onto the membrane, or by serologic identification of virus isolated by this procedure. Viral isolation may be accomplished also by means of chicken embryo kidney cell monolayer cultures. The presence of virus is indicated by giant cell formation, focal necrosis, and the presence of inclusion bodies. A rapid diagnosis, based on the demonstration of inclusions in thin sections of trachea, can be made histologically by special techniques which enable rapid fixation and dehydration of the tissues (Sevoian, 1960). Preparation of the slides requires about 3 hours. Other diagnostic methods include the inoculation of tracheal exudates into LT immune and susceptible birds and the demonstration of specific neutralizing antibody in sick birds.

G. Prevention and Control

VACCINATION

Vaccination is indicated in areas where the disease is endemic but is contraindicated in those areas free of infection because of the hazard created by carrier birds resulting from vaccination. Various types of vaccine and different routes of application have been employed since the inception of the first vaccination procedure for LT 40 years ago, after it was found that the inactivated virus was not immunogenic (Hudson and Beaudette, 1932a,b). The procedure then consisted of applying live, virulent virus to the mucosa of the cloaca. The use of virulent virus was continued until the early 1950's under the mistaken impression that mild strains of the virus fail to produce a satisfactory immunity (Gibbs, 1933; Hart, 1946). At the present time vaccines consisting of virus attenuated by passage in cell culture or feather follicle are available for administration via the conjunctival sac, the nasal route, the feather follicle, or the cloaca. The most satisfactory results are obtained when the vaccine is applied to the cloacal mucosa, possibly because of the important role played by the bursal tissues in the immune response.

Ideally, vaccination should be carried out when the birds are approximately 10 weeks of age, since the parenteral immunity has waned or disappeared by this time. Occasionally postvaccinal infection simulating LT occurs (Laurie-Rhodes, 1955; Raggi and Lee, 1965). Paralysis has also been reported in a small percentage of birds vaccinated by cloacal exposure, possibly as a result of the pressure exerted on the sciatic nerve by the cloacal edema (Furness, 1945).

Evidence for the effectiveness of LT immune serum, used either prophylactically or therapeutically, is conflicting (Graham *et al.*, 1931; Gibbs, 1933; Brandly, 1935). Regardless of its effectiveness, the use of immune serum would not be indicated because of economic considerations.

References

Afshar, A., and Tadjbakhsh, H. (1970). *J. Comp. Pathol.* **80**, 307.

Alexander, R. A., Plowright, W., and Haig, D. A. (1957). *Bull. Epiz. Dis. Afr.* **5**, 489.

Andersen, A. C. (1970). *In* "The Beagle as an Experimental Dog" (A. C. Andersen, ed.), p. 35 Iowa State Univ. Press, Ames.

Andrewes, C. H. (1962). *Advan. Virus Res.* **9**, 271.

Armstrong, J. A., Pereira, H. G., and Andrewes, C. H. (1961). *Virology* **14**, 276.

Atherton, J. G., and Anderson, W. (1957). *Aust. J. Exp. Biol.* **35**, 335.

Aujeszky, A. (1902). *Zentralbl. Bakteriol., Parasitenk., Infektionskr. Hyg., Abt. 1: Orig.* **32**, 353.

Aurelian, L. (1968). *Proc. Soc. Exp. Biol. Med.* **127**, 485.

Baker, J. A. (1942). *Science* **96**, 475.

Baker, J. A., McEntee, K., and Gillespie, J. H. (1960). *Cornell Vet.* **50**, 156.

Bang, F. B. (1942). *J. Exp. Med.* **76**, 263.

Barenfus, M., Delli Quadri, C. A., McIntyre, R. W., and Schroeder, R. J. (1963). *J. Amer. Vet. Med. Ass.* **143**, 725.

Beach, J. R. (1926). *J. Amer. Vet. Med. Ass.* **68**, 570.

Beach, J. R. (1930). *Science* **72**, 633.

Beach, J. R. (1931). *J. Exp. Med.* **54**, 809.

Beach, J. R. (1932). *Science* **76**, 260.

Beaudette, F. R. (1930). *N. J. Agr. Exp. Sta., Annu. Rep.* **51**, 286.
Beaudette, F. R. (1937). *Poultry Sci.* **16**, 103.
Beaudette, F. R. (1949). *J. Amer. Vet. Med. Ass.* **115**, 232.
Benton, W. J., Cover, M. S., and Krauss, W. C. (1960). *Avian Dis.* **4**, 491.
Beveridge, W. I. B., and Burnet, F. M. (1946). *Med. Res. Counc. (Gt. Brit.), Spec. Rep. Ser.* **SRS–256**.
Binn, L. N., Eddy, G. A., Lazar, E. E., Helms, J., and Murnane, T. (1967). *Proc. Soc. Exp. Biol. Med.* **126**, 140.
Bitsch, V., and Dam, A. (1971). *Acta Med. Vet. Scand.* **12**, 134.
Bittle, J. L. (1969). *J. Amer. Vet. Med. Ass.* **155**, 312 (Discussion 314).
Bittle, J. L. (1972). Pitman-Moore, Inc. Washington Crossing, New Jersey (Personal communication).
Bittle, J. L., and Peckham, J. C. (1971). *J. Amer. Vet. Med. Ass.* **158**, 927.
Bittle, J. L., York, C. J., Newberne, J. W., and Martin, M. (1960). *Amer. J. Vet. Res.* **21**, 547.
Bracken, E. C. (1960). *AMA Amer. J. Dis. Child.* **100**, 535.
Brandly, C. A. (1934). *J. Amer. Vet. Med. Ass.* **84**, 588.
Brandly, C. A. (1935). *J. Infec. Dis.* **57**, 201.
Brandly, C. A. (1936). *J. Amer. Vet. Med. Ass.* **88**, 587.
Bryans, J. T. (1968). *Proc. Annu. Amer. Ass. Equine Practitioners Conv.* p. 119.
Bryans, J. T. (1969). *J. Amer. Vet. Med. Ass.* **155**, 294.
Bürki, F. (1963). *World Vet. Congr., Proc., 17th. 1963* p. 559.
Burnet, F. M. (1936). *J. Exp. Med.* **63**, 685.
Burnet, F. M., Lush, D., and Jackson, A. V. (1939). *Aust. J. Exp. Biol. Med. Sci.* **17**, 41.
Burrows, R. (1970). *Proc. Int. Conf. Equine Infec. Dis., 2nd, 1969* pp. 1–12.
Buthala, D. A., and Mathews, J. (1957). *Cornell Vet.* **47**, 143.
Carmichael, L. E. (1965). "Fifteenth Gaines Symposium," p. 24. University of Missouri, Columbus.
Carmichael, L. E. (1970). *J. Amer. Vet. Med. Ass.* **156**, 1714.
Carmichael, L. E. (1972). New York State Veterinary College, Cornell University, Ithaca, New York (personal communication).
Carmichael, L. E., and Barnes, F. D. (1961). *Proc. 65th Annual Meeting U.S. Livestock Sanit. Ass.* p. 384.
Carmichael, L. E., Fabricant, J., and Squire, R. A. (1964). *Proc. Soc. Exp. Biol. Med.* **117**, 826.
Carmichael, L. E., Squire, R. A., and Krook, L. (1965a). *Amer. J. Vet. Res.* **26**, 803.
Carmichael, L. E., Strandberg, J. D., and Barnes, F. D. (1965b). *Proc. Soc. Exp. Biol. Med.* **120**, 644.
Carmichael, L. E., Barnes, F. D., and Percy, D. H. (1970). *J. Infec. Dis.* **120**, 669.
Castrucci, G., Gattaponi, P., and Giuloni, A. (1966). *Arch. Vet. Ital.* **17**, 185.
Castrucci, G., Pedini, B., Cilli, V., and Arancia, G. (1972). *Vet. Rec.* **90**, 325.
Chanock, R. M. (1969). *In* "The Secretory Immunoglobulins" (D. H. Dayton *et al.*, eds.), pp. 83–92. US Govt. Printing Office, Washington, D.C.
Cheatham, W. J., and Crandell, R. A. (1957). *Proc. Soc. Exp. Biol. Med.* **96**, 536.
Chomiac, T. W., Luginbuhl, R. E., and Helmboldt, C. F. (1960). *Avian Dis.* **4**, 235.
Chow, T. L. (1972). *J. Amer. Vet. Med. Ass.* **160**, 51.
Chow, T. L., and Davis, R. W. (1964). *Amer. J. Vet. Res.* **25**, 518.
Cornwell, H. J. C., Wright, N. G., Campbell, R. S. F., Roberts, R. J., and Reed, A. (1966). *Vet. Rec.* **79**, 661.
Crandell, R. A. (1971). *J. Amer. Vet. Med. Ass.* **158**, 922.
Crandell, R. A., and Maurer, F. D. (1958). *Proc. Soc. Exp. Biol. Med.* **97**, 487.

Crandell, R. A., Cheatham, W. J. and Maurer, F. D. (1959). *Amer. J. Vet. Res.* **20**, 505.
Crandell, R. A., Ganaway, J. R., Niemann, W. H., and Maurer, F. D. (1960). *Amer. J. Vet. Res.* **21**, 504.
Crandell, R. A., Rehkemper, J. A., Niemann, W. H., Ganaway, J. R., and Maurer, F. D. (1961). *J. Amer. Vet. Med. Ass.* **138**, 191.
Cruickshank, J. G., Berry, D. M., and Hay, B. (1963). *Virology* **20**, 378.
Deas, D. W., and Johnson, W. S. (1966). *Vet. Rec.* **78**, 828.
Delaplane, J. P. (1945). *J. Amer. Vet. Med. Ass.* **106**, 83.
deRatuld, Y., and Werner, G. H. (1965). *C. R. Acad. Sci.* **261**, 5725.
Dimock, W. W. (1940). *J. Amer. Vet. Med. Ass.* **96**, 665.
Dimock, W. W., and Edwards, P. R. (1932). *Suppl. Ky. Agr. Exp. Sta. Bull.* **333**.
Ditchfield, J., and Grinyer, I. (1965). *Virology* **26**, 504.
Dobson, N. (1935). *Vet. Rec.* **15**, 1467.
Doll, E. R. (1952). *Cornell Vet.* **42**, 505.
Doll, E. R. (1961). *J. Amer. Vet. Med. Ass.* **139**, 1324.
Doll, E. R. (1963). *In* "Equine Medicine and Surgery" (J. F. Bone *et al.*, eds.), pp. 158–165. Amer. Vet. Publ., Santa Barbara, California.
Doll, E. R., and Bryans, J. T. (1962a). *Amer. J. Vet. Res.* **23**, 843.
Doll, E. R., and Bryans, J. T. (1962b). *J. Amer. Vet. Med. Ass.* **141**, 351.
Doll, E. R., and Bryans, J. T. (1963a). *Cornell Vet.* **53**, 24.
Doll, E. R., and Bryans, J. T. (1963b). *Cornell Vet.* **53**, 249.
Doll, E. R., and Bryans, J. T. (1963c). *J. Amer. Vet. Med. Ass.* **142**, 31.
Doll, E. R., and Kintner, J. H. (1954). *Cornell Vet.* **44**, 355.
Doll, E. R., and Wallace, M. E. (1954). *Cornell Vet.* **44**, 453.
Doll, E. R., Richards, M. G., and Wallace, M. E. (1953). *Cornell Vet.* **43**, 551.
Doll. E. R., Wallace, M. E., and Richards, M. G. (1954). *Cornell Vet.* **44**, 181.
Doll, E. R., Wallace, M. E., Bryans, J. T., and McCollum, W. H. (1955). *Cornell Vet.* **45**, 387.
Doll, E. R., Bryans, J. T., McCollum, W. H., and Crowe, M. E. W. (1956a). *Cornell Vet.* **46**, 68.
Doll, E. R. McCollum, W. H., Bryans, J. T., and Crowe, M. E. W. (1956b). *Cornell Vet.* **46**, 97.
Doll, E. R., Bryans, J. T., McCollum, W. H., and Crowe, M. E. W. (1957). *Cornell Vet.* **47**, 3.
Fox, F. H. (1972). New York State Veterinary College, Cornell University, Ithaca, New York (personal communication).
French, E. L. (1962a). *Aust. Vet. J.* **38**, 216.
French, E. L. (1962b). *Aust. Vet. J.* **38**, 477.
French, E. L. (1962c). *Aust. Vet. J.* **38**, 555.
Fritzsche, K., and Gerriers, E. (1959). *In* "Geflügel Krankheiten," pp. 77–81. Parey, Berlin.
Furness, T. L. (1945). *Aust. Vet. J.* **21**, 142.
Galloway, I. A. (1938). *Vet. Rec.* **50**, 745.
Gardiner, M. R., Nairn, M. E., and Sier, A. M. (1964). *Aust. Vet. J.* **40**, 225.
Gaskin, J. M. (1970). Quoted by Scott (1971).
Geldard, H., Geering, W. A., and Bagust, T. J. (1971). *Aust. Vet. J.* **47**, 286.
Gibbons, W. J. (1944). *Cornell Vet.* **34**, 235.
Gibbs, C. S. (1932). *J. Amer. Vet. Med. Ass.* **34**, 651.
Gibbs, C. S. (1933). *Mass., Agr. Exp. Sta., Bull.* **295**, 1.
Gilbert, Y., and Saurat, P. (1970). *In* "Les Maladies Animales à Virus" (P. Lepine and P. Goret, eds.), pp. 17–71. L'Expansion Scientifique Française, Paris.
Gillespie, J. H., Lee, K. M., and Baker, J. A. (1957). *Amer. J. Vet. Res.* **18**, 530.
Gillespie, J. H., Judkins, A. B., and Scott, F. W. (1971). *Cornell Vet.* **61**, 159.
Girard, A., Greig, A. S., and Mitchell, D. (1963). *Cornell Vet.* **53**, 88.
Girard, A., Greig, A. S., and Mitchell, D. (1968). *Can. J. Comp. Med. Vet. Sci.* **32**, 603.

Graham, R., Thorp, F., and James, W. A. (1930). *J. Infec. Dis.* **47**, 83.
Graham, R., Thorp, F., and James, W. A. (1931). *J. Amer. Vet. Med. Ass.* **78**, 506.
Gustafson, D. P. (1967). *Proc. 71st Annual Meeting U.S. Livestock Sanit. Ass.* p. 349.
Gustafson, D. P. (1970). *In* "Diseases of Swine" (H. W. Dunne, ed.), 3rd ed., pp. 337–355. Iowa State Univ. Press, Ames.
Gwatkin, R. (1925). *Ont. Vet. Coll. Rep.* p. 54.
Hahnefeld, H., and Hahnefeld, E. (1962). *Arch. Exp. Veterinaermed.* **16**, 1115.
Haig, D. A. (1967). *Vet. Rec.* **80**, 311.
Hanson, R. P. (1954). *J. Amer. Vet. Med. Ass.* **124**, 259.
Hart, L. (1946). *Aust. Vet. J.* **22**, 125.
Hatzolios, B. C., and Reagan, R. L. (1960). *Amer. J. Vet. Res.* **21**, 856.
Henning, M. W. (1946). *Onderstepoort J. Vet. Res.* **21**, 17.
Hinshaw, W. R. (1931). *Calif., Agr. Exp. Sta., Bull.* **520**, 1.
Hinshaw, W. R., Jones, E. C., and Graybill, H. W. (1931). *Poultry Sci.* **10**, 375.
Hinze, H. C. (1968). *Bacteriol. Proc.* p. 149.
Hinze, H. C. (1969). *Bacteriol. Proc.* p. 157.
Hinze, H. C. (1971a). *Infection Immunity* **3**, 350.
Hinze, H. C. (1971b). *Int. J. Cancer* **8**, 514.
Hitchner, S. B., and Winterfield, R. W. (1960). *Avian Dis.* **4**, 291.
Hitchner, S. B., Shea, C. A., and White, P. G. (1958). *Avian Dis.* **2**, 258.
Hoover, E. A. (1970). College of Veterinary Medicine, Ohio State University, Columbus (unpublished data).
Hoover, E. A., and Griesemer, R. A. (1971). *J. Amer. Vet. Med. Ass.* **158**, 929.
Horvath, Z., Bartha, A., Papp, L., and Juhasz, M. (1965). *Acta Vet.* (*Budapest*) **15**, 415.
Howarth, J. A. (1969). *J. Amer. Vet. Med. Ass.* **154**, 1583.
Howarth, J. A. (1970). *Proc. 74th Annual Meeting U.S. Anim. Health Ass.* p. 371.
Howarth, J. A., and DePaoli, A. (1968). *J. Amer. Vet. Med. Ass.* **152**, 1114.
Huck, R. A. (1964). *Vet. Bull.* **34**, 239.
Hudson, C. B., and Beaudette, F. R. (1932a). *Cornell Vet.* **23**, 63.
Hudson, C. B., and Beaudette, F. R. (1932b). *Science* **76**, 34.
Hughes, J. P., Olander, J. H., and Wada, E. M. (1964). *J. Amer. Vet. Med. Ass.* **145**, 32.
Hupbauer, A. (1938). *Deut. Tieraerztl. Wochenschr.* **46**, 745.
Hurst, E. W. (1934). *J. Exp. Med.* **59**, 729.
Huxsoll, D. L., and Hemelt, I. E. (1970). *J. Amer. Vet. Med. Ass.* **156**, 1706.
Huygelen, C. (1960). *Zentralbl. Veterinaermed.* **7**, 664.
Johnson, R. H., and Thomas, R. E. (1966). *Vet. Rec.* **79**, 188.
Jones, F. S., and Little, R. B. (1927). *J. Exp. Med.* **45**, 519.
Jones, T. C., and Maurer, F. D. (1943). *Amer. J. Vet. Res.* **4**, 15.
Jones, T. C., Gleiser, C. A., Maurer, F. D., Hale, M. W., and Roby, T. O. (1948). *Amer. J. Vet. Res.* **9**, 243.
Jordan, F. T. W. (1963). *J. Comp. Pathol.* **73**, 253.
Kaplan, A. S. (1969). *Virol. Monogr.* **5**, 7.
Karpas, A., Garcia, F. G., Calvo, F., and Cross, R. E. (1968). *Amer. J. Vet. Res.* **29**, 1251.
Kaschula, V. R., Beaudette, F. R., and Byrne, R. J. (1957). *Cornell Vet.* **47**, 137.
Kawakami, Y., Kaji, T., Ishizaki, R., Shimizu, T., and Matumoto, M. (1962). *Jap. J. Exp. Med.* **32**, 211.
Kendrick, J. W. (1971). School of Veterinary Medicine, University of California, Davis (personal communication).
Kendrick, J. W. (1972). School of Veterinary Medicine, University of California, Davis (personal communication).

Kendrick, J. W., and Straub, O. C. (1967). *Amer. J. Vet. Res.* **28**, 1269.
Kendrick, J. W., Gillespie, J. H., and McEntee, K. (1958). *Cornell Vet.* **48**, 458.
Kennedy, P. C., and Richards, W. P. C. (1964). *Pathol. Vet.* **1**, 7.
Kernohan, G. (1931). *J. Amer. Vet. Med. Ass.* **78**, 196.
Kingsbury, F. W., and Jungherr, E. L. (1957). *Poultry Sci.* **36**, 1133.
Komarov, A., and Beaudette, F. R. (1931). *Poultry Sci.* **10**, 391.
Komarov, A., and Beaudette, F. R. (1932). *Poultry Sci.* **11**, 335.
Kretzschmar, C. (1964). *Monatsh. Veterinaermed.* **19**, 248.
Laurie-Rhodes, L. J. (1955). *Aust. Vet. J.* **31**, 194.
Lepper, A. W. D., Haig, D. A., and Wilcox, J. (1969). *J. Comp. Pathol.* **79**, 489.
Ley, K. D., and Burger, D. (1970). *Appl. Microbiol.* **19**, 549.
Lin, Y. C. (1947). *Chin. J. Anim. Husb.* **6**, 6.
Lin, Y. C. (1948). *Abst. Vet. Bull.* **18**, 200.
Lindt, S., Muhlethaler, E., and Bürki, F. (1965). *Schweiz. Arch. Tierheilk.* **107**, 196.
Ljubashenko, S. J., Tjulpanova, A. F., and Grishin, V. M. (1958). *Veterinariya (Moscow)* **35**, 37.
Lukashev, I. I., and Rotov, V. I. (1939). *Sov. Vet.* **7**, 51.
Lundgren, D. L., and Clapper, W. E. (1969). *Amer. J. Vet. Res.* **30**, 479.
McCollum, W. H., Doll, E. R., Wilson, J. C., and Johnson, C. B. (1962). *Cornell Vet.* **52**, 164.
McFerran, J. B., and Dow, C. (1965). *Amer. J. Vet. Res.* **26**, 631.
McKercher, D. G. (1962). School of Veterinary Medicine, University of California, Davis (unpublished data).
McKercher, D. G. (1963). *Amer. J. Vet. Res.* **24**, 501.
McKercher, D. G., and Crenshaw, G. L. (1971). *J. Amer. Vet. Med. Ass.* **159**, 1362.
McKercher, D. G., and Wada, E. M. (1964). *J. Amer. Vet. Med. Ass.* **144**, 136.
McKercher, D. G., Moulton, J. E., and Jasper, D. E. (1954). *Proc. 58th Annual Meeting U.S. Livestock Sanit. Ass.* p. 260.
McKercher, D. G., Moulton, J. E., Kendrick, J. W., and Saito, J. (1955). *Proc. 59th Annual Meeting U.S. Livestock Sanit. Ass.* p. 151.
McKercher, D. G., Saito, J. K., Wada, E. M., and Straub. O. C. (1958). *Proc. 62nd Annual Meeting U.S. Livestock Sanit. Ass.* p. 136.
McKercher, D. G., Straub, O. C., Saito, J. K., and Wada, E. M. (1959). *Can. J. Comp. Med.* **23**, 320.
McKercher, D. G., Wada, E. M., Straub, O. C. (1963). *Amer. J. Vet. Res.* **24**, 510.
McKercher, D. G., Bibrack, B., and Richards, W. P. C. (1970). *J. Amer. Vet. Med. Ass.* **156**, 1460.
McKercher, P. D. (1964). *Can. J. Comp. Med.* **28**, 77.
Madin, S. H., York, C. J., and McKercher, D. G. (1956). *Science* **124**, 721.
Magnusson, H. (1940). *Skand. Veterinaer Tidskr.* **30**, 629.
Mahaffey, L. W. (1962). *Vet. Rec.* **74**, 1295.
Manninger, R., and Csontos, J. (1941). *Deut. Tieraerztl. Wochenschr.* **49**, 105.
Marek, K. (1948). *Med. Wet.* **4**, 767.
Martin, W. B., Martin, B., and Lauder, I. M. (1964). *Vet. Rec.* **76**, 15.
Martin, W. B., Martin, B., Hay, D., and Lauder, I. M. (1966a). *Vet. Rec.* **78**, 494.
Martin, W. B., Hay, D., Crawford, L. V., LeBouvier, G. L., and Crawford, M. (1966b). *J. Gen. Microbiol.* **45**, 325.
Martin, W. B., James, Z., Lauder, I. M., Murray, M., and Pirie, H. M. (1969). *Amer. J. Vet. Res.* **30**, 2151.
Matumoto, M., Ishizaki, R., and Shimizu, T. (1965). *Arch. Gesamte Virusforsch.* **15**, 609.
May, H. G., and Tittsler, R. P. (1925). *J. Amer. Vet. Med. Ass.* **67**, 229.
Mayr, A. (1970). *Proc. Int. Conf. Equine Infec. Dis., 2nd., 1969* pp. 41–45.
Mayr, A., Böhm, H. O., Brill, J., and Woyciechowska, S. (1965). *Arch. Gesamte Virusforsch.* **17**, 216.

Meissner, H., and Harms, F. (1937). *Deut. Tieraerztl. Wochenschr.* **45**, 685.
Mermerski, G., Haralambiev, H., Simeonov, S., Yotov, M., and Peshev, S. (1968). *Vet. Med. Nauki* **5**, 23.
Miller, N. J. (1955). *J. Amer. Vet. Med. Ass.* **126**, 463.
Mitchell, M. V., and Gustafson, D. P. (1971). *Bacteriol. Proc.* p. 187.
Mohanty, S. B., Hammond, R. C., and Lillie, M. G. (1971). *Arch. Gesamte Virusforsch.* **34**, 394.
Mohanty, S. B., Lillie, M. G., Corselius, N. P., and Beck, J. D. (1972). *J. Amer. Vet. Med. Ass.* **160**, 879.
Mondino, G., Cupi, R. M., and Orfei, Z. (1964). *Vet. Ital.* **15**, 664.
Motohashi, T., and Tajima, M. (1966). *Jap. J. Vet. Sci.* **28**, 307.
Newberne, J. W., Robinson, V. B., and Alter, M. L. (1961). *Vet. Med.* **56**, 395.
Nikitin, M. G. (1960). *Sb. Tr. Kharkov Vet. Inst.* **24**, 291.
Olander, H. J., Saunders, J. R., Gustafson, D. P., and Jones, R. K. (1966). *Pathol. Vet.* **3**, 64.
Onstad, O., and Saxegaard, F. (1967). *Nord. Veterinaer Med.* **19**, 49.
O'Reilly, K. J. (1971). *J. Amer. Vet. Med. Ass.* **158**, 920.
Pascoe, R. R., Spradbrow, P. B., and Bagust, T. J. (1968). *Aust. Vet. J.* **44, 485.**
Pascoe, R. R., Spradbrow, P. B., and Bagust, T. J. (1969). *Aust. Vet. J.* **45**, 166.
Pepper, T. A., Stafford, L. P., Johnson, R. H., and Osborne, A. D. (1966). *Vet. Rec.* **78**, 569.
Percy, D. H., Olander, H. J., and Carmichael, L. E. (1968). *Pathol. Vet.* **5**, 135.
Percy, D. H., Carmichael, L. E., Albert, D. M., King, J. M., and Jonas, A. M. (1971). *Vet. Pathol.* **8**, 37.
Persechino, A., Merucci, P., and Orfei, Z. (1965). *Nuova Vet.* **41**, 213.
Petzoldt, K. (1967a). *Arch. Exp. Veterinaermed.* **21**, 115.
Petzoldt, K. (1967b). *Zentralbl. Bakteriol., Parasitenk., Infektionskr. Hyg., Abt. Ref.* **206**, 540.
Piercy, S. E., and Prydie, J. (1963). *Vet. Rec.* **75**, 86.
Pierson, R. A., and Vair, C. A. (1965). *J. Amer. Vet. Med. Ass.* **147**, 350.
Pleva, V., and Goiš, M. (1964). *Arch. Exp. Veterinaermed.* **18**, 737.
Plummer, G. (1964). *Brit. J. Exp. Pathol.* **45**, 135.
Plummer, G., and Waterson, A. P. (1963). *Virology* **19**, 412.
Plummer, G., Bowling, C. P., and Goodheart, C. R. (1969). *J. Virol.* **4**, 738.
Popescu, A. (1962). *Lucr. Inst. Cercet. Vet. Bioprep. Pasteur* **1**, 279.
Poste, G. (1972). *Arch. Gesamte Virusforsch.* **36**, 147.
Poste, G., and King, N. (1971). *Vet. Rec.* **88**, 229.
Povey, R. C., and Johnson, R. H. (1967). *Vet. Rec.* **81**, 486.
Prickett, M. E. (1970). *Proc. Int. Conf. Equine Infec. Dis., 2nd, 1969* pp. 24–33.
Prydie, J., Harrison, M. J., and Graham, J. (1966). *Vet. Rec.* **79**, 660.
Pulsford, M. F. (1953). *Nature (London)* **172**, 1193.
Pulsford, M. F. (1954). *World's Poultry Congr., Proc., 10th., 1954* p. 242.
Pulsford, M. F. (1957). *Inst. Med. Vet. Sci., Adelaide, 19th Annu. Rep.* p. 56.
Pulsford, M. F. (1958). *Inst. Med. Vet. Sci., Adelaide, 20th Annu. Rep.* p. 62.
Pulsford, M. R. (1960). *Aust. J. Exp. Biol. Med. Sci.* **38**, 153.
Pulsford, M. F. (1961). *Aust. Vet. J.* **37**, 97.
Pulsford, M. F., and Watts, P. S. (1961). *Aust. Vet. J.* **37**, 314.
Raggi, L. G., and Lee, G. G. (1965). *Avian Dis.* **9**, 559.
Raggi, L. G., Brownell, J. R., and Stewart, G. F. (1961). *Poultry Sci.* **40**, 134.
Randall, C. C. (1955). *Proc. Soc. Exp. Biol. Med.* **90**, 176.
Randall, C. C., and Lawson, L. A. (1962). *Proc. Soc. Exp. Biol. Med.* **110**, 487.
Randall, C. C., Ryden, F. W., Doll, E. R., and Schell, F. S. (1953). *Amer. J. Pathol.* **29**, 139.

Randall, C. C., Stevens, W. C., and Bracken, E. C. (1954). *Amer. J. Pathol.* **30**, 654.
Rislakki, V. (1965). *Avian Dis.* **9**, 339.
Roberts, S. J. (1949). *Cornell Vet.* **39**, 435.
Rosenquist, B. D., and Loan, R. W. (1969). *Amer. J. Vet. Res.* **39**, 1305.
Rweyemamu, M. M. (1970). *Nature (London)* **225**, 738.
Rweyemamu, M. M., and Johnson, R. H. (1967). *Brit. Vet. J.* **123**, 482.
Rweyemamu, M. M., and Johnson, R. H. (1969). *Res. Vet. Sci.* **10**, 419.
Rweyemamu, M. M., Johnson, R. H., and Tutt, J. B. (1966). *Vet. Rec.* **79**, 810.
Rweyemamu, M. M., Johnson, R. H., and McCrea, M. R. (1968a). *Brit. Vet. J.* **124**, 317.
Rweyemamu, M. M., Johnson, R. H., and Osborne, A. D. (1968b). *Vet. Rec.* **82**, 85.
Rweyemamu, M. M., Johnson, R. H., and Lauriland, R. E. (1969). *Brit. Vet. J.* **125**, 317.
Sabin, A. (1934). *Brit. J. Exp. Pathol.* **15**, 372.
Sabo, A., and Grunert, Z. (1971). *Acta Virol. (Prague), Engl. Ed.* **15**, 87.
Satriano, S. F., Luginbuhl, R. E., Helmboldt, C. F., and Jungherr, E. L. (1957). *Poultry Sci.* **36**, 1155 (Abstr.).
Saunders, J. R., and Gustafson, D. P. (1964). *Proc. 68th Annual Meeting U.S. Livestock Sanit. Ass.* p. 256.
Saunders, J. R., Gustafson, D. P., Olander, H. J., and Jones, R. K. (1963). *Proc. 7th Annual Meeting U.S. Livestock Sanit. Ass.* p. 331.
Saxegaard, F. (1966). *Nord Veterinaermed.* **18**, 504.
Schroeder, R. J., and Moys, M. D. (1954). *J. Amer. Vet. Med. Ass.* **125**, 471.
Schwartz, W. L., and Martin, W. D. (1966). *Vet. Med. & Small Anim. Clin.* **61**, 1171.
Scott, F. W. (1971). *J. Amer. Vet. Med. Ass.* **158**, 946.
Scott, F. W., Kahn, D. E., and Gillespie, J. H. (1970). *Amer. J. Vet. Res.* **31**, 11.
Seddon, H. R., and Hart, L. (1935). *Aust. Vet. J.* **11**, 212.
Seddon, H. R., and Hart, L. (1936). *Aust. Vet. J.* **12**, 13.
Sedlmeier, H. (1938). *Muenchen Tieraerztl. Wochenschr.* **89**, 37.
Seifried, O. (1931). *J. Exp. Med.* **56**, 817.
Semerdjiev, B., and Christov, S. (1958). *Arch. Exp. Veterinaermed.* **12**, 802.
Sevoian, M. (1960). *Avian Dis.* **4**, 474.
Sharma, J. M., and Raggi, L. G. (1969). *Avian Dis.* **13**, 268.
Sharma, J. M., Burger, D., and Kenzy, S. G. (1972). *Infection Immunity* **5**, 406.
Shibley, G. P., Luginbuhl, R. E., and Helmboldt, C. F. (1962). *Avian Dis.* **6**, 59.
Shimizu, T., Ishizaki, R., Ishii, S., Kawakami, Y., Kaji, T., Sugimura, K., and Matumoto, M. (1959). *Jap. J. Exp. Med.* **29**, 643.
Shope, R. E. (1931). *J. Exp. Med.* **54**, 233.
Shope, R. E. (1932). *Proc. Soc. Exp. Biol. Med.* **30**, 308.
Shope, R. E. (1935a). *J. Exp. Med.* **62**, 85.
Shope, R. E. (1935b). *J. Exp. Med.* **62**, 101.
Skoda, R., Grunert, A., and Zubaj, J. (1970). *Arch. Exp. Veterinaermed.* **24**, 167.
Snowdon, W. A. (1965). *Aust. Vet. J.* **41**, 135.
Spertzel, R. O., Huxsoll, D. L., McConnel, S. J., Binn, L. N., and Yager, R. H. (1965). *Proc. Soc. Exp. Biol. Med.* **120**, 651.
Spradbrow, P. B. (1968). *Aust. Vet. J.* **44**, 410.
Stevens, J. G., and Groman, N. B. (1964). *J. Bacteriol.* **87**, 446.
Stewart, S. E., David-Ferreira, J., Lovelace, E., and Landon, J. (1965). *Science* **148**, 1341.
Studdert, M. J., Barker, C. A. V., and Savan, M. (1964). *Amer. J. Vet. Res.* **25**, 303.
Tajima, M., Shimizu, T., and Ishizaki, R. (1961). *Amer. J. Vet. Res.* **22**, 250.
Thorp, F., and Graham, R. (1934). *Poultry Sci.* **30**, 102.
Todd, J. D. (1969). *J. Amer. Vet. Med. Ass.* **155**, 272.

Todd, J. D., Volenec, F. J., and Paton, I. M. (1971). *J. Amer. Vet. Med. Ass.* **159**, 1370.
Todd, J. D., Volenec, F. J., and Paton, I. M. (1972). *Infection Immunity* **5**, 699.
Turner, A. J., Studdert, M. J., and Peterson, J. E. (1970). *Aust. Vet. J.* **46**, 90.
Van Heelsbergen, T. (1929). *In* "Handbuch der Geflügel Krankheiten und der Geflügelzucht" pp. 262–264. Enke, Stuttgart.
Van Roekel, H. V. (1955). *Advan. Vet. Sci.* **2**, 64.
von Hartung, J., and Fritsch, W. (1964). *Monatsh. Veterinaermed.* **19**, 422.
Walton, T. E., and Gillespie, J. H. (1970). *Cornell Vet.* **60**, 232.
Weiss, K. E. (1963). *In* "Emerging Diseases of Animals," pp. 179–201. United Nations (FAO), New York.
Winterfield, R. W., and So, I. G. (1968). *Avian Dis.* **12**, 186.
Woyciechowska, S. (1962). *Ann. Inst. Pasteur, Paris* **102**, 353.
Yedloutschnig, R. J., Breese, S. S., Hess, W. R., Dardiri, A. H., Taylor, W. D., Barnes, B. M., Page, R. W., and Ruebke, H. J. (1970). *Proc. 74th Annual Meeting U.S. Anim. Health Ass.* p. 208.
Zuffa, A. (1963). *Arch. Exp. Veterinaermed.* **17**, 593.
Zwart, D. (1966). *Bull. Epiz. Dis. Afr.* **14**, 405.

Chapter 15

Herpesviruses of Lower Vertebrates

Ken Wolf

I. Introduction

The other contributors to this book have provided authoritative material on comparative aspects of all herpesviruses and on the pathology and other considerations. The role of these agents in human and veterinary medicine, especially in induction or possible induction of malignant tumors is of great interest to researchers in many fields of science. It is more than appropriate, therefore, to restrict this introductory material to general comments on the more specific subject of herpesviruses from two classes of vertebrates, the reptiles and teleost fishes.

In essence, most of the rather limited literature on reptile and teleost herpesviruses deals with two agents that have been isolated and partially characterized: the iguana virus isolated from a terrestrial reptile, and the channel catfish virus isolated from a freshwater teleost. There is fragmentary literature on three other agents whose morphology makes them likely candidates for the herpesvirus group; two are found in snakes and might possibly be a single virus, the third occurs in European carp.

The existence of four or five herpesviruses from reptiles and fishes is not to be compared numerically with the many avian and mammalian members of the group. A better picture might be obtained by comparing the numbers of homeotherm vertebrates (about 8600 avian species and 4500 mammalian species) with the number of poikilotherms (23,000 fishes, 2000 amphibians, and 5000 reptiles). Assuming that herpesviruses are uniformly distributed among animals, the use of host numbers suggests a potential for the existence among poikilotherm vertebrates of more than twice as many herpesviruses as are found among homeotherms.

Although herpesviruses were isolated from a reptile and from a fish, only the fish agent has had unequivocal evidence relating it to specific disease. It is likely that fish health-related research will pursue investigations leading to information that will be useful in achieving control of the disease. Scientific interest and funding are assured, because the host animal is an important food source, and millions of pounds are raised annually for stocking purposes and more importantly for the commercial market. Other investigators from human and veterinary medicine, virology, and oncology also find the catfish virus to be of basic interest. The agent and a susceptible line of cells (CCL-59) are both available from the American Type Culture Collection.

From the more basic considerations of oncogenesis, the herpesvirus seen in hyperplastic lesions of carp with *Epithelioma papulosum*, the so-called "carp pox" merit scientific interest. It seems likely that the virus is causally related to the benign tumor, but the agent itself has not yet been isolated. When this is accomplished, the first question to be asked is does the virus cause the proliferation. If this proves to be the case, proposed mechanisms of viral-dependent changes can then be examined on an easily obtainable animal. Moreover, environmental factors such as temperature, oxygen levels, osmolarity, and other properties of water can be manipulated experimentally. Such work could provide useful clues and perhaps some fundamental information concerning the induction of virus-related tumors and possibly oncogenesis in general.

The state of knowledge of the properties and the occurrence of herpesviruses in fishes and reptiles will now be discussed.

II. Reptilian Hosts

A. Snake Herpesvirus

Herpesvirus has been found in venom from two snakes, the Indian cobra (*Naja naja*) and the banded krait (*Bungarus fasciatus*). At this time, it is not known whether the agents are actually the same virus. The snakes themselves are both native to the Indian subcontinent. Other than the source animals and the size and gross morphology of the particles, little is known about the snake herpesvirus.

Virological research on snake herpesvirus began with the work of Padgett and Levine (1966) who sought to employ crude enzymes in snake venom in an attempt to elucidate substructural details of the Rauscher leukemia virus. In brief, their work showed capsomeres and herpesvirus-like details not previously known for the Rauscher virus. Undoubtedly somewhat skeptical, Monroe *et al.* (1968) wished to check the validity of the snake venom work. They repeated the experiments and found that the herpesvirus structures were actually contaminating virions present in the venom.

Monroe *et al.* (1968) used negative staining and thin sectioning of pellets which had been sedimented from reconstituted, lyophilized snake venom samples. Virus was found in all samples —three from cobras and one from the banded krait.

Enveloped and nonenveloped particles were observed, and in some instances there were aggregates containing up to 100 virions. Capsomeres were clearly evident, but in no case could a capsid be resolved clearly enough to determine critically the capsomere number. Capsids were, however, sufficiently intact to determine that their diameters ranged from 100 to 125 nm. Thin sections of cobra venom pellets were found to contain apparently empty (immature or incomplete) herpesvirus particles which were thought to correspond to the nonenveloped particles seen with negatively stained materials.

B. *Iguana Herpesvirus*

1. History

The original report of isolation of the iguana herpesvirus was made by Clark *et al.* (1968) who had investigated spontaneous degeneration of primary monolayer cultures of green iguana (*Iguana iguana*) cells. They described temperature tolerance of the new agent, cytologic features of infected cells, some basic biophysical properties, and measurement data from electronmicroscopy. Later, descriptive and illustrated details of the original research and findings of new and more comprehensive study of biophysical properties and morphological features were published (Clark and Karzon, 1972; Zeigel and Clark, 1972).

2. Clinical Features of Infection

Thus far the iguana virus has not been clearly related to disease. Culture-grown virus ($\sim 10^{4.9}$ $TCID_{50}$) inoculated into 20 young iguanas by various routes did not produce a recognizable pattern of pathologic change. Seven of twelve animals died during a 15-day observation period, and only one of six control animals died during the same period. Virus was not recovered from organ suspensions from the dead test animals, and histologic preparations were not made. Clark and Karzon (1972) therefore considered that death among inoculated iguanas might not have been due to virus. Supporting their interpretation was the fact that on day 15, ten survivors were killed and virus was recovered from the homogenized spleen of only one of them. The rather common feature of difficulty in recovering herpesviruses from anything less than obviously diseased animals may have played a role in the work. Five iguanas that had been inoculated with virus and subsequently died were used for culture of tissues; with that method both liver and kidney cell cultures of four of the animals yielded virus. Liver and kidney cell cultures from the fifth virus-inoculated animal remained normal for 100 days and for three subculturings.

3. Morphology

Zeigel and Clark (1972) have clearly established the herpesvirus morphology of the iguana agent. The virus has cubic symmetry and hollow capsomeres. They found suggestive evidence for five capsomeres on each capsid edge, therefore a probable complement of 162. Within the nucleus, naked nucleocapsids have an approximate diameter of 115 nm. Enveloped virions are 225 $\pm$ 75 nm. Some seemingly aberrant encapsidation was found wherein virions enclosed unusual 35-nm hexagonal forms, forms that were also found in nuclear aggregates. Envelopment of virions included, at times, material of nuclear origin.

4. Biophysical Properties

The known characteristics of iguana virus suggest that they are members of the herpesvirus group. Exposure to 20% ether for 16 hours at 4° C caused a decrease of at least 99.9% of the initial infectivity. Differential filtration showed that passage through 220-nm membranes greatly reduced infectivity, but that 100-nm membranes retained the virus quantitatively; the findings agree with electron microscopic measurements.

Direct chemical determinations of viral nucleic acid type were not made, but indirect evidence obtained with bromodeoxyuridine (BUdR) gave presumptive evidence of DNA. In controlled work with known RNA and DNA virus systems, a concentration of 20 μg/ml BUdR effected of 10^4-fold reduction of iguana virus yield. The inhibition was reversed when excess thymidine was added to the medium.

Iguana virus is relatively labile at 37° C and has a half-life of approximately 13 hours. There was no detectable loss of infectivity over a period of 40 days at 23° and 4° C.

Serologic comparisons of iguana virus with other herpesviruses have shown the reptile virus to be distinct. By plaque reduction-neutralization tests, iguana virus was not neutralized by 1:4 dilutions of serum against herpes simplex, herpes B, herpes tamarinus, simian virus 8, pseudorabies, equine rhinopneumonitis, infectious bovine rhinotracheitis, or avian laryngotracheitis. Similarly, iguana virus neutralizing activity was not detected in sera from animals hyperimmunized with P-3 Burkitt lymphoma antigen nor in human serum containing Burkitt lymphoma membrane antigen. Rabbit serum prepared against frog renal adenocarcinoma that contained herpesvirus and serum from rabbits immunized with herpesvirus containing cobra venom were also without iguana virus neutralizing activity.

Iguana virus was inoculated, via several routes, into newborn mice without causing disease, and virus could not be recovered from brain tissue 1 week later. The chorioallantoic membrane of hen eggs was also unable to replicate the agent. Various poikilothermic vertebrates were inoculated; they included the following number of species: one toad, one frog, two lizards, three snakes, two turtles, and one alligator. In all, 32 lower vertebrate animals were used; none showed disease, and all were cultured for virus after about 2 weeks at 23° C. Heart cultures of the single tokay gecko (*Gekko gecko*) and spleen cultures of one box turtle (*Terrapene carolina*) yielded virus on outgrowth, but other tissues that had been inoculated onto susceptible cell cultures did not.

5. Replication

Iguana virus was found to replicate only in certain cells or cell lines of reptilian origin. Mammalian cells that were tested and found to be refractory were primary rhesus monkey kidney, and WISH, HEp-2, GMK, and BSC cell lines. Chick embryo fibroblasts, turtle cell lines TS 5 and PH 1, snake cell lines VSW and VH, amphibian cell lines RPH 67.132 and BA 68.1, and fish cell lines FHM (CCL-42) and BF-2 (CCL-91) all failed to show cytopathic effects (CPE). Limited induction of giant cell formation that was not amenable to passage occurred in gecko cell lines GH 1, GH 2, and GL 1 and in primary kidney cultures from an alligator and snake.

Reptilian cell lines which supported replication were iguana lines IgH2, IgVA, IgVB, and IgK17 and turtle lines TH 1, TH 4, TH 4W, and TH 5.

Replication occurred at temperatures of 23°–36° C, but CPE and virus yield differed somewhat at temperatures within this range. At 36° C, CPE consisted of syncytia having up to several hunderd nuclei, whereas at 30° C and below, there were only occasional but more organized syncytia, and the CPE was more cytolytic.

At 36° C, IgK17 cells produced nearly 10^7 $TCID_{50}$ of cell-associated virus (CAV) and virtually no released virus (RV). At 30° C CAV was slightly greater than 10^7 $TCID_{50}$ but RV was about 10^5 $TCID_{50}$. Both CAV and RV were lower at 23°C, but CAV was still about 10^2 $TCID_{50}$ greater than RV.

An incubation temperature of 30°C was used for routine work. With a multiplicity of infection of 5, CPE was first observed on the second day and total virus was about 10^4 $TCID_{50}$. On the third day, the amount had risen to nearly 10^5 $TCID_{50}$, by the seventh it was more than 1×10^6 $TCID_{50}$, and peak titer of more than 10^7 $TCID_{50}$ was reached on the tenth day. At 23°C, attainment of peak titer required 2 weeks incubation.

Cytopathic effects were also maximal on the tenth day, and the agent induced both nuclear and cytoplasmic inclusions. Eosinophilic intranuclear inclusions were common in multinucleated cells of susceptible kinds through the range of 23° to 36°C. Turtle cells showed peculiar hexagonal inclusions but only at 36°C. These unique inclusions were seen first near nuclei of syncytia, but later during the cycle, they were found throughout the cytoplasm.

6. Pathogenesis

The pathologic effects, systemic or histologic, have yet to be determined.

7. Immunity

At concentrations of less than 1:4 iguana virus neutralizing activity was not found in terminal sera from any of the coldblooded vertebrates that had been inoculated. Because of incompatibility of poikilotherm vertebrate antibodies with mammalian reagents, complement fixation was not carried out.

8. Epizootiology

The original isolation was made in 1965 from an adult male green iguana obtained from the zoo in Buffalo, New York. Liver, spleen, kidney, and heart cell cultures all yielded virus. A second iguana was obtained from the same source in 1966, and virus was obtained by culture of kidneys and lung tissue only; other tissues were cultured, and they remained normal. The second isolate was lost during passage. A young iguana was held for about 2 months in the source cage at the zoo, then killed and its tissues cultured, but virus was not found.

Little else is known about iguana virus, but the preponderance of the data suggests that the agent is a natural pathogen for the iguana. It seems likely that it could be highly pathogenic for the young, and it may be transmitted vertically. Experimental infection of very young animals should shed light on many aspects of virus–host relationships.

III. Teleostean Fish Hosts

A. Channel Catfish Virus

Channel catfish virus (CCV) is the only herpesvirus thus far isolated from a fish. It is the etiologic agent of an acute hemorrhagic disease which usually produces high mortality among certain ictalurid fish species. Channel catfish virus has been partially characterized, and in 1971, a plaque-purified stock of virus was deposited in the Collection of Animal Viruses and Rickettsiae of the American Type Culture Collection. The CCV has been designated VR-665 and is available for distribution.

1. History

During the past decade, husbandry of the channel catfish (*Ictalurus punctatus*) and related ictalurid fishes has increased by a factor of at least ten. Current production is slightly over 40 million pounds of live fish annually. With increased and intensified husbandry there have been attendant disease problems; among these problems were severe summer epizootics of young-of-the-year channel catfish. Outbreaks erupted swiftly, and mortality was characteristically high. A cause for such acute disease and death eluded researchers for several years, but Fijan (1968) isolated a virus and showed that it produced the characteristic clinical signs and mortality. He applied the name channel catfish virus disease.

Fijan *et al.* (1970) investigated seven epizootics and isolated virus from four out of five outbreaks among the very young, but they could not isolate virus from epizootics among older fish. These investigators described clinical features of CCV disease, fulfilled Rivers' postulates, and gave data which showed that CCV was highly specific not only for its host but also for cell cultures from ictalurid fishes. Their work included the first features of the biophysical properties of the virus. Plumb (1971a) used experimental infections to determine which fish tissues yielded infectious virus and found that the kidneys were the most productive. In related work, Plumb (1971b) reported on the failure, to date, of anyone to isolate CCV from adult fish using methods which were widely employed for isolating other fish viruses. He showed, however, that serum from suspect carrier fish had significant levels of CCV neutralizing activity and that there was a trend towards higher levels in serum from males than from females. Thus far, the research emphasis had been primarily on the host and secondarily on the pathogen.

Biological and morphological aspects of CCV in cell culture systems were described and illustrated in the report of Wolf and Darlington (1971). Viral morphology, capsomere number, and sequential stages in viral replication were those of a herpesvirus. Microscopic findings and the biological properties that were examined also supported classification of CCV into the herpesvirus group.

More recently, the histopathologic changes in young catfish with experimental CCV infections have been described and illustrated by Wolf *et al.* (1972).

Various aspects of epizootiology, pathogenesis, immunity, and biophysical studies of the virus are currently underway in different laboratories. Reports on such work are expected in the near future, but some of the early findings are already known and will be discussed.

2. Clinical Features of Infection

Natural outbreaks have usually followed periods of elevated temperature (25°C or higher), handling, stress, and/or depressed oxygen levels in the water. Fry or fingerling fish are the most susceptible. Since such young animals are seasonally most abundant during the summer, one could be misled to think that CCV was a problem when hosts were numerous and available. The temperature phenomenon however is real, and experimental trials bear out the fact that infection is easily achieved at 25°C or higher. Lower temperatures generally favor host survival, and replication *in vitro* is also significantly reduced at 20°C and lower.

Infected fish become distressed, and some of them rise to the surface, where they maintain a head high posture with their body hanging at an angle. Affected fry and fingerlings tend to concentrate along pond and trough edges and especially at the outlet end of troughs. Fijan *et al.* (1970) reported that the hanging posture was found in 20–50% of the epizootics and is a specific sign of infection. The same abnormality of behavior also occurs in catfish fry that are distressed by other causes and from which CCV has not been isolated.

With CCV disease, affected fish are typically lethargic, but some may swim convulsively and in spirals. Such agonal swimming may be triggered by reaction to alarm or to feeding, but the obviously affected fry themselves generally refuse to feed.

Moribund and severely affected fish show signs of hemorrhagic disease and fluid or electrolyte metabolic dysfunction. Hemorrhages may be visible externally in fin bases, on the abdomen, and in the caudal peduncle. The gills are usually pale, and in some there may also be hemorrhages. Unilateral or bilateral exophthalmus is common, and the abdomen is generally distended. The anal area of some may protrude and be hemorrhagic.

External parasites, a common finding among pond-raised fishes, may be present. Myxobacterial infection of fin tissues also may occur with CCV disease. Either the parasites or bacterial erosion of fins may contribute to the deterioration of the sick fry, but they are not invariable findings, and the virus alone can produce disease and death.

Gross internal findings typically show the absence of food in the digestive tract, enlarged and pale kidneys, and an accumulation of pale yellowish fluid in the body cavity. The digestive tract itself is usually flaccid, and it too may contain pale yellow fluid, although the fluid tends to be mucoid. Liver and spleen may be pale and enlarged, and internal organs in general may show petechiation or be ecchymotic. Skeletal musculature may show petechiae.

Thus far, the histopathologic findings of CCV disease have been described only for experimental infections (Wolf *et al.*, 1972), and a comparison is needed with specimens taken from natural epizootics. Channel catfish virus produced a hemorrhagic and edematous disease with greatest damage in the internal organs. Renal hematopoietic and excretory tissues show edema and necrosis, the latter in some areas approaching obliteration. The liver shows similar, although not generally as extensive, degenerative and necrotic changes. Tissues of the digestive tract also show edema, and stomach mucosa may separate and slough into the lumen. Macrophages occur in focal concentrations in gut tissue. Skeletal muscle bundles show edematous separation and extravasation of blood. The histopathologic findings agree with gross signs and with the levels of virus in the various tissues reported by Plumb (1971b). Preliminary work with material from a natural epizootic shows a pattern similar to that found in experimental infections, but the changes in skeletal muscle are minimal and extravasation of blood seems to be the exception (M. Landolt, personal communications, 1972).

Hematological and other clinical findings have not yet been reported; they will be difficult to determine, because the usual victim is a very small animal.

When outbreaks of acute disease occur among young catfish during summer and other causes of death can be ruled out, CCV can be suspected. The above behavioral changes, signs, and histopathologic changes can be used as presumptive evidence of CCV, but to be certain of the cause, the virus must be isolated and identified.

3. Morphology

Negatively stained preparations of CCV show enveloped particles having a diameter of 175–200 nm (Wolf and Darlington, 1971). The nucleocapsid is an icosahedron with a diameter of 95–105 nm, and core diameter is 40–50 nm. Hollow capsomeres comprise the capsid, and they number 162.

Plumb (1972) has carried out electron microscopy of tissues from fish infected with CCV. Cellular changes and details of apparent stages in virus replication were described and illustrated, but size determinations were not reported. The two studies are in agreement.

4. Biophysical Properties

Channel catfish virus is ether-labile, being completely inactivated by exposure to 20% (v/v) ether for 24 hours at 4°C or by 5% chloroform for 5 minutes at room temperature. Infectivity is also destroyed by 50% glycerol and by drying.

Compared with other fish viruses, CCV is among the more stable in storage. At −80°C, infectivity has shown no loss during a period of 9 months, and at −20°C infectivity also persists for months. It should be noted, however, that successive cycles of freezing and thawing have each inactivated a significant amount of the initial infectivity.

Stability of CCV in several liquids was tested at 4°C. As shown in Fig. 1, infectivity was maintained at highest levels in cell culture medium with fetal bovine serum (Wolf and Quimby, 1970). Hanks' balanced salt solution containing 0.5% lactalbumin hydrolysate and sterile distilled water gave poorer virus survival, but at least 10% of the original infectivity persisted through 2 months storage, and it is likely that virus could have been recovered for at least 6 months.

Based upon its morphology, mode off replication, and its induction of intranuclear inclusions and syncytia, CCV is a herpesvirus. Indirect evidence has been obtained that indicates CCV is a DNA virus. *In vitro*

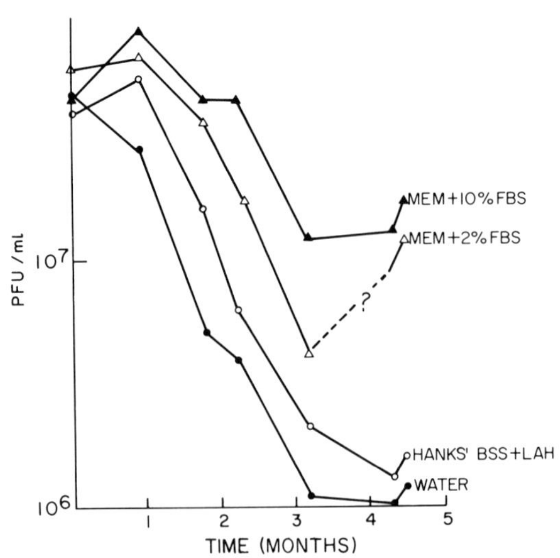

Fig. 1. Comparative stability at 4°C of CCV in water and three physiological solutions.

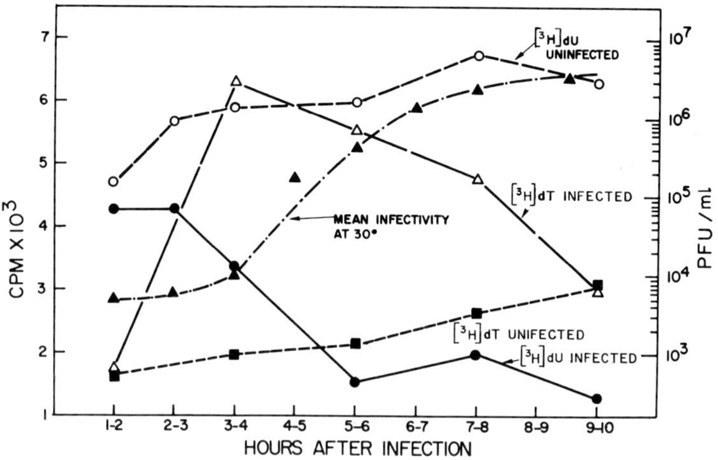

FIG. 2. A comparison at 30°C of uptake of [^{3}H]uridine and [^{3}H]thymidine by uninfected CCL-59 cultures and by comparable cultures infected with CCV. An average one-step growth curve is included as a reference for replication of infectious virus.

replication is inhibited in the presence of 10^{-4} *M* iododeoxyuridine. Metabolic studies using ^{3}H-labeled nucleic acid precursors show that uptake of uridine by CCL-59 cells* is depressed by infection with CCV and conversely that there is a rapid increase in the uptake of thymidine. The work employed 1-hour pulses with [^{3}H]uridine (1 μCi/ml; specific activity 23 Ci/mmole) and [^{3}H]thymidine (1 μCi/ml; specific activity 58 Ci/mmole). Labeled compounds were used in tenfold greater amounts of unlabeled precursor in order to maintain them in an excess and prevent their depletion.

As shown in Fig. 2, uptake of uridine and thymidine by uninfected cells was slow and linear during the 10-hour test period (Wolf and Quimby, 1970). In CCV-infected cultures, uridine uptake was depressed from the start and that depression was accentuated from the third hour onward. The uptake of thymidine by infected cells showed a five- to sixfold increase during the first 3 hours; thereafter it declined until the end of the test period when it equalled that of uninfected cultures. Utilization of thymidine preceded the period of exponential viral replication in cultures under the same conditions. These results can be interpreted as showing the uptake of thymidine presumably for the replication of viral DNA.

Exploratory work in related areas support the above interpretation. When CCV was grown in the presence of [^{3}H]thymidine and put through

* CCL-59 is a certified cell line from the brown bullhead (*Ictalurus nebulosus*) in the collection of Animal Cell Lines of the American Type Culture Collection, Rockville, Md.

sucrose gradient (Fig. 3) peak counts coincided with optical density and peak infectivity at the released virus and the cell-associated virus bands (K. Wolf, unpublished research 1970).

Exploratory autoradiographic studies also support an hypothesis that CCV has DNA. Virus which had been labeled with [^{3}H]thymidine then used to infect coverslip cultures of CCL-59 cells resulted in preferential concentrations of exposed silver grains over cell nuclei (K. Wolf, unpublished research, 1970).

In spite of electron micrographic evidence of an envelope and data from

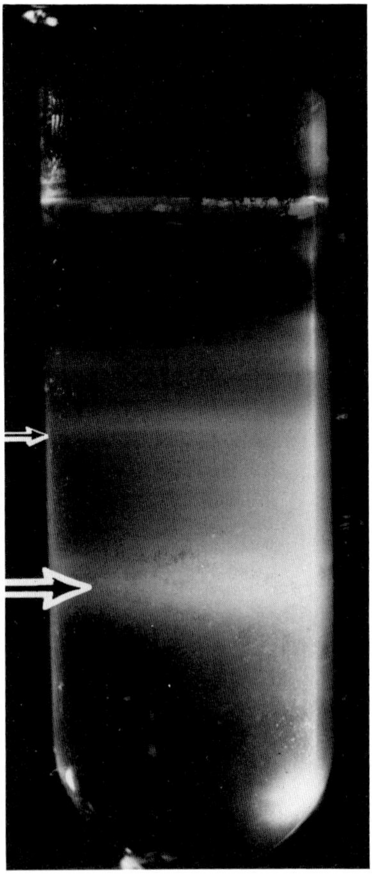

FIG. 3. Sucrose gradient (30–50% w/v) centrifugation of CCV for 30 minutes at an average of 51,000 *g* separates a broad flocculent band of cell-associated virus (large arrow) and an upper homogeneous band of released virus (small arrow).

ether-sensitivity testing that showed an essential lipid component, CCV has shown no ability to agglutinate erythrocytes. The virus, however, can be coated onto tanned sheep erythrocytes and these in turn can be used in passive hemagglutination (D. Allen, unpublished research, 1971).

Rabbit antiserum has been prepared against CCV, but neutralization tests show that a small but non-neutralizable persistent fraction remains even when serum is used without dilution (K. Wolf, unpublished research, 1970). Antigenic relationship of CCV to other herpesviruses has not been investigated.

The density of the DNA of CCV, determined by analytical ultracentrifugation in CsCl density gradients, was found to be 1.715 gm/ml compared to density marker DNA from *Clostridium perfringens* (1.691 gm/ml) and *Micrococcus lysodeikticus* (1.731 gm/ml). This density corresponds to a base composition of 56.1 mole % G + C. Thus, the base composition of CCV is slightly less than that of several horse herpesviruses (C. R. Goodheart, personal communication, 1972).

Differential filtration has shown that infectious CCV will pass through membrane filters of 220 nm and larger mean pore diameter, but that it will be retained by membranes of 100 nm porosity. The findings agree with size determinations made by electron microscopy.

5. Replication

The *in vitro* replication of CCV has been reported by Wolf and Darlington (1971). That study emphasized the results of cultures that were incubated at 30° C. Regarding the exclusive specificity of CCV for ictalurid fish cells, the original work of Fijan *et al.* (1970) was confirmed and extended. Wolf and Darlington (1971) tested four cell lines from fishes, two from amphibians, chick embryo primary cultures, and eight primary or cell line cultures from mammals and found that only CCL-59 cells replicated CCV.

Cells of the CCL-59 line proved to be capable of replicating CCV at temperatures of 10°–33° C but not at 37° C. Representative one-step growth curves for several temperatures are shown in Fig. 4.

At 25° C, the initial level of residual infectivity declined somewhat during the several hours required for penetration and initiation of the replicative cycle. Thereafter, new infectivity appeared, and it reached a plateau at about 20 hours. At 30° and 33° C, infectivity peaked at about 12 hours, but the yield was slightly less than at 25° C. It is interesting to note that virus was replicated to a high level at 33° C, a temperature that is too high for sustained growth of the cells themselves. As could be expected, lower temperatures greatly increased the replicative cycle. At 16° C the cycle was over 40 hours, and yielded only about 50 times the amount of residual infectivity

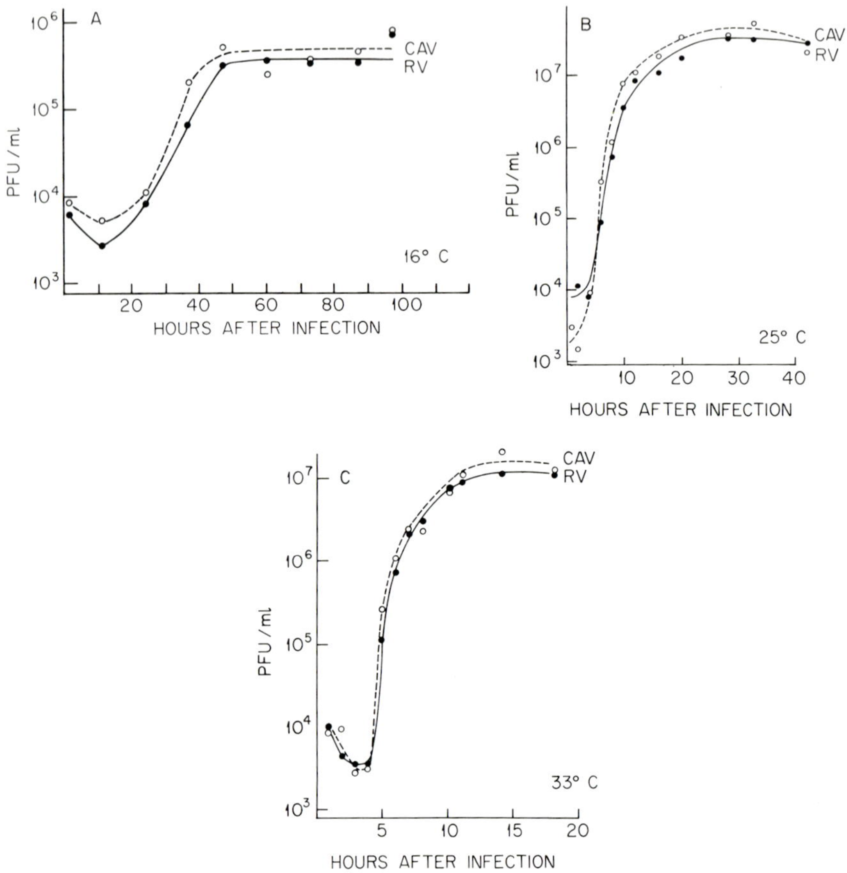

FIG. 4. Representative one-step growth curves of CCV in CCL-59 cells at three different temperatures.

found at the start of the cycle. At 10° C, CCV produced a slowly forming and atypical CPE; cells became pyknotic and formation of syncytia was equivocal in unstained cultures. Even after 18 days, some cells remained attached to the vessel. In one trial, a 13-fold virus increase occurred, and in a second trial, the gain was only twice the input.

Virus replication can be correlated with microscopic changes in the cells themselves. During the period of adsorption, there is little visible change in the cultures. Thereafter, they become pyknotic and basophilic and show aggregation and intranuclear inclusions. These visible changes precede the appearance of new infectivity. As one index, the development of intranuclear inclusions marks the onset of imminent appearance of new infectivity. Karyorrhexis, syncytial contraction, and lysis generally coincide with the period of exponential virus replication.

At the ultrastructural level, electron microscopy can be similarly related to replication. Wolf and Darlington (1971) reported that some cells showed margination of chromatin at 3 hours, but virus itself was not found until 4 hours. At that time, nuclei showed virus in various stages of development, and there was evidence of greater synthesis around a small granular intranuclear body. In some places, the nuclear membrane could not be resolved, and there were unenveloped particles with dense nucleoids in the cytoplasm.

As time progressed, vacuoles appeared at the periphery of nuclei, and they contained mostly enveloped particles. Still later, nuclear disintegration was more extensive, and virions, enveloped and otherwise, were present in vacuolated cytoplasm. Envelopment itself apparently takes place when virions encounter membranes—nuclear, cytoplasmic, or vacuolar.

A peculiar feature of CCV-infected CCL-59 cells is the appearance at about 4 hours of electron-dense lamellar structures within the nucleus. Lamellae were 10–15 nm in width; they varied in number from two to ten and occupied large areas of the nucleus late in the infection. As far as could be determined, they do not occur in other herpesvirus infections. The lamellar structures are not peculiar to CCL-59 cells, since Plumb (1972) has described them in organ tissues of channel catfish that were experimentally infected with CCV. He interpreted them to be paramyelin and found them in spleen and liver cells but not in kidney cells.

6. Pathogenesis

Thus far, the sequence in development of CCV disease has received only slight attention. There are several reasons for this. The disease is one of the newly identified infections, and research laboratories for fishes are few in number. Moreover, an urgent mission in such laboratories is that of determining the source of epizootics and of learning how the virus is transmitted to the young. The object, of course, being to implement a rational approach to reliable viral or carrier detection and avoidance of the disease.

In vitro studies (Wolf and Darlington, 1971) showed cellular basophilia, margination of chromatin, and syncytium formation, presumably due to cell recruitment and fusion at 2 hours postinfection. Intranuclear inclusions, similar in appearance to Cowdry type A, appeared in some cells by 3 hours and were present in most of the cells at 4 hours (Fig. 5). Syncytia increased in size and number of nuclei contained, but at 6 hours postinoculation nuclear disintegration appeared and dense basophilic material, presumably coming from the nucleus, was present in cytoplasm. Curiously, nucleoli were

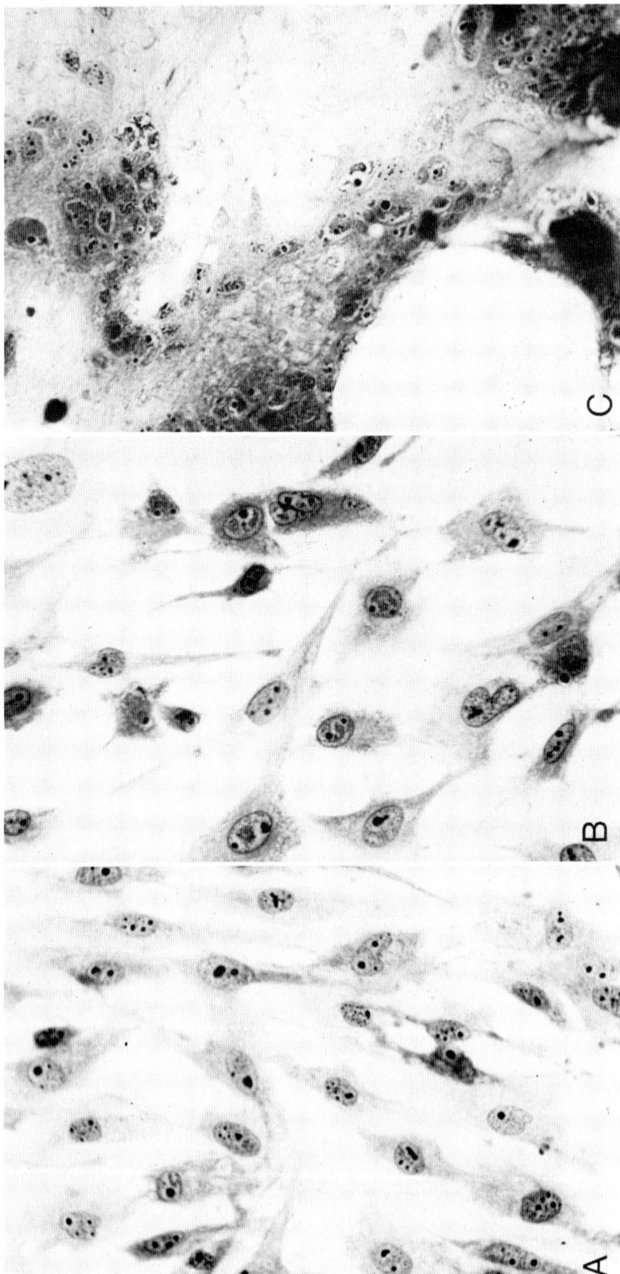

FIG. 5. Sequential effects of CCV in CCL-59 cultures. (A) Uninoculated control. (B) Margination of chromatin, Cowdry type A intranuclear inclusions and beginning syncytium formation are evident several hours postinoculation. (C) Karyorrhexis and contraction of the extensive syncytia are present after about 12 hours incubation. ×360. Hematoxylin and eosin stain.

seemingly unaffected throughout the cycle of infection. Syncytia showed contraction by 8 hours, and at 10 hours there was cytoplasmic fragmentation or lysis. Degenerative changes in the nuclei and cytoplasm were progressive and peaked at 12–14 hours.

The foregoing sequence can be seen in plaques on CCL-59 cells; the earliest changes are evident at the outermost edge of plaques, and the final degenerative contraction and lysis occur in plaque centers (Fig. 6).

The described changes relate to histopathologic findings only insofar as they are probably the sequence that has led to the terminal condition in the fish. Sequential histopathologic study has not been carried out on CCV *in vivo*. Advanced degenerative and lytic change is similar *in vivo* and *in vitro*, but there are important exceptions. Although they have been sought with some diligence, neither intranuclear inclusions nor syncytia have been reported in sections of infected fish tissues.

Plumb (1972) followed the development of viral infectivity in fingerling channel catfish experimentally infected with CCV and kept at 30°C. Each day for 1 week, three fish were taken and some of their tissues were assayed for virus. Because of their small size, the spleens were pooled, but other tissues were handled on an individual basis from each fingerling. At 24 hours, virus was recovered from blood, kidneys, liver, or intestine of two of the specimens. By the second day, all three of the sampled fish had virus in blood and kidneys, and virus was found in the spleen pool and in the brain of one fish. Average infectivity for tissues generally was higher than on the first day. On the third day, all fish showed virus in liver tissue, and mean titers continued to rise. Peak levels of virus were found on the third and fourth days (Table I), but thereafter infectivity generally declined. When the study was terminated on the seventh day, some of the tissues assayed had very little virus, and virus was not detected in others. Additional assays were not carried out because available fish had all either been taken for assay or had died as a consequence of the infection.

Plumb (1972) stated that histologic aspects of CCV disease were under

TABLE I
MEAN PEAK LEVELS OF INFECTIVITY OF SOME TISSUES FROM CHANNEL CATFISH FINGERLINGS INJECTED WITH CCV AND ASSAYED AT 72 AND 96 HOURS[a]

	Kidneys	Intestine	Liver	Brain[b]	Blood	Spleen
Number of fish	6	6	6	3	3	2
Titer[c]	5.9	5.6	4.8	4.4	4.3	4.1

[a] Adapted from Plumb (1972).
[b] Only 96-hour data—virus not recovered at 72 hours.
[c] Expressed as exponent $\log_{10}$ ($TCID_{50}$ – 50% end point) per gram of tissue.

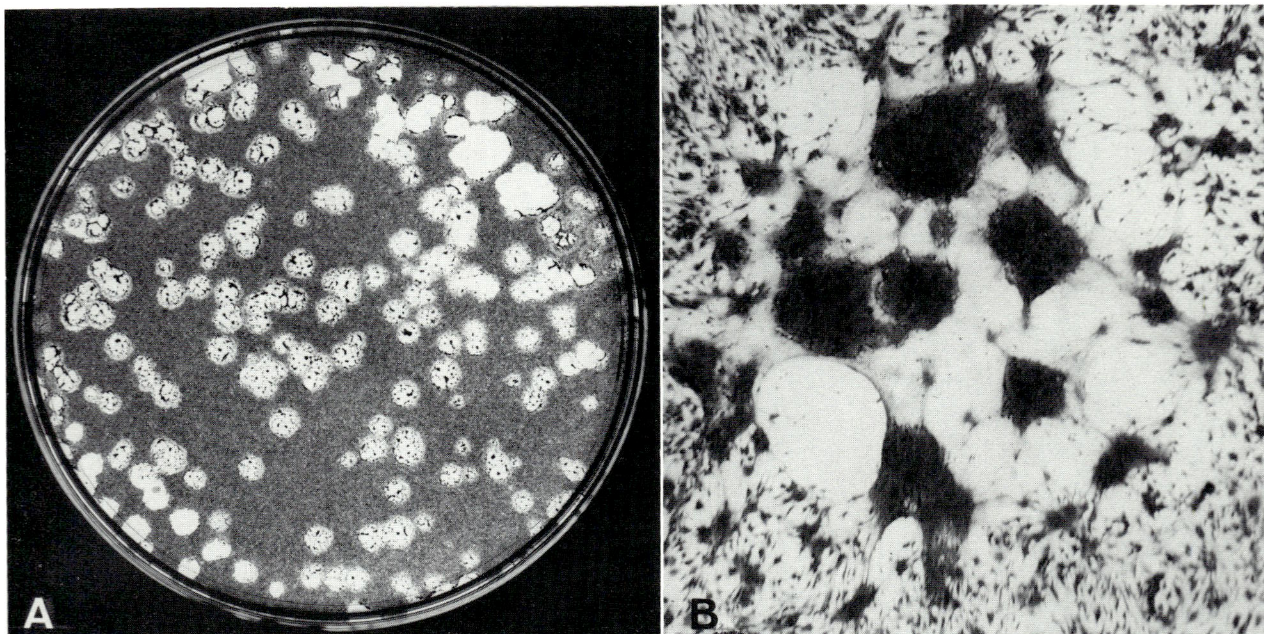

FIG 6. Channel catfish virus plaques on CCL-59 cells. (A) Plaques are mature and sharply defined at 40 ± 4 hours. (B) Plaque shows peripheral syncytia and internal contraction and lysis.

study and that early results showed that infectivity was correlating with pathologic findings. At 24 hours postinoculation, focal pathologic changes were present both in liver and in the kidneys, and maximum damage in these tissues was found on the third day. It should be noted than an early viremia assures rapid distribution of CCV. Based upon early recovery, highest infectivity, and the most virions visualized therein, the kidneys were the initial target organs and the principal site of virus replication.

7. Immunity

There are very few facts concerning the immune response evoked in catfish by CCV. McGlamery *et al.* (1971) showed that channel catfish had an immune capability and that they responded to injection of either bovine serum albumin (BSA) or vesicular stomatitis virus (VSV). The response to BSA was quantified at intervals using passive hemagglutination, and serum neutralization was also used to measure the response to VSV. Sera used were heated at 56° C for 30 minutes. Chemical identification of the serum activity was not made, therefore its nature is presumed to have been antibody.

Plumb (1972) compared the response of subadult channel catfish to live CCV and to virus which had been heat-inactivated for 1 hour at 60° C. Sera taken prior to inoculation were not heat-inactivated, and some showed CCV neutralizing activity. Specific procedures used to quantify that activity were not detailed but the results were expressed as neutralization indices (NI). Of 20 fish used, seven had an NI of 10 or less, seven were in the range of 10–50, and six had values over 50. Though critical points were lacking, five control fish (injected with cell culture medium) failed to show an increase in CCV neutralizing activity during a period of up to 180 days; initial levels of two actually declined. Heat-killed CCV similarly did not evoke an increase in neutralizing activity. In contrast, nine of ten fish given live CCV showed a significant increase in CCV neutralization in the day 30 samples. Activity reached a peak at 60 days and declined in the 90 day and 120 day samples. Two fish were then given booster inoculations of CCV, and within 30 days the titers rose to and exceeded the previous 60 day peaks.

Whether or not prior antigenic experience provides functional protection to channel catfish is not known. The answer to that question may be difficult to determine for the consensus of observation is that channel catfish, like other fishes, sustain highest mortality to viral infection while they are very young. As fish become fingerlings, their increased age and size is accompanied with an apparent acquisition of resistance, for disease and mortality due to viruses decline and older fish are completely resistant.

Whereas it has not yet been possible to show that adult catfish are in fact carriers of CCV, the presence of viral neutralizing activity in their serum is presumptive evidence that they could well be the source. At present, such serum activity at least provides a clue that such fish should not be used for brood stock purposes; instead, until it is shown to be otherwise, brood stock should be taken from populations which show no evidence of CCV neutralizing activity.

8. Epizootiology

Thus far, CCV disease is known to occur only in North America and principally from the Midsouth and South where the host is under intensive husbandry. As of 1972, Plumb (1972) reported a total of 23 epizootics from which virus had been isolated. The channel catfish is the only host in which natural infection is known to occur, but Plumb (1972) stated that one epizootic among blue catfish (*I. furcatus*) had been diagnosed and that a "CCV-like" pathogen had been isolated. Experimentally, both the blue catfish and the white catfish (*I. catus*) have been shown to have some susceptibility. Channel catfish are apparently the most susceptible and mortality can exceed 90%, but it has been lower in some outbreaks.

Channel catfish virus disease has shown a pattern of occurring among progeny of some brood stock populations, but there has been some inconsistency in that it has not shown up every year among the young of all such stocks. A considerable amount of circumstantial evidence favors the hypothesis that some brood stocks harbor carriers, but that has yet to be demonstrated.

Contact transmission is readily demonstrated during an epizootic, and healthy fry or fingerlings readily contract the infection if they are held in raceways but below fish with active disease. Virus is also readily transmitted by feeding and by intraperitoneal or intramuscular injection. An effective transmission can be achieved by holding susceptible fish for 30 minutes or more in water to which CCV has been added.

There are no firm data, but there is circumstantial evidence for vertical transmission of CCV with eggs. With viruses from North American salmonid fishes, their transmission is effected by shedding with feces, eggs, and with seminal fluid. At one time or another during a year, such shed virus is readily demonstrated. In contrast, the same materials from suspected carrier catfish have not been found to have virus.

As cited by Plumb (1972), Fijan and Naftel found a correlation between temperature and virulence of CCV. At temperatures of 30°C or higher, mortality was acute and reached 85–100%. At 20°–25°C mortality was chronic, but little or no mortality occurred below 15°C. The role of environmental factors in diseases of fishes is well known; it is likely that factors other than temperature may also have an influence.

Plumb (1972) tested the effect of temperature manipulation on the expression of disease and mortality among channel catfish fingerlings. At about

19°C, mortality averaged 14%, whereas at about 27°C the mean mortality was 94%. Fish which had been infected at 19°C but warmed to 27°C after 24 hours showed a 98% mortality. Conversely, when fish were infected at 27°C and the temperature was lowered after 24 hours, the mortality was only 24%. Later reduction of temperature also effected a lowering of mortality, but it was 68–78%—closer to that of constant warm temperature than to constant low temperature.

At present, the most effective control consists of avoiding the infection. Stocks of brood fish having no known history of the disease can be propagated in water from wells or other supplies that do not harbor feral ictalurids. The concept of specific-pathogen-free fish husbandry is growing in acceptance.

The consequences of an epizootic include the immediate mortality, and the possibility of future disease. In addition, survivors seem to have somewhat reduced growth potential, and they do not show as good feed conversion as do fish which have always been healthy.

On the occasion of one confirmed viral epizootic where mortality was low, the fish were destroyed and the pond was disinfected by adding a soluble hypochlorite compound to the equivalent of 20 ppm chlorine. After the chlorine had dissipated, susceptible channel catfish were held as sentinels in a live-car in the treated pond and they remained healthy. The disinfection apparently was successful, and similar or greater levels of chlorine could be tried elsewhere. Since CCV is inactivated by drying, that too has application in clean-up after outbreaks do occur.

B. Epithelioma papillosum-*Associated Virus*

As early as the sixteenth century benign epidermal tumors have been reported from the cultured carp (*Cyprinus carpio*) and several other cyprinids in Europe.

The lesions are superficial, smooth, and somewhat glassy in appearance. Individually, they are localized, but they can occur over rather extensive areas of the skin. Structurally, they are papillomatous and owe their size to a thickening of the epidermis. Necrosis is not common, but the lesions usually slough in time, and pigmented scars follow (see Fig. 7).

The condition is also known as *variola*, hyperplastic epidermal disease, cutaneous warts, fish pox, and perhaps most commonly as carp pox. Whereas "chicken pox" in man has been inappropriate for reasons of host and etiology, carp pox in the fish is inappropriate because the lesion is not a pock nor is a pox virus involved. *Epithelioma papillosum* has long been thought to have a viral cause, but it has not been until the last decade that unequivocal evidence of even an associated virus has been reported.

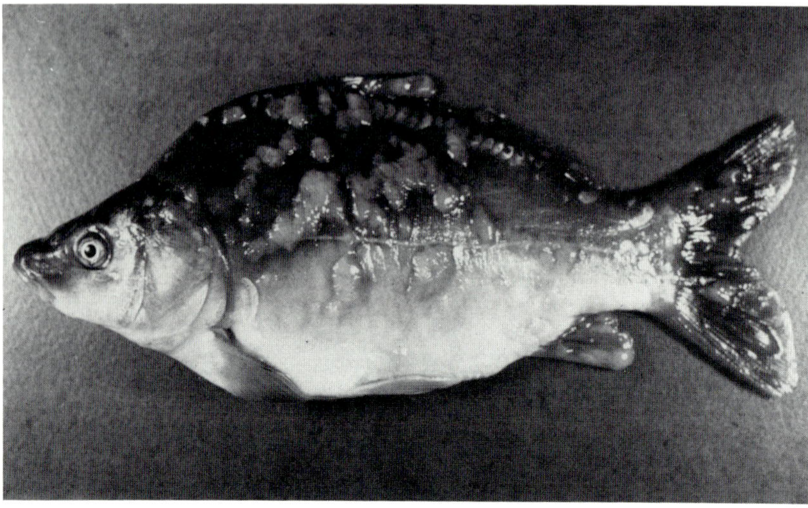

FIG. 7. Carp with multiple dermal lesions of *Epithelioma papulosum* or "carp pox." Photo courtesy Dr. N. N. Fijan, Vet. Faculty U. Zagreb, Yugoslavia.

Whether or not the herpesvirus-like agent visualized in cells of the lesions is the etiologic agent remains to be established.

Carp have been introduced into North America from Europe, but to date, neither *Epithelioma papillosum* nor anything like it has been found in this fish in its new environment. As discussed by Nigrelli (1948, 1952, 1954) and Wolf (1966), lesions having a similar appearance and structure have been found in the bluegill (*Lepomis macrochirus*), a North American centrarchid fish, but electron microscopy has thus far failed to show any indication of virus. Thus, the balance of the discussion will be confined to the carp. The most recent reviews of *Epithelioma papillosum* are the clinically oriented works of Schäperclaus (1969) and Ghittino (1970). The only extant virological data consist of reports on electron microscopy by Schubert (1964, 1966).

Schubert (1964, 1966) examined ultrathin sections of lesions from carp and described and illustrated intracellular virus. He noted that its morphology and the features of its apparent mode of replication were similar to the general pattern of the herpesvirus group. Without equivocation he believed the carp agent to be a herpesvirus and postulated that it was the cause of the tissue proliferation.

Within cell nuclei there were areas of "clustered chromatin" which could be distinguished from nucleoli. What appeared to be very dense nucleoids occurred at the margins of such chromatin masses. Predominantly oval "shells" were also present in the nuclei; their overall size was about 110 nm. Some of the "shells" were empty but others had within them a dense nucleoid ringlike, circular, and, in some, elongated structure, with or without a central constriction. In a few particles, the nucleoid appeared to be passing through the membrane of shell, but it was not possible to determine its direction. It seems valid to equate "shell" as used by Schubert with capsid. Virus appeared to bud from the nuclear membrane and in so doing, a second membrane was acquired and the final diameter was 140–150 nm. In some cells, virus appeared to be leaving the nucleus by way of enlarged pores. Such particles were enclosed in a single membrane; but within the cytoplasm particles within a single membrane were found budding into the endoplasmic reticulum and thereby acquiring the double membrane of mature particles. Desmosomes in the micrographs were credible evidence of the kind of cell being examined.

Cells showing virus were generally in an advanced state of degeneration, and there was some slight margination of chromatin. Though not illustrated in his 1966 report, Schubert alludes to cytoplasmic inclusion bodies that could be demonstrated by conventional microscopy using the fluorescent stain, thioflavine S. At the ultrastructural level, ctyoplasmic cysts were found and were believed to be homologous with those seen by light microscopy. Aggregations of small numbers of virus were found in the cytoplasm of infected cells.

Although it is unsightly, *Epithelioma papillosum* is not a significant health hazard to the carp. This fact probably accounts for the scant attention it has received from researchers. In this regard, methods for transmission are not known. A well-planned experimental approach, using methods of fish tissue culture and concurrent inoculation of established fish cell lines of epithelial-like morphology, is very likely to be productive.

IV. Specific Pathogen-Free Test Animals

In research and diagnostic work with homeotherm vertebrates, availability of test animals that are suitable for experimental or test use is so common that it is often taken for granted. Admittedly somewhat oversimplified, one may order embryonated eggs, young chicks, and a wide variety of laboratory mammals with reasonable assurance of getting a high-quality animal. For some work, specific-pathogen-free warm-blooded animals are essential, and they too are available from commercial sources. Even germ-free animals of a variety of species can be purchased. It goes almost without saying that genetically characterized stock provides the foundation for most laboratory homeotherm populations.

Quite a different situation exists regarding research and diagnostic work with poikilotherm vertebrates, and a discussion of the relevant facts is important to a better understanding of the preceding material on herpesviruses and for that matter on work dealing with any of the parasites and pathogens of cold-blooded vertebrates. Interestingly and understandably enough, there is a great paucity of poikilotherm vertebrates that are suited for laboratory work. Although poor in contrast with homeotherms, the best situation exists among propagated teleost fishes, the availability of experimental amphibians is more seriously limited and confined to a few anurans. The worst restrictions are among the reptiles where the user is generally dependent upon captive stock which has been collected from the wild and is indiscriminately held under crowded conditions which facilitate the transfer of pathogens.

Although some strains of certain species of teleost fishes come close, there is as yet no true counterpart to the laboratory white mouse, guinea pig, etc. Some brood stock populations of propagated fishes are under regular health surveillance by competent specialists in fishery biology. Since the best stocks are kept in water from wells or other protected sources, such fishes are in fact free of the most troublesome parasites and pathogens. Freshwater salmonids comprise the great bulk of such quality fishes, ictalurids probably rank second, and a few cyprinids occupy a questionable third place. Although a number of other species are propagated, the conditions of husbandry are just a step removed from the wild. From time to time, the stock is supplemented from the wild; introductions are made from other populations; and water supplies usually harbor feral and/or wild fishes. The researcher or diagnostician must always be on the alert to the possibility of latent infection which can create problems. Such infection may coexist with a test pathogen and thereby complicate clinical signs with nonrelated pathologic change. Prior infection with the organism may interfere with or even entirely prevent the response to a test virus, bacterium, or parasite. Still other organisms, chronic in nature, may stress the host and trigger latent but more virulent pathogens, and the latter can quickly overcome host defenses. The animals may be lost before results are obtained. All of these types of problems are known among those who work with fishes, and although some certified quality type fishes are available, there is still an occasional need for the researcher to rear his own fish—at least from the egg.

Virus work with amphibians has also been complicated by unknown currrent or prior disease entities in the lives of the test animals. With little doubt, failures in some virus inoculation work have been due to an existing or earlier antigenic experience. Certified specific-pathogen-free amphibians are not available in sufficient numbers to come anywhere near meeting the needs of the investigator. Again, the conscientious worker may have to rear his own stock—at least from the egg.

The problem with reptiles is worse than with amphibians and fishes, since breeding populations are virtually nonexistant. Reptile eggs are relatively few in number and difficult to obtain, and not all reptiles are oviparous or ovoviviparous; some are viviparous.

The picture is not altogether hopeless, and the investigator can apply a number of quality checks. For one, test animals may be acquired in numbers sufficient for preexperimental assay to determine whether or not the population already harbors an entity which could interfere with the proposed work. Direct virological examination or culture of appropriate tissues can be done rather easily. This approach has been particularly useful in work with small salmonid, ictalurid, and centrarchid fishes. When larger animals are involved, and it becomes feasible to draw blood, serological methods are more sensitive and reliable.

An alternate approach is that of employing a surrogate host, phylogenetically related but from a distinctly different and preferably geographically distant area.

The rather high or exclusive host specificity of herpesviruses poses added problems in the use of test or experimental work; there may well be only a single animal species that can be infected by a specific herpesvirus.

References

Clark, H. F., and Karzon, D. T. (1972). *Infect. Immunity* **5**, 559–569.

Clark, H. F., Zeigel, R. F., Fabian, F. B., and Karzon, D. T. (1968). *Bacteriol. Proc.* pp. 149–150.

Fijan, N. (1968). *Bull. Off. Int. Epizoot.* **69**, 1167–1168.

Fijan, N. N., Wellborn, T. L., Jr., and Naftel, J. P. (1970). *U.S., Bur. Sport Fish. and Wildl., Tech. Pap.* **43**, 1–11.

Ghittino, P. (1970). *In* "Ittiopatologia" (Edizioni Rivista di Zootecnia), Vol. 2, p. 420. Stampa Strada–Sesto S. G. Italy.

McGlamery, M. H., Dawe, D. L., and Gratzek, J. B. (1971). *J. Wildl. Dis.* **7**, 299–306.

Monroe, J. H., Shibley, G. P., Schidlovsky, G., Nakai, T., Howatson, A. F., Wivel, N. W., and O'Connor, T. E. (1968). *J. Nat. Cancer Inst.* **40**, 135–139.

Nigrelli, R. F. (1948). *Zoologica (New York)* **33**, 133–137.

Nigrelli, R. F. (1952). *Ann. N. Y. Acad. Sci.* **54**, 1076–1092.

Nigrelli, R. F. (1954). *Trans. Amer. Fish. Soc.* **83**, 262–296.

Padgett, F., and Levine, A. S. (1966). *Virology* **30**, 623–630.

Plumb, J. A. (1971a). *J. Wildl. Dis.* **7**, 213–216.

Plumb, J. A. (1971b). *Ala., Agr. Exp. Sta., Progr. Rep. Ser.* **95**, 1–3.

Plumb, J. A. (1972). Doctoral Dissertation, Auburn University, Auburn, Alabama.

Schäperclaus, W. (1969). *In* "Handbuch der Virusinfektionen bei Tieren" (H. Röhrer, ed.), pp. 1067–1141. Fischer, Jena.
Schubert, G. (1964). *Z. Naturforsch. B.* **19**, 675–682.
Schubert, G. H. (1966). *Bull. Off. Int. Epizoot.* **65**, 1011–1022.
Wolf, K. (1966). *Advan. Virus Res.* **12**, 35–101.
Wolf, K., and Darlington, R. W. (1971). *J. Virol.* **8**, 525–533.
Wolf, K., and Quimby, M. C. (1970). *U.S., Bur. Sport Fish. Wildl., Resour. Publ.* **106**, 86–95.
Wolf, K., Herman, R. L., and Carlson, C. P. (1972). *J. Fish. Res. Bd. Can.* **29**, 149–150.
Zeigel, R. F., and Clark, H. F. (1972). *Infect. Immunity* **5**, 570–582.

Chapter 16
The Epstein-Barr Virus*

George Klein

I. History

The Epstein-Barr (EB) virus was discovered in the course of an intense search for viruses associated with Burkitt's lymphoma that was initiated by Burkitt's suggestion that the climate-related geographical distribution of the high-endemic disease was best explained by the transmission of an insect-vectored virus (Burkitt, 1962, 1963). The involvement of an infectious agent was strongly supported by the time-space clustering of the disease (Pike, *et al.*, 1967).

An electron microscopic search for viral particles in tumor specimens gave no positive findings, and attempts were therefore made to detect viruses in cultured cells derived from Burkitt's lymphoma (Epstein *et al.*,

*This chapter was written while the author was a Fogarty Scholar at the Fogarty International Center, National Institutes of Health, Bethesda, Maryland.

1964b). Stationary suspension cultures of lymphoblastoid cells were derived from Burkitt's lymphoma biopsies and propagated as continuous lines (Pulvertaft, 1964; Epstein and Barr, 1964). Cells of one line (EB1) contained virus particles with a herpes-like morphology (Epstein *et al.*, 1964). The number of particles was large in each positive cell, but only a small fraction of the cell population was positive. Tests for known herpesviruses gave negative results (Epstein *et al.*, 1965), and it was therefore assumed that this was a previously unidentified virus. This was definitely confirmed by the serological studies of Henle and Henle (1966a). They found that a small proportion of acetone-fixed cells of several, but not all Burkitt's lymphoma (BL)-derived cell lines showed an intensely brilliant immunofluorescence when exposed to the sera of Burkitt's lymphoma patients and of certain normal individuals. All positive lines carried the herpes-like virus described by Epstein *et al.* (1964b), whereas negative lines contained no detectable virus. There was no relationship between the reactivity of different sera against the virus-positive BL lines and their antibody titer against a large number of other herpesviruses or against viruses of other families. The relationship between the Henle reaction and the EB virus was confirmed by several findings. The percentage of virus-carrying cells detected by electron microscopy corresponded to the percentage of fluorescent cells in each line. In the course of serial passage, the virus became undetectable in some lines that were shown to be originally positive by electron microscopy. The proportion of immunofluorescence (IF)-positive cells decreased in parallel. In another study (zur Hausen *et al.*, 1967), the same cells were examined by IF and electron microscopy. Only IF-positive cells contained herpes-like particles. Another link was established between the virus and the fluorescent antibody when it was found that only IF-positive sera led to the visible coating and agglutination of viral particles (Henle *et al.*, 1966; Mayyasi *et al.*, 1967). A variety of efforts to identify EB virus with some previously known member of the herpes group produced negative results (Henle and Henle, 1966b). Similar findings were reported by investigators using complement fixation (Armstrong *et al.*, 1966; Henle and Henle, 1966a; Gerber and Birch, 1967) and immunoprecipitation tests (Old *et al.*, 1966; Oettgen *et al.*, 1967) for EB virus antigens. This has led to the unanimous conclusion that EB virus is a previously unknown member of the herpes group.

The association between Burkitt's lymphoma and the EB virus was established by yet another series of findings. Lymphoma cells of fresh BL biopsy specimens carry a distinctive membrane antigen, absent from normal lymph node or bone marrow cells and from various leukemias (G. Klein *et al.*, 1966; E. Klein *et al.*, 1967). Established, EB virus-producing lymphoblastoid cell lines have a similar, if not identical membrane antigen (G. Klein *et al.*, 1967b). It is not identical with the viral antigen detected by the Henle test (G. Klein *et al.*, 1968b, 1969b), but is is induced by the virus, since it appears promptly when EB virus antigen-negative lymphoblastoid lines are exposed to irradiated, virus-yielding cells (G. Klein *et al.*, 1967a) or to viral concentrates (Gergely *et al.*, 1971a; W. Henle and Henle, 1970; Horoszіewicz *et al.*, 1970).

II. Virus–Cell Relationships

Cells productively infected with herpesviruses degenerate and die. The EB virus is no exception. Virus containing cells show a variety of cytopathological changes (Epstein *et al.*, 1965; Rabson *et al.*, 1966; Pope *et al.*, 1968a). The virus can also enter a nonpermissive proliferation stimulating interaction with certain lymphoid cells, however. Henle *et al.* (1967) exposed peripheral white cells of newborn female children to lethally X-irradiated cells of the EB-virus producing, BL-derived P3HR-1 line of male origin. Permanent lymphoblastoid lines emerged; they had a female karyotype and a small proportion of the cells produced EB virus. No such "transformation" was observed when irradiated cells of a nonproducer line (Raji) were substituted instead of P3HR-1 (Diehl *et al.*, 1969).

Gerber *et al.* (1969b) exposed buffy coat leukocytes of healthy, EB-virus seronegative donors to EB virus concentrates and obtained a permanent EB-virus carrying lymphoblastoid lines. Miller *et al.* (1969) were also successful in converting normal adult lymphocytes into established lines, by exposing them to X-irradiated cells of an EB virus-producing blastoid line derived from an American leukemic child. Another leukemic cell line that did not produce EB virus failed to transform. Transformation was specifically inhibited by sera that contains antibodies against (Miller *et al.* 1971).

These experiments suggested that EB virus was somehow required for the conversion of peripheral lymphocytes into established lymphoid lines with an unlimited life span. This impression was strengthened by the finding of several groups that EB virus-carrying lymphoblastoid lines could often be established from the peripheral blood of seropositive donors but not, or only very rarely, from seronegative donors (for review, see Miller, 1971; Nilsson, 1971). Perhaps the most significant fact was that fetal or neonatal lymphocytes never converted into lines unless EB virus or EB virus-containing filtrates were added. Pope *et al.* (1968b) showed that cell-free filtrates prepared from an EB virus-carrying line derived from a leukemic donor induced continuous growth of fetal thymic or spleen lymphocytes. Fetal lymphocytes did not proliferate in the absence of EB virus-containing filtrates. Sera containing anti-EB virus antibodies inhibited transformation, whereas negative sera had no effect (Pope *et al.*, 1969a). Chang *et al.* (1971) converted umbilical cord leukocytes into permanent lines by adding extracts of EB virus-producing lines derived from healthy individuals. Uninfected, cord blood cells failed to convert into lines in a large number of control experiments. Closely similar findings were reported by Nilsson *et al.* (1971). The inability of Nilsson to establish lines from fetal lymphoid tissues in the absence of EB virus was in strong contrast to his high success rate in growing lines from seropositive adults. Recently, a microplate assay has been designed to assess the biological activity of EB virus in transforming cord blood lymphocytes (Moss and Pope, 1972). This test is also suitable to measure virus neutralization.

Attempts to transmit the EB virus to cells of other than human species were largely unsuccessful in spite of the numerous attempts (Stewart, 1969). Recently, Miller *et al.* (1972b) have found, however, that the human EB virus can be transmitted to squirrel monkey and marmoset leukocytes *in vitro*. Werner *et al.* (1973) obtained similar results with Gibbon leukocytes. It was also shown (Landon *et al.*, 1968) that cells cultured from the peripheral blood of chimpanzees carried a herpes-type virus that was morphologically indistinguishable from EB virus and cross reacted in complement-fixation (CF) tests (Gerber and Birch, 1967).

The proliferation-stimulating role of EB virus for human lymphoid cells contrasts with the cytopathic effect of virus production and shows the existence of different virus–cell interactions. The presence of viral genetic information in virus-negative lymphoblastoid cells was suggested by the finding of Pope *et al.* (1969b) that the BL-derived Raji line contained an EB virus-determined CF antigen and a soluble antigen, demonstrated by immunodiffusion (Pope *et al.*, 1971). The EB virus association of these antigens was shown by their reactivity with EB virus-positive but not with EB virus-negative sera. Similar observations were made by Vonka *et al.* (1970) concerning three other lymphoid lines that showed no evidence of EB virus by electron microscopy or by the Henle test. They suggested that an EB virus-coded nonstructural protein was responsible for the CF activity. Analogous findings were made by Gerber and Deal (1970).

Recently an EB virus-determined nuclear antigen could be visualized in 85–95% of the cells in all EB virus genome-carrying producer and nonproducer lines by anticomplementary immunofluorescence (Reedman and Klein, 1973). Designated as EBNA, this antigen shows, a striking similarity with the T antigens of the small oncogenic DNA virus systems, although it remains associated with the chromosome during mitosis. It is also present in the BL biopsies.

The finding that nonproducer lines of human lymphoblastoid origin contained EB virus genetic information gave support to the notion that the virus-negative majority of the producer lines also contained the viral genome. This implies the periodic activiation of virus production "from within" in a small number of cells, as contrasted to a carrier culture with a continuous horizontal reinfection cycle between originally virus-free cells. This notion received decisive experimental support from cloning experiments (Miller, 1971; Zajac and Kohn, 1970; Maurer and Wilberg, 1970; Miller *et al.*, 1970). When single-cell clones were derived from various established EB virus-producing lymphoblastoid lines, in the presence of antiviral serum, each clone behaved like the parental line, showing approximately the same frequency of EB virus-positive cells, suggesting that the virus was associated with all cells of the original culture in some repressed form and that the activation frequency of the viral cycle was characteristic for each line.

The presence of the EB viral genome in human lymphoblastoid lines, including "nonproducers", was confirmed by nucleic acid hybridization. This approach became feasible after methods were developed to isolate and purify EB virus DNA in suitable quantities (Weinberg and Becker, 1969; Schulte-Holthausen and zur Hausen, 1970; Wagner *et al.*, 1970). The buoyant density of EB virus DNA in CsCl was defined at 1.718 gm/cm^3, allowing good separation from cellular DNA. By using purified, radioactive EB virus DNA for DNA–DNA hybridization studies, zur Hausen and Schulte-Holthausen (1970) found significant hybridization between the viral DNA and the DNA of the "virus-free" Raji line. A number of human lines of nonlymphoblastoid origin were negative. Epstein-Barr virus DNA did not cross hybridize with herpes simplex virus-infected cells. Raji cell RNA showed an increased annealing with EB virus DNA, compared to controls, suggesting the transcription of EB virus-specific RNA.

Experiments involving DNA–DNA hybridization also demonstrated the presence of EB virus DNA in biopsy materials derived from Burkitt's lymphoma (BL) and nasopharyngeal carcinoma (NPC), but in not a number of other tumors growing in EB virus-seropositive patients (zur Hausen *et al.*, 1970). This "control tumor" category included cases of Hodgkin's disease, lymphosarcomas, and carcinomas of the head and the neck region other than NPC.

Deoxyribonucleic acid from multiple tumors of the same BL donor annealed with EB virus DNA within a similar range, whereas the extent of hybridization varied considerably between tumors of different patients. The behavior of multiple tumors of the same patient is in line with the isozyme marker study of Fialkow *et al.* (1970), demonstrating that single or multiple tumors of BL patients originate from a single clone. This approach was based on the *G6PD* mosaicism of heterozygous African females. Since *G6PD* is an X-linked marker and only one X chromosome is functional in each female cell, normal tissues of heterozygous females consist of two cell populations, and the two isozyme types are present in approximately equal proportions. Burkitt's lymphomas of such patients always contained one enzyme type only, however, leading to the conclusion that the tumor was uniclonal (for review, see Fialkow, 1972).

Hybridizations of DNA–DNA are technically difficult, and the relatively low specific radioactivities of the viral DNA preparations thus far obtained can introduce various sources of error. More recent studies (zur Hausen, 1972; Nonoyama and Pagano, 1971), therefore have shifted to hybridization between *in vitro* synthesized RNA complementary to viral DNA (cRNA) and cellular DNA. Using this method, zur Hausen (1972) found that eight lymphoblastoid lines of human origin, that failed to produce detectable virus or any of the viral antigens detectable by immunofluoresence, all contained significant amounts of hybridizable DNA. This material included the Raji line of BL origin, the SKL-1 and 6410 lines derived from leukemia patients, the LY1 and LY2 lines derived from NPC patients, the NC37 line from a normal donor, and the S84 and S94 lines originating from Hodgkin's disease patients. The average number of EB virus genome equivalents per cell ranged between 3–4 (SKL1) and 121 (NC37) in the different lines. Zur Hausen pointed out that these calculations were approximate and may represent overestimates. Nevertheless, the data clearly confirmed that non-producer lymphoblastoid lines contain EB virus DNA and that the EB virus genome "load" varies from line to line. Similar findings were reported by Nonoyama and Pagano (1971). They estimated approximately 65 EB virus genome equivalents per cell for the Raji line, 45 for 6410, 100 for F-265 (derived from a healthy donor), 80 for NC 37, and none detectable for HeLa and HEP monolayer cultures.

The cRNA–DNA hybridization technique was also applied to BL and NPC biopsies. Zur Hausen (1972) found that 23 BL and 6 NPC samples hybridized significantly above the background of various controls, including 21 other tumors of the head and neck and the lymphatic system. Preparations of DNA derived from eight cases of chronic lymphatic leukemia and from leukocytes of some EB virus seropositive adult donors (but not cord blood leukocytes) showed a somewhat increased annealing as well. Significant cRNA–DNA hybridization of BL and NPC biopsies was also found by Nonoyama *et al.* (1973).

The regular demonstrability of the EB virus genome in established human lymphoblastoid lines, including all nonproducers that have been tested so far, together with the evidence that fetal lymphocytes cannot be grown into established lines unless EB virus is added suggest that the viral genome may be necessary for the unlimited multiplication of human lymphoid cells and/or their growth under *in vitro* conditions. It is obviously important to examine the state of the viral genome in the transformed cells, particularly the nature of its association with the genetic material of the host cell, the regulation of viral transcription and translation, and the events leading to the activation of an abortive or productive cycle. Studies on these problems are in their earliest stage.

Zur Hausen performed (1972) *in situ* cRNA–DNA hybridization experiments in cytological preparations and found that EB virus DNA is associated with the chromosomes of the nonproducer Raji cell. This is in line with the demonstration of Nonoyama and Pagano (1971) that chromosomes isolated from metaphase-arrested Raji cells contained as much hybridizable viral DNA as total cell DNA. A relatively stable association between viral and cellular DNA is also suggested by the finding that continuous lines preserved their "EB virus load" at a relatively constant level from year to year. On the other hand, noncovalently bound viral DNA has been recently found in Raji cells, and it has been suggested that the viral genome may be carried in a plasmidlike state (Nonoyama and Pagano, 1972). This finding does not exclude, however, that some part of the viral DNA may exist in a covalently linked form in addition.

More recent evidence (Adams *et al.*, 1973) indicates that EB virus DNA is linearly integrated with the Raji host cell DNA, in a pronase- and phenol-resistant, but alkali-labile, form.

The presence of relatively, if not fully, complete viral genomes in nonproducer lines was confirmed by the recent demonstration (Hampar *et al.*, 1972a; Gerber, 1972) that bromodeoxyuridine (BUdR) could induce the production of viral antigens in the Raji and the NC37 line. In addition to early antigens, viral capsid antigens and virus particles were produced as well, after release from the drug treatment.

It is possible that the cell-associated viral genome exerts some repressor-like function that restricts viral transcription in nonproducer cells. Superinfection of the Raji line with EB virus concentrates (Horosziewicz *et al.*, 1970; Henle *et al.*, 1970b; Gergely *et al.*, 1971a) has led to the appearance of EB virus-associated membrane antigens (MA) and early antigens (EA), demonstrated by immunofluorescence. Both antigens appeared 10–16 hours after infection and were not inhibited by cytosine arabinoside (Ara-C), or iododeoxyuridine (IUdR), given in doses that completely stopped DNA synthesis (Gergely *et al.*, 1971a). Viral capsid antigens appeared later, in a smaller minority of the cells and only after infection with high viral multiplicities. The viral cycle induced by the superinfection eventually aborted in most reported experiments and nonproducer lines did thus not convert into producers, as a rule. The number of genome equivalents, demonstrable by nucleic acid hybridization, could be raised permanently by superinfection, however (H. zur Hausen, personal communication).

Virus-producer and nonproducer lymphoblastoid lines were compared with regard to their ability to adsorb virus and to respond to superinfection by the appearance of early antigen (EA)-positive cells 48 hours after infection (G. Klein *et al.*, 1972). All 11 nonproducer lines tested adsorbed the virus but only 7 responded with significant EA development. Viral function appeared to be blocked in four lines, either due to some function of the resident viral genome, e.g., the production of a repressor, or to nonpermissive properties of the host cell. Eighteen virus-producer lines were also studied in the same way. Only 9 showed good virus adsorption; 4 of the 9 responded with a significant increment of EA-positive cells, whereas 5 failed to do so. These two categories thus behaved similarly to the corresponding nonproducer groups. There was a third major category, consisting of 9 producer lines, however, that showed no significant virus adsorption. There was no significant EA increment after the superinfection of these lines either. Conceivably, their viral receptors may have been blocked by viral products from the inside. These experiments thus demonstrate that resistance to EB virus superinfection may due to a block at the receptor level or to some postreceptor, presumably intracellular mechanism.

Different "producer lines" show great variations in their permissiveness when compared with regard to the relationship between the frequencies of early (EA) and late (VCA) viral antigen-positive cells and their release of infectious virus. Lines that release sufficient virus to induce EA-positive cells in a suitable indicator line, e.g., Raji, are exceptional. So far there is only a single clonal derivative of the Jijoye line, P3HR1, established by Hinuma and Grace (1967), that regularly yields infectious supernatants, if Judged by the EA test. Most other producer lines contain a significant number of VCA-positive cells, some of them comparable to or higher than P3HR1, but release little or no infectious virus. Still other show an accumulation of cells containing early viral products (MA or EA), but with few or no VCA-positive cells. This suggests that the viral cycle which becomes activated in a minority of the cells in producer lines tends to abort at different stages, depending on the line. Most EA-positive cells show a progressive inhibition of macromolecular synthesis in certain producer lines and in superinfected cells (Gergely *et al.*, 1971b,c) and only some can proceed to the DNA synthesis that is a prerequisite of VCA and virus particle formation (Gergely *et al.*, 1971c; Hampar *et al.*, 1972b). Those that do not produce VCA and viral particles probably die soon after they developed EA. The appearance of MA, without EA is, on the other hand, compatible with continued host cell macromolecular synthesis (Gergely *et al.*, 1971b).

The frequency of viral antigen-positive cells can be increased in some producer lines by cultivating the cells on arginine-deficient medium or at 32°C (Hinuma *et al.*, 1967; Henle and Henle, 1968), whereas other lines failed to respond to these treatments. Small doses of mitomycin C, actinomycin D, X rays, or methotrexate increased the frequency of MA-positive cells in some lines, whereas cytosine arabinoside treatment or growth at 31°C had no such effect (Yata *et al.*, 1970). Puromycin decreased the frequency of MA-positive cells in producer lines (Yata *et al.*, 1970) and prevented the appearance of MA and EA in superinfected cells (Gergely *et al.*, 1971a).

Although the mechanisms by which these various treatments affect viral antigen expression are unknown, it may be speculated that they alter the relationship between viral DNA and cellular controls. The remarkable differences in the sensitivity of different lines to the same treatment indicate that qualitatively or quantitatively different controls may be involved, or, alternatively, that the viral genome is more or less complete.

Recent findings (Klein and Dombos, 1973) favor the idea that differences in control mechanisms are more likely to be responsible than differences in viral defectiveness. We have compared the superinfectability of various lymphoblastoid lines, as assessed by the EA-induction test, with the activability of viral antigen (EA) expression in the corresponding uninfected line, by BUdR and IUdR treatment. Superinfection-sensitive lines were readily activable, as a rule; IUdR treatment was somewhat more efficient than BUdR treatment. Viral receptor-positive lines that failed to respond to superinfection, i.e., showed no significant increment of EA–positive cells, were also refractory to induction by BUdR and IUdR. Viral receptor-negative lines showed a wide range of inducibility. These findings suggest the existence of negative controls of variable strength that limit the production of viral antigens and can affect incoming, superinfecting viral genomes and activated resident genomes to a similar extent.

In view of the large size of the viral genome, the number of antigens defined by the serological reactions so far described, is no doubt strongly understated. Recently, the EA complex was subdivided into two subclasses, designated R (restricted) and D (diffuse), that differ with respect to antigenic specificity and localization (G. Henle *et al.*, 1971b). The R component is assembled into dense cytoplasmic clumps and is alcohol sensitive. The D antigen is finely dispersed over both nucleus and cytoplasm and is resistant to alcohol. Both antigens appear at the same time during the virus cycle. Surprisingly, antibody formation against the two antigens is not always concordant, and the discordances show some interesting disease relationships, as discussed in Section IV.

The membrane antigen (MA) was divided into three subsites distinguished on the basis of antigenic specificity (Svedmyr *et al.*, 1970). Sera containing anti-MA antibodies may react with one, two, or three subsites. All three components appeared to be parts of the same macromolecular complex, since they appeared on the same cellular structures simultaneously in superinfection experiments and fluctuated in parallel during growth cycle-related changes in antigen expression. This could be visualized by two-color immunofluorescence (G. Klein *et al.*, 1971).

All three MA subsites mentioned appeared early in the course of the viral cycle and were uninfluenced by DNA inhibitors. Preliminary experiments indicate that there may exist other, late MA components as well, only expressed on the surface of VCA-positive cells in producer lines (Ernberg and Klein, 1973). Surprisingly, the early MA components are also expressed on the viral envelope (Silvestre *et al.*, 1971). This appears paradoxical at first sight, since it is hard to understand why viral envelope components become inserted into the plasma membrane, while the virus buds from the nuclear membrane, and why this happens at an early stage of the viral cycle in spite of the fact that envelopment is a late step in viral maturation. It is conceivable, however, that the virus inserts some envelope components into all cell membranes. Alternatively, plasma membrane changes may appear as a secondary consequence of virally determined enzyme action, such as in the antigenic conversion of *Salmonella* (Luria and Darnell, 1968) or, alternatively, as a requirement for viral DNA replication (cf. Klein 1971b). If this were the case, the appearance of early, virally determined membrane antigens on the envelope of the mature virus would be merely a consequence of their presence on a variety of cellular membranes, including those involved in virus budding.

III. EB Virus and Infectious Mononucleosis

It is now established beyond reasonable doubt that EB virus is the causative agent of the heterophil-positive, classical form of infectious mononucleosis (IM), a disease with predilection for adolescents and young adults in the higher socioeconomic groups. The first clue that EB virus was involved in its etiology came when it was observed (Henle *et al.*, 1968) that one of the EB virus-seronegative technicians converted to seropositive after she developed infectious mononucleosis. Her peripheral lymphocytes yielded lymphoblastoid lines harboring EB virus during the next 2 months, but not prior to or 4 months after the illness. A similar tendency was manifested by the peripheral lymphoid cells of other IM patients (Pope, 1967; Glade *et al.*, 1968; Diehl *et al.*, 1968). These initial observations were followed by a retrospective study on the sera of college students, preserved in the Yale serum bank (Henle *et al.*, 1968; Niederman *et al.*, 1968). Pre-illness sera were available from 24 students, sampled 1 month to 5 years prior to the onset of mononucleosis: they were all negative for EB virus-antibodies.

In the course of the disease, anti-EB virus antibodies appeared in all cases and rose to titers between 1:40 and 1:640 within a few weeks. There was no correlation between EB virus and heterophile antibody titers. High anti-EB virus antibody levels were maintained for several months after the disease and were still demonstrable at lower levels one or several years later, long after heterophile antibodies disappeared. Confirmatory evidence was reported by several groups (Pereira *et al.*, 1969; Banatvala *et al.*, 1969; Hirshaut *et al.*, 1969). Analogous findings were made with regard to anti-MA antibodies (G. Klein *et al.*, 1968a), CF antibodies (Gerber *et al.*, 1968), and virus-neutralizing antibodies (Miller *et al.*, 1972a): they were all absent from preillness sera, appeared regularly in mononucleosis patients, and were demonstrable many years after the disease. Antibodies reacting with EB virions, demonstrated by the immunoferritin technique, were mainly of the IgM class when they appeared in heterophile-positive sera in the course of the disease, whereas the corresponding activity of seropositive normal donors resided in the IgG class (Hampar *et al.*, 1971). This was interpreted as evidence the anti-EB virus antibodies found in the course of IM reflect a primary immunogenic exposure to the virus. Recently, 200 patients with heterophil-positive IM and 60 with heterophile-negative IM-like disease were examined for anti-EA (early antigen) antibodies (W. Henle *et al.*, 1971). All patients in the acute phase of the disease had titers of anti-VCA between 1:40 and 1:64. Only 75% of these patients developed anti-EA antibody at titers between 1:5 and 1:320. Anti-EA antibody titers reached peaks later than anti-VCA titers and disappeared again with a few months. It was concluded that the presence of anti-EA antibody at titers of 1:20 or above probably denotes a current primary infection in most cases. The delay in anti-EA antibody development and its early disappearance were found useful for the serodiagnosis of IM, in that fourfold or greater increments or declines in titer, indicative of a current EB-virus infection, were observed with greater frequency than corresponding changes in anti-VCA titers. This was particulary helpful for the diagnosis of EB virus mononucleosis in patients without heterophile antibody responses. After the two subcomponents of the EA system, D and R were distinguished (G. Henle *et al.*, 1971b), it was found that the anti-EA responses in IM are anti-D antibody, as a rule, like the antibody found in anti-EA antibody-positive NPC cases. In contrast, anti-R antibody reactivity pre-dominates in the BL and also in the rare anti-EA positive healthy individuals (*vide infra*).

There is some evidence that anti-EA responses in IM are related, to some extent, to the severity of the illness. Patients with anti-VCA titers of 1:160 or more and anti-EA titers of 1:80 or more, as one extreme, tended to have more severe illness than patients with anti-VCA titers of 1:40 to 1:80 and no detectable anti-EA, taken as the other extreme.

Decisive evidence for the etiological role of EB virus in IM came from prospective studies (Niederman *et al.*, 1968, 1970; Evans *et al.*, 1968; Wahren *et al.*, 1970; Sawyer *et al.*, 1971; Evans, 1971). A summarizing report (Evans, 1971) states that 100 cases of IM appeared among 977 adults observed for periods of 9 months to 8 years whose sera lacked anti-EB virus (VCA) antibody at dilutions of 1:5 to 1:10. Not a single case appeared in the corresponding seropositive group of 1141 individuals. This can only be interpreted to mean that anti-EB virus antibodies indicate immunity to infectious mononucleosis. This leads to the logical conclusion that EB virus causes mononucleosis, and no rational alternative interpretation has been put forward to explain these findings. Glade and Hirschhorn (1970) have suggested that the disease is caused by another, as yet unidentified agent. This hypothesis implies the assumption that EB virus is either transmitted vertically from mother to child, without any antibody response, or that antibodies formed after early primary infections decline subsequently to nondetectable levels. However, there is no evidence either for vertical transmission of EB virus, nor loss of antibodies to VCA, once acquired. The assumption that the unidentified virus would cause a lymphoproliferative response and thereby activate latent EB virus infections is not confirmed, furthermore, by the study of known virus infections that are accompanied by an increase in lymphocyte levels, such as rubella (Sawyer *et al.*, 1971); infectious lymphocytosis (Blacklow and Kapikian, 1970); hepatitis (Henle *et al.*, 1968), cytomegalovirus infection (Klemola and Kaariainen, 1965); or coxsackievirus, adenovirus, or myxovirus infections (Niederman *et al.*, 1968).

The age-dependent distribution of anti-EB virus titers in relation to socioeconomic groups, has been studied in normal populations in various countries by numerous investigators (Armstrong *et al.*, 1966; Henle *et al.*, 1969; Evans and Niederman, 1972; Niederman *et al.*, 1970; Porter *et al.*, 1969; Hirshaut *et al.*, 1969; Gerber and Birch, 1967; Gerber and Rosenblum, 1968; Gerber *et al.*, 1968; Old *et al.*, 1966, Stevens *et al.*, 1970; G. Henle and Henle, 1970). These studies have elucidated the reasons that infectious mononucleosis is essentially a "college disease." Anti-EB virus titers are present in the newborn, due to the passive transfer of antibody from the mother. This is followed by a rapid decline during the first 6–12 months. The first major rise in the incidence of seropositive children occurs around the age of 4–5 years. In the low socioeconomic groups seroconversion continues progressively, and 70–80% of the population becomes positive before puberty. In the high socioeconomic groups, there is a plateau, and a second rise occurs in the later teens or in early adolescents is required to produce the symptoms typical of classical, heterophile-positive infectious mononucleosis, although "silent" seroconversions, without recognized disease, can be registered in adolescents, however with a lower frequency (Niederman *et al.*, 1970; Evans, 1971; G. Henle and Henle, 1970). It is not known whether the infection of young children leads to any particular disease syndrome; relatively mild, noncharacteristic forms of infectious disease may well occur, but typical infectious mononucleosis is relatively rare.

It is possible that EB virus is not the sole agent that induces IM or IM-like diseases. Certain clinical cases of heterophile-negative disease that resembled IM, but were distinguished by the absence of sore throat and widespread lymphadenopathy were accompanied by rise of CF antibody titers to cytomegalovirus (Klemola and Kaariainen, 1965). A closer study of 44 heterophile-negative IM cases showed (Klemola *et al.*, 1970) that both CMV and EB virus could give rise to cases diagnosed as heterophile-negative IM. Cytomegalovirus-induced cases were not associated with a seroconversion against EB virus.

Cases of EB virus transmission through blood transfusion, with IM-like symptoms, have been documented (Gerber *et al.*, 1969a; Blacklow *et al.*, 1971; Henle *et al.*, 1970b). In the largest series by Henle *et al.* (1970c) 18 patients without preoperative anti-EB virus antibodies received multiple blood transfusions for heart surgery. Six of these acquired anti-EB virus antibody titers, although none of them developed any IM-like illness.

It is noteworthy that although IM is a self-limiting disease, an extensive lymphoid infiltration of the major parenchymatous organs occurs, resembling neoplastic proliferation (Carter, 1972). This, together with the demonstrated ability of EB virus to transform normal lymphoid cells into established lines with an unlimited life span raises the question of how the EB virus-induced lymphoproliferative disease, manifested by the IM syndrome, is brought to a standstill eventually. It is reasonable to assume that this is due to the host immune response. The anti-MA and virus-neutralizing antibodies that appear during the course of the disease (G. Klein *et al.*, 1968a; Miller *et al.*, 1972a), may bear the major responsibility for this, alone or together with sensitized lymphoid cells.

The natural transmission of EB virus in causing IM is not definitely known, but the dominating role of close oral contact has been long suspected (Hoagland, 1955). It is therefore of interest that throat washings of IM patients were recently shown to convert cells of an EB virus antigen-negative lymphoblastoid line to antigen positive (Golden *et al.*, 1971) and to transform lymphocytes of an EB virus-negative donor into an EB virus-positive established line (Pereira *et al.*, 1972).

IV. Relationship between EB Virus and Burkitt's Lymphoma (BL)

Burkitt's tumor is a malignant lymphoma of children that occurs in a particularly high frequency in certain areas of Africa (Burkitt, 1962, 1963) and New Guinea (Ten-Seldam *et al.*, 1966). At a low frequency, it has also been found all over the world (Burkitt and Wright, 1970). The relationship between high annual mean temperature and rainfall and the distribution of the high endemic areas led Burkitt (1962, 1963) to suggest that it could be due to a virus with an insect vector.

In about 50% of the cases, the primary disease is localized in the jaws, but it can also start in various internal organs, e.g. the kidneys, adrenals, thyroids, ovaries, testes, or the long bones. The spleen, peripheral lymph nodes, and the bone marrow are rarely involved (O'Connor and Davies, 1960). Tumors are most common in 6–10-year-old children and are rarely seen in older teenagers or adolescents or in children less than 1 year of age (Burkitt and O'Connor, 1961).

Ever since EB virus has been first demonstrated (Epstein *et al.*, 1964b) in an established cell line derived from a case of Burkitt's lymphoma (BL), its relationship to this disease has been under continuous scrutiny. A strong association was suggested by the serological evidence. (Henle and Henle 1966; Henle *et al.*, 1969). All of 139 African Bl patients with histologically confirmed diagnosis were anti-EB virus (VCA) positive, and 87% had high titers ($\geqq$ 1:160). The geometric mean titer was 1:275, higher by a factor of 8 than in an African control population (1:37) that included age and sex matched siblings and other family members of the BL patients. The distribution of anti-MA antibodies showed similar differences between BL patients and African controls (Gunvén *et al.*, 1970).

Patients with many other neoplastic diseases, including lympho- and myeloproliferative malignancies failed to show similarly regular or high anti-EB virus antibody titers, with the possible exception of the lymphocyte-depleted form of Hodgkin's disease (Johansson *et al.*, 1970; Levine *et al.*, 1971), poorly differentiated lymphocyte-lymphoblast lymphoma (Johansson *et al.*, 1971), and, the most notable exception of all, nasopharyngeal carcinoma (Old *et al.*, 1968; W. Henle *et al.*, 1970a; de Schryver *et al.*, 1969). Hypo- and oropharyngeal carcinomas or other head and neck malignancies, including tumors localized to the nasopharynx, showed no significant elevation of anti-EB virus antibody titers (de Schryver *et al.*, 1972). The same was true for a large number of other malignancies of ecto- and endodermal or mesenchymal origin (de Schryver *et al.*, 1972). With regard to sarcoidosis, the evidence is conflicting; there is clearly some elevation of titers, but it is less regular and more moderate than in BL (Hirshaut *et al.*, 1970; Wahren *et al.*, 1971; Gergely, 1973). Acute leukemias show no elevation of anti-EB virus antibody titers; on the contrary, the mean titers are lower than that expected in a control population (Gahrton *et al.*, 1971).

The serological reactivity of "Burkitt's lymphoma" diagnosed outside the high endemic regions showed less regular patterns. Their evaluation presents a more difficult problem however, since histopathology alone does not allow a sharp distinction between BL and other lymphomas. The combined clinical and pathological picture has readily recognizable features in the high-endemic areas, but they are less characteristic in other regions, and the classification becomes more arbitrary. Serological findings on Burkitt-like lymphomas outside Africa are partly in line with African BL's (Ahlström *et al.*, 1967; G. Klein *et al.*, 1970) and are partly different, i.e., have no distinctively high EB virus-associated reactivity (defined as a high anti-EB virus antibody titer and/or a high level of membrane-reactive antibodies) and, thus, resemble ordinary lymphosarcomas rather than "true" BL's. At present, this picture cannot be interpreted meaningfully, since pathology cannot unequivocally guide any decision as to whether non-African cases are African Burkitt-like or not. It is quite possible, of course, that the non-African Burkitt-like cases are heterogeneous. Some of them may be "true Burkitt's", i.e., have the same etiology as the African cases, whereas others would be different and comparable to ordinary lymphosarcomas. Whether a classification can be built on the EB virus-associated serological pattern will, of course, depend on whether the relationship of EB virus to BL is of an essential or of an accidental nature.

An unusually firm association between EB virus and African BL is also suggested by nucleic acid hybridization experiments. Both DNA–DNA (zur Hausen *et al.*, 1970) and cRNA–DNA (zur Hausen, 1972; Nonoyama *et al.*, 1973) hybridization revealed the consistent presence of EB virus DNA in BL tumor biopsies, whereas a number of "control tumors", derived from EB virus-seropositive patients with other malignancies, gave no evidence of detectable tumor associated EB virus DNA. Nasopharyngeal carcinoma was the outstanding exception, as discussed in Section V.

Corroborative evidence, indicating a more regular association of the virus with BL and NPC than with other tumors that occur in seropositive patients, has come from a study on the effect of local tumor irradiation on various EB virus-associated antibody titers (Einhorn, 1972; Einhorn *et al.*, 1972). Irradiation of BL and NPC *in vivo* has led to an increase of antibody titers against the EB virus-determined MA and VCA, whereas the irradiation of various other tumors has failed to do so. Viral activation followed by antigen release or simple antigen release due to tumor disintegration may be possible explanations of this effect.

What is the relationship between the virus and the Burkitt's lymphoma cell *in vivo*? Virus particles and viral capsid antigens are not found in biopsy specimens. After explantation, capsid antigens regularly appear in 3–5 days (Nadkarni *et al.*, 1970). In the majority of the established BL-derived cell lines, a small number of cells continue to produce EA, VCA, and viral particles, although there are a number of BL-derived lines (prototype: Raji) that do not produce any of the viral antigens that are detectable by immunofluorescence. However, all such lines, when studied, have been found to contain EB virus DNA and/or EB virus-determined antigens detected by CF, however (Pope *et al.*, 1969b, 1971; Vonka *et al.*, 1970; Gerber and Deal, 1970; zur Hausen and Schulte-Holthausen, 1970; zur Hausen, 1972; Nonoyama and Pagano, 1971). Furthermore, all clones isolated in the presence of antiviral sera from cultured BL lines contained the EB virus genome, in spite of the fact that the parent cultures only contained a small proportion of cells with detectable viral antigens (Hinuma *et al.*, 1967, Zajac and Kohn, 1970; Maurer *et al.*, 1970).

In principle, the noncytocidal interaction of the EB viral genome with its host cell is compatible with an oncogenic potential (without proving it), since an oncogenic herpesvirus must obviously remain "silent" in its target cells while replicating its nucleic acid regularly.

In certain lines, the frequency of cells making viral proteins could be increased by arginine deficiency (Henle and Henle 1968), X irradiation, or small doses of certain synthetic inhibitors, such as mitomycin C, IUdR, BUdR, actinmycin D, or cytosine arabinoside (Yata *et al.*, 1970; Gergely, *et al.*, 1971c). Recently, production of viral antigens and of viral particles could be induced in nonproducer lines by treatment with BUdR and IUdR (Hamper *et al.*, 1972a; Gerber, 1972; Klein and Dombos, 1973). This suggested that the viral genome carried by the "silent" lines is probably more or less complete. This is directly supported by the recent demonstration of a close correspondence between the DNA reassociation kinetics obtained with purified EB virus DNA, as compared to the viral DNA found in "nonproducer" lines and in BL biopsies (Nonoyama *et al.*, 1973).

Obviously, the only truly representative malignant BL cell is the *in vivo* tumor cell itself. It is, therefore, very important to consider its viral antigen status. As already mentioned, early antigen (EA) and viral capsid antigen (VCA) are not found in biopsy cells (Nadkarni *et al.*, 1970), whereas EB virus-associated membrane antigens (MA) are regularly found (G. Klein *et al.*, 1966, 1967b, 1968b). Since they appear on the majority of the cells, it may be assumed that they are compatible with continuous cell proliferation. The findings described in Section II of this chapter showed that the appearance of MA on EB virus-superinfected cells did not inhibit continued synthesis of host cell macromolecules. Therefore, it is possible that the MA plays a role analogous to the membrane-associated antigens on virally induced experimental neoplasms. Such antigens are regularly exposed on the outer surface of tumor cells induced by both RNA and DNA viruses. They are virus-specific, i.e., identical or cross reactive for all tumors induced by the same virus; they can induce rejection reactions *in vivo* capable of dealing with at least a limited number of syngeneic tumor cells induced by the same virus (for review, see G. Klein, 1966; Old and Boyse, 1964; Pasternak, 1969; Sjögren, 1965).

The possible importance of virus-induced membrane changes for the oncogenic function of herpesviruses has been emphasized by Roizman (1972). Long before any herpesviruses were suspected of any such function, he showed (Roizman and Spring, 1967) that different mutants of herpes simplex virus, characterized by slightly different envelope proteins, insert their distinctive proteins into the outer plasma membrane of the infected cell. At the same time, the "social behavior" of the infected cells changes in a way that is characteristic for each mutant. Mixed infection with two mutants may lead to the predominance of membrane proteins from one virus type; the change in social behavior follows the corresponding pattern.

Cells infected with lytic herpesviruses, such as herpes simplex virus, invariably die. It is noteworthy, however, that UV-inactivated herpes simplex virus type 2 was recently reported to induce malignant transformation in hamster fibroblasts (Duff and Rapp, 1971). The transformants grew as highly malignant tumors after inoculation into hamsters. The sera of the tumor-bearing animals contained antibodies that neutralized the virus and reacted with the membrane of the transformed cells (Rapp and Duff, 1972). Indirectly at least, this suggests that part of the viral genome may be present in the cells and is perhaps responsible for their malignant behavior. It may be recalled that UV-inactivated herpes simplex virus was also found capable of introducing a virally determined enzyme (thymidine kinase) into an enzyme-deficient cell line maintained on selective medium (Munyon *et al.*, 1971).

There are other reasons why membrane changes in tumor cells deserve attention, particularly when they are due to an oncogenic virus or to a virus regularly associated with the tumor. Growth-regulating impulses, including humoral, long-range and contact short-range signals, have to be transmitted through membrane-associated receptors. The outer membrane of tumor cells is reportedly changed in a number of ways. A disruption of normal membrane architecture due to the insertion of viral-determined products may, if compatible with continued cell life and proliferation, create a state of decreased responsiveness to growth control, i.e., neoplasia.

Suggestive as these arguments may be, they are obviously inconclusive as far as the etiology of BL is concerned. The possibility remains that EB virus is merely a passenger in the tumor, although it is difficult to see, in that case, why it should not show a corresponding association with other malignant lymphoproliferative diseases as well. Also, if EB virus is irrelevant for the genesis of BL, a number of seronegative patients would be expected. In the young age groups at risk, there is a substantial proportion (10–15%) of seronegative children, even in the high endemic regions of Africa. These considerations, together with the proven ability of the virus to cause at least a self-limiting lymphoproliferative disease *in vivo* and its remarkable tendency to stimulate lymphoid cell proliferation *in vitro*, are at least in line with an oncogenic potential. The regular presence of viral nucleic acid in the tumor cells is also consistent with this possibility. Perhaps the most important argument comes from the analogies with the oncogenic animal herpesviruses, particularly herpesvirus saimiri and Marek's disease, discussed in Chapters 17 and 18.

If EB virus is involved in BL in a more important capacity than that of accidental passenger, it will be necessary to understand the difference between the infectious process that leads to seroconversion, without disease, or to infectious mononucleosis or malignant lymphoma. One possibility is that different virus subtypes are responsible. There is no evidence for or against this; the absence of fully permissive target cells *in vitro* has inhibited a search for viral mutants, and the antigenic studies thus far performed tended to emphasize the common features of the virus carried in lymphoblastoid lines of different origin. There was no effort to look specifically for subtype differences.

Another alternative is that the same virus is associated with the benign and malignant diseases, and the difference depends on genetic and/or environmental cofactors. Burkitt, who originally interpreted his findings concerning distribution of the high endemic regions as suggestive of an oncogenic virus transmitted by an insect (Burkitt, 1963), has more recently modified his view to accommodate an ubiquitous virus, such as EB virus associated with an insect-transmitted cofactor required for the manifestation of a malignant potential, such as chronic holoendemic malaria (Burkitt, 1969). Conceivably, malaria might act by providing additional stimulus for lymphoid proliferation or as an immunosuppressive influence permitting a self-limiting disease to turn into a malignant tumor (O'Connor, 1970). At the moment, there is no factual basis for distinguishing between these alternatives. The prospective study recently initiated in the West Nile district of Uganda (Geser and de Thé 1972) may provide more definite epidemiological answers for the involvement of EB virus in BL.

Before leaving the subject of EB virus and BL, it may be appropriate to comment on the remarkable immunological behavior of the tumor *in vivo*. It is quite clear that the tumor is relatively highly antigenic in the human patient (Klein, 1971a). This is manifested in the documented occurrence of spontaneous regressions (Burkitt and Kyalwazi, 1967) and the substantial proportion (15–30%) of long-time survivors after chemotherapy, some of them perhaps permanently cured (Burkitt, 1967; Clifford *et al.*, 1967; Ngu, 1967). The different EB virus-associated antibodies relate to the course of the disease in individual patients in different ways. Antibodies to early antigens (G. Henle, *et al.*, 1971a,b) and possibly to soluble, immunoprecipitating antigens as well (G. Klein *et al.*, 1969a, 1970) are more frequently present and have a higher titer in tumor-bearing patients than in regressors. In remission patients, the risk of recurrence is higher in anti-EA antibody-positive than in antibody-negative patients (G. Henle *et al.*, 1971a,b).

In approximately 80% of 124, seropositive BL patients, anti-EA titers were usually lower but sometimes equal to the anti-VCA titers (although never higher) (G. Henle *et al.*, 1971a). Among African control children of comparable age and sex, anti-EA antibody titers were rarely found, and, if detected, the titers did not exceed 1:20, as a rule, even in donors with high anti-VCA titers. In a retrospective study of the relationships between anti-EA titers and the clinical course of the BL patients, it was found (G. Henle *et al.*, 1971a) that patients admitted with a negative anti-EA titer had a better chance of survival than patients admitted with high anti-EA titers, unless they were in a very advanced stage of the disease at the time of admission. The mortality within 1 year of patients with high anti-EA titers was nearly twice that of patients admitted without anti-EA antibody titers. The majority of dying patients had high anti-EA titers, whereas more than half of the long-time survivors (at least 2 years) had no or only low levels of anti-EA antibody, in spite of often, very high anti-VCA titers. In the survivors that had residual high anti-EA titers, tumor recurrences were substantially more frequent (60%) that among comparable survivors with no or low levels of anti-EA antibody (18%). Antibodies against the R component of the EA complex were considerably more frequent in anti-EA-positive BL patients than in IM or NPC cases (where antibodies against the D component were more common) (G. Henle *et al.* 1971b).

Epstein-Barr virus-associated CF antibodies were also studied in relation to the course of the BL disease. Sohier and de Thé (1972) found that CF antibodies, tested against antigen prepared from an EB virus producer cell line, were at a relatively low level in the sera of BL patients after tumor regression and during the remission period, but rose to a high level in patients with advancing or progressive tumors. They suggested that this situation may be similar to acute viral infection, where CF antibodies disappeared rapidly when the infection was controlled. There is a curious discordance between this report and a recent study of Vonka *et al.* (1972). These authors tested the sera of IM patients and normal controls of corresponding age groups for anti-VCA antibodies, assessed by the Henle IF test, and for CF antibodies against a soluble (S) antigen extracted from a "nonproducer" line, NC37. Sera of all IM patients taken during the acute stage of the disease or up to 9 years thereafter contained anti-VCA antibody, whereas the sera taken during the acute stage of the disease were virtually free of complement-fixing anti-S antibody. However, after the seventh month following IM, the majority of the patients developed anti-S antibody. The authors concluded that anti-S antibody appears much later in the course of EB virus infection than the VCA antibody. The majority of the VCA-positive normal subjects who had no history of IM had S antibody as well. Since Sohier and de Thé used an EB virus producer cell line to prepare their antigen, whereas Vonka *et al.* used a nonproducer line, the question arises whether they may have measured responses to different antigens. Since producer lines have a substantial proportion of EA-positive cells, detected by immunofluorescence (the WIL line used by Sohier and de Thé is a particularly good example of this) while the nonproducer lines have no EA antigen, it is conceivable that the antibody measured by Sohier and de Thé (but not by Vonka *et al.*) was related to EA. This is suggested by the parallel between the findings by Sohier and de Thé and those obtained by Henle *et al.*, concerning the relationship between anti-EA antibody and tumor load of BL patients (G. Henle *et al.*, 1971a). This interest of the system described by Vonka *et al.* lies in the fact that the antibody titers against the S antigen extracted from the nonproducer line were maintained for many years after the disease. In this respect, there is at least a superficial similarity between anti-S, anti-MA (*vide infra*), and anti-VCA antibodies since they all tend to remain high for long periods after tumor regression in BL patients (Gunvén *et al.*, 1970) and in post-IM cases or healthy anti-VCA positive persons (G. Klein *et al.*, 1968a; Hewetson *et al.*, 1972a). The persistently high anti-MA and anti-S titers may be indicative of antigens present in latent, nonproducer cells, presumably restricted in their proliferative capacity by the immune response, or, alternatively, may reflect the periodic activator of virus production that may occur in analogy with other perpesvirus infections.

Membrane-reactive (anti-MA) antibodies also show disease-related changes in BL, although they are of a different nature. In BL patients with recurring tumors, which continue to grow in spite of chemotherapy, membrane-reactive antibody levels that may decrease at or around the time of recurrence can rise again (G. Klein *et al.*, 1969a). Subsequently, the lymphoma cells become coated with IgG, as a rule if the tumor persists. It is conceivable that such cells represent immunoresistant variants (Fenyö *et al.*, 1968). This is supported, indirectly at least, by the history of two patients whose tumors recurred after several years of total regression and contained a high frequency of near-tetraploid cells (Clifford *et al.*, 1968). This is in contrast to a large number of BL tumor biopsies examined, with a shorter clinical history, which were all in the near-diploid range. Tetraploid cells can frequently outgrow host responses that efficiently reject diploid cells of the same lineage (Hauschka *et al.*, 1956).

The immunoglobulin coat acquired by tumors that persist in spite of therapy contains antibodies directed against cell surface antigens. Eluted IgG shows anti-MA specificity: it can block the direct radioactive-labeled MA reaction (Hewetson *et al.*, 1972a) and has EB virus neutralizing activity as well (G. Klein, unpublished results). It may represent the equivalent of enhancing of blocking antibody in Hellström's sense (Hellström and Hellström, 1969) and is not necessarily an alternative to the possibility that membrane-reactive antibodies may have a growth inhibitory action, but is rather another facet of the same complex picture. An antibody that is cytotoxic for or inhibits the growth of immunosensitive cells may enhance the growth of immunoresistant cells, i.e., protect them against the cell-mediated immune response. In addition, different antibodies no doubt differ; some can be cytotoxic and others enhancing toward the same target cell. In the course of chemotherapy that falls short of a total tumor kill, and the subsequent regrowth of the residual tumor with more antigen release and antibody binding, the immunosensitivity of the tumor cell population and the killing versus enhancing power of the antibody population may obviously change in a complex way.

In addition to the changes in the membrane-reactive antibody levels brought about by the tumor itself (due to absorption, antigen release, effect of tumor growth on the immune response, etc.), the antibody titer may change for other, tumor-unrelated reasons, and this may, in turn, influence tumor growth. This possibility has been brought into focus by the history of a BL patient (G. Klein *et al.*, 1969a) who was in total tumor regression for a period of 4½ years and subsequently developed widespread abdominal metastases. Her membrane-reactive antibody level fell abruptly, more than 6 months prior to recurrence, at a time when there was no reason to suspect presence of any metastases. When the abdominal tumor recurrence became obvious 6 months later, the membrane-reactive antibody level was still low, and the tumor cells were not yet coated with IgG. In the course of the subsequent 2 months, the serum antibody level increased again and the lymphoma cells became IgG-coated. The antibodies against EA were at a moderately high level while the tumor was in regression, but increased to a very high level after the recurrence. At the same time, immunoprecipitating antibodies appeared, reacting against the soluble antigen described by Old *et al.* (1968).

This sequence of events does not lend much support to the possibility that the fall of the membrane-reactive antibody level 6 months prior to recurrence was merely due to absorption by a cryptic tumor. In that case, a period of slow tumor growth would have occurred during the subsequent 6 months period, and the secondary increase in antibody level, as well as the immunoglobulin coating of the lymphoma cells should have taken place in the interim, appearing already at the time of clinical recurrence. Indirect as this reasoning is, it serves to raise the question of whether a fall in membrane-reactive antibody levels may be the cause and not merely the consequence of tumor recurrence in facilitating the outgrowth of "dormant" neoplastic cells.

The analysis of the MA-reactive antibody patterns of other BL patients, presently in progress (Gunvén *et al.*, 1973) is in line with this picture, indicating that longtime survivors have a consistently maintained and often relatively high level of antibody, whereas cases of tumor recurrence often show a fall of antibody titer prior to the reappearance of clinically diagnosed tumor.

V. Relationship between EB Virus and Other Lymphoproliferative Diseases

On the whole, the serological association between EB virus and lymphoproliferative diseases other than Burkitt's lymphoma is unimpressive (G. Henle *et al.*, 1969; de Schryver *et al.*, 1972; Gahrton *et al.*, 1971) but there are certain exceptions (Johansson *et al.*, 1970, 1971; Levine *et al.*, 1971; Hirshaut *et al.*, 1970; Wahren *et al.*, 1971; Evans *et al.*, 1971). Hodgkin's disease is a particularly intriguing case in point (Johansson *et al.*, 1970; Levine *et al.*, 1971). The lymphocyte rich, relatively benign form shows no regular elevation of anti-EB virus antibody, compared to controls. The lymphocyte-depleted or sarcomatous form that has a different age distribution and takes a highly malignant course is, on the other hand, associated with high anti-VCA and anti-MA titers. A simple passenger hypothesis would have predicted the opposite, i.e., a parellel between anti-EB virus antibody titers and lymphocytic infiltration. Moreover, epidemiological data have been interpreted to indicate that Hodgkin's disease may have a multiple etiology (MacMahon, 1966). One cannot dismiss the possibility that EB virus, or some of its subtypes, is involved in one form of Hogkin's disease. It is equally possible, however, that the high antibody titers associated with the lymphocyte-depleted form are merely a consequence of the disease. Specifically, it has been suggested (W. Henle, personal communication) that the impairment of cell-mediated immunity, particularly pronounced in the lymphocyte-depleted form, may promote the proliferation of EB virus-carrying lymphoid clones, with a subsequent increase of antigen load and humoral antibody formation. In view of the neoplastic potential of EB virus-carrying lymphoblastoid cell lines, demonstrated by their ability to grow into frank lymphomas upon heterotransplantation to immunosuppressed animals (Southam *et al.*, 1969; Adams *et al.*, 1967, 1970; Levine, *et al.*, 1969), it may be questioned whether the postulated mechanism would be capable of leading to an appropriately limited lymphoid proliferation. A study of anti-EB virus antibody titers in immunosuppressed patients, e.g., kidney transplant recipients, would be of interest in this connection.

A study of chronic lymphatic leukemia (CLL) and lymphocytic lymphoma (LL) (Johansson *et al.*, 1971) has shown a certain elevation of anti-VCA and anti-MA titers. In CLL, 40% of the patients has relatively high serological reactivities, although the mean anti-VCA and anti-MA titers did not differ significantly from the control group. There was no significant rise of anti-EA reactivity, as a rule (Henle, 1971). The LL sera showed significantly higher reactivities than the controls. This was particularly pronounced in patients with poorly differentiated tumors.

In sarcoidosis, the evidence is conflicting. Some authors reported a significant increase of anti-EB virus antibody titers (Hirshaut *et al.*, 1970). Others found some patients with elevated titers, but no regular increase in titers (Wahren *et al.*, 1971). Still others failed to find any significant change (Gergely, 1973). Some elevation has also been noted in systemic lupus erythematosus (Evans *et al.*, 1971). All these increases fall far below what has been observed for Burkitt's lymphoma, and their significance, if any, remains to be established.

VI. Relationship between EB Virus and Nasopharyngeal Carcinoma

The serological relationship between nasopharyngeal carcinoma (NPC) and EB virus was first demonstrated by Old *et al.* (1966) using immunodiffusion tests with soluble extracts of EB virus producing cell lines. A strong association was also found using immunofluorescence tests with VCA (W. Henle *et al.*, 1970a) and MA-type antigens (de Schryver *et al.*, 1969). Histologically confirmed NPC's were as regularly associated with high antibody titers as BL, irrespective of geographic origin. In a large group of 235 African and Chinese NPC patients, 84% had high anti-EB virus antibody titers (≧ 1:160), with a geometric mean titer of 1:348 (W. Henle *et al.*, 1970a). Patients with carcinomas arising in head and neck areas other than the nasopharynx exceeded the 1:160 titer level in only 13% of the cases, and their geometric titer was 1:36, nearly a tenfold difference. Similar differences were reported in relation to anti-MA antibodies (de Schryver *et al.*, 1969, 1972) and precipitating antibodies (Oettgen *et al.*, 1967). As in BL, some NPC patients did not have antibodies against EA, but 75% were anti-EA positive, often with very high titers (G. Henle, 1971). Unlike BL, however, and similar to IM, the anti-EA antibodies were most frequently of the anti-D type (G. Henle *et al.*, 1971b).

It seems particularly significant that carcinomas localized to the hypopharynx or the oropharynx, and malignant tumors other than NPC that were localized to the nasopharynx, were not associated with high anti-EB virus antibody titers (de Schryver *et al.*, 1969).

There was a certain relationship between anti-VCA and anti-EA titers in NPC and the stage of the disease (G. Henle, 1971). Antibody levels were lowest in stage I and increased gradually as the disease progressed to stage V. This apparent relationship to the tumor burden, particularly when considered together with the pronounced lymphoid infiltration of the carcinoma tissue, suggests that EB virus may be a mere passenger in NPC. It is noteworthy, on the other hand, that the same high EB virus-associated antibody titers were found in NPC patients of Chinese, African, American, Swedish, and French origin. This consistency is particularly significant in view of the fact that NPC represents a clear pathological entity and is not readily confused with other conditions. Furthermore, EB virus DNA could be regularly demonstrated in NPC biopsies (zur Hausen *et al.*, 1970; Nonoyama *et al.*, 1973). Also, local irradiation of NPC has led to a temporary rise of anti-EB virus antibody titers, as in BL, and in contrast to other irradiated tumors of EB virus-seropositive patients (Einhorn, 1972; Einhorn *et al.*, 1972). While this evidence indicates an unusually firm association between the tumor tissue and EB virus in NPC, it is not known whether the virus is associated with the lymphoid or the epidermal cells.

At this time, the possibility that EB virus may play a more important role in the pathogenesis of NPC than a harmless passenger cannot be dismissed entirely. To maintain the passenger hypothesis, it is necessary to postulate that EB virus grows preferentially in the kind of lymphoid cell that is present in NPC, but not in the various "control tumors." This is possible, but there is no evidence for or against it.

For a comprehensive discussion of the various hypotheses related to the etiology of NPC the reader is referred to a recent review by de Thé (1972).

VII. Cell-Mediated Immunity

The study of cell-mediated immunity in EB virus-associated conditions and/or against EB virus-carrying target cells is in an early stage of its development, but it is already clear that important findings can be expected.

Delayed hypersensitivity reactions have been found in BL patients exposed to autologous tumor cell extracts (Fass *et al.*, 1970a,b), but it is not known whether these reactions are directed against EB virus-induced antigens or not.

Interesting findings have been made recently on established lymphoblastoid cell lines in mixed leukocyte culture (MLC)-type experiments (Hewetson *et al.*, 1972b; Golub *et al.*, 1972a,b; Junge *et al.*, 1971; Steel and Hardy, 1970; Han *et al.*, 1970; Flier *et al.*, 1970). All lines tested exerted a remarkably powerful stimulating effect on the DNA synthesis of allogeneic and, more surprisingly, autologous lymphocytes, after their own DNA synthesis had been inhibited by mitomycin C or X-irradiation. Since all lymphoblastoid cell lines tested were found to carry the EB viral genome, as already discussed, it cannot be decided whether the autologous reaction is directed against EB virus-determined antigens. Blocking experiments with suitable batteries of EB virus antibody-positive and -negative sera have not yet been reported. It is at least conceivable that the reaction reflects the role of cell-mediated immunity in checking the proliferation of EB virus-transformed lymphoid cell clones *in vivo*. It may be relevant to recall, in this context, that BL is a uniclonal disease (Fialkow *et al.*, 1970). If EB virus is involved in etiology of BL, this would mean that the disease arises by the occasional escape of an EB virus-transformed clone from the normal surveillance mechanism. Surveillance may fail for a number of reasons, including immunosuppression alone or combined with overwhelming lymphoproliferative stimuli. Chronically immunosuppressed patients, e.g., kidney graft recipients, are known to develop an unexpectedly high number of tumors, predominantly lymphomas and reticulum cell sarcomas (reviewed by Penn, 1970). It would be important to investigate the possible role of EB virus-transformed clones in the origin of these diseases.

VIII. Discussion

Perhaps the most unique feature of EB virus is its extreme host specificity. In spite of extensive attempts of many laboratories to force the species or the tissue barrier, the host cell range is still restricted to the human lymphoid cell, and, possibly, some primate lymphoid cells as well. Human cells of nonlymphoid origin are resistant to EB virus infection and do not carry detectable viral genome, as a rule. Of course, it cannot be excluded that an unknown reservoir of EB virus exists in some human tissue that perpetuates the production of infectious virus, in analogy with the role of the feather follicle in Marek's disease (Calnek *et al.*, 1970). Alternatively, it is conceivable that the viral genome is restricted to lymphoid cells. This would be an essentially nonpermissive interaction, with occasional production of viral antigens in a small minority of the cells, sometimes proceeding to the formation of viral particles, as in the established cell lines *in vitro*. Considering these alternatives, it must be remembered that EB virus is a remarkably successful, horizontally transmitted virus. Its mode of transmission is largely unknown, although the evidence that IM is transmitted by what Evans and Niederman (1972) termed as "cellular kissing" is quite convincing. In that situation, transmission of the viral genome may occur between cells, without the actual production of viral particles, perhaps in analogy with the passage of EB virus from X-irradiated, virus-carrying cell lines to normal peripheral lymphocytes (Henle *et al.*, 1967). Transmission of the HVS (Herpesvirus saimiri) genome after the transplantation of HVS-induced, nonproducer lymphoma cells to susceptible recipients is another case in point (see Chapter 18). It is questionable, however, whether this type of intercellular transmission could account for the relatively more frequent, early EB virus infections that are particularly prevalent in low socioeconomic groups and are not linked to the clinical entity known as IM.

The maintenance of fairly constant anti-VCA titers in EB virus-infected individuals through many years and the frequent isolation of permanent EB virus-carrying lymphoblastoid lines from their blood, suggests that EB virus, like other herpesviruses, can remain latent in infected organisms through very long periods of time. Occasional activation and virus release could account for the persistently positive antibody titers.

Antibodies directed against the early antigen (EA) behave in a different way. In IM, they decline and, as a rule, disappear after the acute infection and are only exceptionally found in normal, EB virus-positive individuals. They persist, however, in tumor-bearing patients with EB virus-associated neoplastic diseases, particularly BL and NPC. In long-term survivors anti-EA antibodies tend to disappear; their persistence after chemotherapeutically induced regression of BL is correlated with a relatively high risk of recurrence.

Curiously enough, a different type of anti-EA (anti-R) antibody tends to be associated with most cases of BL than with IM and NPC, where it is predominantly anti-D (G. Henle *et al.*, 1971b). This suggests some difference in the virus–cell–host interaction but its significance is obscure.

The relatively consistent relationship between positive anti-EA titers and continuing proliferation of EB virus-carrying lymphoid clones may be viewed in relation to the finding on *in vitro* systems (Gergely *et al.*, 1971c) that a large number of EA-positive cells die before they have entered the late viral cycle. Such cells may release EA, whereas others that proceed to the late, VCA productive, stage may consume much of the EA and not release it in quantity and/or the form required to induce antibody formation. Conceivably, an excess of EA-positive, VCA-negative cells that die may be characteristic for the pathological lymphoproliferation expressed in IM and the EB virus-associated neoplastic diseases. It is possible that the EB virus-harboring cells of the normal organism are different and perhaps more permissive.

In spite of the ubiquitousness of EB virus, and in contrast to the equally, if not more ubiquitous C-type viruses, there is no evidence of vertical transmission. Several tissue culturists, who were regularly able to establish permanent lymphoblastoid lines from the peripheral blood or the lymph nodes of EB virus-infected individuals, were uniformly unsuccessful in their attempts to establish lines from uninfected fetal or neonatal lymphoid tissue. However, addition of EB virus or filtrates from EB virus-carrying lines has led to the prompt conversion of fetal lymphoid cells into lines. This appears to refute the possibility of vertical transmission. The same conclusion can be drawn from the characteristic age-incidence distribution of the antibody titers. Initial postnatal fall in antibody titers can be related to the disappearance of passively transmitted maternal antibody. The rise in titer beginning in infancy and the subsequent characteristic patterns, related to age and socioeconomic group, are best explained by horizontal transmission. It may be added that there is strong evidence against the vertical transmission of some other herpesviruses as well, including the oncogenic MDHV (Purchase, 1972).

The experiments on fetal cells have also shown that EB virus can convert lymphoid cells with a limited life span into potentially "immortal" cell lines. This is independently supported by the finding that all established lymphoblastoid cell lines thus far tested contained the EB viral genome, as judged by nucleic acid hybridization, and one or several types of EB virus-associated antigens, with soluble CF antigen as the minimum common denominator. No evidence was obtained for the presence of the EB viral genome or EB virus antigen in human cell lines of nonlymphoblastoid origin.

Lymphoid cells are very heterogeneous with regard to structure, and function, and the number of distinguishable subpopulations is increasing continuously as methods become more discriminating. The EB virus-susceptible subclass or subclasses have not yet been defined; not even the major subdivision between the T and B cell kingdoms has been made. Many (although not all) EB virus-carrying lines secrete small amounts of immunoglobulin. Furthermore, a substantial number of EB virus-carrying BL-derived lines have remarkably large amounts of surface-associated IgM (E. Klein *et al.*, 1968, 1972; Eskeland and Klein, 1971). This is suggestive of a B-cell involvement. Recent findings indicate, however, that T cells may have membrane-associated immunoglobulin receptors as well, in particular IgM, although they are less well exposed on the outer cell surface than the corresponding B-cell receptors (Marchalonis *et al.*, 1972). It is hard to exclude the possibility that an EB virus-induced transformation of T cells might change the distribution or the surface exposure of IgM sites.

Among the EB virus-associated *in vivo* conditions, IM is perhaps most closely analogous to the EB virus-induced transformation of lymphoid cells *in vitro*. This is also the disease where the etiological role of EB virus can be regarded to be established conclusively. Peripheral lymphoid cells of IM patients turn readily into established lines *in vitro* (Diehl *et al.*, 1968; Junge *et al.*, 1971) and can often be cloned directly, without preadaptation to tissue culture, in soft plasma clot substrates (J. Hewetson, personal communication). A recent, unique autopsy material of acute IM patients who died for unrelated reasons showed extensive lymphoid infiltration of most major parenchymatous organs (Carter, 1972). This raises the question of how the EB virus-induced lymphoproliferation is abruptly stopped in IM, rather than progressing into a malignant disease.

Peripheral lymphocytes of EB virus-positive recipients undergo lymphoblast transformation and DNA synthesis when exposed to autologous lymphoblastoid lines (Hewetson *et al.*, 1972b; Golub *et al.*, 1972a,b; Junge *et al.*, 1971; Steel and Hardy, 1970; Han *et al.*, 1970; Flier *et al.*, 1970). It is possible that this response is the expression of a relatively powerful cell-mediated immunity against EB virus-carrying cells. Together with the membrane-reactive antibodies that appear during IM (G. Klein *et al.*, 1968a), this provides a potential mechanism that may turn IM into a self-limiting disease. One test of this hypothesis would be to show that the lymphocytes of EB virus-negative donors are not as readily stimulated by autologous, *in vitro* EB virus-converted lymphoblastoid cells as the lymphocytes of EB virus-positive donors.

The relationship between EB virus and BL raises many fascinating problems. One conspicuous difference between IM and BL lies in the fact that IM represents, in all probability, a polyclonal proliferation of lymphoid cells (Glade and Chessin, 1968), whereas Burkitt's lymphoma is a uniclonal disease *in vivo*, and its cells give rise to corresponding uniclonal lines *in vitro* (Fialkow *et al.*, 1970; Fialkow, 1972). The polyclonal nature of IM is in line with expectations, provided that virally induced conversion of resting lymphocytes into clones with a high proliferative capacity and their outgrowth into relatively large populations are highly probable events. It is interesting to recall in this connection that the uniformly lethal lymphoreticular neoplasia induced by herpesvirus saimiri in the marmoset is also a polyclonal disease (Chu and Rabson, 1972).

Although these findings show that polyclonal transformation can be induced by an oncogenic herpesvirus in monkeys and by EB virus in man, the uniclonality of BL does not exclude viral etiology or the involvement of EB virus. It may be recalled, in this connection, that virally induced neoplastic transformation is by no means synonymous with the outgrowth of transformed cells into a frank tumor *in vivo*. Polyomavirus transforms appropriate target cells *in vitro* with a high efficiency, for instance, and there is evidence of many incipient neoplastic foci in neonatally inoculated animals, but only one or a few manage eventually to grow into a tumor. Concomitant immunity (demonstrable as the resistance of animals with progressively growing antigenic tumors against the new implantation of small tumor inocula with the same antigenicity) provides an efficient mechanism that can explain how the successful emergence of one virally transformed, antigenic clone may lead to the suppression of all others induced by the same virus (for review, see Klein, 1969). The peculiar distribution of BL, with well-localized solid tumors and the lack of lymph node involvement, would also be in line with this view. In fact, the only conceivable reason why a lymphoma would remain restricted to solid lumps, in spite of the demonstrated ability of its cells to spread freely throughout the body, lies in the restricting influence of a host response.

If immune mechanisms can restrict the growth of all but one virally transformed clone in the tumor patient, it is reasonable to postulate that, in many similarly infected individuals, they will restrict neoplastic growth altogether, or make it self-limiting, as in IM. The spontaneous regressions described (Burkitt and Kyalwazi, 1967) are the rare, visible manifestations of what must happen at the microscopic level with a much higher frequency. It becomes very important to understand the difference, in terms of immune mechanisms and/or cellular susceptibility to them, between the self-limiting and the malignant disease.

In Marek's disease, self-limiting and malignant forms are known to occur, and their relative proportions are influenced by genetic factors, age, sex, previous virus exposure, social stress, etc. In genetically resistant strains, thymectomy increases the incidence of the malignant form, indicating that resistance is determined by thymus-dependent, presumably cell-mediated immunity (Payne, 1972). In genetically susceptible strains with a high incidence, thymectomy has no effect.

Thus far, in this discussion, it has been assumed that EB virus converts normal lymphocytes into potentially neoplastic cells, and only host forces prevent them from growing into frank tumors. This assumption is included in what I previously referred to as the *cofactor hypothesis* (Klein, 1971a; 1972). In the broader sense, this hypothesis implies that the realization of the neoplastic potential depends on genetic and/or environmental factors. Burkitt (1969) has recently formulated this in more explicit terms. After analyzing the geographical distribution of BL, he specified chronic holoendemic malaria as the cofactor that would convert a benign viral infection into a malignant disease (see also O'Connor, 1970). Heavy malarial infections have strong immunosuppressive and lymphoproliferative components, and this may play an important role. One may also consider other vector-transmitted cofactors, however, and variations in the genetic susceptibility of the host provides further alternatives within the cofactor hypothesis.

A somewhat different kind of explanation is provided by the *multiple virus hypothesis*. Biologically different virus subtypes are postulated, with wide variations in their oncogenic potential. In the EB virus system, discriminative studies to identify different viral subtypes are yet to be performed. In Marek's disease, biological variation in viral pathogenicity is a well-established fact (Nazerian, 1972). The most dramatic demonstration is the recent, successful isolation of an MDHV-related, apathogenic herpesvirus from turkeys (HVT) (Kawamura *et al.*, 1969; Witter *et al.*, 1970) that can protect chicks from the oncogenic effect of MD herpesvirus (Okafaki *et al.*, 1970) without reducing viral maturation of infectivity.

Differences in viral pathogenicity must always be viewed in relation to host susceptibility. The existence of MD-susceptible and MD-resistant chicken strains is a case in point. This is even more clearly illustrated by the herpesvirus saimiri system (Chapter 18). Depending on the species, the virus can cause a 100% lethal lymphoproliferative malignancy or no disease at all.

The third main alternative that must be considered in relation to the role of EB virus in BL is the *passenger hypothesis*. It implies that the virus is a relatively innocuous inhabitant of lymphoid tissues, even though it may cause IM under certain conditions. Lymphoma develops because of other, unrelated causes, but the virus is carried along by the neoplastic cells, with a corresponding increase in viral nucleic acid, antigens, and antibodies. This possibility cannot be critically excluded on the basis of any existing evidence, but it appears less likely than a few years age. This is due to (a) the regular association of high anti-EB virus antibody titers with BL; (b) the lack of a similarly consistent association with most other lymphoproliferative diseases; (c) the association of viral nucleic acid with BL (and NPC) but not with other malignancies in EB virus-seropositive individuals; (d) the fact that EB virus can convert lymphocytes with a limited life span into proliferating clones with an unlimited growth potential; (e) the fact that it can cause a violent lymphoproliferative disease *in vivo* in the form of IM; and (f) the increasing knowledge on the involvement of herpesviruses in the causation of animal lymphomas.

References

Adams, A., Lindahl, T., and Klein, G. (1973) *Proc. Nat. Acad. Sci. U.S.*, in press.
Adams, R. A., Foley, G. E., Uzman, B. G., Farber, S., Lazarus, H., and Kleinma, L. (1967). *Cancer Res.* **27**, 772.
Adams, R. A., Foley, G. E., Farber, S., Flowers, A., Lazarus, H., and Hellerstein, E. (1970). *Cancer Res.* **30**, 338.
Ahlström, C. G., Andersson, T., Klein, G., and Åkerman, M. (1967). *Int. J. Cancer* **2**, 583.
Armstrong, D., Henle, G., and Henle, W. (1966). *J. Bacteriol.* **91**, 1257.
Banatvala, J. E., Path, M. C., and Grylls, S. G. (1969). *Brit. Med. J.* **3**, 444.
Blacklow, N. R., and Kapikian, A. Z. (1970). *Lancet* **1**, 647.
Blacklow, N. R., Watson, B. K., Miller, G., and Jacobson, B. M. (1971). *Amer. J. Med.* **51**, 549.
Burkitt, D. (1962). *Nature* (*London*) **194**, 232.
Burkitt, D. (1963). *Int. Rev. Exp. Pathol.* **2**, 67.
Burkitt, D. (1967). *In* "Treatment of Burkitt's Tumours" (J. H. Burchenal and D. P. Burkitt, eds.), UICC Monogr., pp. 94–101. Springer-Verlag, Berlin and New York.
Burkitt, D. (1969). *J. Nat. Cancer Inst.* **42**, 19.
Burkitt, D. and Kyalwazi, S. K. (1967). *Brit. J. Cancer* **21**, 14.
Burkitt, D., and O'Connor, G. T. (1961). *Cancer* **14**, 258.
Burkitt, D. P., and Wright, D. H., eds. (1970). "Burkitt's Lymphoma." Livingstone, Edinburgh.
Calnek, B. W., Adlinger, H. K., and Kahn, D. E. (1970). *Avian Dis.* **14**, 219.
Carter, R. L. (1972). *In* "Oncogenesis and Herpesviruses" (R. M. Biggs, G. de Thé, and L. N. Payne, eds.), pp. 230–238 Int. Agency Res. Cancer, Lyon.
Chang, R. S. (1971). *Nature* (*London*) *New Biol.* **233**, 124.
Chang, R. S., Hsieh, M. W., and Blankenship, W. (1971). *J. Nat. Cancer Inst.* **47**, 479.

Chen, J. H., and Purchase, H. G. (1970). *Virology* **40**, 410.
Chu, E. W., and Rabson, A. S. (1972). *J. Nat. Cancer Inst.* **48**, 271.
Clifford, P. (1970). *Int. J. Cancer* **5**, 185.
Clifford, P., Singh, S., Stjernswärd, J., and Klein, G. (1967). *Cancer Res.* **27**, 2578.
Clifford, P., Gripenberg, N., Klein, E., Fenyö, E. M., and Manolov, G. (1968). *Lancet* **2**, 517.
de Schryver, A., Friberg, S., Jr., Klein, G., Henle, W., Henle, G., de Thé, G., Clifford, P., and Ho, H. C. (1969). *Clin. Exp. Immunol.* **5**, 443.
de Schryver, A., Klein, G., Henle, G., Henle, W., Cameron, H. M., Santesson, L., and Clifford, P. (1972). *Int. J. Cancer* **9**, 353.
de Thé, G. (1972). *In* "Pathobiology Annual," New York (in press).
Diehl, V., Henle, G., Henle, W., Kohn, G. (1968). *J. Virol.* **2**, 663.
Diehl, V., Henle, G., Henle, W., and Kohn, G. (1969). *In Vitro* **4**, 92.
Duff, R., and Rapp, P. (1971). *Nature (London) New Biol.* **233**, 48.
Durr, F. E., Monroe, J. H., Schmitter, R., Traul, K. A., and Hirschaut, Y. (1970). *Int. J. Cancer* **6**, 436.
Einhorn, N. (1972). *Cancer* **29**, 714.
Einhorn, N., Henle, G., Henle, W., Klein, G., and Clifford, P. (1972). *Int. J. Cancer* **9**, 182.
Epstein, M. A., and Barr, Y. M. (1964). *Lancet* **1**, 252.
Epstein, M. A., Achong, B. G., and Barr, Y. M. (1964a). *Lancet* **1**, 702.
Epstein, M. A., Barr, Y. M., and Achong, B. G. (1964b). *Nat. Cancer Inst., Monogr.* **17**, 637.
Epstein, M. A., Henle, G., Achong, B. G., and Barr, Y. M. (1965). *J. Exp. Med.* **121**, 761.
Ernberg, I., and Klein, G. (1973). To be published.
Eskeland, T., and Klein, E. (1971). *J. Immunol.* **107**, 1368.
Evans, A. S. (1960). *Amer. J. Hyg.* **71**, 342.
Evans, A. S. (1971). *J. Infec. Dis.* **124**, 330.
Evans, A. S. and Niederman, J. C. (1972). *In* "Oncogenesis and Herpesviruses" (P. M. Biggs, G. de Thé, and L. N. Payne, eds.), pp. 351–356. Int. Agency Res. Cancer, Lyon.
Evans, A. S., Niederman, J. C., and McCollum, R. W. (1968). *N. Engl. J. Med.* **279**, 1121.
Evans, A. S., Rothfield, N. F., and Niederman, J. C. (1971). *Lancet* **1**, 167.
Fass, L., Herberman, R. B., and Ziegler, J. (1970a). *N. Engl. J. Med.* **282**, 776.
Fass, L., Herberman, R. B., Ziegler, J., and Morrow, R. H. (1970b). *J. Nat. Cancer Inst.* **44**, 145.
Fenyö, E. M., Klein, E., Klein, G., and Swiech, K. (1968). *J. Nat. Cancer Inst.* **40**, 69.
Fialkow, P. J. (1972). *Advan. Cancer Res.* **15**, 191.
Fialkow, P. J., Klein, G., Gartler, S. M., and Clifford, P. (1970). *Lancet* **1**, 384.
Flier, J. S., Glade, P. R., Broder, S. W., and Hirschhorn, K. (1970). *Cell. Immunol.* **1**, 596.
Gahrton, G., Wahren, B., Killander, D., and Foley, G. E. (1971). *Int. J. Cancer* **8**, 242.
Gerber, P. (1972). *Proc. Nat. Acad. Sci. U.S.* **69**, 83.
Gerber, P., and Birch, S. M. (1967). *Proc. Nat. Acad. Sci. U.S.* **58**, 478.
Gerber, P., and Deal, D. R. (1970). *Proc. Soc. Exp. Biol. Med.* **134**, 748.
Gerber, P., and Rosenblum, B. N. (1968). *Proc. Soc. Exp. Biol. Med.* **128**, 541.
Gerber, P., Hamre, D., Moy, R. A., and Rosenblum, B. N. (1968). *Science* **161**, 173.
Gerber, P., Walsh, G. H., Rosenblum, B. N., and Purell, R. H. (1969a). *Lancet* **1**, 593.
Gerber, P., Whang-Peng, J., and Monroe, J. H. (1969b). *Proc. Nat. Acad. Sci. U.S.* **63**, 740.
Gergely, L. (1973). *Klin. Wochenschr.* (in press).
Gergely, L., Klein, G., and Ernberg, I. (1971a). *Virology* **45**, 10.
Gergely, L., Klein, G., and Ernberg, I. (1971b). *Virology* **45**, 22.
Gergely, L., Klein, G., and Ernberg, I. (1971c). *Int. J. Cancer* **7**, 293.
Geser, R., and de Thé, G. (1972). *In* "Oncogenesis and Herpesviruses" (P. M. Biggs, G. de Thé, and L. N. Payne, eds.), pp. 372–375. Int. Agency Res. Cancer, Lyon.
Glade, P. R., and Chessin, L. N. (1968). *J. Clin. Invest.* **47**, 2391.

Glade, P. R., and Hirschhorn, K. (1970). *Cell. Immunol.* **1**, 359.
Glade, P. R., Kasel, J. A., Moses, H. L., Whang-Peng, J., Hoffman, P. F., Hammermeyer, J. K., and Chessin, L. N. (1968). *Nature (London)* **217**, 564.
Golden, H. O., Chang, R. S., Lou, J. J., and Cooper, T. Y. (1971). *J. Infec. Dis.* **124**, 422.
Golub, S. H., Hewetson, J. S., Svedmyr, E. A. J., and Singh, S. (1972a). *Int. J. Cancer* **10**, 150.
Golub, S. H., Svedmyr, E. A. J., Hewetson, J. S., Klein, G., and Singh, S. (1972b). *Int. J. Cancer* **10**, 157.
Gunvén, P., Klein, G., Henle, G., Henle, W., and Clifford, P. (1970). *Nature (London)* **228**, 1053.
Gunvén, P., Klein, G., Henle, W., and Henle, G. (1973). To be published.
Hampar, B., Hsu, K. C., Martos, L. M., and Walker, J. L. (1971). *Proc. Nat. Acad. Sci. U.S.* **68**, 1407.
Hampar, B., Derge, J., Martos, L. M., and Walker, J. L. (1972a) *Proc. Nat. Acad. Sci. U.S.* **69**, 78.
Hampar, B., Derge, J. G., Martos, L. M., Tagamets, M. A., and Burroughs, M. A. (1972b). *Proc. Nat. Acad. Sci. U.S.* **69**, 2589.
Han, T., Moore, G. E., and Sokal, J. E. (1970). *Proc. Soc. Exp. Biol. Med.* **136**, 976.
Hauschka, T. S., Kvedar, B. J., Grinnel, S. T., and Amos, D. B. (1956). *Ann. N.Y. Acad. Sci.* **63**, 683.
Hellström, K. E., and Hellström, I. (1969). *Advan. Cancer Res.* **12**, 167.
Henle, G. (1971). *In* "Princess Takamatsu Cancer Research Fund" (W. Nakahara *et al.*, eds.), pp. 343–349. Tokyo Press, Tokyo.
Henle, G., and Henle, W. (1966a). *J. Bacteriol.* **91**, 1248.
Henle, G., and Henle, W. (1966b). *Trans. N.Y. Acad. Sci.* [2] **29**, 71.
Henle, G., and Henle, W. (1970). *J. Infec. Dis.* **121**, 303.
Henle, G., Henle, W., and Diehl, V. (1968). *Proc. Nat. Acad. Sci. U.S.* **59**, 94.
Henle, G., Henle, W., Clifford, P., Diehl, V., Kafuko, G. W., Kirya, B. B., Klein, G., Morrow, R. H., Munube, G. M. R., Pite, P., Tukei, P. M., and Ziegler, J. L. (1969). *J. Nat. Cancer Inst.* **43**, 1147.
Henle, G., Henle, W., Klein, G., Gunvén, P., Clifford, P., Morrow, R. H., and Ziegler, J. L. (1971a). *J. Nat. Cancer Inst.* **46**, 861.
Henle, G., Henle, W., and Klein, G. (1971b). *Int. J. Cancer* **8**, 272.
Henle, W., and Henle, G. (1968). *J. Virol.* **2**, 182.
Henle, W., and Henle, G. (1970). *In* "Comparative Leukemia Research 1969" (R. M. Dutcher, ed.), pp. 706–713. Karger, Basel.
Henle, W., and Henle, G. (1972). *In* "Oncogenesis and Herpesviruses" (P. M. Biggs, G. de Thé, and L. N. Payne, eds.), pp. 269–274. Int. Agency Res. Cancer, Lyon.
Henle, W., Hummeler, K., and Henle, G. (1966). *J. Bacteriol.* **92**, 269.
Henle, W., Diehl, V., Kohn, G., zur Hausen, H., and Henle, G. (1967). *Science* **157**, 1064.
Henle, W., Henle, G., Burtin, P., Cachin, Y., Clifford, P., de Schryver, A., de Thé, G., Diehl, V., Ho, H. C., and Klein, G. (1970a). *J. Nat. Cancer Inst.* **44**, 225.
Henle, W., Henle, G., Zajac, B., Pearson, G., Waubke, R., and Scriba, M. (1970b). *Science* **169**, 188.
Henle, W., Henle, G., Scriba, M., Joyner, G. R., Harrison, F. S., von Essen, R., Paloheimo, J., and Klemola, E. (1970c). *N. Engl. J. Med.* **282**, 1068.
Henle, W., Henle, G., Niederman, J. C., Klemola, E., and Healti, K. (1971). *J. Infec. Dis.* **124**, 58.
Hewetson, J., Gothoskar, B., and Klein, G. (1972a). *J. Nat. Cancer Inst.* **48**, 87.
Hewetson, J., Golub, S. H., Klein, G., and Singh, S. (1972b). *Int. J. Cancer* **10**, 142.
Hinuma, Y., and Grace, J. (1967). *Proc. Soc. Exp. Biol. Med.* **124**, 107.
Hinuma, Y., Konn, M., Yamaguchi, J., Wudarski, D. J., Blakeslee, J. R., Jr., and Grace, J. T., Jr. (1967). *J. Virol.* **1**, 1045.

Hirshaut, Y., Glade, P., Moses, H., Manaker, R., and Chessin, L. (1969). *Amer. J. Med.* **47**, 520.

Hirshaut, Y., Glade, P., Otavo, L., Vier, B. D., Ainbender, E., Dvorak, B., and Siltzbach, L. E. (1970). *N. Engl. J. Med.* **283**, 502.

Hoagland, R. J. (1955). *Amer. J. Med. Sci.* **229**, 262.

Horosziewicz, J. S., Dunkel, V. C., Avila, L., and Grace, J. T. (1970). *In* "Comparative Leukemia Research 1969" (R. M. Dutcher, ed.), pp. 722–738, Karger, Basel.

Johansson, B., Klein, G., Henle, W., and Henle, G. (1970). *Int. J. Cancer* **6**, 450.

Johansson, B., Klein, G., Henle, W., and Henle, G. (1971). *Int. J. Cancer* **8**, 475.

Junge, U., Hoekstra, J., and Deinhardt, S. (1971). *J. Immunol.* **106**, 1306.

Kawamura, M., King, D. J., and Anderson, D. P. (1969). *Avian Dis.* **13**, 853.

Klein, E., Clifford, P., Klein, G., and Hamberger, C. A. (1967). *Int. J. Cancer* **2**, 27.

Klein, E., Klein, G., Nadkarni, J. S., Nadkarni, J. J., Wigzell, H., and Clifford, P. (1968). *Cancer Res.* **28**, 1300.

Klein, E., van Furth, R., Johansson, B., Ernberg, I., and Clifford, T. (1972). *In* "Oncogenesis and Herpesviruses" (P. M. Biggs, G. de Thé, and L. N. Payne, eds.), pp. 253–257. Int. Agency Res. Cancer, Lyon.

Klein, G. (1966). *Annu. Rev. Microbiol.* **20**, 223.

Klein, G. (1969). *Fed. Proc., Fed. Amer. Soc. Exp. Biol.* **28**, 1739.

Klein, G. (1971a). *Advan. Immunol.* **14**, 187.

Klein, G. (1971b). *Strategy Viral Genome, Ciba Found. Symp.* pp. 295–315.

Klein, G. (1972). *Proc. Nat. Acad. Sci. U.S.* **69**, 1056.

Klein, G., and Dombos, L. (1973). *Int. J. Cancer* **11**, 327.

Klein, G., Clifford, P., Klein, E., and Stjernswärd, J. (1966). *Proc. Nat. Acad. Sci. U.S.* **55**, 1628.

Klein, G., Klein, E., and Clifford, P. (1967a). *Cancer Res.* **27**, 2510.

Klein, G., Clifford, P., Klein, E., Smith, R. T., Minowada, J., Kourilsky, F. M., and Burchenal, J. H. (1967b). *J Nat. Cancer Inst.* **39**, 1027.

Klein, G., Pearson, G., Henle, G., Henle, W., Diehl, V., and Niederman, J. C. (1968a). *J. Exp. Med.* **128**, 1021.

Klein, G., Pearson, G., Nadkarni, J. S., Nadkarni, J. J., Klein, E., Henle, G., Henle, W., and Clifford, P. J. (1968b). *J. Exp. Med.* **128**, 1011.

Klein, G., Clifford, P., Henle, G., Henle, W., Old, L. J., and Geering, G. (1969a). *Int. J. Cancer* **4**, 416.

Klein, G., Pearson, G., Henle, G., Henle, W., Goldstein, G., and Clifford, P. J. (1969b). *J. Exp. Med.* **129**, 697.

Klein, G., Geering, G., Old, J. J., Henle, G., Henle, W., and Clifford, P. (1970). *Int. J. Cancer* **5**, 185.

Klein, G., Gergely, L., and Goldstein, G. (1971). *Clin. Exp. Immunol.* **8**, 593.

Klein, G., Dombos, L., and Gothoskar, B. (1972). *Int. J. Cancer* **10**, 44.

Klemola, E., and Kaariainen, L. (1965). *Brit. Med. J.* **2**, 1099.

Klemola, E., von Essen, R., Henle, G., and Henle, W. (1970). *J. Infec. Dis.* **121**, 608.

Landon, J. C., Ellis, L. B., Zeve, V. H., and David, P. A. (1968). *J. Nat. Cancer Inst.* **40**, 181.

Levin, A., Friberg, S., and Klein, E. (1969). *Nature (London)* **222**, 997.

Levine, P. H., Ablashi, D. V., Berard, C. W., Carbone, P. P., Waggoner, D. E., and Malan, L. (1971). *Cancer* **27**, 416.

Luria, S. E., and Darnell, J. E. (1968). "General Virology." 2nd ed. Wiley, New York.

MacMahon, B. (1966). *Cancer Res.* **26**, 1189.

Marchalonis, J. J., Cone, R. E., Atwell, J. L., and Rolley, R. T. (1972). *In* "The Biochemistry of Gene Expression in Higher Organisms" (J. W. Lee and J. K. Pollak, eds.). Australia and New Zealand Book Co., Sydney (in press).

Maurer, B. A., and Wilberg, S. M. (1970). *Bacteriol. Proc.* p. 195.

Maurer, B. A., Glick, J. L., and Minowada, J. (1970). *Proc. Soc. Exp. Biol. Med.* **133**, 1026.
Mayyasi, S. A., Schidlovsky, G., Bulfone, L. M., and Buscheck, F. T. (1967). *Cancer Res.* **27**, 2020.
Miller, G. (1971). *Yale J. Biol. Med.* **43**, 358.
Miller, G., Lisco, H., Kohn, H. L., and Stitt, D. (1971). *Proc. Soc. Exp. Biol. Med.* **137**, 1459.
Miller, G., Niederman, J. C., and Stitt, D. A. (1972a). *J. Infec. Dis.* **125**, 403.
Miller, G., Shope, T., Lisco, H., Stitt, D., and Lipman, M. (1972b). *Proc. Nat. Acad. Sci. U.S.* **69**, 383.
Miller, K., Endes, J. F., Lisco, H., and Kohn, H. L. (1969). *Proc. Soc. Exp. Biol Med.* **132**, 247.
Miller, M. H., Stitt, D., and Miller, G. (1970). *J. Virol.* **6**, 699.
Moss, D. J., and Pope, J. H. (1972). *J. Gen. Virol.* **17**, 233.
Munyon, W., Kvasielburd, E., Davis, D., and Manu, J. (1971). *J. Virol* **7**, 813.
Nadkarni, J. S., Nadkarni, J. J., Klein, G., Henle, W., Henle, G., and Clifford, P. (1970). *Int. J. Cancer* **6**, 10.
Nazerian, K. (1972). *Advan. Cancer Res.* **17**.
Ngu, V. A. (1967). *In* "Treatment of Burkitt's Tumours" (J. H. Burchenal and D. P. Burkitt, eds.), UICC Monogr., pp. 71–76. Springer-Verlag, Berlin and New York.
Niederman, J. C., McCollum, R. W., Henle, G., and Henle, W. (1968). *J. Amer. Med. Ass.* **203**, 205.
Niederman, J. C., Evans, A. C., Subrahmanyan, L., and McCollum, R. W. (1970). *N. Engl. J. Med.* **282**, 361.
Nilsson, K. (1971). *Int. J. Cancer* **8**, 432.
Nilsson, K., Klein, G., Henle, W., and Henle, G. (1971). *Int. J. Cancer* **8**, 443.
Nonoyama, M., and Pagano, J. (1971). *Nature (London), New Biol.* **233**, 103.
Nonoyama, M., and Pagano, J. (1972). *Nature (London), New Biol.* **238**, 169.
Nonoyama, M., Pagano, J., Klein, G., and Singh, S. (1973). *Proc. Nat. Acad. Sci. U.S.* (in press).
O'Connor, G. T. (1970). *Amer. J. Med.* **48**, 279.
O'Connor, G. T., and Davies, J. N. P. (1960). *J. Pediat.* **56**, 526.
Oettgen, H. F., Aoki, T., Geering, G., Boyse, E. A., and Old, L. J. (1967). *Cancer Res.* **27**, 2532.
Okafaki, W., Purchase, H. G., and Burmester, B. R. (1970). *Avian Dis* **14**, 413
Old, L. J., and Boyse, E. A. (1964). *Annu. Rev. Med.* **15**, 167.
Old, L. J., Boyse, E. A., Oettgen, H. F., de Harven, E., Geering, G., Williamson, B., and Clifford, P. (1966). *Proc. Nat. Acad. Sci. U.S.* **56**, 1699.
Old, J. J., Boyse, E. A., Geering, G., and Oettgen, H. F. (1968). *Cancer Res.* **28**, 1288.
Pasternak, G. J. (1969). *Advan. Cancer Res.* **12**, 1.
Payne, L. N. (1972). *In* "Oncogenesis and Herpes-type Viruses," pp. 21–37 Cambridge Univ. Press, London and New York.
Pearson, G., Dewey, S., Klein, G., Henle, G., and Henle, W. (1970). *J. Nat. Cancer Inst.* **45**, 989.
Penn, J. (1970). *Recent Results Cancer Res.* **35**, 1–51.
Pereira, M. S., Blake, J. M., and Macrae, A. D. (1969). *Brit. Med. J.* **4**, 526.
Pereira, M. S., Field, A. M., Blake, J. M., Rodgers, F. G., Bailey, L. A., and Davies, J. R. (1972). *Lancet* **1**, 710.
Pike, M. C., Williams, E. H., and Wright, B. (1967). *Brit. Med. J.* **2**, 396.
Pope, J. H. (1967). *Nature (London)* **216**, 810.
Pope, J. H., Achong, B. G., and Epstein, M. A. (1968a). *Int. J. Cancer* **3**, 171.
Pope, J. H., Horne, M. K., and Scott, W. (1968b). *Int. J. Cancer* **3**, 857.
Pope, J. H., Horne, M. K., and Scott, W. (1969a). *Int. J. Cancer* **4**, 255.
Pope, J. H., Horne, M. K., and Wetters, E. J. (1969b). *Nature (London)* **222**, 186.
Pope, J. H., Scott, W., Reedman, B. M., and Walters, M. K. (1971). *In* "Princess Takamatsu Cancer Research Fund" (W. Nakahara *et al.*, eds.), pp. 177–188. Tokyo Press, Tokyo.

Porter, D. D., Wimberly, I., and Benyesh-Melnick, M. (1969). *J. Amer. Med. Ass.* **208**, 1675.
Pulvertaft, R. J. V. (1964). *Lancet* **1**, 238.
Purchase, G. (1972). *In* "Oncogenesis and Herpesviruses" (P. M. Biggs, G. de Thé, and L. N. Payne, eds.), pp. 95–98. Int. Agency Res. Cancer, Lyon.
Rabson, A. S., O'Connor, G. T., Baron, S., Whang, J. J., and Legallais, F. Y. (1966). *Int. J. Cancer* **1**, 89.
Rapp, F., and Duff, R. (1972). *In* "Oncogenesis and Herpesviruses" (P. M. Biggs, G. de. Thé and L. N. Payne, eds.), pp. 447–450. Int. Agency Res. Cancer, Lyon.
Reedman, B., and Klein, G. (1973). *Int. J. Cancer* **11**, 499.
Roizman, B. (1972). *In* "Oncogenesis and Herpesviruses" (P. M. Biggs, G. de Thé, and L. N. Payne, eds.), pp. 1–20. Int. Agency. Res. Cancer, Lyon.
Roizman, B., and Spring, S. B. (1967). *In* "Proceedings of the Conference on Cross Reacting Antigens and Neo-Antigens" (J. J. Trentin, ed.), pp. 85–97. Williams & Wilkins, Baltimore, Maryland.
Sawyer, R. N., Evans, A. S., Niederman, J. C., and McCollum, R. W. (1971). *J. Infec. Dis.* **123**, 263.
Schulte-Holthausen, H., and zur Hausen, H. (1970). *Virology* **40**, 776.
Silvestre, D., Kourilsky, F. M., Klein, G., Yata, J., Neuport-Sautes, C., and Levy, J. P. (1971). *Int. J. Cancer* **8**, 222.
Sjögren, H. O. (1965). *Progr. Exp. Tumor Res.* **6**, 289.
Sohier, R., and de Thé G. (1972). *Int. J. Cancer* 9, 524.
Southam, C. M., Burchenal, J. H., Clarkson, B., Tanzi, A., Mackey, R., and McComb, V. (1969). *Cancer* **23**, 281.
Steel, C. M., and Hardy, D. A. (1970). *Lancet* **1**, 1322.
Stevens, D. A., Pry, T. W., and Blackham, E. A. (1970). *Blood* **35**, 263.
Stewart, S. E. (1969). *Advan. Virus Res.* **15**, 291.
Svedmyr, A., Demissie, A., Klein, G., and Clifford, P. (1970). *J. Nat. Cancer Inst.* **44**, 595.
Ten-Seldam, R. E. J., Cooke, R., and Atkin, L. (1966). *Cancer* **19**, 437.
Vonka, V., Benyesh-Melnick, M., Lewis, R. T., and Wimberly, I. (1970). *Arch. Gesamte Virusforsch.* **31**, 113.
Vonka, V., Vlckova, I., Zavadova, H., Kouba, K., Lazovska, J., and Duber, J. (1972). *Int. J. Cancer* **9**, 529.
Wagner, E. K., Roizman, B., Savage, T. H., Mizell, M., Durr, F. E., and Sypowicz, D. (1970). *Virology* **42**, 251.
Wahren, B., Lantorp, K., Sterner, G., and Espmark, Å. (1970). *Proc. Soc. Exp. Biol. Med.* **133**, 934.
Wahren, B., Carlens, E., Espmark, Å., Lundbeck, H., Löfgren, S., Madar, E., Henle, G., and Henle, W. (1971). *J. Nat. Cancer Inst.* **47**, 347.
Weinberg, A., and Becker, Y. (1969). *Viorlogy* **39**, 712.
Werner, J., Pinto, C., Hult, R. E., Henle, G., and Henle, W . (1973). *Int. J. Cancer* (in press).
Witter, R. L., Nazerian, K., Purchase, H. G., and Burgoyne, H. G. (1970). *Amer. J. Vet. Res.* **31**, 525.
Yata, J., Klein, G., Hewetson, J., and Gergely, L. (1970). *Int. J. Cancer* **5**, 394.
Zajac, B. A., and Kohn, G. (1970). *J. Nat. Cancer Inst.* **45**, 399.
zur Hausen, H. (1972). *Progr. Exp. Tumor Res.* (in press).
zur Hausen, H., and Schulte-Holthausen, H. (1970). *Nature (London)* **227**, 245.
zur Hausen, H., Henle, W., Hummeler, K., Diehl, V., and Henle, G. (1967). *J. Virol.* **1**, 830.
zur Hausen, H., Schulte-Holthausen, H., Klein, G., Henle, W., Henle, G., Clifford, P., and Santesson, L. (1970). *Nature (London)* **228**, 1056.

Chapter 17
Marek's Disease

P. M. Biggs

I. Introduction

Marek's disease is a lymphoproliferative disease of the domestic chicken caused by a herpesvirus. Almost any organ or tissue can be involved, but the disease has an unusual predilection for nervous tissue. In its acute form the proliferation of lymphoid tissue is most apparent in visceral organs, whereas in the less acute disease, or classical form, the changes are most commonly associated with peripheral nerves. When the disease is chronic, inflammatory changes confined to the nervous system predominate.

Marek's disease was first described during the first decade of this century in Hungary (Marek, 1907) and has now been recognized throughout the world. The disease that was present in both Europe and the United States during the first two decades of the century was confined to the nervous system (Kaupp, 1921; van der Walle and Winkler-Junius, 1924). However, Pappenheimer *et al.* (1929) noted that about 10% of chickens with the disease had lymphoid tumors principally involving the ovary. In the late 1920's and throughout the 1930's Marek's disease became a serious cause of mortality in commercial poultry in the United States and in Europe. This increase in the incidence of the disease appeared to be associated with the increase in the intensive systems of farming poultry. The next landmark in the history of the disease was the appearance of a highly pathogenic form which was first recognized in the United States (Benton and Cover, 1957). This form was epizootic in nature and was soon seen in most, if not all, countries with intensively run poultry industries. This form is known as the acute form of the disease, and it has been responsible for serious economic loss to the poultry industries of many countries. It is still a serious cause of mortality in chickens in many countries, although in some it is now being controlled by vaccination.

In this chapter no attempt is made to review fully the literature on Marek's disease but rather to point out the salient features and facts known about the disease and its cause. For more detailed coverage of the literature the reader is referred to papers by Biggs (1967, 1968, 1971), Payne (1969), Calnek and Witter (1972), and Purchase (1972).

II. Clinical Disease

Clinically Marek's disease may be manifest by evidence of involvement of the nervous system. In these cases the most common symptom is a degree of paralysis varying from slight paresis to spastic or rarely flaccid paralysis of the legs and wings. Any of the peripheral nerves including autonomic nerves can be affected, resulting in other symptoms such as difficulty in breathing, torticollis, and paralysis of the tail and eyelids. In other cases nervous symptoms are not present, and chickens may die suddenly in good condition or sometimes with a wasting preceding death.

Marek's disease affects chickens from about 6 weeks of age, although it is most frequent between 12 and 24 weeks of age. Two forms have been described: the classical form which is characterized primarily by neural involvement, and the acute form by visceral lymphoid tumors as the prominent feature. In the classical form symptoms of paresis and paralysis are common. In this form there is usually a lower incidence of disease than in the acute form, and in individuals the disease takes a more chronic course. Mortality in the acute form is usually higher, and there may be no specific symptoms in birds dying early in an outbreak. Birds dying later often show symptoms of paresis and paralysis and on postmortem examination are seen to have enlarged nerves.

The incubation period in the natural disease is difficult to estimate because the time of infection is not usually known. However the limited number of investigations that have been undertaken would suggest that the incubation period is very variable even among a single group of chickens. It probably varies from as short a period as 3 or 4 weeks up to several months.

Mortality varies from a few to 70–80%. Usually the classical form affects a small percent of the flock (up to 10%) and the acute form between 20 and 30%. Sporadic cases may also be seen, particularly in flocks of adult chickens.

Chicks experimentally infected in the absence of maternally derived antibody may die within 10 to 17 days of infection after a period of depression and stunted growth (see Section III,B,1) (Calnek, 1972a).

III. Pathology

The pathology and pathogenesis of Marek's disease has recently been reviewed by Payne (1972).

A. *Morbid Anatomy*

1. Macroscopic Changes

Macroscopic changes that occur in Marek's disease are due to proliferative lymphoid lesions, inflammatory lesions in the peripheral nerves, and the presence of lymphomas in visceral organs and other tissues. Peripheral nerves may be enlarged up to several times their normal thickness. The enlargement may be nodular but is more usually diffuse (Fig. 1). All nerves

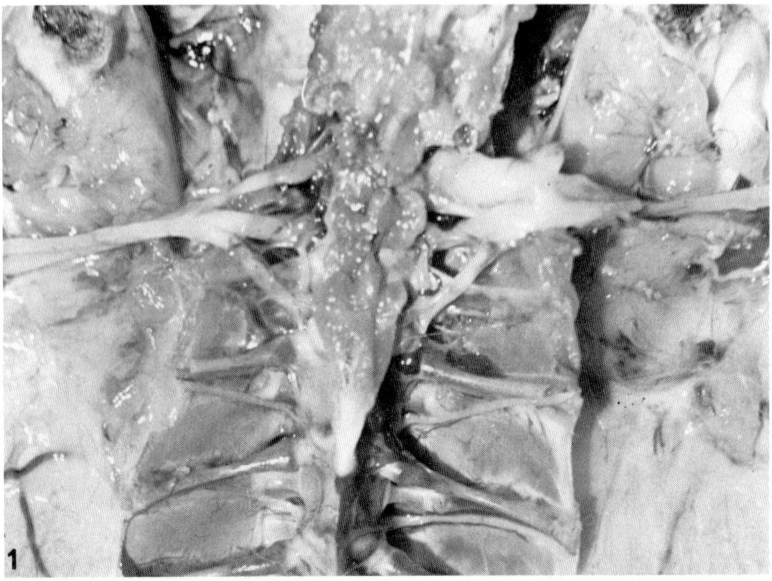

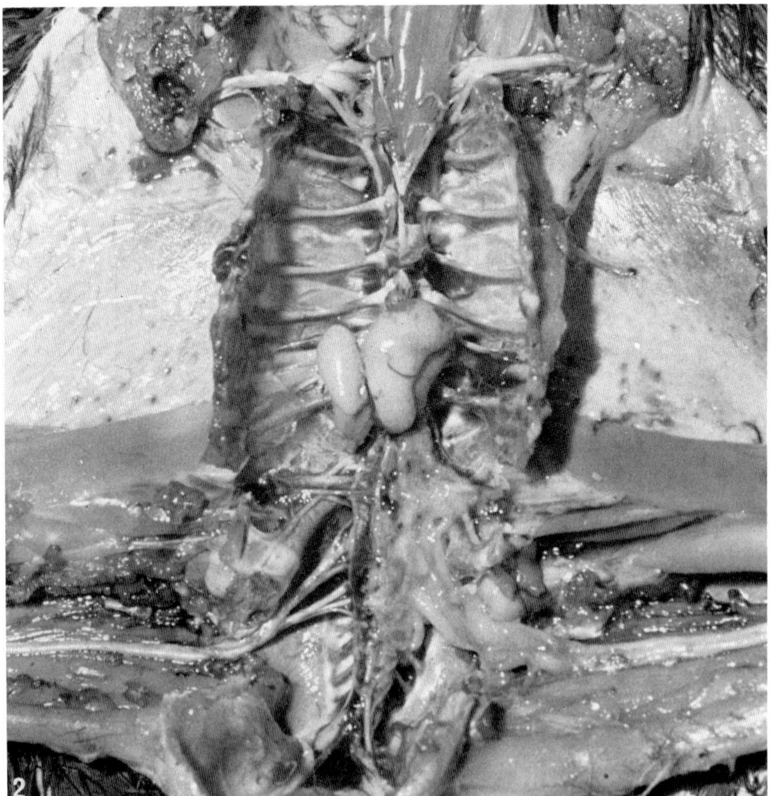

may be enlarged including those of the autonomic system. However those commonly affected and easily seen at autopsy are the brachial and sciatic plexuses, celiac plexus, and vagus and intercostal nerves (Gibbs, 1934; Goodchild, 1969). Dorsal route ganglia are also enlarged (Sevoian and Chamberlain, 1964). Nerve enlargement is more common in the classical form of the disease than in the acute form.

Lymphomas may be present in any organ or tissue. They are most common in the gonads (Figs. 2 and 3) and are frequently seen in the liver, spleen, kidneys, lungs, and heart. Lymphomas may also occur in muscle, in the proventriculus, and in the feather follicles. These sites are not as common as the first mentioned, but they are characteristic of Marek's disease. The lymphoid neoplasia usually involves the organ in a diffuse proliferative response, although in some cases discrete tumor nodules may be seen. The lymphoid response in the feather follicles forms small nodules which are only easily seen after the chicken has been plucked and dressed.

2. Microscopic Changes

a. Peripheral Nerves. The majority of chickens affected with Marek's disease have lesions in the peripheral nerves. They may be affected by proliferative, inflammatory, or chronic but minor lesions. These have been described by Biggs and Payne (1967) as type A, B, and C lesions, respectively. This terminology will be used; however, type A lesions correspond with lesions of types I and III of Wight (1962a), type T of Fujimoto *et al.* (1971), and type B with type II and type R of the same authors.

The type A lesion consists of proliferating lymphoid cells which include primitive and activated reticulum cells, lymphoblasts, and small and medium lymphocytes. Aberrant cells which have been called "Marek's disease cells" (Payne and Biggs, 1967) may be present in some type A lesions, particularly in the classical form of the disease. These cells appear to be degenerating blast cells. Type A proliferative lesions may vary in extent and degree of development. They may vary from small focal lesions to lesions which diffusely involve the whole nerve (Fig. 4). However, even in the latter case, extension through the perineurium of the nerve is rare. In the more rapidly developing lesions, the less mature lymphoid cells are more common than in lesions that proliferate more slowly. Where there is widespread and diffuse involvement of the nerve (Fig. 4), demyelination and some loss of axons is present (Wight, 1962a, 1964; Payne and Biggs, 1967; Ubertini and Calnek,

Figs. 1 and 2. Fig. 1, diffuse enlargement of the left brachial plexus in a chicken infected with the HPRS-16 strain of Marek's disease herpesvirus. Fig. 2, tumor of the left testis and enlargement with diffuse perineural involvement of the left sciatic plexus in a chicken infected with the HPRS-16 strain of Marek's disease herpesvirus.

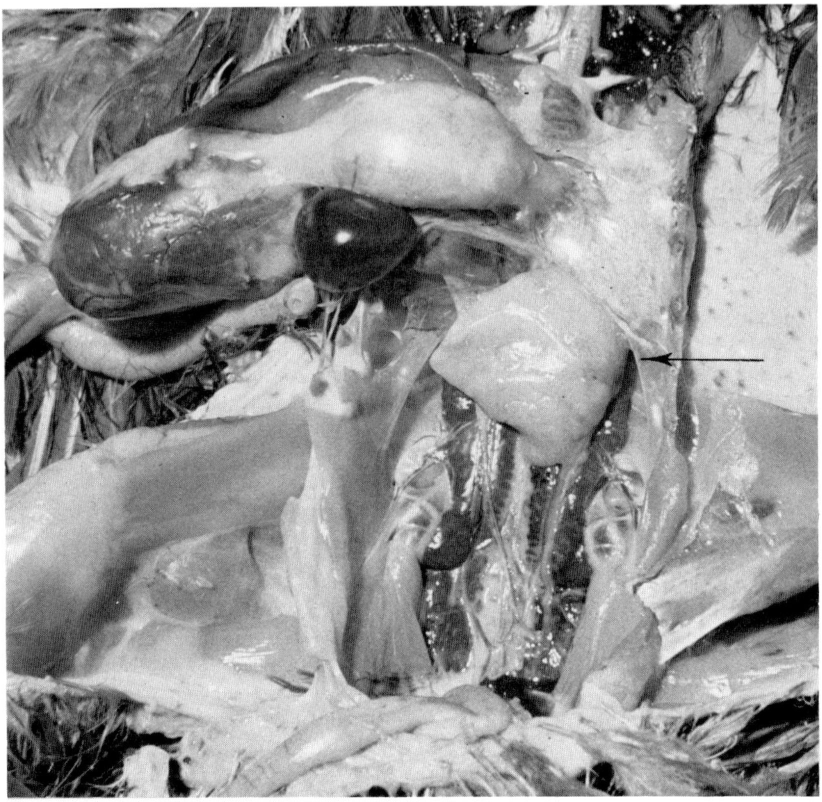

FIG. 3. Tumor of the ovary of a chicken infected with the HPRS-16 strain of Marek's disease herpesvirus.

1970). These changes have been confirmed by ultrastructural studies (Wight, 1969; Prineas and Wright, 1972) where in the severe form of the proliferative type A lesion, complete disintegration of many myelin sheaths together with extensive destruction of axons was noted. Hypertrophy of Schwann cells was also seen although it was more common in the inflammatory type B lesion. Another feature of type A lesions is the presence of nuclear "pockets" in the lymphoblasts (Wight, 1969; Okada, 1970).

The inflammatory type B lesion is characterized by interneuritic edema, Schwann cell proliferation, and hypertrophy with a light to moderate scattering of small lymphocytes and plasma cells (Fig. 5). Ultrastructural studies have confirmed that activation and hypertrophy of Schwann cells are a common feature. Macrophages are also present, and the interneuritic spaces contain thick arrays of collagen fibers (Wight, 1969; Ubertini and Calnek,

1970). Demyelination is characterized by a thinning rather than a complete destruction of the myelin sheath.

The type C lesion consists of small areas of lightly scattered lymphocytes and plasma cells.

According to Payne and Biggs (1967), the type A lesion is seen most commonly in chickens dying early in the disease process and is more frequently seen in association with lymphoid tumors than the type B lesion, which is more commonly present in chickens with disease of longer standing. The type C lesion is seen in infected birds which show no clinical symptoms.

b. CENTRAL NERVOUS SYSTEM. Lesions of the central nervous system may include proliferative lesions of the type A variety, but more commonly inflammatory lesions characteristic of a viral encephalomyelitis are present. The most prominent lesion, both in the brain and spinal cord, is perivascular infiltration with lymphoid cells, but endotheliosis and focal areas of gliosis may also be present (Wight, 1962b; Sevoian and Chamberlain, 1964; Purchase and Biggs, 1967; Fujimoto *et al.*, 1971).

c. LYMPHOMAS. The most common lesion in visceral organs and tissues, other than the nervous system, is a proliferative lymphoid lesion which can vary in size from a microscopic change to a gross tumor. The cellular composition is similar to the type A lesion of peripheral nerves (Fig. 6) and consists of primitive and activated reticulum cells, small and medium lymphocytes, and lymphoblasts. In the slower-growing tumors, the cells are more pleomorphic than in the faster-growing tumors in which blast cells predominate (Biggs and Payne, 1967; Purchase and Biggs, 1967; Fujimoto *et al.*, 1971). No chromosomal abnormalities characteristic of Marek's disease have been noted. A low incidence of tetraploid cells has been described by both Owen *et al.* (1966) and by Bloom (1970). The former also found a 6% incidence of chromatid and isochromatid breaks.

d. BLOOD. Changes in the number of blood cells are not consistently present or very great. However, quite frequently there is a moderate but temporary increase in polynuclear cells early in the disease which is followed by a degree of lymphocytosis. Some individuals have lymphocyte counts as high as 200×10^3 to $300 \times 10^3/mm^3$ or about 10 to 15 times normal (Johnson and Conner, 1933; Seagar, 1933; Furth, 1935; Sevoian and Chamberlain, 1964; Patterson *et al.*, 1969; Evans and Patterson, 1971). Most authors have remarked on the increase of lymphoblasts, and Cho *et al.* (1968) have described the rare presence of atypical lymphocytes which contain cytoplasmic globules. These cells become more frequent after leukocytes of Marek's disease virus-infected chickens have been cultured for 24 hours.

Changes in the serum proteins have been noted (Howard *et al.*, 1967;

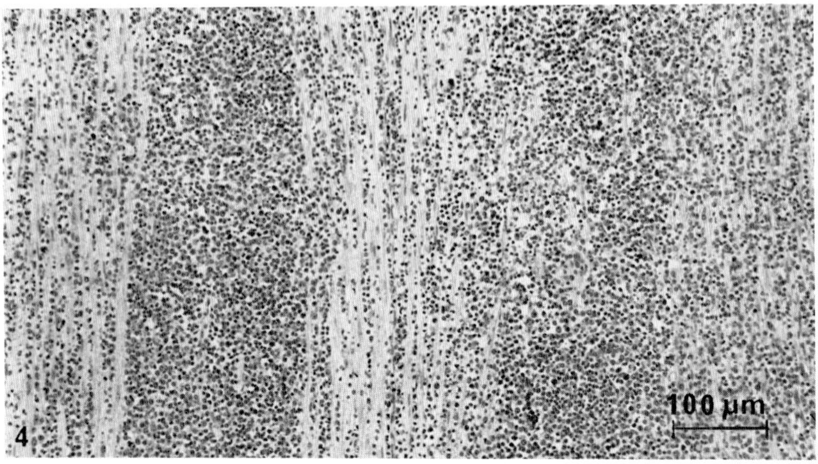

4

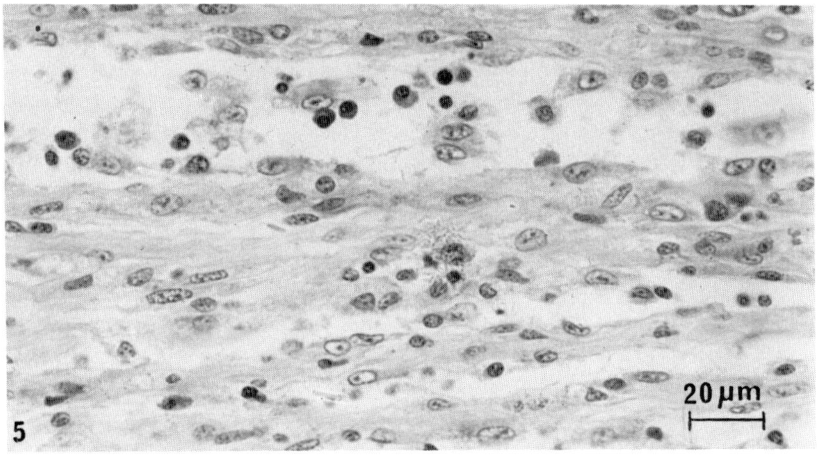

5

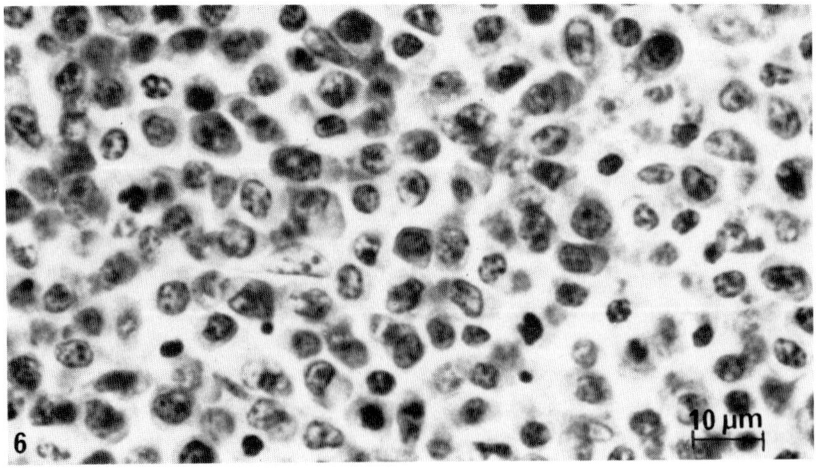

6

Ringen and Akhtar, 1968; Samadieh *et al.*, 1969; Washburn and Eidson, 1970). An increase in plasma proteins has been observed which included a decrease in albumin but an increase in globulins, probably mainly immunoglobulins. These changes occurred mainly during the period of greatest mortality in the chickens.

e. EYE. Blindness and changes in the iris and ciliary body have been associated particularly with the classical form of Marek's disease (see Biggs, 1968). The most common lesion is an infiltration of the iris and ciliary body with lymphocytes and plasma cells, and sometimes myeloid metaplasia may be present (Grundboeck, 1965, 1966; Simpson, 1969).

f. SKIN. Because of the importance of skin in respect to the production of infectious virus and the spread to other chickens, a description of the changes seen in this tissue is particularly relevant. Degenerative changes occur in the transitional, intermediate, and corneus layers of the stratum germinativum of the epithelium lining the feather follicles. In some of the cells of these layers, intranuclear and more rarely intracytoplasmic inclusions are present. These changes are associated with the replication of Marek's disease virus (Calnek and Hitchner, 1969; Nazerian and Witter, 1970; Purchase, 1970; Lapen *et al.*, 1970). The degenerative lesions may be present alone or in association with aggregates of lymphoid tissue in the dermis associated with the feather follicles, which in some cases develop into lymphomas (Helmboldt *et al.*, 1963; Payne and Biggs, 1967; Lapen *et al.*, 1970). A specific relationship between the presence of Marek's disease virus and associated antigens in the feather follicle epithelium and the appearance of lymphoid cells in the dermis and development to lymphomas has been shown by Lapen *et al.* (1971).

g. LYMPHOID ORGANS. Lymphomatous involvement of the spleen is common in the acute form of Marek's disease. Such involvement of the bursa of Fabricius may also occur and is interfollicular. Lymphomatous change occurs less commonly in the thymus.

Degenerative lesions may also be present in the bursa of Fabricius and the thymus together with, or independent of, proliferative lymphoid lesions. The organs in these cases are atrophied with loss of cells; variable degrees of cytolysis and areas of necrosis can also be present. In the bursa of

FIGS. 4–6. Fig. 4, well-developed type A lesion in the peripheral nerve of a chicken infected with the HPRS-B14 strain of Marek's disease herpesvirus. Hematoxylin and eosin, magnification × 120. (From Biggs *et al.*, 1968a.) Fig. 5, type B lesion in peripheral nerve of chicken infected with the HPRS-16 strain of Marek's disease herpesvirus. Hematoxylin and eosin, magnification ×480. (From Biggs *et al.*, 1968.) Fig. 6, ovarian lymphoid tumor from chicken infected with the HPRS-16 strain of Marek's disease herpesvirus. Hematoxylin and eosin, magnification × 940. (From Biggs *et al.*, 1968a.)

Fabricius, the necrosis results in the formation of cysts. Interfollicular proliferation of reticular cells may rarely be present in the bursa of Fabricius (Purchase and Biggs, 1967; Jakowski *et al.*, 1969, 1970; Purchase, 1970; Evans *et al.*, 1971a). In young chicks infected in the absence of maternally derived antibody to Marek's disease, these changes are much more severe, and intranuclear inclusions may be seen in the reticular cells (Jakowski *et al.*, 1969, 1970; Payne, 1972; L. N. Payne and M. Rennie, personal communication).

h. OTHER ORGANS. In young chickens infected in the absence of maternally derived antibodies to Marek's disease, an aplasia of the bone marrow with consequent anemia can be present, together with cytolytic changes resulting in generalized or focal necrosis in the kidneys and many other organs (Jakowski *et al.*, 1970; Fletcher *et al.*, 1971; Calnek, 1972a).

B. Pathogenesis

1. DEVELOPMENT AND REGRESSION OF LESIONS

The development of lesions of Marek's disease can be considered in three phases. In highly susceptible chickens, particularly when infected in the absence of maternally derived antibody soon after hatching, atrophic changes occur in the thymus, bursa of Fabricius, and bone marrow; degenerative changes and necrosis associated with intranuclear inclusions also occur in these and many other organs, including the kidneys, liver, pancreas, proventriculus, spleen, and heart. These changes occur early in the disease process and may result in death 10–17 days after infection (Calnek 1972a).

Accompanying this phase, and extending beyond it in time, is a proliferative, or second phase, which first involves areas of reticular and lymphoid cells. Later only areas of primarily lymphoid cells are involved (Biggs and Payne, 1967; Purchase and Biggs, 1967; Fletcher *et al.*, 1971; L. N. Payne and M. Rennie, personal communication). These early proliferative changes in lymphoid cells may progress to form lymphomas which result in death of the chicken at any time from about 21 days to several months after infection, or alternatively they may regress (Payne and Biggs, 1967; F. G. Aigster and S. C. Schmittle, personal communication). A nonpurulent encephalomyelitis may accompany these changes (Purchase and Biggs, 1967).

The third phase is a chronic inflammatory one and is seen principally in peripheral nerves as a type B lesion. There has been some disagreement over the sequence of changes in peripheral nerves. This has revolved around whether the inflammatory type B change precedes the proliferative type A change or *vice versa* (see Biggs, 1968; Payne, 1972). However, the only sequential studies that have been done have shown the proliferative type

A lesion to precede the inflammatory type B lesion in both classical and acute Marek's disease (Payne and Biggs, 1967; Purchase and Biggs, 1967). No change in the nerves preceding the proliferative A type lesion was noted by these authors who used light microscopy for their studies. However, this does not preclude a primary ultrastructural alteration in the nervous tissue. Wight (1969) and Prineas and Wright (1972) have described changes in Schwann cells and myelin that they have suggested are primary changes. Unfortunately, their studies were on birds showing clinical symptoms or recognizable lesions of Marek's disease. There is a need for an ultrastructural study of nerves prior to the appearance of lymphoid proliferative changes.

The development of pathological changes in the disease can be summarized as follows: In highly susceptible chickens, the initial changes may be cytolytic. This phase may progress or more commonly start with lesions characterized by a multifocal proliferation of lymphoid cells. In some chickens, this proliferative change develops to lymphoma formation in visceral organs, other tissues, and nerves, whereas in others the early proliferative lesions regress or, in nerves, are replaced by inflammatory type B lesions. Death may occur in any one of these three phases of the disease.

2. Distribution of Virus and Antigen

Virus infectivity is present in organs and tissues of the chicken in a cell-associated form, with the exception of the feather follicle epithelium. Cell-associated infectivity appears to be more readily identified in tissues of the chicken after infection than antigen detectable by immunofluorescence or by the agar gel precipitin test. Cell-associated infectivity is present in a number of organs soon after infection. Phillips and Biggs (1972) found that the lungs and/or lymphoid organs are first to show infectivity within 1 to 4 days of infection. They found that leukocytes only became infected subsequently. They suggested that the lungs and lymphoid tissues, particularly the spleen, are the primary sites of infection and that infection is disseminated by the blood leukocytes to many other organs and tissues a few days later. Cell-associated infectivity was detected in leukocytes, spleen, thymus, bursa of Fabricius, nerve plexuses, brain, liver, lungs, kidneys, gonads, skin, and feather follicle epithelium. In most tissues, cell-associated infectivity reached a peak titer within 2 weeks of infection, and in some cases a biphasic response was noted. Thereafter infectivity declined, but was still present at detectable levels in most organs 55 days after infection. Cell-associated infectivity in circulating leukocytes has been shown to persist throughout the commercial life of the chicken, about 75 weeks (Witter *et al.*, 1971; Biggs *et al.*, 1972a,b). The titer was highest in the lungs, spleen, and liver, but cell-associated infectivity is also at a high level in lymphomas (Biggs *et al.*, 1968a). The only site from which virus can be obtained in a cell-free infectious state is the feather follicle epithelium (Calnek *et al.*, 1970a).

Virus-associated antigens have been detected in many tissues by immunofluorescence and precipitation in agar gel (Calnek and Hitchner, 1969; Spencer and Calnek, 1970; Purchase, 1970; von Bülow and Payne, 1970; Calnek, 1972a; L. N. Payne and M. Rennie, personal communication). However, the greatest concentrations have been found in the feather follicle epithelium and medulla of the bursa of Fabricius. Viral-associated antigens are always found in the feather follicle epithelium but only rarely in lymphomas and nerves.

There is an increase in the quantity and distribution of antigen and infectivity, particularly in lymphoid organs, when chicks are infected in the absence of maternally derived antibodies (L. N. Payne and M. Rennie, personal communication; Calnek, 1972a).

In spite of rigorous searching, virus particles have only rarely been seen in tissues of infected chickens except in the feather follicle epithelium where the fully mature enveloped virus is present. Virus has occasionally been seen in gonad tumors, kidneys, bursa of Fabricius, and peripheral nerves (Nazerian and Burmester, 1968; Ahmed and Schidlovsky, 1968; Schidlovsky *et al.*, 1969; Wight, 1969; Nazerian and Witter, 1970; Calnek *et al.*, 1970b). However, in chickens infected in the absence of maternally derived antibodies, intranuclear and intracytoplasmic virions (the latter associated with inclusions similar to those seen in the feather follicle epithelium) are present in necrobiotic cells (Frazier and Biggs, 1972).

3. Nature of the Lymphoid Proliferation

a. Stimulus for Lymphoid Proliferation. There has been discussion on the nature of the lymphoproliferative lesions in Marek's disease for many years. In the past some have considered that the majority of proliferative lesions are essentially inflammatory and others that they are neoplastic. With the appearance of acute Marek's disease, there is now little doubt that the well-developed lymphoproliferative lesions are neoplastic because they fulfill many of the criteria of neoplasia, including progressive proliferation and tissue invasion, qualitative differences from and excessive increases over lymphoid hyperplasia produced by other infections of the domestic chicken, multifocal and diffuse origin, presence of abnormal cells, and deficiency in function of the immune system. The major question that arises, therfore, is not whether Marek's disease is a neoplastic disease, but what is the stimulus for the widespread proliferation of lymphoid tissue. This question has been discussed by Biggs (1968) and Payne (1972). The nature of the stimulus is unknown, but the possibilities can be considered to fall into two groups: (1) those in which the stimulus comes from within the cell, the intrinsic theory and (2) those in which the stimulus is outside the cell, the extrinsic theory. The first theory requires the change to a neoplastic lymphoid cell to be dependent on infection of the cell. This could occur as a direct or indirect result of infection. In the former case, virus infection would directly endow the cell with properties of neoplasia. In the latter case, neoplasia would result from an indirect process such as damage to the lymphocytes "self recognition" mechanism resulting in the production of "forbidden" clones (Burnet, 1969). The extrinsic theory requires that the lymphocytic proliferation is a response to some external stimulus which is most likely to be antigenic. The antigenic stimulus could be provided by the virus or virus-dependent antigens, virus antigen–antibody complexes, or autoantigens released from an immunologically priviledged site by the virus infection.

There is no conclusive proof for any of these possibilities, and for a detailed discussion the reader is referred to Payne (1972). The rarity of fluorescent antigen and virus particles in lymphomas and the low proportion of lymphoma cells which record as infectious units suggest that productive viral infection of lymphocytes does not or only rarely occurs. These observations are evidence against the intrinsic theory. However, lymphoid cells could well be nonproductively infected, a requirement for neoplastic transformation with herpesviruses because productive infections are cytolytic (Roizman, 1972; Biggs, 1972a). Support for a nonproductive infection in lymphocytes comes from the work of Campbell and Woode (1970) who induced productive infections in lymphocytes derived from Marek's disease virus-infected chickens after induction of blastoid transformation in culture by phytohemagglutinin.

At present, there is also little supportive evidence for the extrinsic theory. The greatest concentration of virus, and virus-associated antigens, has been found in the feather follicle epithelium and bursa of Fabricius, yet these are not common sites for lymphomas. The production of Marek's disease in agammaglobulinemic chickens (Payne and Rennie, 1970) is evidence against stimulation by antigen–antibody complexes. The similarity between the neural lesions of Marek's disease and experimental allergic encephalomyelitis and neuritis (Siller, 1960; Petek and Quaglio, 1967) has provided the best evidence for the extrinsic theory. The possibility of an autoimmune response to an antigen of nervous tissue made available to the immune system by the virus infection is suggested by their observations. A theory of this kind would also account for the unusual predilection which the proliferating lymphoid cells have for neural tissue in Marek's disease. However, the question of the stimulus for proliferation of lymphoid cells is far from resolved, and it should be remembered that the intrinsic and extrinsic theories are not mutually exclusive.

b. Composition of Lymphomas and Lymphoproliferative Lesions. Marek's disease affects the immune competence of both the bursa of Fabricius and the thymus-dependent immune systems (Purchase *et al.*, 1968; Payne and Rennie, 1970; Evans and Patterson, 1971).

However, there is no evidence suggesting that the lymphomatous transformation occurs primarily in either the bursa of Fabricius or thymus. These organs are relatively rarely involved in lymphomatous change compared with other organs, and lymphoma induction and other lesions of Marek's disease are not prevented by either bursectomy (Payne and Rennie, 1970; Fernando and Calnek, 1971) or thymectomy (L. N. Payne and M. Rennie, personal communication). The complexity of the lymphoma is evident in most cases from the pleomorphic nature of their cells and the finding that they are formed from both bursa of Fabricius and thymic-derived cells (Biggs, 1962; Payne and Roszkowski, 1972). Recently, Hudson and Payne (1973) have confirmed by an immunofluorescent technique that lymphomas are composed of both bursa- and thymic-derived cells and that the thymic-derived cells are in a majority of between 70 and 80%. The bursectomy studies suggest the bursa-derived cells do not form an essential part of the lymphomas. Recent thymectomy studies by Payne and Rennie (see Payne, 1972) confirm the essential part that the thymic-derived cells play in lymphoma formation. They found that in genetically susceptible chickens, thymectomy decreased the proportion of birds with gross lymphomas and lymphoproliferative lesions in the nerves, and in genetically resistant chickens, thymectomy increased the proportion with gross lymphomas. They have interpreted these findings as suggesting that the thymus-dependent lymphoid system has two roles in the pathogenesis of Marek's disease: (1) providing the target cells for neoplastic transformation and (2) as mediators of an immune response against the transformed cells. They suggest that in susceptible chickens the former property predominates and the latter property is more evident in genetically resistant chickens.

IV. Etiology

A. Experimental Transmission

Attempts to transmit Marek's disease with materials collected from clinically affected chickens have been made repeatedly from the early part of this century. However, unequivocal evidence for the transmissibility of this disease had to await the availability of genetically susceptible chickens and adequate isolation accommodation to keep control chickens free of the disease (Sevoian *et al.*, 1962; Biggs and Payne, 1963). Additional difficulties were associated with the now well-recognized, cell-associated state of the causative herpesvirus in all tissues except the feather follicle epithelium. It was not until spread of the disease to uninfected chickens in direct and indirect contact with infected chickens was conclusively demonstrated (Biggs and Payne, 1963, 1967; Sevoian *et al.*, 1963a) that the disease was unequivocally shown to be due to an infectious and contagious agent. Even the production of the disease by inoculation of materials collected from affected chickens provided difficulties of interpretation. For many years the only material found to be infectious consisted of suspensions of intact living cells which included lymphocytes or lymphoid tumor cells. The question of whether the experimentally produced disease was the result of a cell transplant or the transfer of an infectious agent was not resolved until it was shown, by chromosome labeling techniques, that cell transplants only rarely occurred (Owen *et al.*, 1966; Biggs *et al.*, 1968a). More recently, cell-free preparations of Marek's disease herpesvirus prepared from feather follicle epithelium have been shown to produce Marek's disease (Calnek *et al.*, 1970a; Nazerian and Witter, 1970).

1. Isolates

A large number of isolates of Marek's disease have been made, and many have been well characterized and are regularly used for experimental studies. The isolates most used are JM (Sevoian *et al.*, 1962), HPRS-16 (Biggs *et al.*, 1965; Purchase and Biggs, 1967), HPRS-B14 (Biggs and Payne, 1963, 1967), WSU-GF (Kenzy *et al.*, 1964), GA (Eidson and Schmittle, 1968), Conn A (Chomiak *et al.*, 1967), Cal-1 (Bankowski *et al.*, 1969), and HPRS-27 (Biggs and Milne, 1972; Phillips and Biggs, 1972). These isolates vary greatly in pathogenicity. The HPRS-27 isolate is apathogenic or very mildly pathogenic for the host chicken; HPRS-B14, WSU-GF, and Conn A produce mainly neural lesions characteristic of the classical disease, whereas the remainder are more pathogenic, producing a higher incidence of lymphomas and a disease characteristic of the acute form of Marek's disease. Serological differences between field isolates have not been noted using the indirect immunofluorescence and agar gel precipitin tests (Chubb and Churchill, 1968; Purchase, 1969; Biggs and Milne, 1972).

2. Host

Marek's disease is readily transmitted to the domestic chicken, as already discussed. Reports have been made of experimental transmission to turkeys

(Sevoian *et al.*, 1963b; Witter *et al.*, 1970a), pheasants (Harriss, 1939), and ducks (Baxendale, 1969). In ducks, no disease was produced, but Marek's disease virus could be reisolated and specific antibodies appeared in a few ducks. Attempts to infect hamsters (Churchill, 1968; Calnek and Witter, 1972) and primates have been unsuccessful (Sharma *et al.*, 1972).

B. A Herpesvirus as the Causative Agent of Marek's Disease

The cell-associated nature of the causative agent of Marek's disease was well established before isolation of a putative etiological agent for Marek's disease had been made (Biggs, 1966, 1968; Biggs and Payne, 1967; Biggs *et al.*, 1968a). This is a property commonly associated with the herpesvirus group. When an avidly cell-associated herpesvirus was isolated from cases of Marek's disease (Churchill and Biggs, 1967; Solomon *et al.*, 1968; Nazerian *et al.*, 1968), it was, therefore, an excellent candidate for the causative agent, although paradoxically its cell-associated nature precluded unequivocal proof that this was so. However, both qualitative and quantitative circumstantial evidence has strongly supported the theory that a herpesvirus infection is the cause of Marek's disease (Biggs *et al.*, 1968a; Witter *et al.*, 1969a). More recently, conclusive proof for the herpesvirus etiology of Marek's disease has been provided by the reproduction of the disease with cell-free, filtered preparations of the herpesvirus (Calnek *et al.*, 1970a; Nazerian and Witter, 1970) and from the protection provided by attenuated strains of the Marek's disease herpesvirus and a closely related herpesvirus of turkeys (Churchill *et al.*, 1969a; Okazaki *et al.*, 1970).

The etiology of Marek's disease in its broadest sense is made up of a number of factors. Apart from an infectious causative agent which is the prime requirement, there are factors associated with the host chicken and its environment that are also of importance. There are also factors of importance in relation to the causative virus, in particular the strain of virus and its pathogenicity and the dose at infection. These are discussed in Sections IV,A, and VI,D,1.

C. Host factors Associated with the Etiology of Marek's Disease

1. Genetic Constitution

The genetic constitution of the chicken has been known to influence the incidence of Marek's disease since the pioneering work of Hutt and Cole (1947). Many observations since that time, with a number of strains of Marek's disease herpesvirus, have shown that there are wide differences in genetically controlled susceptibility to the disease between experimental lines and between and within commercial lines of chicken (Biggs *et al.*, 1968b; Cole, 1968; Han *et al.*, 1969; Morris *et al.*, 1970; Hartmann and Sanz, 1971). The relative susceptibility of lines of chickens to different strains of Marek's disease virus appears to be the same (Biggs and Payne, 1963, 1967; Purchase and Biggs, 1967; Schmittle and Eidson, 1968; Crittenden *et al.*, 1972). All chickens, whether genetically susceptible to Marek's disease or not, can be infected, suggesting that resistance to the disease is not a resistance to infection but a resistance to the development of disease after infection. The fluorescent antibody studies of Calnek and Hitchner (1969) and the virus isolation studies of Spencer (1969) suggest that the genetic constitution of the chicken affects the rate of spread of the virus in the host chicken.

2. Age at Infection

An effect of age at infection on the incidence of Marek's disease has been noted by many authors and was first described as early as 1936 (see Biggs, 1968). However, in all these studies, the immune status of the birds was not known, and, therefore, the greater resistance of older birds could have been due to a prior infection with an immunizing apathogenic or mild virus and not to the effect of age alone. More recent studies, where freedom from infection with Marek's disease herpesvirus was ensured before deliberate exposure, have shown some evidence for a decline in susceptibility with age (Vielitz and Landgraf, 1970; Anderson *et al.*, 1971; Ianconescu *et al.*, 1971; P. M. Biggs and D. G. Rootes, unpublished observations). However, the degree and significance of this change is not clear at present. There is no change in susceptibility to infection with age (Anderson *et al.*, 1971).

3. Sex

There is now ample evidence from both experimental and field studies to show that females are, in most circumstances, more susceptible to Marek's disease than males (Biggs and Payne, 1967; Purchase and Biggs, 1967; Cole, 1968; Biggs *et al.*, 1968b; Morris *et al.*, 1970).

D. Environmental Factors Associated with the Etiology of Marek's Disease

Apart from the environmental factors, which allow persistence of the causative virus in the surroundings where young uninfected chickens are to be housed, stress has been the main environmental factor associated with increased incidence of Marek's disease. Such stresses as movement, vaccination against other diseases, handling, debeaking, and changes of food have been considered as affecting the incidence of Marek's disease. It is of interest to note that Gross (quoted by Witter, 1972) found that, in a well-controlled experiment, social stress increased the incidence of Marek's disease. The possible effect of stressing factors in exacerbating a Marek's disease infection is interesting in respect to the well-accepted role stress plays in exacerbating clinical herpes simplex infection (Scott, 1957).

V. Virology

A. Biological Properties

1. Growth in Chickens

What is known of the spread and growth of Marek's disease herpesvirus in chickens has been described in Section III,B,2. Virus infection is established at first in the lungs and lymphoid organs, and within a few days appears to be disseminated by infected leukocytes (presumably lymphocytes) via the blood stream to a very wide range of organs. Some infected cells were found in a wide range of organs and tissues examined by Phillips and Biggs (1972), and viral-associated antigens have been found in many, although in most at low concentration and frequency (Calnek and Hitchner, 1969; Purchase, 1970; L. N. Payne and M. Rennie, personal communication). A productive infection is only consistently present in the feather follicle epithelium (Calnek *et al.*, 1970a; Nazerian and Witter, 1970); a productive, but in most cases abortive infection may occasionally occur in other tissues and organs, but usually only when an acute cytolytic infection is present (Calnek *et al.*, 1970b; Frazier and Biggs, 1972). It would appear that the majority of cells, and in particular lymphoid cells and the cells of lymphomas, are infected nonproductively.

2. Growth in Cultured Cells

Marek's disease herpesvirus has been grown in a wide range of cells cultured from the chicken (Churchill and Biggs, 1967; Churchill, 1968; Witter *et al.*, 1968a; Solomon *et al.*, 1968; Kottaridis *et al.*, 1968; Calnek and Madin, 1969). Cultured embryo cells of many avian species support the growth of Marek's disease herpesvirus and show cytopathic changes (Purchase *et al.*, 1971a). Until recently no mammalian cell or cell line has been found which supports the growth of Marek's disease herpesvirus (Calnek *et al.*, 1969; Esposito *et al.*, 1972). However, Bedigian and Sevoian (1973) have described the growth of Marek's disease herpesvirus in primary hamster kidney cells, although this could not be repeated by Hlozanek and Sovova (1973). Chick kidney cells (CKC) and duck embryo fibroblasts (DEF) have been used and studied more extensively because the herpesvirus of Marek's disease produces a readily recognizable cytopathic change in these cells

(Churchill and Biggs, 1967; Churchill, 1968; Solomon *et al.*, 1968). The virus grows and also produces a cytopathic effect in chick embryo fibroblasts (CEF) (Nazerian, 1968, 1970). Primary isolation is CEF from cells collected from infected chickens has been described (Kottaridis *et al.*, 1968) but this has not been a general experience (Biggs and Payne, 1964; Nazerian, 1970). However, cocultivation of either infected CKC or DEF with CEF results in the transfer of infection to CEF (Nazerian, 1970; Ross *et al.*, 1972). But culture in CEF alters the properties of Marek's disease herpesvirus; even after three passages, a considerable reduction in the concentration of one of the viral-associated antigens (A antigen, see Section V,D) was noted by Ross *et al.* (1973).

The cytopathic changes produced in CKC, DEF, and CEF by infection with Marek's disease herpesvirus are essentially similar. Marek's disease herpesvirus produces plaques of altered cells in all these cell cultures. They consist of groups of altered cells which are rounded in CKC (Figs. 7–9) and more fusiform in DEF. Among the rounded or fusiform cells may be binucleate and polykaryocytes, some of which contain Cowdry type A intranuclear inclusions. In CKC, in particular, as the plaque develops the rounded cells may be drawn to the edge of the plaque leaving a clear space with only a few cells left in the middle. The size and plaque morphology varies for each cell type, for different virus strains, and in each laboratory. Plaques in CKC tend to retract and form clear spaces surrounded by rounded cells, whereas plaques in DEF tend to consist of groups of rounded and fusiform cells. In CKC small, medium, and large plaques have been described (Biggs and Milne, 1972). The small plaques were characterized by small groups of large and small, rounded refractile cells (Fig. 7); medium plaques initially consisted of groups of mainly small, rounded cells which later sometimes retracted around a hole in the monolayer (Fig. 8); and large plaques were larger but otherwise similar to the medium plaques (Fig. 9). Small-plaque viruses grew slowly in culture and were all either apathogenic or only mildly pathogenic. Medium-plaque isolates were all pathogenic and grew more quickly than small-plaque viruses, but more slowly than large-plaque viruses. Large-plaque viruses comprised only attenuated Marek's disease herpesvirus and the herpesvirus of turkeys (see Sections V,E and V,F).

The spread of virus in cultured cells is not by cell-free virus because secondary plaques are not formed (Churchill, 1968; Sharma *et al.*, 1969). The finding that treatment of mixtures of infected and uninfected cells with Sendai virus inactivated with ultraviolet irradiation increased the efficiency of infection, whereas treatment with phytohemagglutinin did not (Hlozanek, 1970) suggests that viral transfer may be achieved via temporary intercellular bridge formation.

In all cell culture systems field virus is cell associated, although small

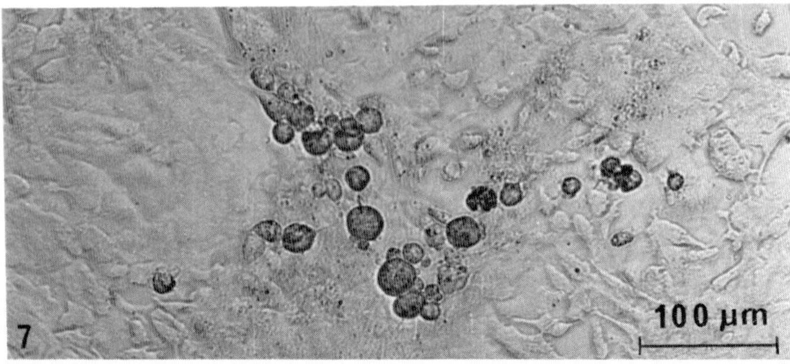
100 μm
7

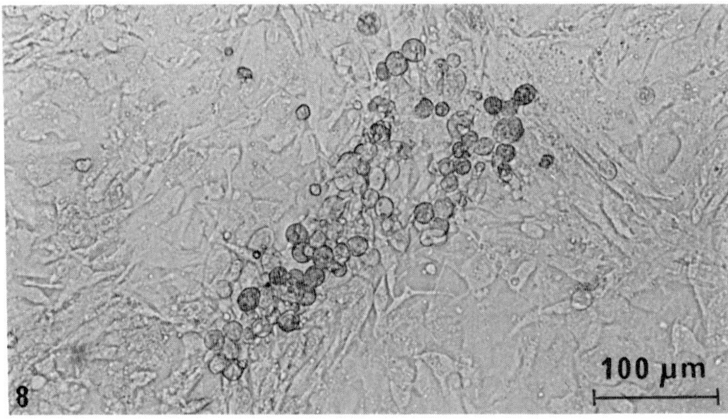
100 μm
8

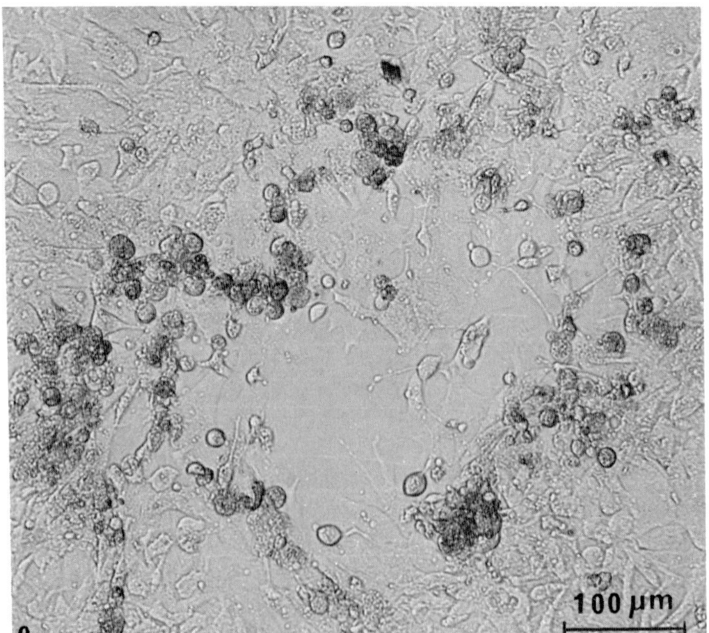
100 μm
9

quantities of cell-free virus can be released by disruption of both infected CKC and CEF (Calnek *et al.*, 1970c; Nazerian, 1970). For this Calnek *et al.*, (1970c) found the stabilizer SPGA (Bavarnick *et al.*, 1950) with 0.2% disodium ethylenediaminetetraacetic acid (EDTA) to be particularly useful. Attenuated Marek's disease herpesvirus is also cell associated, but cell-free virus can more readily be prepared than for field virus (Nazerian, 1970; F. R. W. Shilleto and P. M. Biggs, unpublished results).

Ultrastructural studies of infected CKC and DEF have shown essentially similar results (Epstein *et al.*, 1968; Nazerian and Burmester, 1968; Nazerian, 1971). The main site of development is the nucleus where particles with the characteristics of naked herpesvirus are seen together with smaller, ring-shaped structures which have long been associated with viruses of the herpes group (Morgan *et al.*, 1959). Naked herpesviruses are also present in the cytoplasm. Enveloped particles are mainly present in the nucleus but are also seen in the cytoplasm. These particles are mainly present in the space between the two nuclear membranes or in nuclear vesicles; occasionally they are present in membrane-bound vesicles in the cytoplasm.

Viral-associated antigens have been noted in the nucleus, cytoplasm, and on the cell membrane (Purchase, 1969; von Bülow and Payne, 1970; Nazerian and Purchase, 1970; Chen and Purchase, 1970; Ahmed and Schidlovsky, 1972).

3. Growth in Embryos

Infection of the chick embryo was first shown when Marek's disease developed in young chicks which had been inoculated as embryos (Biggs, 1962; Biggs and Payne, 1967). However, when infected cells which were not immunologically competent became available it was found that infection of the chick embryo with such cells via the chorioallantoic membrane (CAM) or yolk sac route resulted in the formation of pocks on the CAM (Figs. 10 and 11) (von Bülow, 1968, 1969; Churchill, 1968; Biggs and Milne, 1971; Katz and Kohn, 1971). Splenomegaly with white foci of proliferating reticular cells and focal necrosis in the liver occurs after infection via the allantoic cavity (Evans *et al.*, 1971b). Splenomegaly specific to infection with Marek's disease virus has also been noted after infection by the yolk sac route (Biggs and Milne, 1971).

Figs. 7–9. Fig. 7, a small plaque 7 days after inoculation of primary cultured CKC with HPRS-27 infected cells. Magnification × 160. (From Biggs and Milne, 1972.) Fig. 8, a medium plaque 7 days after inoculation of primary CKC with HPRS-16 infected cells. Magnification × 160. (From Biggs and Milne, 1972.) Fig. 9, a large plaque 7 days after inoculation of primary CKC with attenuated HPRS-16 infected cells. Magnification × 160. (From Biggs and Milne, 1972.)

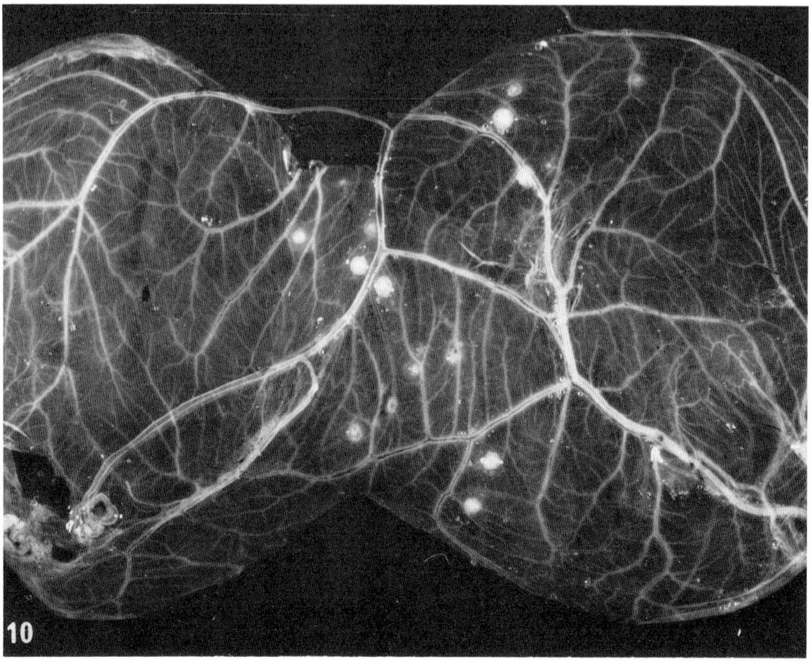
10

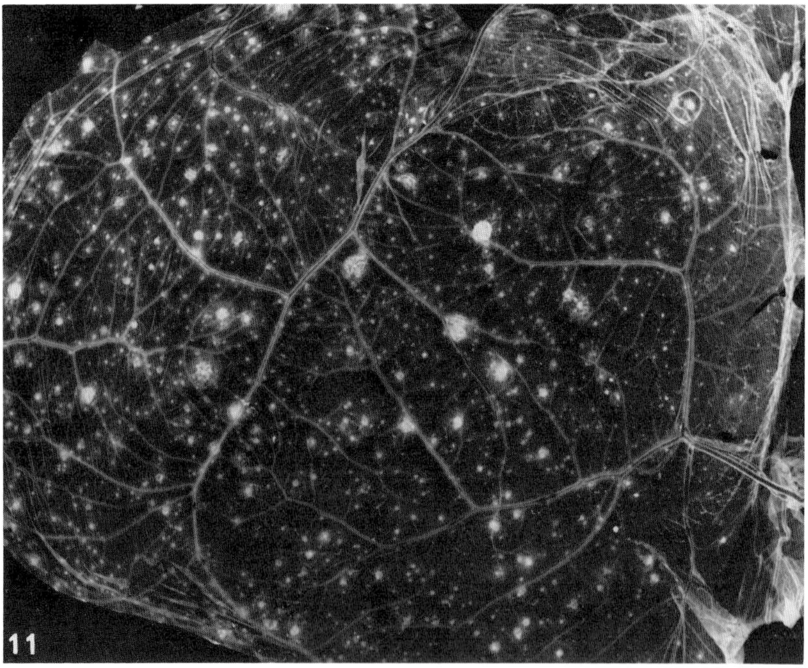
11

4. Pathogenicity

Strains or isolates of Marek's disease virus vary greatly in their pathogenicity (Section IV,A,1). Some isolates are fully pathogenic and produce the acute form of the disease, others are less so and produce the classical form, and still others are nonpathogenic. All apparently possess the A antigen (see Section V,D), and apart from their difference in pathogenicity they can only be distinguished by their plaque size. Biggs and Milne (1972) found that all medium-plaque isolates produced either the acute or the classical form of Marek's disease, whereas 8 out of 9 small-plaque isolates were nonpathogenic, the ninth producing the classical form of Marek's disease.

B. Assay Systems

1. Virus

a. Cell Associated. Chickens, cultured cells, and embryos can be used for assay of Marek's disease herpesvirus. A short-term assay in chickens has been described using histological lesions as the parameter of infection 14–21 days after infection of susceptible 1-day-old chicks (Biggs and Payne, 1967). However this is only useful for fully pathogenic viruses. Nonpathogenic viruses or viruses of low pathogenicity are better assayed using the production of antibody such as precipitins (Chubb, 1969) or the presence of antigens detected by the immunofluorescence test as the parameter of infection.

Both cultured cells and chick embryos can be used for enumerative assays for Marek's disease herpesvirus-infected cells. The CAM and yolk sac route in the chick embryo (Biggs and Milne, 1971) and CKC, DEF, and CEF for cultured cells (Churchill, 1968; Witter *et al.*, 1969b) can be used. There is a linear relationship between the number of pocks or plaques and the dose of infective material. The dose response curve for the CAM route in embryos and the cultured cell systems has a slope of 1, but this is not so for the yolk sac route in embryos. The cell culture systems vary slightly in their sensitivity according to the type of infected cell in the inoculum. The CAM route of embryo assay is of similar sensitivity as the cell culture techniques, but the yolk sac route is more sensitive than cell culture techniques for the assay of infected cells derived from infected chickens. However, the *in vivo* assay in the chicken is the most sensitive for the assay of the latter type of material (Witter *et al.*, 1969b).

Figs. 10 and 11. Fig. 10, pocks on the CAM of a 19-day-old chicken embryo inoculated onto the CAM 8 days previously with HPRS-16 infected cultured CKC. (From Biggs and Milne, 1971.) Fig. 11, pocks on the CAM of an 18-day-old chicken embryo inoculated into the yolk sac 14 days previously with HPRS-16 infected cultured CKC. (From Biggs and Milne, 1971.)

b. Cell-Free. Little is known of the relative merits of possible assay systems for cell-free virus. No studies on the use of the chick embryo have been reported. Cell-free virus can be assayed in cell culture where CKC are the cells of choice. Cultures that are 24 hours old are more sensitive than older cultures, and the inclusion of 5 m*M* EDTA in the inoculum increases the sensitivity of the assay (Adldinger and Calnek, 1971, 1972). Because cell-free virus induces disease in chickens there is no reason why an *in vivo* assay could not be used. Results reported by Calnek and Adldinger (1971) suggest assay in chickens would have about the same sensitivity as assay in cell culture.

2. Antibody

There are a number of techniques that have been described for the detection of antibodies to virus-associated antigens. An indirect hemagglutination test using tanned horse erythrocytes sensitized with an antigen prepared from Marek's disease herpesvirus-infected DEF has been described (Eidson and Schmittle, 1969). This test has not been used extensively, probably because of difficulties in the production of adequate quantities of antigen.

Antibodies to at least three (A, B and C; see Section V,D) virus-associated antigens have been detected using precipitation by double diffusion in agar gel (Churchill *et al.*, 1969b). This has been the most commonly used test for routine detection of antibodies in infected chickens. Antigen preparations most commonly used contain primarily the A antigen and are made from infected cultured cells or the supernatant media (Chubb and Churchill, 1968), skin (Calnek *et al.*, 1970b), and feathers (Haider *et al.*, 1970).

An indirect immunofluorescence test for detecting antibody has been described (Purchase and Burgoyne, 1970; Spencer and Calnek, 1970). Purchase and Burgoyne (1970) found it to be more sensitive than the agar gel precipitin test. Marek's disease herpesvirus grown in cultured chick kidney cells was found to be a superior antigen to the virus grown in duck embryo fibroblasts.

The recent availability of cell-free virus prepared from the feather follicle epithelium of infected chickens (Calnek *et al.*, 1970a) has enabled the use of a neutralization test (Calnek and Adldinger, 1971). Antibodies detected in this test differ from precipitins detected in the agar gel test (Calnek, 1972b; F. R. W. Shilleto and P. M. Biggs, unpublished results).

C. Physical and Chemical Properties

Because cell-free virus has only recently been available for study there is little information on its physical properties. Calnek and Adldinger (1971) have reported that the JM strain is stable at $-65°C$, but loses infectivity at

−20° C. It is inactivated in 2 weeks at 4° C, 4 days at 25° C, 18 hours at 37° C, 30 minutes at 56° C, and 10 minutes at 60° C. Viral infectivity was completely destroyed at a pH below 4 and above 10. The virus was resistant to freeze and thaw cycles and to ultrasonic vibration for up to 5 minutes. The increase in titer found by Nazerian (1972) after 45 seconds sonication, and the removal of infectivity from the supernatant by centrifugation at 5000 *g* for 1 hour suggests that cell-free virus has a tendency to form aggregates or to be absorbed to larger particles. Cell-free Marek's disease herpesvirus can be lyophilized in the presence of an appropriate stabilizer with little loss of infectivity (Calnek *et al.*, 1970c).

The DNA of the JM strain of Marek's disease virus has a molecular weight of 1.0×10^8 daltons (Lee *et al.*, 1971; Bachenheimer *et al.*, 1972). Several estimates of the buoyant density and the guanine + cytosine (G + C) content of Marek's disease herpesvirus have been made with two different results. Lee *et al.* (1969), using DNA extracted from partially purified attenuated JM strain of virus (see Nazerian, 1972), found Marek's disease herpesvirus to have a buoyant density of 1.716 gm cm^3 and G + C content of 56–57%. However, Burg *et al.* (1970), using similar techniques reported for the GA strain a buoyant density of 1.706 gm/cm^3 and G + C content of 46%. These latter figures were later also found for the JM strain (Lee *et al.*, 1971; Bachenheimer *et al.*, 1972).

The structural proteins of the GA strain have been studied using partially purified virus and polyacrylamide gel electrophoresis (Chen *et al.*, 1972). At least eight proteins were described which have been designated VPI–VPVIII. VPI was the major protein, and it was suggested that VPII and VPIV are glycoproteins and therefore probably associated with the viral envelope. The molecular weight of the proteins varied between 33,000 and 126,000 daltons (Nazerian, 1972).

D. *Viral Antigens*

The agar gel precipitin test and immunofluorescent test have been used to study the virus-associated antigens of Marek's disease virus. Up to six antigens were noted by Churchill *et al.* (1969b) in infected cultures of chick kidney cells. However, only three of these were regularly recognized, and and they were termed A, B, and C antigen. All three antigens are present in infected cultured chick kidney cells, but only the A antigen is present in the supernatant. The concentration of the A antigen decreased with passage in infected cultured chick kidney cells and was found to be absent from the highly passaged attenuated Marek's disease herpesvirus (Churchill *et al.*, 1969b). The concentration of the A antigen is rapidly decreased during passage in cultured chick embryo fibroblasts (Ross *et al.*, 1973). The A antigen produced in duck embryo fibroblasts has been purified and found to be a glycoprotein with a molecular weight of between 75,000 and 90,000 daltons and an isoelectric point ranging between pI 4.5 and 5.5 (Ross *et al.*, 1973).

All field isolates examined by Biggs and Milne (1972), whether pathogenic or not, possessed the A antigen. However these studies were not done with cloned virus. Purchase *et al.* (1971b) found that in some pathogenic, cloned virus the A antigen was absent; however, their cloning procedure involved growth in chick embryo fibroblasts, and this may have been responsible for the loss of this antigen.

Morphologically, four different antigens have been noted in cultured cells using immunofluorescence (Purchase, 1969; Nazerian and Purchase, 1970; Chen and Purchase, 1970; Ahmed and Schidlovsky, 1972). These consisted of a diffuse nuclear antigen, diffuse and granular cytoplasmic antigen, and an antigen on the surface of infected cells. Nazerian and Purchase (1970) and Ahmed and Schidlovsky (1972) found that the immunofluorescent antigens were only present in cells containing virus particles.

Purchase (1969) examined seven field isolates of Marek's disease herpesvirus by the indirect fluorescent antibody test and found no differences among them. However, he later described differences between viruses with and without the A antigen (Purchase *et al.*, 1971b). Virus with the A antigen produced antigen in flattened cells surrounding the plaque, whereas virus without the A antigen did not.

Studies using immunofluorescence, precipitation in agar gel, and virus agglutination have shown cross reactions between Marek's disease herpesvirus and Epstein-Barr virus, the herpesvirus of Lucké renal carcinoma, herpes simplex types 1 and 2, and pseudorabies virus (Naito *et al.*, 1970; Ono *et al.*, 1970; Ross *et al.*, 1972; Kirkwood *et al.*, 1972). These cross reactions could be due to the presence of a group-specific antigen suggested by Kirkwood *et al.* (1972).

E. Attenuation

Multiple passage of pathogenic Marek's disease herpesvirus in cultured cells has resulted in a number of changes in the properties of the HPRS-16, JM, GA, and Cal 1 strains (Churchill *et al.*, 1969b; Nazerian 1970; Eidson and Anderson, 1971; Onoda *et al.*, 1971; Phillips and Biggs, 1972). The rate of spread of the virus in culture increases, resulting in larger plaque formation; however the rate of spread in chickens is decreased, and lower levels of infectivity are found. Pathogenicity and the A antigen are lost, and the altered virus grows better in chicken embryo fibroblasts than the parent virus. These results suggested that the A antigen was associated with pathogenicity. However, these two properties are probably unrelated because pathogenic viruses without the A antigen and apathogenic viruses with it have recently been described (Purchase *et al.*, 1971b; Biggs and Milne, 1972).

F. Turkey Herpesvirus

In 1969, Kawamura *et al.* isolated a herpesvirus from turkeys which was later shown to be similar to a herpesvirus isolated from this species by Witter *et al.* (1970a) during investigations on the prevalence of Marek's disease herpesvirus in turkeys. The turkey herpesvirus was shown to be antigenically related to Marek's disease herpesvirus but not to be pathogenic for chickens or turkeys (Witter *et al.*, 1970a). However, more recently, P. M. Biggs and B. S. Milne (unpublished results) have found that many of the turkey herpesviruses will produce minor but characteristic lesions of Marek's disease in nerves of highly susceptible chickens. Infection with the turkey herpesvirus offers excellent protection against the effects of later infection with pathogenic Marek's disease herpesvirus under experimental and field conditions (Okazaki *et al.*, 1970; Purchase *et al.*, 1971c). Although the herpesvirus of turkeys is serologically closely related to Marek's disease herpesvirus, there are differences between them. The turkey herpesvirus grows more quickly in cultured chick kidney cells, producing larger plaques in a shorter time than Marek's disease herpesvirus (Biggs and Milne, 1972). A high proportion of naked virions in cultured cells are morphologically distinct. Many turkey herpesvirus virions lack a central dense core but are characterized by a central electron-lucent cross (Nazerian *et al.*, 1971). Serological differences have been described (Witter *et al.*, 1970a). Neutralization is greater with homologous than with heterologous antisera, and the use of homologous antisera in the immunofluorescent tests results in both nuclear and cytoplasmic fluorescence, whereas usually only nuclear fluorescence occurs when heterologous antisera are used.

VI. Epizootiology

The epizootiology of Marek's disease has recently been reviewed by Witter (1972), and the reader is referred to this publication for a detailed discussion.

A. Distribution of Marek's Disease

Prior to the use of vaccines for Marek's disease (Section VII,B,2) the disease was widespread among the poultry populations of the world. In most countries it is, or was, responsible for serious economic loss to their poultry industry. In spite of widespread infection of the chicken population (Section VI,B) the unpredictable occurrence of the disease has been one of its main features. Mortality is variable between flocks, and also between houses and pens within a house in individual flocks. For example, mortality was found to vary between 0 and 15% in pens of a single house (Biggs *et al.*, 1972b).

B. Distribution of Marek's Disease Virus

Infection with Marek's disease herpesvirus in ubiquitous among the poultry populations of the world. Evidence of infection has been found in all commercial flocks that have been examined, covering many parts of the world. Recently Weiss and Biggs (1972) and Morgan (1971) have found precipitating antibodies to the A antigen in feral jungle fowl in Malaya and in native village chickens in Africa. In commercial flocks all or nearly all adult chicken are, or have been, infected (Chubb and Churchill, 1968; Witter *et al.*, 1970b, 1971; Ianconescu and Samberg, 1971; Biggs *et al.*, 1972b).

Little is known of the relative frequency of apathogenic viruses and viruses which produce the classical and acute forms of Marek's disease. However, viruses of all three degrees of pathogenicity may be present in a single flock, and viruses of more than one level of pathogenicity may be present in small groups of commercial chickens (Biggs *et al.*, 1972b).

The age at which infection occurs may vary, but under commercial conditions it is commonly within the first weeks after hatching (Witter *et al.*, 1970b; Biggs *et al.*, 1972a,b). Once a flock is infected it remains so throughout its commercial life (Witter *et al.*, 1971; Biggs *et al.*, 1972a,b). Infection is persistent and, for most if not all chickens, infection persists throughout life.

C. Cycle of Infection

1. SHEDDING

Because vertical transmission of Marek's disease herpesvirus is unlikely, it must be highly contagious in order to account for the ubiquitous nature of the infection. Oral and nasal washings (Kenzy and Biggs, 1967; Witter and Burmester, 1967), feces (Witter and Burmester, 1967), semen (Sevoian, 1971), and dander (Beasley *et al.*, 1970) have been shown to be infectious. However, the most likely source of infection is desquamated epithelial cells and molted feathers, because the feather follicle epithelium is the only site in which complete, enveloped, and cell-free infectious virus is formed (Calnek *et al.*, 1970a,b; Nazerian and Witter, 1970). Shedding of infection has been reported 2–3 weeks after infection and to continue, in at least a proportion of infected chickens, throughout life (Kenzy and Biggs, 1967; Kenzy and Cho, 1969; Witter *et al.*, 1971).

Evidence for vertical transmission has been reported by Sevoian (1968). However, more recent evidence has suggested that this mode of transmission either does not, or only rarely, occurs. Chicks hatched from presumably infected parents have been kept free of infection when hatched and reared in strict isolation (Rispens *et al.*, 1969; Vielitz and Landgraf, 1970; Witter, 1970; Solomon *et al.*, 1970). Solomon *et al.* (1970) were also unable to detect virus in 72 embryos derived from viraemic hens.

2. Source and Survival of Infection

Infection is probably transmitted by virus produced in the feather follicle epithelial cells either as cell-free virus, desquamated cells, or molted feathers (Calnek *et al.*, 1970a). Dander, poultry dust, and litter contain such material and have been shown to remain infectious for at least 4, 6, and 16 weeks, respectively (Beasley *et al.*, 1970; Jurajda and Klimes, 1970; Witter *et al.*, 1968b). In such a resistant form, infectivity can be moved long distances on inanimate and animate fomites. In this respect, Eidson *et al.* (1966) reported that *Alphitobius diaperinus*, a beetle commonly found in poultry houses, was able to carry Marek's disease herpesvirus. However, there is no evidence to suggest that these or other arthropods are important in the natural transmission of Marek's disease herpesvirus (Beasley and Lancaster, 1971; Witter, 1972).

Airborne transmission of Marek's disease has been clearly shown (Sevoian *et al.*, 1963a; Colwell and Schmittle, 1968), and, therefore, air in the vicinity of infected chickens must be considered to contain Marek's disease herpesvirus. This infectivity is probably due to material originally arising from the feather follicles. It may arise directly from the chicken or indirectly by disturbance of litter or other sites of poultry dust.

D. Factors Affecting the Outcome of Infection

There are a number of factors which affect the severity of Marek's disease in an individual chicken and the severity of an outbreak of disease in a flock. These can be grouped under (1) virus, (2) host, and (3) environment.

1. Virus

The variable pathogenicity of strains of Marek's disease herpesvirus has already been mentioned (Section IV,A,1). The strain with which a chicken or group of chickens is infected will, therefore, influence the outcome of infection. However, the position may not be so simple. Biggs and Milne (1972) have shown that groups of chicken are infected with viruses of more than one degree of pathogenicity. It is probable that individual chickens can be infected with more than one strain of virus because chickens infected with attenuated Marek's disease herpesvirus can be superinfected with field virus (Churchill *et al.*, 1969a; Biggs *et al.*, 1970). Experimentally it has been found that mild or nonpathogenic strains immunize against the effects of later infection with a pathogenic strain (Rispens *et al.*, 1969; P. M. Biggs and B. S. Milne, unpublished results). It has, therefore, been suggested that the important factor is whether a chicken or group of chickens has been infected with a mild or nonpathogenic virus prior to exposure to a fully pathogenic one (Biggs *et al.*, 1972b).

2. Host

The part played by the genetic constitution and sex of the host chicken and the age at infection in influencing the outcome of infection has already been discussed (Section IV,C). The immune status of the host is also of importance. Passively acquired immunity renders young chicks more resistant than antibody-free chicks to the results of infection with Marek's disease herpesvirus (Chubb and Churchill, 1969; Jakowski *et al.*, 1970; Ball *et al.*, 1971). However, immunity provided by infection with a mild or nonpathogenic virus, as discussed in Section VI,D,1, is probably of much greater significance.

3. Environment

The dose of virus affects the outcome of infection, and under field conditions the level of exposure is controlled by the degree of contamination of the environment. The higher the dose the shorter the latent period and greater likelihood of disease. The role stress may play in affecting the outcome of infection has been discussed in Section IV,D.

VII. Control

The control of Marek's disease can be either by prevention of infection or mitigation of its effects.

A. Prevention of Infection

Because vertical transmission of infection either does not occur, or is relatively unimportant, chickens free of infection with Marek's disease herpesvirus can be produced by hatching, rearing, and maintaining them in adequate isolation. Experience has shown that this is not easy, owing to the highly contagious nature of the disease. However, chickens free from infection with Marek's disease herpesvirus have been produced both in isolators (Solomon *et al.*, 1970; Cooper and Timms, 1972a,b) and houses (Drury *et al.*, 1969) maintained under positive pressure with filtered air. Burmester and Witter (1972) have shown that filters with an 80–85% efficiency for retaining particles of about 0.3 μm completely retain naturally occurring Marek's disease infectious particles. These procedures are not economical for the management of commercial poultry at present and are only used for the production and maintenance of chickens free of infection with Marek's disease herpesvirus for experimental use and for providing substrates for vaccine production.

B. Mitigation of the Effects of Infection

1. Selection for Resistance

The recognition that the genetic constitution of the chicken affects its susceptibility to Marek's disease (Section IV,C,1) suggested that selection for resistance by breeders would improve the resistance of commercial chickens. However, before such an approach can be evaluated as a means of control, answers to a number of questions are required. First, is there adequate heterogeneity in commercial poultry in respect of resistance to Marek's disease? Second, does resistance to one strain of Marek's disease convey resistance to all or most strains? The answer to these two questions are in the affirmative and have been discussed in Section IV,C,1. The third question is whether there is an absence of a negative correlation between resistance to Marek's disease and other economic traits. Biggs *et al.* (1968b) have shown that egg number, egg weight, shell strength, and body weight were not correlated with resistance or susceptibility to Marek's disease.

Because the answers to these questions are in the affirmative a selection program for resistance to Marek's disease should be profitable. The methods of selection have been reviewed by Biggs (1972b). Although under experimental conditions progress in selection for resistance can be rapid (Cole, 1968), perhaps because a small number of genes are involved (Cole, 1972), progress in commercial breeding has not been rapid probably because adequate selection pressure was not possible. For this reason the poultry industry at present relies largely on vaccination for the control of Marek's disease.

2. Vaccination

There are theoretically three types of vaccine of use in the control of Marek's disease: (a) modified Marek's disease herpesvirus, (b) turkey herpesvirus, and (c) nonpathogenic field Marek's disease herpesvirus. Although the last viruses provide protection against challenge with pathogenic viruses, it appears that before they can be considered for use as commercial vaccines some modification is necessary either to increase their growth rate in culture or to eliminate their low level of pathogenicity or to do both (Rispens *et al.*, 1972a; Biggs and Milne, 1972).

a. MODIFIED MAREK'S DISEASE HERPESVIRUS. Marek's disease herpesvirus vaccines could be classified according to the pathogenic characteristics of the parent virus. However, it is more useful to classify them according to their characteristics as vaccine viruses. They fall into two groups: those that have lost the A antigen and do not spread naturally from chicken to chicken, and those that have retained the A antigen and do spread naturally.

i. Vaccines without A antigen. These vaccines do not spread from chicken to chicken. Under experimental laboratory and field conditions they have been found to be effective and safe (Churchill *et al.*, 1969a; Biggs *et al.*, 1970, 1972a; Eidson and Anderson, 1971; Meulemans *et al.*, 1971; Eidson *et al.*, 1971; Blaxland *et al.*, 1972; Willemart, 1972). They have been used in the cell-associated form, and although superinfection with field virus can occur, the incidence of Marek's disease is significantly reduced.

ii. Vaccines with A antigen. The protective value of these vaccines has been shown in laboratory trials where adequate isolation was available to allow the use of controls (Rispens *et al.*, 1972a). However, because these viruses spread naturally from chicken to chicken, properly controlled field trials are impossible to design. Nevertheless circumstantial evidence from the use of these vaccines in the field suggests they offer a good degree of protection (Rispens *et al.*, 1972b; Vielitz and Landgraf, 1971).

b. TURKEY HERPESVIRUS (SECTION V,F). Laboratory studies have shown that the turkey herpesvirus in the cell-associated form is safe and protects chickens from challenge with pathogenic virus (Okazaki *et al.*, 1970). Vaccination with the turkey herpesvirus does not prevent superinfection with field Marek's disease herpesvirus, and cell-free field virus is found in the feather follicles and spreads to other chickens, although at a lower rate than in unvaccinated chickens (Purchase and Okazaki, 1971).

Recently, cell-free turkey herpesvirus has been shown to be effective, and turkey herpesvirus in this form has the advantage that it can be stored in the lyophilized state (Eidson and Anderson, 1971; Patrascu *et al.*, 1972).

A number of field trials with turkey herpesvirus have been reported (Purchase *et al.*, 1971c, 1972; Eidson *et al.*, 1971; Dorn and Schindler, 1971; Vielitz and Landgraf, 1971); however, in only one (Willemart, 1972) was the lyophilized form used. In all trials the vaccine proved safe and efficacious.

Each type of vaccine has its own advantages and disadvantages, and the choice of which to use may vary according to the circumstances. Nevertheless, at present, the turkey herpesvirus is most widely used because it has, at least, advantages in production, and, in the lyophilized form in storage and distribution.

C. Conclusions

The three methods of control of Marek's disease are not mutually exclusive. Selection for genetically controlled resistance and the use of vaccination should both reduce the level of field virus in the chicken population. It is, therefore, not a forlorn hope to consider erradication of the Marek's disease herpesvirus from the chicken population as a possibility for the future, since with a reduction in field virus, prevention of infection of flocks by isolation procedures would become practical.

References

Adldinger, H. K., and Calnek, B. W. (1971). *Arch. Gesamte Virusforsch.* **34**, 391–395.

Adldinger, H. K., and Calnek, B. W. (1972). *In* "Oncogenesis and Herpesviruses" (P. M. Biggs, G. de Thé, and L. N. Payne, eds.), pp. 99–105. Int. Agency Res. Cancer, Lyon.

Ahmed, M., and Schidlovsky, G. (1968). *J. Virol.* **2**, 1443–1457.

Ahmed M., and Schidlovsky, G. (1972). *Cancer Res.* **32**, 187–192.

Anderson, D. P., Eidson, C. S., and Richey, D. J. (1971). *Amer. J. Vet. Res.* **32**, 935–938.

Bachenheimer, S. L., Kieff, E. D., Lee, L. F., and Roizman, B. (1972). *In* "Oncogenesis and Herpesviruses" (P. M. Biggs, G. de Thé, and L. N. Payne, eds.), pp. 74–81. Int. Agency Res. Cancer, Lyon.

Ball, R. F., Hill, J. F., Lyman, J., and Wyatt, A. (1971). *Poultry Sci.* **50**, 1084–1090.

Bankowski, R. A., Moulton, J. E., and Mikami, T. (1969). *Amer. J. Vet. Res.* **30**, 1667–1676

Bavarnick, M. R., Miller, J. C., and Snyder, J. C. (1950). *J. Bacteriol.* **59**, 509–522.

Baxendale, W. (1969). *Vet; Rec.* **85**, 341–342.

Beasley, J. N., and Lancaster, J. L. (1971). *Poultry Sci.* **50**, 1552.

Beasley, J. N., Patterson, L. T., and McWade, D. H. (1970). *Amer. J. Vet Res.* **31**, 339–344.

Bedigan, H. G., and Sevoian, M. (1973). *J. Nat. Cancer Inst.* **50**, 129–135.

Benton, W. J., and Cover, M. S. (1957). *Avian Dis.* **1**, 320–327.

Biggs, P. M. (1962). *Proc. Symp. Colston Res. Soc.* **13**, 83–99.

Biggs, P. M. (1966). *World's Poultry Congr., Symp. Pap., 13th, 1966* pp. 91–118.

Biggs, P. M. (1967). *Vet. Rec.* **81**, 583–592.

Biggs, P. M. (1968). *Curr. Top. Microbiol. Immunol.* **43**, 92–125.

Biggs, P. M. (1971). *In* "Poultry Disease and World Economy" (R. F. Gordon and B. F. Freeman, eds.), BEMB Symp. No. 7, pp. 121–133. British Poultry Sci. Ltd.

Biggs, P. M. (1972a). *J. Clin Pathol. Suppl. No 6.* **25**, 65–72.

Biggs, P. M. (1972b). *World's Poultry Congr., Proc., 14th, 1970* **1**, 55–64.

Biggs, P. M., and Milne, B. S. (1971). *Amer. J. Vet. Res.* **32**, 1795–1809.

Biggs, P. M., and Milne, B. S. (1972). *In* "Oncogenesis and Herpesviruses" (P. M. Biggs, G. de Thé, and L. N. Payne, eds.), pp. 88–94. Int. Agency Res. Cancer, Lyon.

Biggs, P. M., and Payne, L. N. (1963). *Vet. Rec.* **75**, 177–179.

Biggs, P. M., and Payne, L. N. (1964). *Nat Cancer Inst. Monogr.* **17**, 83–97.

Biggs, P. M., and Payne, L. N. (1967). *J. Nat. Cancer Inst.* **39**, 237–280.

Biggs, P. M., Purchase, H. G., Bee, B. R., and Dalton, P. J. (1965). *Vet. Rec.* **77**, 1339–1340.

Biggs, P. M., Churchill, A. E., Rootes, D. G., and Chubb, R. C. (1968a). *Perspect. Virol.* **6**, 211–230.
Biggs, P. M., Thorpe, R. J., and Payne, L. N. (1968b). *Brit. Poultry Sci.* **91**, 37–52.
Biggs, P. M., Payne, L. N., Milne, B. S., Churchill, A. E., Chubb, R. C., Powell, D. G., and Harris, A. H. (1970). *Vet. Rec.* **87**, 704–709.
Biggs, P. M., Jackson, C. A. W., Bell, R. A., Lancaster, F. M., and Milne, B. S. (1972a). *In* "Oncogenesis and Herpesviruses" (P. M. Biggs, G. de Thé, and L. N. Payne, eds.), pp. 139–146. Int. Agency Res. Cancer, Lyon.
Biggs, P. M., Powell, D. G., Churchill, A. E., and Chubb, R. C. (1972b). *Avian Pathol.* **1**, 5–25.
Blaxland, J. D., Macleod, A. J., Baxendale, W., and Hall, T. (1972). *Vet. Rec.* **90**, 431–437.
Bloom, S. E. (1970). *Avian Dis.* **14**, 478–490.
Burg, R. W., Morris, C. W., Adler, S. A., and Maag, T. A. (1970). *Bacteriol. Proc.* p. 170.
Burmester, B. R., and Witter, R. L. (1972). *Appl. Microbiol.* **23**, 505–508.
Burnet, M. (1969). "Self and Not Self." Cambridge Univ. Press, London and New York.
Calnek, B. W., (1972a). *Infection Immunity* **6**, 193–198.
Calnek, B. W. (1972b). *In* "Oncogenesis and Herpesviruses" (P. M. Biggs, G. de Thé, and L. N. Payne, eds.), pp. 129–136. Int. Agency Res. Cancer, Lyon.
Calnek, B. W., and Adldinger, H. K. (1971). *Avian Dis.* **15**, 508–517.
Calnek, B. W., and Hitchner, S. B. (1969). *J. Nat. Cancer Inst.* **43**, 935–949.
Calnek, B. W., and Madin, S. H. (1969). *Amer. J. Vet Res.* **30**, 1389–1402.
Calnek, B. W., and Witter, R. L. (1972). *In* "Diseases of Poultry" (M. S. Hofstad, ed.), 6th ed., pp. 470–502. Iowa State Univ. Press, Ames.
Calnek, B. W., Madin, S. H., and Kniazeff, A. J. (1969). *Amer. J. Vet Res.* **30**, 1403–1412.
Calnek, B. W., Adldinger, H. K., and Kahn, D. E. (1970a). *Avian Dis.* **14**, 219–233.
Calnek, B. W., Ubertini, T., and Adldinger, H. K. (1970b). *J. Nat. Cancer Inst.* **45**, 341–351.
Calnek, B. W., Hitchner, S. B., and Adldinger, H. K. (1970c). *Appl. Microbiol.* **20**, 723–726.
Campbell, J. G., and Woode, G. N. (1970). *J. Med. Microbiol.* **31**, 463–473.
Chen, J. H., and Purchase, H. G. (1970). *Virology* **40**, 410–412.
Chen, J. H., Lee, L. F., Nazerian, K., and Burmester, B. R. (1972). *Virology* **47**, 434–443.
Cho, B. R., Kenzy, S. G., and Kim, U. H. (1968). *Can. J. Comp. Med.* **32**, 562–567.
Chomiak, T. W., Luginbuhl, R. E., Helmboldt, C. F., and Kottaridis, S. D. (1967). *Avian Dis.* **11**, 646–653.
Chubb, R. C. (1969). *Brit. Vet. J.* **125**, XVI–XVII.
Chubb, R. C., and Churchill, A. E. (1968). *Vet. Rec.* **83**, 4–7.
Chubb, R. C., and Churchill, A. E. (1969). *Vet. Rec.* **85**, 303–305.
Churchill, A. E. (1968). *J. Nat. Cancer Inst.* **41**, 939–950.
Churchill, A. E., and Biggs, P. M. (1967). *Nature* (*London*) **215**, 528–530.
Churchill, A. E., Payne, L. N., and Chubb, R. C. (1969a). *Nature* (*London*) **211**, 744–747.
Churchill, A. E., Chubb, R. C., and Baxendale, W. (1969b). *J. Gen. Virol.* **4**, 557–564.
Cole, R. K. (1968). *Avian Dis.* **12**, 9–28.
Cole, R. K. (1972). *In* "Oncogenesis and Herpesviruses" (P. M. Biggs, G. de Thé, and L. N. Payne, eds.), pp. 123–128. Int. Agency Res. Cancer, Lyon.
Colwell, W. M., and Schmittle, S. C. (1968). *Avian Dis.* **12**, 724–729.
Cooper, D. M., and Timms, J. R. (1972a). *Avian Pathol.* **1**, 47–57.
Cooper, D. M., and Timms, J. R. (1972b). *Avian Pathol.* **1**, 59–67.
Crittenden, L. B., Muhn, R. L., and Burmester, B. R. (1972). *Poultry Sci.* **51**, 261–267.
Dorn, von P., and Schindler, P. (1971). *Deut. Tieraerztl. Wochenschr.* **78**, 389–392.
Drury, L. N., Patterson, W. C., and Beard, C. W. (1969). *Poultry Sci.* **48**, 1640–1646.
Eidson, C. S., and Anderson, D. P. (1971). *Avian Dis.* **15**, 68–81.
Eidson, C. S., and Schmittle, S. C. (1968). *Avian Dis.* **12**, 467–476.

Eidson, C. S., and Schmittle, S. C. (1969). *Avian Dis.* **13**, 774–782.
Eidson, C. S., Schmittle, S. C., Goode, R. B., and Lal, J. B. (1966). *Amer. J. Vet. Res.* **27**, 1053–1057.
Eidson, C. S., Anderson, D. P., Kleven, S. H., and Brown, J. (1971). *Avian Dis.* **15**, 312–322.
Epstein, M. A., Achong, B. G., Churchill, A. E., and Biggs, P. M. (1968). *J. Nat. Cancer Inst.* **41**, 805–820.
Esposito, J., Lukert, P. D., and Eidson, C. S. (1972). *Amer. J. Vet Res.* **33**, 171–175.
Evans, D. L., and Patterson, L. T. (1971). *Infection Immunity* **4**, 567–574.
Evans, D. L., Beasley, J. N., and Patterson, L. T. (1971a). *Avian Dis.* **15**, 680–687.
Evans, D. L., Patterson L. T., and Beasley, J. N. (1971b). *Appl. Microbiol.* **21**, 321–326.
Fernando, W. W. D., and Calnek, B. W. (1971). *Avian Dis.* **15**, 467–476.
Fletcher, O. J., Eidson, C. S., and Page, R. K. (1971). *Amer. J. Vet Res.* **32**, 1407–1416.
Frazier, J. A., and Biggs, P. M. (1972). *J. Nat. Cancer Inst.* **48**, 1519–1524.
Fujimoto, Y., Nakagawa, M., Okada, K., Okada, M., and Matsukawa, K. (1971). *Jap. J. Vet. Res.* **19**, 7–26.
Furth, J. (1935). *Arch. Pathol.* **20**, 379–428.
Gibbs, C. S. (1934). *Mass., Agr. Exp. Sta., Bull.* **308**, 1–31.
Goodchild, W. M. (1969). *Vet. Rec.* **84**, 87–89.
Grundboeck, M. (1965). *Bull Vet. Inst. Pulawy* **9**, 137–139.
Grundboeck, M. (1966). *Bull. Vet. Inst. Pulawy* **10**, 1–24.
Haider, S. A., Lapen, R. F., and Kenzy, S. G. (1970). *Poultry Sci.* **69**, 1654–1657.
Han, F., Smyth, J. R., Jr., Sevoian, M., and Dickinson, F. M. (1969). *Poultry Sci.* **48**, 76–87.
Harriss, S. T. (1939). *Brit. Vet. J.* **95**, 104–106.
Hartmann, W., and Sanz, M (1971). *Arch. Gefluegelk* **35**, 1–6.
Helmboldt, C. F., Wills, F. K., and Frazier, M. N. (1963). *Avian Dis.* **7**, 402–411.
Hlozanek, I. (1970). *J. Gen. Virol.* **9**, 45–50.
Hlozanek, I., and Sovova, V. (1973). *Folia Biol.* (in press).
Howard, E. B., Jannke, C., Vickers, J., and Kenyon, A. J. (1967). *Cornell Vet.* **57**, 183–194.
Hudson, L., and Payne, L. N. (1973). *Nature* (*New Biology*) **241**, 52–53.
Hutt, F. B., and Cole, R. K. (1947). *Science* **106**, 379–384.
Ianconescu, M., and Samberg, Y. (1971). *Avian Dis.* **15**, 177–186.
Ianconescu, M., Purchase, H. G., Okazaki, W., and Burmester, B. R. (1971). *Avian Dis.* **15**, 745–752.
Jakowski, R. M., Fredrickson, T. N., Luginbuhl, R. E., and Helmboldt, C. F. (1969). *Avian Dis.* **13**, 215–222.
Jakowski, R. M., Fredrickson, T. N., Chomiak, T. W., and Luginbuhl, R. E. (1970). *Avian Dis.* **14**, 374–385.
Johnson, E. P., and Conner, B. V. (1933). *J. Amer. Vet. Med. Ass.* **83**, 325–343.
Jurajda, V., and Klimes, B. (1970). *Avian Dis.* **14**, 188–190.
Katz, D., and Kohn, A. (1971). *Avian Dis.* **15**, 187–198.
Kaupp, B. F. (1921). *J. Amer. Ass. Poultry Husb.* **7**, 25.
Kawamura, H., King, D. J., Jr., and Anderson, D. P. (1969). *Avian Dis.* **13**, 853–863.
Kenzy, S. G., and Biggs, P. M. (1967). *Vet. Rec.* **80**, 565–568.
Kenzy, S. G., and Cho, B. R. (1969). *Avian Dis.* **13**, 211–214.
Kenzy, S. G., McLean, G., Mathey, W. J., and Lee, H. C. (1964). *Nat. Cancer Inst., Monogr.* **17**, 121–130.
Kirkwood, J., Geering, G., and Old, L. J. (1972). *In* "Oncogenesis and Herpesviruses" (P. M. Biggs, G. de Thé, and L. N. Payne, eds.), p. 479. Int. Agency Res. Cancer, Lyon.
Kottaridis, S. D., Luginbuhl, R. E., and Fredrickson, T. N. (1968). *Avian Dis.* **12**, 246–258.
Lapen, R. F., Piper, R. C., and Kenzy, S. G. (1970). *J. Nat. Cancer Inst.* **45**, 941–950.

Lapen, R. F., Kenzy, S. G., Piper, R. C., and Sharma, J. M. (1971). *J. Nat. Cancer Inst.* **47**, 389–399.
Lee, L. F., Roizman, B., Spear, P. G., Kieff, E. D., Burmester, B. R., and Nazerian, K. (1969). *Proc. Nat. Acad. Sci. U.S.* **64**, 951–956.
Lee, L. F., Kieff, E. D., Bachenheimer, S. L., Roizman, B., Spear, P. G., Burmester, B. R., and Nazerian, K. (1971). *J. Virol.* **7**, 289–294.
Marek, J. (1907). *Deut. Tieraerztl. Wochenschr.* **15**, 417–421.
Meulemans, G., Halen, P., Schyns, P., and Bruynooghe, D. (1971). *Vet. Rec.* **89**, 325–329.
Morgan, C., Rose, H. M., Holden, M., and Jones, E. P. (1959). *J. Exp. Med.* **110**, 643–656.
Morgan, H. R. (1971). *Avian Dis.* **15**, 611–613.
Morris, J. R., Ferguson, A. E., and Jerome, F. N. (1970). *Can. J. Anim. Sci.* **50**, 69–81.
Naito, M., Ono, K., Tanabe, S., Doi, T., and Kato, S. (1970). *Biken J.* **13**, 205–212.
Nazerian, K. (1968). *Proc. Electron Microsc. Soc., 26th Annu. Meet.* pp. 222–223.
Nazerian, K. (1970). *J. Nat. Cancer Inst.* **44**, 1257–1267.
Nazerian, K. (1971). *J. Nat. Cancer Inst.* **47**, 207–217.
Nazerian, K. (1972). *In* "Oncogenesis and Herpesviruses" (P. M. Biggs, G. de Thé, and L. N. Payne, eds.), pp. 59–73. Int. Agency Res. Cancer, Lyon.
Nazerian, K., and Burmester, B. R. (1968). *Cancer Res.* **28**, 2454–2462.
Nazerian, K., and Purchase, H. G. (1970). *J. Virol.* **5**, 79–90.
Nazerian, K., and Witter, R. L. (1970). *J. Virol.* **5**, 388–397.
Nazerian, K., Solomon, J. J., Witter, R. L., and Burmester, B. R. (1968). *Proc. Soc. Exp. Biol. Med.* **127**, 177–182.
Nazerian, K., Lee, L. F., Witter, R. L., and Burmester, B. R. (1971). *Virology* **43**, 442–452.
Okada, M. (1970). *Jap. J. Vet Res.* **18**, 97.
Okazaki, W., Purchase, H. G., and Burmester, B. R. (1970). *Avian Dis.* **14**, 413–429.
Ono, K., Tanabe, S., Naito, M., Doi, T., and Kato, S. (1970). *Biken J.* **13**, 213–217.
Onoda, T., Koyama, K., Konobe, T., Takaku, K., Ono, K., and Kato, S. (1971). *Biken J.* **14**, 167–176.
Owen, J. J. T., Moore, M. A. S., and Biggs, P. M. (1966). *J. Nat. Cancer Inst.* **37**, 199–209.
Pappenheimer, A. M., Dunn, L. C., and Cone, V. (1929). *J. Exp. Med.* **49**, 63–86.
Patrascu, I. V., Calnek, B. W., and Smith, M. W. (1972). *Avian Dis.* **16**, 86–93.
Patterson, L. T., Wade, S. K., Evans, D. L., and Beasley, J. N. (1969). *Poultry Sci.* **48**, 1857.
Payne, L. N. (1969). *In* "Veterinary Annual" (C. S. G. Grunsell, ed.), pp. 49–61. Wright, Bristol.
Payne, L. N. (1972). *In* "Oncogenesis and Herpesviruses" (P. M. Biggs G. de Thé, and L. N. Payne, eds.), pp. 21–37. Int. Agency Res. Cancer, Lyon.
Payne, L. N., and Biggs, P. M. (1967). *J. Nat. Cancer Inst.* **39**, 281–302.
Payne, L. N., and Rennie, M. (1970). *J. Nat. Cancer Inst.* **45**, 387–397.
Payne, L. N., and Roszkowski, J. (1972). *Avian Pathol.* **1**, 27–34.
Petek, M., and Quaglio G. L. (1967). *Pathol. Vet.* **4**, 464–476.
Phillips, P. A., and Biggs, P. M. (1972). *J. Nat. Cancer Inst.* **49**, 1367–1373.
Prineas, J. W., and Wright, R. G. (1972). *Lab. Invest.* **26**, 548–557.
Purchase, H. G. (1969). *J. Virol.* **3**, 557–565.
Purchase, H. G. (1970). *Cancer Res.* **30**, 1898–1908.
Purchase, H. G. (1972). *Advan. Vet. Sci.* **16**, 223–258.
Purchase, H. G., and Biggs, P. M. (1967). *Res. Vet. Sci.* **8**, 440–449.
Purchase, H. G., and Burgoyne, M. S. (1970). *Amer. J. Vet. Res.* **31**, 117–123.
Purchase, H. G., and Okazaki, W. (1971). *Avian Dis.* **15**, 391–397.
Purchase, H. G., Chubb, R. C., and Biggs, P. M. (1968). *J. Nat. Cancer Inst.* **40**, 583–592.
Purchase, H. G., Burmester, B. R., and Cunningham, C. H. (1971a). *Amer. J. Vet. Res.* **32**, 1811–1823.

Purchase, H. G., Burmester, B. R., and Cunningham, C. H. (1971b). *Infection Immunity* **3**, 295–303.

Purchase, H. G., Okazaki, W., and Burmester, B. R. (1971c). *Poultry Sci.* **50**, 775–783.

Purchase, H. G., Okazaki, W., and Burmester, B. R. (1972). *Avian Dis.* **16**, 57–71.

Ringen, L. M., and Akhtar, A. S. (1968). *Avian Dis.* **12**, 4–9.

Rispens, B. H., van Vloten, J., and Maas, H. J. L. (1969). *Brit. Vet. J.* **125**, 445–453.

Rispens, B. H., van Vloten, H., Mastenbroek, N., Maas, H. J. L., and Schat, K. A. (1972a). *Avian Dis.* **16**, 108–125.

Rispens, B. H., van Vloten, H., Mastenbroek, N., Maas, H. J. L., and Schat, K. A. (1972b). *Avian Dis.* **16**, 126–138.

Roizman, B. (1972). *In* "Oncogenesis and Herpesviruses" (P. M. Biggs, G. de Thé, and L. N. Payne, eds.), pp. 1–17. Int. Agency Res. Cancer, Lyon.

Ross, L. J. N., Frazier, J. A., and Biggs, P. M. (1972). *In* "Oncogenesis and Herpesviruses" (P. M. Biggs, G. de Thé, and L. N. Payne, eds.), pp. 480–484. Int. Agency Res. Cancer, Lyons.

Ross, L. J. N., Biggs, P. M., and Newton, A. A. (1973). *J. Gen. Virol.* **18**, 291–304.

Samadieh, B., Bankowski, R. A., and Carroll, E. J. (1969). *Amer. J. Vet Res.* **30**, 837–846.

Schidlovsky, G., Ahmed, M., and Jenson, K. E. (1969). *Science* **164**, 959–961.

Schmittle, S. C., and Eidson, C. S. (1968). *Avian Dis.* **12**, 571–576.

Scott, T. F. McN. (1957). *Amer. J. Ophthamol.* [5] **43**, 134–147.

Seagar, E. A. (1933). *Brit. Vet. J.* **89**, 557–561.

Sevoian, M. (1968). *Poultry Sci.* **47**, 1644–1648.

Sevoian, M. (1971). *Poultry Sci.* **50**, 1530–1532.

Sevoian, M., and Chamberlain, D. M. (1964). *Avian Dis.* **8**, 281–310.

Sevoian, M., Chamberlain, D. M., and Counter, F. (1962). *Vet. Med.* **57**, 500–501.

Sevoian, M., Chamberlain, D. M., and Larose, R. N. (1963a). *Avian Dis.* **7**, 102–105.

Sevoian, M., Chamberlain, D. M., and Larose, R. N. (1963b). *World Vet. Congr., Proc.*, 17th *1963* Vol. 2, pp. 1475–1476.

Sharma, J. M., Kenzy, S. G., and Rissberger, A. (1969). *J. Nat. Cancer Inst.* **43**, 907–916.

Sharma, J. M., Witter, R. L., Shramek, G., Wolfe, L. G., Burmester, B. R., and Deinhardt, F. (1972). *J. Nat. Cancer Inst.* **49**, 1191–1197.

Siller, W. G. (1960). *J. Pathol. Bacteriol.* **80**, 43–53.

Simpson, C. F. (1969). *Cancer Res.* **29**, 33–39.

Solomon, J. J., Witter, R. L., Nazerian, K., and Burmester, B. R. (1968). *Proc. Soc. Exp. Biol. Med.* **127**, 173–177.

Solomon, J. J., Witter, R. L., Stone, H. A., and Champion, L. R. (1970). *Avian Dis.* **14**, 752–762.

Spencer, J. L. (1969). *Avian Dis.* **13**, 753–761.

Spencer, J. L., and Calnek, B. W. (1970). *Amer. J. Vet. Res.* **31**, 345–358.

Ubertini, T., and Calnek, B. W. (1970). *J. Nat. Cancer Inst.* **45**, 507–514.

van der Walle, N. and Winkler-Junius, E. (1924). *Tijdschr. Vergelijk. Geneesk.* **10**, 34–50.

Vielitz, E., and Landgraf, H. (1970). *Deut. Tieraerztl. Wochenschr.* **77**, 537–562.

Vielitz, E., and Landgraf, H. (1971). *Deut. Tieraerztl. Wochenschr.* **78**, 617–648.

von Bülow, V. (1968). *Deut. Tieraerztl. Wochenschr.* **81**, 365–367.

von Bülow, V. (1969). *Zentralbl, Veterinaer Med.* **16**, 97–114.

von Bülow, V., and Payne, L. N. (1970). *Zentralbl. Veterinaer Med.* **17**, 460–478.

Washburn, K. W., and Eidson, C. S. (1970). *Poultry Sci.* **49**, 784–793.

Weiss, R. A., and Biggs, P. M. (1972). *J. Nat. Cancer Inst.* **49**, 1713–1725.

Wight, P. A. L. (1962a). *J. Comp. Pathol. Ther.* **72**, 40–48.

Wight, P. A. L. (1962b). *J. Comp. Pathol. Ther.* **72**, 348–359.

Wight, P. A. L. (1964). *Res. Vet. Sci.* **5**, 46–55.

Wight, P. A. L. (1969). *J. Comp. Pathol. Ther.* **79**, 563–570.
Willemart, J. P. (1972). *Rec. Med. Vet.* **148**, 203–216.
Witter, R. L. (1970). *World's Poultry Sci. J.* **26**, 755–762.
Witter, R. L. (1972). *In* "Oncogenesis and Herpesviruses" (P. M. Biggs, G. de Thé, and L. N. Payne, eds.), pp. 111–122. Int. Agency Res. Cancer, Lyon.
Witter, R. L., and Burmester, B. R. (1967). *Proc. Soc. Exp. Biol. Med.* **124**, 59–62.
Witter, R. L., Burgoyne, G. H., and Solomon, J. J. (1968a). *Avian Dis.* **12**, 169–185.
Witter, R. L., Burgoyne, G. H., and Burmester, B. R. (1968b). *Avian Dis.* **12**, 522–530.
Witter, R. L., Burgoyne, G. H., and Solomon, J. J. (1969a). *Avian Dis.* **12**, 171–184.
Witter, R. L., Solomon, J. J., and Burgoyne, G. H. (1969b). *Avian Dis.* **13**, 101–118.
Witter, R. L., Nazerian, K., Purchase, H. G., and Burgoyne, G. H. (1970a). *Amer. J. Vet. Res.* **31**, 525–538.
Witter, R. L., Moulthrop, J. I., Burgoyne, G. H., and Connell, H. C. (1970b). *Avian Dis.* **14**, 255–267.
Witter, R. L., Solomon, J. J., Champion, L. R., and Nazerian, K. (1971). *Avian Dis.* **15**, 346–365.

Chapter 18
Herpesvirus saimiri

Friedrich Deinhardt

I. Introduction

Herpesvirus saimiri (HVS), a simian oncogenic herpesvirus, was first isolated by Melendez *et al.* (1968) from cell cultures of apparently healthy squirrel monkey kidneys. Focal cell degeneration, with the formation of intranuclear inclusion bodies, occurred about 13–28 days after cultivation *in vitro*, and herpesvirus-like particles were observed in the degenerating cells. Similar particles observed in the cell-free supernatants of such cultures were propagated serially in several types of simian primary cell cultures and established simian cell lines, and propagation in human cells was also reported by one laboratory (Ablashi *et al.*, 1971a). From its physical and chemical properties the virus was identified as a typical herpesvirus (Melendez *et al.*, 1969a,b, 1970b,d; Falk *et al.*, 1970, 1971; Goodheart, 1970; Morgan *et al.*, 1970; Barahona and Melendez, 1971; Deinhardt *et al.*, 1972; Heine *et al.*, 1971).

Although it seems that HVS does not induce overt disease in squirrel monkeys, it induces lymphomas in several other New World nonhuman primate species (Hunt and Melendez, 1969; Hunt *et al.*, 1970, 1972a; Melendez *et al.*, 1970a,b,c, 1971b; Ablashi *et al.*, 1971b; Wolfe *et al.*, 1971). These were important observations because the relationships between some herpesviruses (including those of man) and malignant tumors have been a subject of intense debate. Herpesviruses are known to be associated with the Lucké frog carcinoma (Granoff, Chapter 19), neurolymphomatosis in chickens (Marek's disease) (Biggs, Chapter 17), and lymphomas in rabbits (Hinze, 1971); the causal relationship of herpes simplex virus type II and Epstein–Barr virus (EB virus) with human malignancies, still an undecided question, has been considered by Rawls (Chapter 10) and Klein (Chapter 16). The discovery of a simian herpesvirus with established oncogenicity for primates was, therefore, particularly interesting, quite apart from providing an excellent model for studying oncogenicity of a herpesvirus in primates.

II. Studies *in Vitro*

A. Growth in Cell Cultures

Herpesvirus saimiri grows in various cell cultures (Table I) with the development of a typically herpesvirus-like cytopathic effect (CPE), which generally develops in foci, progresses relatively slowly, and consists initially of small clusters of rounded and multinucleated giant cells. Later, foci develop into holes in the cell sheet, with clusters of rounded cells and some multinucleated cells in the periphery. Degenerating cells develop typical, type A inclusion bodies. Under optimal conditions, CPE may be detected first at 48–72 hours after infection, and final virus titers are usually determined after 21 days.

Multiplication of HVS in human cells has been reported by only one laboratory, and only low virus titers were obtained. Pretreatment of the human cell cultures with diethylaminoethyl dextran apparently enhances their susceptibility to HVS (Ablashi *et al.*, 1971a).

Virus harvested from cell-free supernatants or from infected cells may be quick frozen, usually with less than 0.5 $\log_{10}$ loss in titer, and is stable

TABLE I
CELLS SUSCEPTIBLE TO HERPESVIRUS SAIMIRI

Origin	Cell Type	Reference
Primary cell cultures		
African green monkey (*Cercopithecus* sp.)	Kidney	Ablashi *et al.*, 1971b
Marmoset (*Saguinus* sp.)	Kidney	L. A. Falk, unpublished data
Owl monkey (*Aotus* sp.)	Kidney	Ablashi *et al.*, 1971b
Continuous cell lines		
Squirrel monkey (*Saimiri sciureus*)	Kidney	Melendez *et al.*, 1968
	Fetal heart, lung, and intestine	Daniel *et al.*, 1971
Marmoset (*Saguinus* sp.)	Kidney	Wolfe *et al.*, 1971
	Muscle	L. A. Falk, unpublished data
	Fetal lung	L. A. Falk, unpublished data
African green monkey (*Cercopithecus* sp.)	Kidney (Vero)	Melendez *et al.*, 1969a
	Kidney (BSC-1)	Daniel *et al.*, 1971
Owl monkey (*Aotus* sp.)	Kidney	Melendez *et al.*, 1969a
Human	Embryonic skin and muscle (Wi-38)	Ablashi *et al.*, 1971a

during storage at $-65°$ or $-120°$ C for months or even years, a characteristic similar to other herpesviruses.

B. *Plaque Assay and Morphology*

Under agar, methylcellulose, or starch overlays (Falk *et al.*, 1970, 1971; Deinhardt *et al.*, 1972; Daniel *et al.*, 1971), HVS forms small (0.5–1 mm) and large (2–3 mm) plaques. Attempts to plaque-purify HVS in order to obtain pure "small-" or "large-plaque" forming variants have failed. Even after five plaque purification passages, during which single large or small plaques were picked for passage, no pure clones were obtained. In each passage the same mixture of small and large plaques appeared, regardless whether the inoculum was obtained from a large or small plaque of the previous passage.

C. *Rate of Virus Multiplication*

The rate of multiplication of HVS in cell cultures has been studied (1) by means of standard growth curves, by assaying infectious HVS; (2) by fluorescent antibody (FA) techniques measuring the development of viral antigens in the infected cells; and (3) by formation of viral particles by electron microscopy. A typical growth curve of HVS in marmoset kidney cells is given in Fig. 1.

Viral antigens are first detectable by FA techniques in nuclei of individual infected cells 24–48 hours after inoculation. By 72 hours antigen is present in the cytoplasm, and surrounding cells show nuclear staining. Later, larger foci of stained cells are observed; cells closer to the center of the foci show nuclear and cytoplasmic or predominantly cytoplasmic staining, whereas peripheral cells show predominantly nuclear staining (Falk *et al.*, 1970, 1972d). When studied by electron microscopy (Morgan *et al.*, 1970; Heine *et al.*, 1971) the development of viral particles followed a pattern typical of other herpesviruses, and the temporal sequence and spatial arrangement agreed with the results of the growth curve experiments in which infectious virus and the development of viral antigens were assayed.

D. *Assay for Neutralizing Antibodies and Antigenic Characteristics*

Neutralizing serum antibodies to HVS can be measured in neutralization tests in which approximately 100 $TCID_{50}$ of virus are mixed and incubated for 12–18 hours at 4° C with serial serum dilutions in the presence of guinea pig complement. Surviving virus was assayed in susceptible cells by the inoculation of the mixtures into tube cultures or plaque bottles. Antibodies to HVS may also be assayed by indirect FA techniques, and the titers obtained by both techniques are comparable, except that titers of marmoset sera obtained early during the disease are usually higher by FA than by neutralization tests.

Comparison of the antigenic characteristics of HVS with other herpesviruses is given in Table II. Herpesvirus saimiri does not cross react in

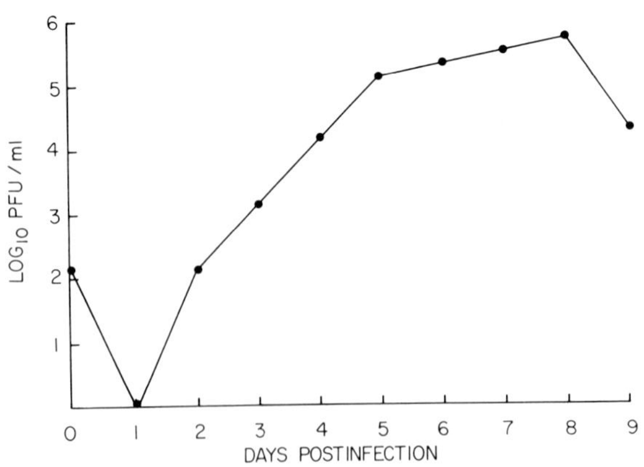

FIG. 1. Growth curve of HVS in marmoset kidney cell cultures.

TABLE II

ANTIGENIC CROSS REACTIVITY BETWEEN SOME HERPESVIRUSES[a]

Antigen	Herpes simplex virus	Herpes-virus platyrrhi-nae	Spider monkey herpes virus[b]	Epstein–Barr virus	Herpes-virus saimiri	Marek's disease virus	Herpes-virus of turkeys	Rabbit lymphoma virus
Herpes simplex virus	+	±	±	−	−	−	−	−
Herpesvirus platyrrhinae	±	+	±	−	−	−	−	−
Spider monkey herpesvirus	±	±	+	−	−	−	−	−
Epstein–Barr virus	−	−	−	+	−	−	−	−
Herpesvirus saimiri	−	−	−	−	+	−	−	−
Marek's disease virus	−	−	−	−	−	+	±	−
Herpesvirus of turkeys	−	−	−	−	−	±	+	−
Rabbit lymphoma virus	−	−	−	−	−	−	−	+

[a]All tested by FA. Herpesvirus saimiri, Herpesvirus platyrrhinae, and herpes simplex virus also tested by neutralization tests.

[b]Similar to but antigenically distinct from Herpesvirus platyrrhinae. Host range and pathogenicity are the same (from Holmes *et al.*, 1964, 1966; Hull *et al.*, 1972).

neutralization tests with any other primate herpes simplex type viruses (which cross react among themselves), and in this respect it is similar to Epstein-Barr virus (EB virus) which also fails to cross react in neutralization tests with other primate herpes simplex type viruses. However, no cross reactivity exists between HVS and EB virus. Similarly neither HVS nor EB virus share antigenic specificities (detectable by neutralization tests) with the avian oncogenic herpesviruses [Marek's disease virus (MDV) and herpesvirus of turkeys (HVT)] or with the herpesvirus causing lymphomas in rabbits (Hinze, 1971).

III. Natural History

A. *Virus Isolations*

1. Squirrel Monkeys (*Saimiri sceiureus*)

a. Original Isolations from Squirrel Monkey Tissues. Herpesvirus saimiri was first isolated from six kidneys obtained for the preparation of kidney cell cultures from ten apparently healthy squirrel monkeys (Melendez *et al.*, 1968). A focal herpes-like CPE appeared between 13 to 23 days of cultivation in monolayer kidney cell cultures prepared by standard techniques. Affected cells develop intranuclear inclusion bodies, and the harvests from these cultures were used as inocula for the further propagation and identification of HVS.

b. Isolations of HVS from Lymphocytes of Healthy Squirrel Monkeys. Later studies (Falk *et al.*, 1972a,b) showed that HVS could be isolated from the circulating lymphocytes of squirrel monkeys in two small zoo colonies and a larger experimental colony. Fresh or frozen whole blood, viable or frozen Ficoll-Hypaque (FH) purified lymphocytes or polymorphonuclear leukocytes, or plasma were cocultivated or inoculated into cultures of Vero cells. Herpesvirus saimiri was isolated from cultures cocultivated with fresh whole blood or viable, purified lymphocytes but not from polymorphonuclear leukocytes or from the cultures inoculated with frozen samples. Table III indicates the frequency of isolation and the presence or absence of antiviral, circulating, serum antibodies in the same animals. All squirrel monkeys in this study were clinically healthy with normal hematological values. Fifty of these animals continue under observation and their bloods examined for antibodies and virus. To date, virus has been isolated up to 3 times each from 33 animals over a period of 6 months, and levels of circulating antibodies have essentially remained stable (L. A. Falk, T. Clarkson, L. G. Wolfe, and F. Deinhardt, unpublished observation).

TABLE III
ISOLATION OF HERPESVIRUS SAIMIRI FROM THREE GROUPS OF SQUIRREL MONKEYS

Squirrel monkey group	Virus isolation		Antibodies to HVS
	Whole blood	FH-lymphocytes	
A			
First bleeding	2/3	3/3	2/3[a]
Second bleeding	6/10	5/6	4/6[a]
B	39/129	23/35	108/126[b]
C	NT[c]	6/8	5/8[b]

[a]Determined by virus neutralization tests.
[b]Determined by indirect FA tests.
[c]Not tested.

2. SPIDER MONKEYS

A herpesvirus (Herpesvirus ateles) (HVA) similar to HVS was isolated recently from tissues of healthy spider monkeys (Melendez *et al.*, 1971a, 1972; Hunt *et al.*, 1972b). This agent has biologic characteristics apparently similar to HVS but has been reported to be antigenically different.

B. Epidemiology

1. DISTRIBUTION OF ANTIBODIES

The distribution of antibodies to HVS in various species of New World monkeys is given in Table IV. It appears that squirrel monkeys and perhaps also spider monkeys are natural hosts to HVS, but at this time it cannot be said whether the antibodies in spider monkeys are caused by infection with HVS or with HVA of spider monkeys since there may be a partial antigenic overlap between the two agents.

The antibodies detected in the sera of 2 of 19 marmosets (*Saguinus geoffroyi*) and the failure to induce disease in one common marmoset (*Callithrix jacchus*) reported by Rabin (1971), may indicate that infection of wild marmosets does occur occasionally and that some marmoset species may be more resistant to infection than others (*S. oedipus, S. fuscicollis, S. nigricollis*) which invariably succumbed to infection with HVS. Antibodies in the two seropositive owl monkeys were demonstrated by FA only; because insufficient serum prevented confirmation by neutralization tests, the most that may be said about these results is that either wild owl monkeys may survive occasional infections or, more probably, that these particular sera gave some nonspecific staining, unrelated to anti-HVS antibodies.

TABLE IV
SERUM ANTIBODIES TO HERPESVIRUS SAIMIRI IN NEW WORLD MONKEYS

Species	Positive/total
Black spider monkeys (*Ateles fusciceps*)	4/9
Red spider monkeys (*Ateles geoffroyi*)	2/2
White face monkeys (*Cebus capucinus*)	0/6
Marmoset monkeys (*Saguinus sp.*)	
S. geoffroyi	2/19
S. oedipus, S. fuscicollis	0/49
S. nigricollis	
Owl monkeys (*Aotus trivirgatus*)[a]	2/23
Squirrel monkeys (*Saimiri sciureus*)	167/196

[a]Not confirmed by neutralization tests.

2. TRANSMISSION OF DISEASE IN NATURAL HOST SPECIES

From the distribution of antibodies and the incidence of virus isolation in squirrel monkeys (Table V), it is probable that the transmission of HVS in squirrel monkeys is horizontal, and primary infection occurs usually early in life, at least among those animals living in a closed colony. Animals were born with low titers or undetectable maternal antibodies, which disappeared between 6 to 12 weeks of age; between 6 months and 2 years a rapidly increasing number of animals became infected and converted to an antibody-positive status. Simultaneously, the animals became virus-positive, i.e., HVS was isolated from their circulating lymphocytes by cocultivation techniques.

Transmission of HVS by arthropods from experimentally infected and "viremic" (having circulating virogenic lymphocytes) marmosets to uninfected marmosets was evaluated in a collaborative study between our laboratory, the University of North Dakota (Dr. Robert Fischer), and the National Cancer Institute, National Institutes of Health, U.S. Public Health Service (Dr. George Burton). The disease was not transmitted in interrupted feeding experiments with stable flies (*Stomoxys calcitrans*), mosquitoes (*Anopheles quadrimaculatus* and *Aedes aegypti*), or cat fleas (*Ctenocephalides felis*). Experimentally, HVS was recovered from the arthropods after a meal of blood containing HVS-infected lymphocytes only for as long as viable lymphocytes could be recovered from the arthropods alimentary canal (i.e., about 6 hours).

No information is yet available on natural or experimental transmission of HVS or HVA in spider monkeys, but it is unlikely that the behavior of HVS or HVA in spider monkeys is different in principle from that of HVS in squirrel monkeys.

TABLE V
ISOLATION OF HERPESVIRUS SAIMIRI AND DETERMINATION OF ANTIBODIES IN A COLONY OF SQUIRREL MONKEYS

Origin	Age	Virus Isolation from lymphocytes	Antibodies[a] to HVS
Colony born	≤ 2 months	0/7	0/7
	≤ 1 year	6/15	6/16 (1:9)
	≥ 2 years	4/5	19/19 (1:16)
	≥ 3 years	10/11	67/67 (1:36)
Wild-caught	Adult	14/18	16/22 (1:24)

[a]Determined by indirect FA tests; geometric mean titers are given in parentheses.

IV. Pathogenesis of Diseases Caused by Herpesvirus saimiri

A. Natural Disease in Squirrel Monkeys

The high incidence (90%) of anti-HVS antibodies in juvenile and adult squirrel monkeys indicated that the disease induced by HVS in squirrel monkeys must be relatively mild and not usually fatal. Melendez *et al.* (1970d) reported that HVS did not induce disease in experimentally inoculated adult squirrel monkeys; but since these squirrel monkeys had anti-HVS antibodies before inoculation and no antibody rise was observed after inoculation, these animals were probably completely immune to HVS before experimental inoculation. H. Rabin and R. Cooper (personal communication, 1972) infected 4 antibody-free adult squirrel monkeys; no disease developed although successful infection was demonstrated by the development of neutralizing antibodies in the inoculated animals. Most recently, Falk *et al.* (1972c) identified a small number of infant squirrel monkeys (12–16 weeks old) which were free of antibodies and whose lymphocytes did not yield virus when cocultivated with Vero cells on four different occasions over an 8-week period. Three of these animals, 4–6 months old, were inoculated intramuscularly (im) with $10^{4.7}$ $TCID_{50}$ of HVS; they were caged with control animals of the same age. The animals were observed regularly for clinical signs of disease; blood was taken at intervals for hematological examination and virus isolation; and throat and stool swabs were obtained for virus isolation. The animals exhibited no signs of clinical disease; no virus was isolated from throat or stool swabs; and their hematological values remained normal but virus was isolated from viable lymphocytes by cocultivation and the inoculated animals developed neutralizing HVS antibodies (Table VI). One uninoculated cage-contact animal became virus-positive 60 days and one 78 days after inoculation of its cagemate. These studies are continuing.

TABLE VI
ISOLATION OF HERPESVIRUS SAIMIRI FROM PERIPHERAL LYMPHOCYTES OF YOUNG, EXPERIMENTALLY INFECTED SQUIRREL MONKEYS

Group	Inoculum	Virus isolation from lymphocytes[a]	Antibody titers to HVS[a]
I	$10^{4.7}$ $TCID_{50}$ of HVS	0/3 (-15,-7,0)	0/3 (-15,-7,0,7,14)
		2/3 (17)	1/3 (17)
		3/3 (24,31,42,52)	3/3 (24,31,42,52)
		2/3 (60,78)	
II	None (Cage contact controls)	0/2 (-15,-7,0,17,24,31,42, 52)	0/2 (-15,-7,0,7,14,17,24,31, 52)
		1/2 (60)	
		2/2 (78)	
III	None (controls, kept isolated from groups I and II)	0/2 (-15,-7,0,17,24,31, 42)	0/2 (-15,-7,0,10,17,24,31, 42,52)
		0/2 (60,78)	

[a] Number virus positive/number tested, or number with HVS antibodies/number tested. Numbers in parentheses are those pre- and postinoculation days when tests were performed.

B. Malignant Lymphoproliferative Diseases in Other Nonhuman Primates

1. TYPES OF SUSCEPTIBLE SPECIES

In contrast to the low pathogenicity of HVS for squirrel monkeys, inoculation of a number of other New World and one African nonhuman primate species is followed by the development of malignant lymphoproliferative diseases. Fatal lymphomas of reticulum cell types following inoculation of HVS were reported first in cotton-topped marmosets (CT) (*S. oedipus*) and owl monkeys (*Aotus trivirgatus*) (Melendez *et al.*, 1969b). These observations were later confirmed (Hunt *et al.*, 1970; Ablashi *et al.*, 1971b; Wolfe *et al.*, 1971) and induction of malignant lymphomas by HVS was reported also to occur in white-lipped marmosets (WL) (*S. nigricollis*, *S. fuscicollis*) (Falk *et al.*, 1970; Wolfe *et al.*, 1971), a white-moustached marmoset (*S. mystax*) (Rabin, 1971), cinnamon ringtail monkeys (*Cebus albifrons*) (Melendez *et al.*, 1970a,c), spider monkeys (*Ateles geoffroyi*) (Hunt *et al.*, 1972a), and African green monkeys (*Cercopithecus aethiops*) (Melendez *et al.*, 1970d). Induction of lymphocytic leukemia rather than lymphomas has been described recently in owl monkeys (Melendez *et al.*, 1971b; Ablashi *et al.*, 1971b) and WL marmosets (Falk *et al.*, 1971; Wolfe *et al.*, 1971). In contrast, im inoculation of juvenile galagos (*Galago crassicaudatus*) (Wolfe *et al.*, 1971), rhesus monkeys (*Macaca mulatta*) (Hunt *et al.*, 1972a), a talapoin monkey (*Cercopithecus talapoin*), and a common marmoset (*C. jacchus*) (Rabin, 1971) with HVS was not followed by any clinical disease or hematologic abnormalities, and animals remained antibody negative. Induction of malignant lymphomas in rabbits has been reported (Melendez *et al.*, 1970d; Daniel *et al.*, 1970), but we have been unable to confirm this in studies in our laboratory.

2. Experimental Infection and Clinical Disease

The following description of the pathogenicity of HVS (Wolfe *et al.*, 1971) in experimentally inoculated CT and WL marmosets agrees in all major points with other published descriptions (see above for references). Animals inoculated im with $10^{3.9}$ to $10^{4.9}$ $TCID_{50}$ of HVS were observed daily for clinical signs of disease.

Blood was obtained at weekly or biweekly intervals for hematologic evaluation, isolation of virus, and determination of antibodies. Throat and stool swabs were collected for virus isolation at the same time intervals, and serial percutaneous liver biopsies were obtained from some animals every 7–14 days. The animals were sacrificed when *in extremis*; complete autopsies were performed; and tissues were obtained for light and electron microscopic evaluation, for FA studies, and for virus isolation.

The inoculated animals appeared clinically healthy until hours or at most a few days before death when inactivity, weakness, anorexia, and subnormal rectal temperatures were observed. Mild peripheral lymphadenopathy was detected in CT and WL marmosets as early as 10 days postinoculation (PI) and was always present to varying degrees by 25 days PI. During the terminal stages of the disease, lymph nodes were two to four times normal size, and splenomegaly was consistently present only in CT marmosets. All CT marmosets were dead or *in extremis* by 35 days PI, whereas the disease was more protracted (up to 116 days) in WL marmosets.

Both CT and WL marmoset developed, usually after 25 days PI, a leukocytosis and absolute lymphocytosis. The course of the hematological disease of one WL marmoset is given in detail in Table VII. In approximately 50% of both CT and WL marmosets, a mild absolute neutrophilia without a shift to the left accompanied the absolute lymphocytosis, and 5–50% of the circulating lymphocytic cells were classified as either lymphoblasts or atypical cells. The atypical cells had deeply basophilic, vacuolated cytoplasm with coarsely clumped nuclear chromatin and sometimes closely resembled the Downey cells frequently found in human patients with infectious mononucleosis (Fig. 2). In several experiments uninoculated animals were caged with experimentally infected animals, but none of them, including

TABLE VII
DEVELOPMENT OF LEUKEMIA INDUCED BY HERPESVIRUS SAIMIRI IN A WHITE-LIPPED MARMOSET

Days PI	Leuko-cytes per mm^3	Lymphocytes (%)	Infectivity of whole blood (log 10 $TCID_{50}$/ml)[a]	Minimum number of lymphocytes yielding infectious HVS
0	6,600	44	negative	negative
5	8,800	60	negative	negative
12	2,850	35	negative	negative
14	7,205	48	negative	negative
21	7,150	39	1.2	10^6
28	8,250	46	1.2	10^6
35	33,450	81	6.5	162
48	170,000	93	7.5	17
58	282,000	95	8.0	14
61	340,000	97	8.0	17

[a]Determined by cocultivation of whole blood with susceptible indicator cells.

one animal which was housed together with several infected animals consecutively for a period of 10 months, developed either disease or anti-HVS antibodies.

3. Macroscopic Lesions

The distribution of macroscopic lesions is remarkably consistent in CT marmosets. The findings in animals dying > 25 days postinfection (PI) are as follows: hepatosplenomegaly (Fig. 3), generalized lymphadenopathy, enlarged adrenal glands with hemorrhagic thickened cortices, enlarged hemorrhagic thymuses, enlarged tonsils and Peyer's patches, focal grayish mottling throughout the kidney cortices, enlarged salivary glands with hemorrhagic mottling, and the reddish-gray stippling at the im inoculation sites. Animals sacrificed at shorter intervals after inoculation show mild generalized lymphadenopathy and splenomegaly at 10 days PI, and the other manifestations of disease are not usually found until 21 or more days PI.

Macroscopic lesions in WL marmosets were much more varied. An occasional WL marmoset develops lesions very similar to those observed in CT marmosets but most develop no hepatomegaly, only a mild enlargement of the spleen, and often a more prominent peripheral and visceral lymphadenopathy (Fig. 4).

4. Microscopic Lesions

Microscopic lesions compatible with a proliferative lymphoreticular disease are found both in CT and WL marmosets (Hunt and Melendez, 1969;

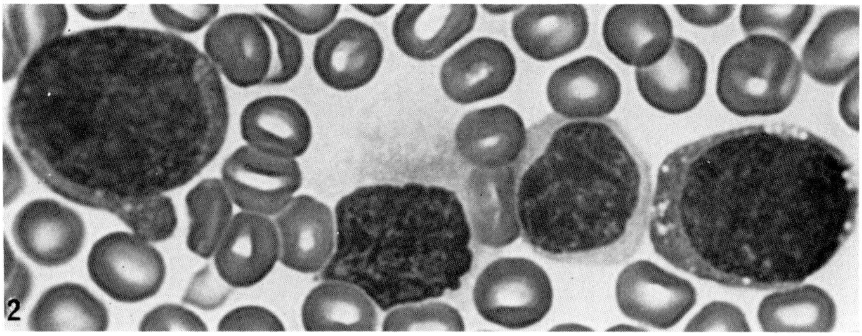

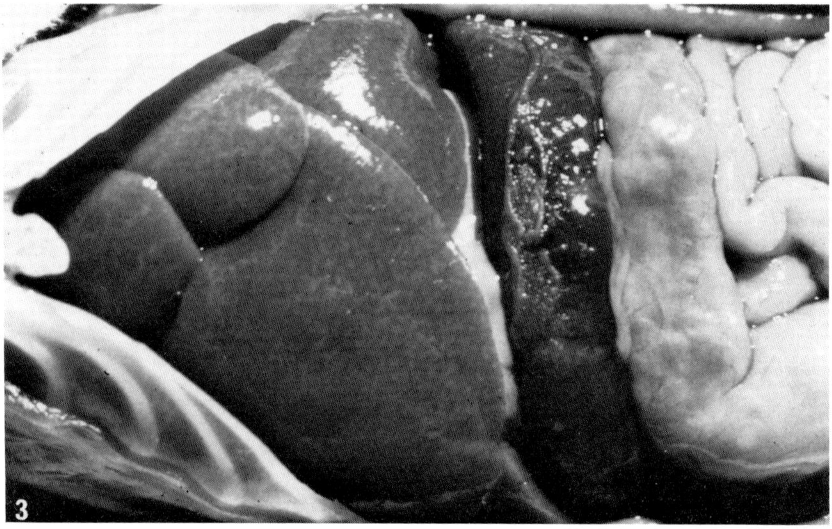

FIGS. 2 and 3. Fig. 2, peripheral blood from marmoset, with lymphoblast and a smaller, atypical cell with cytoplasmic vacuoles or globules. Wright-Giemsa, ×450. Fig. 3, hepatosplenomegaly in CT marmoset 35 days after inoculation, with spleen enlarged to ten times normal size and extending completely across ventral abdomen. Liver with prominent reticular pattern caused by severe periportal infiltration of lymphoreticular cells.

Hunt *et al.*, 1970, 1972a; Wolfe *et al.*, 1971). Cotton-topped marmosets consistently develop a widely disseminated disease characterized by massive infiltration of tissues by reticulum cells and by immature cells of the lymphocytic series. The distribution and density of the cellular infiltrates are remarkably similar from animal to animal at specific PI intervals, especially late in the course of the disease. In contrast, the disease induced in WL marmosets is highly variable from animal to animal. Some develop widely disseminated lesions, whereas the characteristic feature in others is a pro-

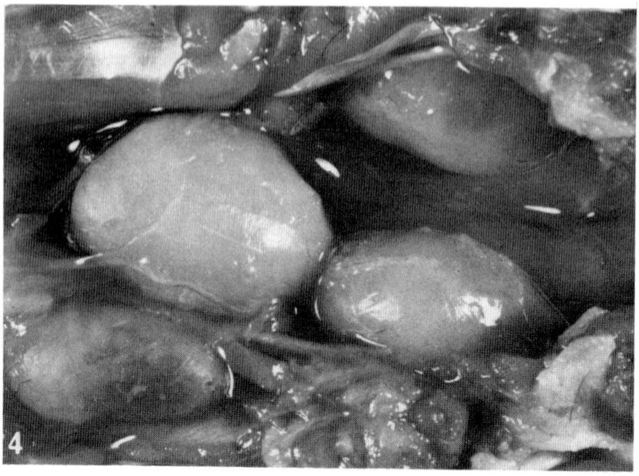

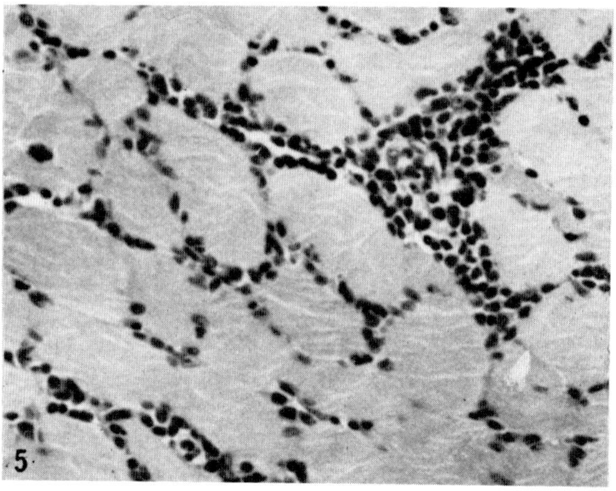

FIGS. 4 and 5. Fig, 4, pelvic lymph nodes (1.0–1.5 cm long) of WL marmoset with severe, generalized peripheral and visceral lymphadenopathy. Fig. 5, lymphoreticular cells at im inoculation site of CT marmoset 7 days after inoculation. Hematoxylin and eosin, ×60.

nounced lymphocytosis with little cellular infiltration of limited distribution. Intranuclear inclusion bodies have never been found in the tissues of either WL or CT marmosets nor in any of those studies using other susceptible primate species.

By 25 days PI, cellular infiltrates are already widely disseminated throughout the tissues in CT marmosets. The cellular infiltrates, morphologically very similar in each tissue, are composed of reticulum cells and lymphoblasts, the former being the predominant cell type. Mitotic figures, including bizarre forms, are numerous. Marginated chromatin clumps, pyknosis, and karyorrhexis have been observed.

The distribution of lesions in CT marmosets remains basically unchanged between 25 to 35 days PI, but the amount of cellular infiltrate increases with time. During the terminal stages of the disease, microscopic lesions are particularly severe in visceral and peripheral lymph nodes, thymus, spleen, liver, adrenal glands, and kidneys. The normal cytoarchitecture of these tissues is replaced by the cellular infiltrates, with capsular invasion usually demonstrable in the lymphoid tissues. The lesions are identical in peripheral and visceral nodes, without a particular lymph node chain being more severely involved than any other; lesions in tonsils and Peyer's patches are similar to those observed in the lymph nodes although usually less severe. Tissue sections of bone marrow are consistently hypercellular, owing to generally reactive marrows and perivascular accumulations of lymphoblasts and reticulum cells. The evaluation of bone marrow smears confirms the presence of stem cells, lymphoblasts, and increased numbers of lymphocytes in the terminal stages of the disease. Skeletal muscle at the inoculation site is completely replaced by neoplastic cells, and perivascular cuffs of lymphoblasts and recticulum cells are present in nearly all tissues of every CT marmoset studied during the terminal stages of the disease. Hemorrhage has often been observed at the inoculation site and in the spleen, lungs, salivary glands, thymus, and lymph nodes.

In a study of the sequential development of the disease (Wolfe *et al.*, 1971) in CT marmosets the first lesion that was found to be unequivocally associated with the experimentally induced disease was observed at the im inoculation site at 7 days PI and was represented by a few reticulum cells and lymphoblasts surrounding vessels and muscle fibers and by a relative increase in the numbers of sarcolemmal nuclei (Fig. 5). It was found that the cellular infiltrate at the inoculation site increases in amount as the PI interval progresses, making it the most consistent and prominent feature of the disease through 22 days PI (Fig. 6). At 10 days PI, lesions are either still restricted to the inoculation site or are already more generalized. In the latter case mild reticular cell infiltrates in the portal tracts of the liver, mild parafollicular proliferation of mononuclear cells in the spleen, and lymphoid hyperplasia in peripheral and visceral lymph nodes are found in addition to the cellular infiltrates at the inoculation site. In lymph nodes, hyperplasia is evident in the cortical regions but the subcapsular sinuses are not obliterated. By 22 days PI, lesions are more generalized but still relatively mild. They include a mild proliferative response in the medullary areas of the thymus, mild cellular infiltrations in the adrenal cortices and in portal tracts of the liver, parafollicular proliferations in the spleen, and mild perivascular infiltrates in kidneys, lungs, and salivary glands. A slight increase in the numbers of lymphocytes is also observed in the bone marrow. The lymph nodes at 20–22 days PI intervals are characterized by diffuse cortical lymphoid hyperplasia, by partial obliteration of subcapsular sinuses, and by

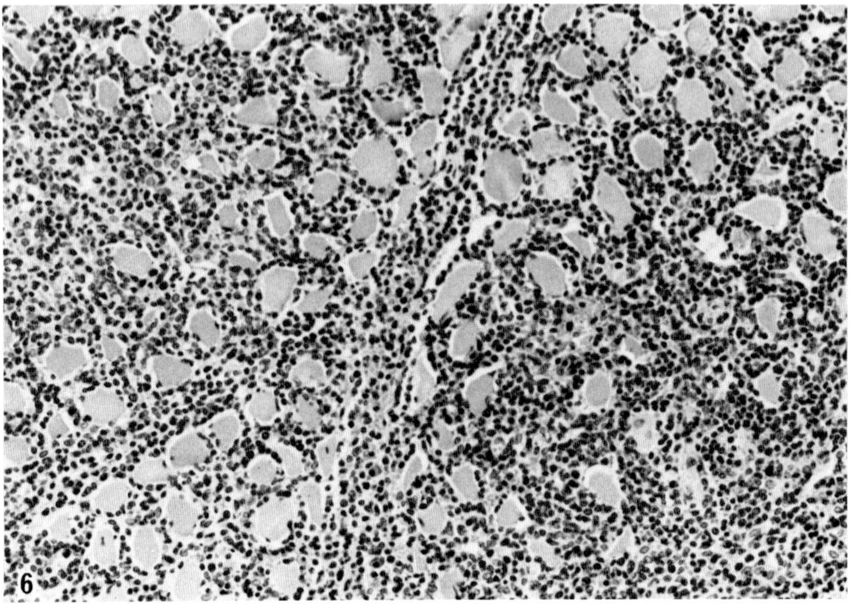

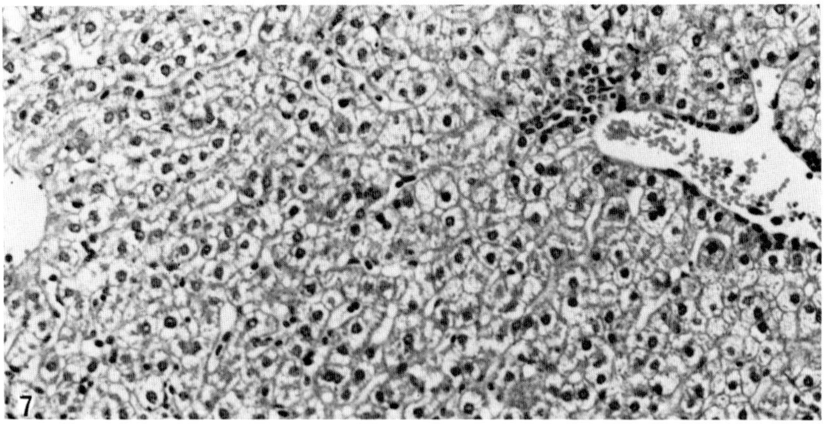

FIGS. 6 and 7. Fig. 6, severe lymphoreticular cell infiltrate surrounding and replacing skeletal muscle bundles at im inoculation site of CT marmoset 35 days after inoculation. Hematoxylin and eosin, ×40. Fig. 7, liver biopsy of marmoset 20 days after inoculation with a few lymphoreticular cells in portal tract. Hematoxylin and eosin, ×40.

prominent mantles surrounding the postcapillary venules. Compared to the relatively mild lesions observed between 7 to 22 days PI, all CT marmosets that were studied between 25 to 35 days PI had pronounced, widely disseminated cellular infiltrates. The widespread distribution of massive cellular infiltrates and the detection of abnormal circulating cells in the peripheral blood have been observed at about the same PI intervals (Figs. 7–9).

The ultrastructural features of the mononuclear cellular infiltrates are similar, irrespective of the tissue or the PI interval. The nuclei are round or oval and sometimes indented. Clumps of nuclear chromatin are present throughout the nuclei, although margination of chromatin along the nuclear membranes may be especially prominent. The nucleoli are enlarged but their fine structure appears normal. There are oval-to-round mitochondria, granular endoplasmic reticulum, Golgi complexes, and numerous free ribosomes in the cytoplasm; lysosomes are rarely found. Most cells were surrounded by relatively smooth plasma membranes. Viral particles are not observed either in the neoplastic cells or in the adjacent parenchymal cells.

In contrast to CT marmosets, the microscopic lesions in WL marmosets are highly variable from animal to animal. The lesions in some animals are compatible with lymphomas of a poorly differentiated type. The normal cytoarchitecture of the peripheral and visceral lymph nodes is completely replaced by diffuse sheets of lymphoblasts, obliterating the subcapsular sinuses and invading through the capsules into perinodal tissues. The tonsils and Peyer's patches in these animals are similarly affected. A marked lymphocytosis is reflected by pronounced hypercellularity in hepatic and splenic sinusoids, in alveolar lining capillaries of the lung, and in the vascular spaces of the adrenal glands. The bone marrow contains increased numbers of lymphocytic cells, with lymphocytes and lymphoblasts among them. In contrast to CT marmosets, the normal cytoarchitecture of the spleen and adrenal glands is retained, and there are only mild portal infiltrates in the liver. Mild perivascular lymphocytic infiltrates are present at the im inoculation sites and widely disseminated throughout the body, but are less pronounced than those observed during the terminal stages of the disease in CT marmosets. Electron microscopically, the infiltrating cells in lymph nodes, spleen, and bone marrow have similar morphologic features as those previously described for CT marmosets. In other WL marmosets the distribution of the lesions is similar to the animals described above, but the predominant cell type and the character of the lymph node lesions are different. Small- and medium-sized lymphocytes comprise the majority of the infiltrating cells in these animals. In the lymph nodes, wide lymphocytic cuffs surrounding the postcapillary venules and a diffuse lymphoid hyperplastic response replacing well-defined lymphoid follicles are present, but the subcapsular and medullary sinuses are intact and capsular invasion is not evident. Large numbers of small lymphocytes are observed in the bone marrow smears.

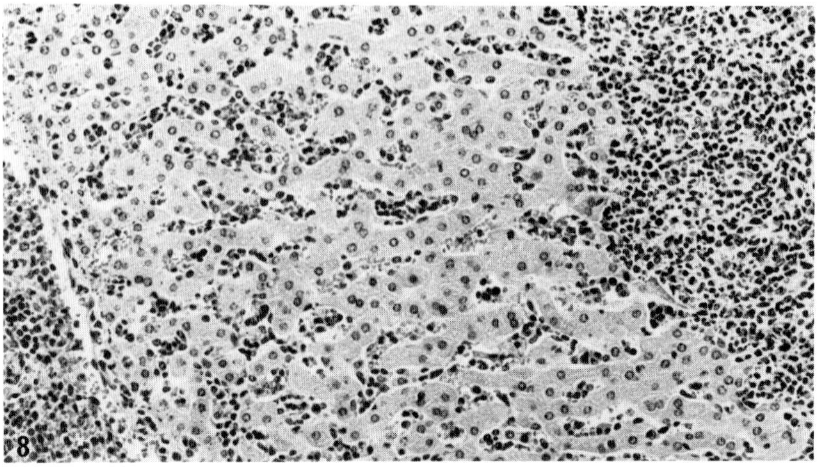

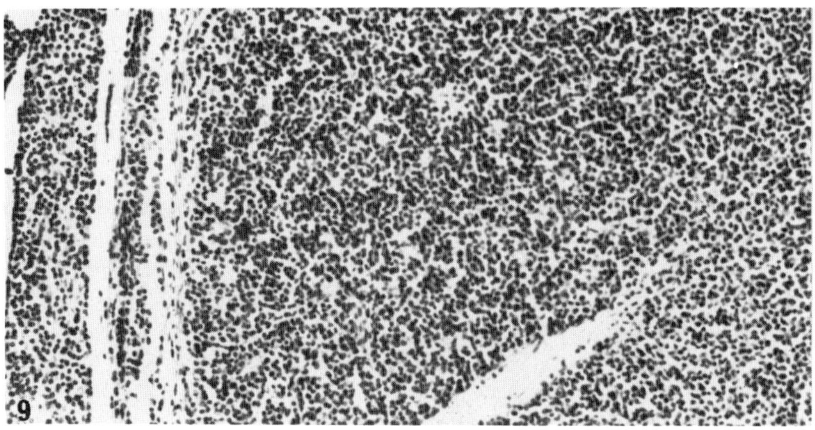

FIGS. 8 and 9. Fig. 8, liver biopsy of same marmoset shown in Fig. 7, 7 days later. Severity of disease remarkably increased, with portal tract and surrounding parenchyma replaced by dense lymphoreticular cell infiltrate, diffuse hypercellularity in sinusoids, and central vein packed with cells. Hematoxylin and eosin, ×40. Fig. 9, lymph node, also shown in Fig. 4, with normal cytoarchitecture replaced by diffuse sheet of lymphoreticular cells, capsular invasion, and numerous cells in perinodal tissue. Hematoxylin and eosin, ×40.

Nonspecific lesions have been observed in all CT and WL marmosets caught in the wild, and other lesions, of questionable specificity, have been observed only in CT marmosets. The lesions of questionable specificity were observed 7–22 days PI and included single-cell necrosis of hepatocytes, focal hepatic granulomas, and necrosis of scattered cells lining the venous sinusoids of the spleen. In the later stages of the disease, such subtle lesions, if present, were obliterated or masked by the massive cellular infiltrates and accompanying compression necrosis. Inclusion bodies were never observed at any stage of the disease. Extramedullary hematopoiesis, observed in the liver of some animals, was probably secondary to periodic collection of blood (Tischendorf and Wolfe, 1970) rather than replacement of bone marrow.

5. Reisolation of Virus from Infected Animals

In the study by Wolfe *et al.* (1971), as well as in later studies in our laboratory, virus has never been isolated from throat and stool swabs of diseased animals when the swabs are handled in a manner that excludes the presence of viable cells. In contrast HVS has been recovered from unclarified rectal specimens which probably contained viable lymphocytic cells. Herpesvirus saimiri was also isolated from an oral swab of an infected owl monkey which had developed a serious nasal discharge (Ablashi *et al.*, 1971b), and it is likely that this specimen, too, contained some viable cells.

Similarly virus could not be isolated from frozen blood or tissue extracts free of viable cells in any of the studies reported by various laboratories, nor could viral particles be detected in any blood cells or other tissues immediately after their removal from the animal, and viral antigens were not detected in the cells of such tissues. However, virus has been readily recovered when tissues of the diseased animals were cultured in cell culture either by themselves or in cocultivation cultures together with susceptible indicator cells (Falk *et al.*, 1970; Melendez *et al.*, 1970a,b; Wolfe *et al.*, 1971; Ablashi *et al.*, 1971b). If tissue of solid organs is cultured by either method, herpesvirus-like CPE develops between 5 to 28 days, the affected cells develop intranuclear inclusion bodies, virus antigens can be demonstrated by FA techniques, virus particles are seen by electron microscopy, and infectious virus can be demonstrated in such cultures by passage to susceptible indicator cells. Virus has been isolated from explant cultures of inoculation sites which had been removed surgically as early as 3 days PI. At 10 days PI, virus could be recovered from thymus, spleen, inguinal and mesenteric lymph nodes, kidneys, and lungs; at 14 days, virus was recovered from most of 22 examined tissues (including whole blood), and from 17 days on, HVS has always been recovered from whole blood and from all or nearly all examined tissues. The course of the disease and isolation of HVS from blood obtained at various stages of the disease and cocultivated with Vero cells is given in Table VII. During the terminal stages HVS was isolated from as few as 14 lymphocytic cells. Later studies showed that the virus genome was carried specifically by the lymphocytic cells and that all or nearly all lymphocytic cells were infected during the late stages of the disease. However, inclusion bodies, viral particles, viral antigens, or infectivity could never be demonstrated in the infected cells *in vivo* or immediately after removal from the animal.

C. *Herpesvirus saimiri* in Lymphocyte Cell Cultures

As discussed above HVS is carried by overtly normal lymphocytes of squirrel monkeys and by altered lymphocytes of experimentally infected and diseased animals of other susceptible nonhuman primate species. Viral functions are repressed in these cells *in vivo*, but derepression occurs rapidly when the lymphocytes are cultured *in vitro*.

Falk *et al.* (1972d) showed that when lymphocytes of infected and diseased marmosets were examined immediately after removal from the animal, they did not contain inclusion bodies; they were free of virus particles when examined by electron microscopy; extracts of the lymphocytes did not yield infectious virus; and the cells contained no viral antigens detectable by FA techniques. However, when such cells were cultured alone or when they were cocultivated with susceptible indicator cells, viral antigen became detectable in the lymphocytes as early as 24 hours after explantation.

In lymphocytes cultured alone, the most common observation was that of an intense, diffuse, fluorescence suggesting both nuclear and cytoplasmic staining of viral antigens, although in some lymphocytes specific nuclear and cytoplasmic staining could be clearly distinguished. In smears made after 24 hours of cultivation, the percentage of positive cells varied between 1 and 5%, although in smears from one marmoset up to 40% of the cells were positive. Smears prepared at 48 and 72 hours after incubation showed no increase in the number of positive cells or in the intensity of FA staining.

Of the fluorescent foci observed in coverslip preparations of lymphocytes cocultivated with Vero cells and fixed after 24 hours of incubation, 85–90% were small, individual cells which, by their morphology, could be clearly identified as lymphocytes that had attached to the underlying sheet of Vero cells. However, already at this time, 10–15% of the fluorescent foci contained a fluorescing lymphocyte surrounded by positive Vero cells, suggesting that the viral genome had already been transferred in some form from the latently infected lymphocytes to the susceptible Vero cells (Fig. 10). Cultures examined at 48 hours showed that 90–95% of the fluorescent foci contained multiple, positive cells and only a few single fluorescing cells. In the multiple-cell foci it was no longer possible to identify the originally infected lymphocyte.

Unsuccessful attempts were made to isolate HVS from supernatants and from cell-free extracts of lymphocyte suspensions of short-term cultures at

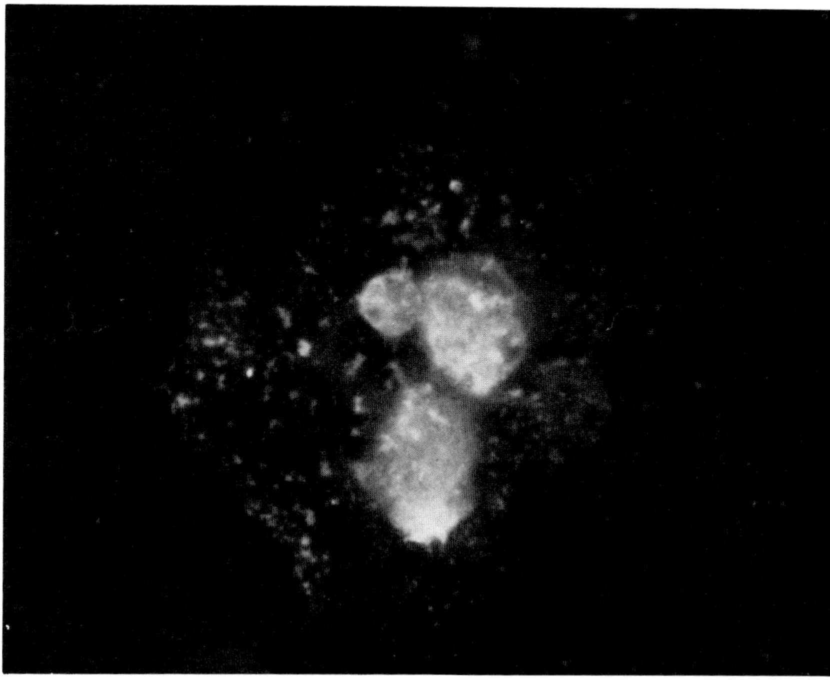

FIG. 10. Focus of small, fluorescing lymphocyte with two adjacent Vero cells showing intense nuclear staining and some granular cytoplasmic staining, × 500.

24, 48, and 72 hours of incubation. However, infectious HVS was recovered regularly from supernatants and from cell-free extracts of cocultivation cultures (lymphocytes and Vero cells), and at 120 hours titers of $10^{2.0}$ and $10^{4.5}$ $TCID_{50}$/ml, respectively, were obtained.

Some short-term lymphocytic cultures from lymph nodes or the peripheral circulation of WL or CT marmosets gave rise to cell lines which have been maintained in serial cell culture passages indefinitely (Deinhardt *et al.*, 1972; Falk *et al.*, 1972e). A lymphocytic cell line has also been established by Rabson *et al.* (1971) from lymph nodes of a CT marmoset, and another by Ablashi *et al.* (1971b) from enlarged and fused retroperitoneal lymph nodes of an owl monkey, both of which were infected experimentally with HVS. Some of these cell lines grow as pure suspension cultures of round cells, others grow as monolayers with a cellular morphology resembling reticulum cells, or cultures consist of both types of cells, in varying proportions from passage to passage. Viral antigen could be detected in 0.1–5% of the cells. Virus could be recovered regularly by cocultivation of the cells with susceptible indicator cells, but it could be recovered from cell extracts or cell-free supernatants usually only after prolonged cultivation (40 days) of the cell lines and in low concentrations. Incomplete virus particles have been observed by Rabson *et al.* (1971) in their cell line, and an occasional incomplete and complete virion has also been observed in our cell lines, but the electron microscopic evaluation of these cell lines is still incomplete.

Infectivity of HVS-carrying cell lines was also evaluated by transplantation of live cells between unrelated marmosets (Marczynska *et al.*, 1973). The malignant cells of marmosets experimentally infected with cell-free HVS preparations were often male and female (marmosets usually give birth to twins which are hematopoietic chimeras), and this indicated that the HVS disease in marmosets must be multiclonal, consistent with the recently reported observation that a cell line derived from an infected CT marmoset contained male and female cells (Chu and Rabson, 1972). Cell lines were established from HVS-inoculated marmosets of male–male or female–female twins born in captivity, and such cells lines were transplanted to animals of the opposite sex from male–male or female–female twins (Table VIII). All inoculated animals developed typically lymphoproliferative disease, and chromosome analysis showed that although the malignant cells were initially of both donor and recipient origin, as the disease progressed, fewer and fewer donor cells were observed, and they were usually absent in preparations obtained from blood or tissue samples more than 30 days PI. This showed that the transplanted cells, before they were rejected by the recipients, transferred the viral genome in some form to the recipient's cells.

V. Discussion

Under natural conditions HVS is an inapparent, persistent infection of squirrel monkeys and possibly also of spider monkeys. More than 90% of adult squirrel monkeys have antibodies to HVS and carry the HVS genome in their lymphocytes. Infection spreads by horizontal transmission, and primary infection (at least under the conditions of a closed colony) usually occurs between 6 months and 2 years of age, without causing overt disease. Similarly disease was not observed in a few experimentally infected, antibody-free infant and adult squirrel monkeys, although these animals developed antibodies, became virus carriers, and transmitted the disease to their two cagemates. Once infected, squirrel monkeys carry HVS in a latent form in the lymphocytes for thé remainder of their lives. The site of virus multiplication after initial infection is unknown, and most viral functions are depressed once the infection reaches the chronic carrier stage. However, viral genome is almost immediately derepressed when the latently infected lymphocytes are cultured *in vitro*. A minimum of 10^4–10^5 circulating

TABLE VIII

CHROMOSOMAL ANALYSIS OF CIRCULATING LYMPHOCYTIC CELLS OF ANIMALS INOCULATED WITH CELL-FREE *HERPESVIRUS SAIMIRI* OR *HERPESVIRUS SAIMIRI*-INFECTED LIVE CELLS

	Recipient animal		Days	Chromosomal analysis of circulating lymphocytic cells	
Inoculum	Sex	Chimeric state	PI	% female	% male
Cell-free HVS	Female	Female + male	0	65	35
			14	50	50
			32	46	54
Cell-free HVS	Female	Female + male	14	75	25
			32	79	21
HVS-infected, male lymphocytic cells	Female	Female	20	100	0
HVS-infected, female lymphocyte cells	Male	Male	35	0	100
HVS-infected, female lymphocytic cells	Male	Female + male	35	10	90

lymphocytes is needed to detect virus, indicating that at least one cell in 10^4–10^5 circulating lymphocytes contains virus, but it is not known whether this is the true percentage of infected cells or if all lymphocytes are infected but only a few can be persuaded to yield viral antigens or infectious virus at any given time. Similarly, it is unclear whether transmission of the disease occurs at the same high rate as that observed in experimental colonies in the early life of wild squirrel monkeys because insufficient numbers of serum specimens from wild, living animals have been tested. The results of the few experimental infections of squirrel monkeys must also be interpreted with caution, since the parenteral route of inoculation obviously differs from the natural route and the number of experimentally infected animals is very small. Nonetheless, it is reasonable to assume from available data that infection of squirrel monkeys in the wild occurs early in life and is followed at most by a very mild and insignificant disease. A life-long carrier state follows the primary infection, but it is unknown whether this chronic infection could cause a lymphoproliferative disease later in life, perhaps in conjunction with some other chronic stimulation of the lymphoreticular system. If this occurs, it is unlikely to have been detected, and experimental chronic stimulation of the lymphoreticular stystem, or immunosuppression of chronically infected squirrel monkeys, may lead to observations of great interest and far-reaching implication.

In contrast to squirrel monkeys, some other nonhuman primate species respond to inoculation with HVS by the development of malignant and always fatal lymphoproliferative diseases, ranging from lymphomas of reticulum cell type to lymphomas of poorly differentiated cell type or lymphocytic leukemias. Animals of all ages, including newborns, are equally susceptible, and studies in marmosets that are hematopoietic chimeras show that the disease is multiclonal. While the pathogenesis of the malignant diseases induced by HVS is still not entirely understood, available experimental data make the following course probable: After parenteral inoculation. of susceptible animals, HVS infects lymphoreticular cells at the site of inoculation. The infected cells develop neither inclusion bodies, infectious virus, nor detectable amounts of viral antigens, but the cells transform and proliferate as multiple malignant clones. Whether the virus genome spreads from the transformed cells to still normal, uninfected lymphoreticular cells at local or distant sites or whether virus multiplication occurs in any other type of cells remains unknown. No evidence for virus multiplication has been found anywhere in infected animals, i.e., no virus inclusion bodies have been observed, no virus particles demonstrated by electron microscopy, no infectious virus recovered from tissue extracts, and no viral antigens demonstrated by FA techniques. However, this failure to identify a site does not exclude the possibility that virus multiplication occurs in an overlooked site. The way in which viral spread occurs among lymphoreticular cells has been partially resolved by transplantation experiments, i.e., the direct transfer (without culture *in vitro*) of circulating malignant lymphocytic cells of one sex to an animal of the opposite sex and the demonstration that the disease in the recipient was caused by recipient cells from which HVS could in turn be isolated. However, it is unclear whether transfer of HVS between lymphoreticular cells also occurs within the virus inoculated animals (without transfer to another animal) or if the transfer of HVS to recipient animal cells occurs only while transplanted cells are undergoing rejection. It is possible either that brief derepression of viral functions produces just enough infectious virus to infect recipient animal cells or that some form of direct cell-to-cell contact allows transfer of the viral genome. Establishment of transformed, non-virus-producing cell lines by infection of lymphocytes of chimeric animals *in vitro*, the cloning of such lines until they contain only cells of one sex, and reinoculation back into the animal from which the cells were originally obtained may clarify our understanding of the process of virus spread. Transplantation antigen incompatibility should not affect survival of these cell lines *in vivo*, or it should be limited to those cell membrane antigens altered by the HVS infection, a situation similar to the condition existing in animals inoculated with cell-free HVS preparations.

Another, and extremely puzzling, aspect of HVS-induced disease is the development of high-titered neutralizing antibodies without detectable formation of viral antigens, both in latently infected squirrel monkeys and in infected animals with lymphoproliferative disease. It is possible that viral antigens are produced at an unidentified site, but it is equally possible that those lymphocytic cells which first become infected and carry the virus genome are also those cells which produce antiviral antibodies. The various cell lines established from diseased animals are being tested for the production of antiviral antibodies, but no immunoglobulins have been detected on the cell surface by FA techniques, a negative "finding" which does not exlude the possibility that globulins are excreted by these cells. Even if globulin production cannot be detected in the cell cultures by concentration of culture media, cells may produce globulins when they are growing under the much more optimal conditions *in vivo*.

The mechanism responsible for repression of most viral functions in infected lymphoreticular cells *in vivo* and the almost immediate, partial derepression *in vitro* poses another puzzle. Preliminary experiments indicate that a temperature effect is unlikely to be responsible because cells grown at temperatures ranging from 35° to 40° C behave similarly, nor is control of viral function brought about by the presence per se of circulating antibodies to HVS because viral expression is also suppressed in HVS-infected cells early after infection when no circulating antibodies are detectable. Evidence that cells other than lymphoreticular cells are susceptible to infection with HVS *in vivo* is lacking, and the isolation of HVS from explant cultures of tissues from all organs of infected animals is probably due to the presence of infected lymphoreticular cells in these explant cultures. The resistance of the tissue cells *in vivo* and their susceptibility *in vitro* is probably the result of cell surface changes that occur during *in vitro* culture, similar to the change in susceptibility of kidney cells to enteroviruses after explantation into *in vitro* culture (Casto and Hammon, 1969).

Last, but not least, an understanding is needed of the reasons why HVS causes a latent persistent infection in squirrel monkeys and a rapidly progressing malignant lymphoproliferative disease in some other nonhuman primate species. The reasons may lie at the cellular level, i.e., infection of squirrel monkey cells usually results in inapparent infection without cell transformation, whereas infection of cells of those animals which develop malignant disease in response to HVS infection is generally followed by cell transformation. Knowledge of the reasons for this difference in virus–host cell interaction by the cells from the various primate species should provide a much better understanding of the transformation process. Is the HVS genome integrated into the host cell genome at different sites, and does this direct the outcome either to an inapparent or a transforming infection? Or do cells transform in both types of animals (squirrel monkeys and those primate species which develop overt disease) to be eliminated by squirrel monkeys but not by animals of other species? Or is the infection age dependent, i.e., does primary infection in early life induce an inapparent infection with ensuing immunity (i.e., wild squirrel monkeys) whereas primary infection of adult animals (most experimental studies) causes malignant disease? However, in at least some experiments, the outcome of experimental infection of marmosets is uninfluenced by the age of the animals, and adult, antibody-free squirrel monkeys in one study were as resistant to infection with HVS as infants. It would be necessary to assume that animals of susceptible species have a specific immunological paralysis to tumor-specific, nonviral transplantation antigens of the HVS-transformed cells (the animals produce good antiviral neutralizing antibodies) or that squirrel monkeys possess specific sensitivity to these antigens in order to explain the difference in response of animals of these different species to infection with HVS. It would be interesting to know whether the cell membrane antigens of cells infected persistently with HVS are altered and whether viral antigens similar to the early antigens of EBV develop in superinfected or primary infected cells (Klein, Chapter 16). It is hoped that current studies of these antigens and of the circulating antibody and cell-mediated immune responses of the infected animals will answer some of these questions in the near future.

Whether any of the herpesviruses associated with malignant diseases are the actual cause of these diseases or whether they act only as activators for ubiquitous "oncogenes" in form of C-type RNA virus has been questioned. For HVS the postulates of Koch for an association of an infectious agent with a disease have been fulfilled, and few infectious agents induce their corresponding disease with as much regularity as HVS induces malignant disease in susceptible animal species. In addition, the fact that HVS-infected animals do not develop antibodies to the interspecies group-specific (GS) antigen(s) of mammalian C-type viruses, that GS antigen could not be detected in HVS-induced lymphoma tissues, and that no C-type virions have been seen in these tissues by electron microscopy speaks against the oncogene activation theory. However, the presence of classes of RNA in Burkitt's lymphoma cells, which can be hybridized with the DNA product of mouse leukemia virus RNA-dependent DNA polymerase, as demonstrated recently by Kufe *et al.* (1973), is suggestive evidence for the activation of a C-type RNA virus oncogene in Burkitt's lymphoma cells. Similar studies with the HVS carrier cell lines and lymphoma tissues are incomplete, and until current hybridization experiments yield clear results, the question of a possible activation of an RNA oncogene by HVS, although unlikely, must be left open.

Herpesvirus saimiri is similar in some respects to other herpesviruses which have been associated with neoplasia and which all, in contrast to the RNA tumor viruses, appear to be transmitted horizontally. As in Marek's disease, EB virus-associated Burkitt's lymphoma or carcinoma of the retropharyngeal space, virus cannot be found in the actual tumor tissue. In contrast to Marek's disease, but as in EB virus-induced infectious mononucleosis or EB virus-associated neoplasias, a site of multiplication *in vivo* of HVS has not been identified. Both EB virus and HVS appear to infect only lymphoreticular cells *in vivo*, resulting either in a completely inapparent or a transforming infection of the cells. The lymphoproliferative disease following primary EB virus infections is self-limiting, probably through rejection of the transformed cells by immunological mechanisms (Junge *et al.*, 1971), but it is followed by persistence of the virus genome in normal lymphocytic cells. The causal association of EB virus to Burkitt's lymphoma or to carcinoma of the retropharyngeal space, which occur long after the primary infection, remains an open question. In contrast, primary HVS infection in its natural host does not seem to be associated with transformation of the infected cells, but, like EB virus in man, HVS infection of squirrel monkeys leads to a chronic carrier state similar to the carrier state of EB virus in man. Herpesvirus saimiri regularly produces malignant lymphoproliferative diseases in a number of animal species other than its natural host, and this may also prove to be true for EB virus (T. Shope and G. Miller, personal communication). The HVS-induced experimental disease, in its frequency of occurrence and rapidity of progression, is similar to neurolymphomatosis induced by MDV in chickens. It is interesting to note that, whereas in HVS infections it is the species of animal which decides the outcome of the infection, in Marek's disease two almost identical herpesviruses have been isolated, one of which, MDV, causes neurolymphomatosis, whereas the other, HVT, only causes an inapparent infection in either species: chicken or turkey. Infection with HVT renders chickens immune to subsequent tumor induction by MDV, providing an ideal means for stimulating natural protection against a neoplastic disease.

Too little is known about other mammalian "oncogenic" herpesviruses, i.e., the rabbit lymphoma virus (Hinze, 1971) or guinea pig herpesvirus (Hsiung and Kaplow, 1970), to compare them with HVS.

VI. Addendum

1. Herpesvirus Ateles

Additional herpesviruses with characteristics similar to HVS and HVA have been isolated recently from blood lymphocytes of healthy spider monkeys (Deinhardt *et al.*, 1973). It now appears that there are at least 3 groups of oncogenic simian herpesviruses [all isolates of HVS, isolates of HVA (Melendez *et al.*, 1971a, 1972), and HVA isolates (Deinhardt *et al.*, 1973)] all of which, although sharing some antigenic characteristics, are antigenically distinct from each other.

2. Natural Disease in Squirrel Monkeys

In recent studies HVS was isolated from cell-free throat swabs of experimentally or naturally infected squirrel monkeys (L. A. Falk, L. G. Wolfe, and F. Deinhardt, unpublished observation). Virus excretion from the oropharynx was demonstrated persistently or intermittently over prolonged periods of time (> 6 months) making oral or nasal transmission of HVS in nature highly probable.

3. Herpesvirus saimiri in Lymphocyte Cell Cultures

All lymphoblastoid cell lines derived from HVS-induced lymphomas or leukemias examined so far have T cell characteristics (Wallen *et al.*, 1973; G. Klein, personal communication; L. A. Falk, L. G. Wolfe, and F. Deinhardt, unpublished observation). This is interesting because all EB virus-transformed simian cell lines have B cell characteristics. Why, despite all the other close similarities that link HVS and EB virus, the 2 viruses have such a narrow tropism for T or B cells, respectively, is puzzling. However, marmosets and owl monkeys are not the natural hosts for HVS and the disease caused by HVS in these species is much more generalized and explosive than EB virus in man. It will be important to establish whether HVS or HVA cause any disease in their natural hosts and whether the lymphoproliferative cells in such instances have B or T cell characteristics. Lymphomas induced by another herpesvirus, Marek's disease virus of chickens, have recently been shown to be of T cell origin, whereas lymphomas induced by the RNA leukosis viruses appear to be of B cell origin. Yet the cells of many of the murine leukemias induced by RNA viruses have T cell markers, and only few have the characteristics of B cells. It was also shown that radiation-induced murine lymphatic leukemias were probably of T cell origin, whereas chemical carcinogen-induced disease appeared to be caused by malignant proliferation of B cells. These interrelationships need much further study and a more definitive characterization of B and T cells, but they may hold important clues to understanding chemical carcinogenesis and the pathogenicity and oncogenicity of herpesviruses and of C-type RNA viruses acting alone or in concert.

4. Antigens of HVS

Antigens similar to the early antigens (EA) and viral capsid antigens (VCA) of EB virus have recently been demonstrated for HVS (Klein *et al.*, 1973). The appearance of these antigens in HVS-infected cells and the antibody responses of naturally or experimentally infected animals are very similar to EB virus in man, and further study of the antigen–antibody relationships in the HVS model should yield further insights into the rôle of immune responses in the development of latent carrier states or malignant lymphoproliferative diseases.

References

Ablashi, D. V., Armstrong, G. R., Heine, U., and Manaker, R. A. (1971a). *J. Nat. Cancer Inst.* **47**, 241–244.

Ablashi, D. V., Loeb, W. F., Valerio, M. G., Adamson, R. H., Armstrong, G. R., Bennett, D. G., and Heine, U. (1971b). *J. Nat Cancer Inst.* **47**, 837–855.

Barahona, H. H., and Melendez, L. V. (1971). *Proc. Soc. Exp. Biol. Med.* **136**, 1163–1167.

Casto, B. C., and Hammon, W. McD. (1969). *Proc. Soc. Exp. Biol. Med.* **132**, 154–160.

Chu, E. W., and Rabson, A. S. (1972). *J. Nat. Cancer Inst.* **48**, 771–775.

Daniel, M. D., Melendez, L. V., Hunt, R. D., King, N. W., and Williamson, M. E. (1970). *Bacteriol. Proc.* p. 195.

Daniel, M. D., Rabin, H., Barahona, H. H., and Melendez, L. V. (1971). *Proc. Soc. Exp. Biol. Med.* **136**, 1192–1196.

Deinhardt, F., Falk, L., Marczynska, B., Shramek, G., and Wolfe, L. (1972). *In* "Comparative

Leukemia Research 1971" (R. M. Dutcher, ed.), pp. 416–427. Karger, Basel.

Deinhardt, F., Falk, L., and Wolfe, L. G. (1973). *Cancer Res.* **33**, 1924–1936.

Falk, L. A., Wolfe, L. G., Shramek, G., and Deinhardt, F. (1970). *Proc. Cent. Soc. Clin. Res.* **43**, 80–81.

Falk, L. A., Wolfe, L. G., and Deinhardt, F. (1971). *Fed. Proc., Fed. Amer. Soc. Exp. Biol.* **30**, 514.

Falk, L. A., Wolfe, L. G., and Deinhardt, F. (1972a). *Fed. Proc., Fed. Amer. Soc. Exp. Biol.* **31**, 806.

Falk, L. A., Wolfe, L. G., and Deinhardt, F. (1972b). *J. Nat. Cancer Inst.* **48**, 1499–1505.

Falk, L. A., Wolfe, L. G., and Deinhardt, F. (1972c). *In* "Medical Primatology, 1972" (E. I. Goldsmith and J. Moor-Jankowski, eds.), Part 3, pp. 151–159. Karger, Basel.

Falk, L. A., Wolfe, L. G., Hoekstra, J., and Deinhardt, F. (1972d). *J. Nat. Cancer Inst.* **48**, 523–530.

Falk, L. A., Wolfe, L. G., Marczynska, B., and Deinhardt, F. (1972e). *Bacteriol. Proc.* p. 191.

Goodheart, C. R. (1970). *J. Amer. Med. Ass.* **211**, 91–96.

Heine, U., Ablashi, D. V., and Armstrong, G. R. (1971). *Cancer Res.* **31**, 1019–1029.

Hinze, H. C. (1971). *Infection Immunity* **3**, 350–354.

Holmes, A. W., Caldwell, R. G., Dedmon, R. E., and Deinhardt, F. (1964). *J. Immunol.* **92**, 602–610.

Holmes, A. W., Devine, J. A., Nowakowski, E., and Deinhardt, F. (1966). *J. Immunol.* **90**, 668–671.

Hsiung, G. D., and Kaplow, L. S. (1970). *In* "Comparative Leukemia Research 1969" (R. M. Dutcher, ed.), pp. 578–583. Karger, Basel.

Hull, R. N., Dwyer, A. C., Holmes, A. W., Nowakowski, E., Deinhardt, F., Lennette, E. H., and Emmons, R. W. (1972). *World Health Organ., Sci. Publ.* **235**, 137–144.

Hunt, R. D., and Melendez, L. V. (1969). *Lab. Anim. Care* **19**, 221–234.

Hunt, R. D., Melendez, L. V., King, N. W., Gilmore, C. E., Daniel, M. D., Williamson, M. E., and Jones, T. C. (1970). *J. Nat. Cancer Inst.* **44**, 447–465.

Hunt, R. D., Melendez, L. V., King, N. W., and Garcia, F. G. (1972a). *J. Med. Primatol.* **1**, 114–128.

Hunt, R. D., Melendez, L. V., and Trum, B. F. (1972b). *In* "Medical Primatology, (E. I. Goldsmith and J. Moor-Jankowski, eds.), Part 3, pp. 159–162. Karger, Basel.

Junge, U., Hoekstra, J., and Deinhardt, F. (1971). *J. Immunol.* **106**, 1306–1315.

Klein, G., Pearson, G., Rabson, A., Ablashi, D. V., Falk, L., Wolfe, L., Deinhardt, F., and Rabin, H. (1973). *Int. J. Cancer* **11**, (to be published).

Kufe, D., Magrath, I. T., Ziegler, J. L., and Spiegelman, S. (1973). *Proc. Nat. Acad. Sci. U.S.* **70**, 737–741.

Marczynska, B., Falk, L., Wolfe, L., and Deinhardt, F. (1973). *J. Nat. Cancer Inst.* **50**, 331–337.

Melendez, L. V., Daniel, M. D., Hunt, R. D., and Garcia, F. G. (1968). *Lab. Anim. Care* **18**, 374–381.

Melendez, L. V., Daniel, M. D., Garcia, F. G., Fraser, C. E. O., Hunt, R. D., and King, N. W. (1969a). *Lab. Anim. Care* **19**, 372–377.

Melendez, L. V., Hunt, R. D., Daniel, M. D., Garcia, F. G., and Fraser, C. E. O. (1969b). *Lab. Anim. Care* **19**, 378–386.

Melendez, L. V., Daniel, M. D., and Hunt, R. D. (1970a). *In* "Comparative Leukemia Research 1969" (R. M. Dutcher, ed.), pp. 751–753. Karger, Basel.

Melendez, L. V., Daniel, M. D., Hunt, R. D., Fraser, C. E. O., Garcia, F. G., King, N. W., and Williamson, M. E. (1970b). *J. Nat. Cancer Inst.* **44**, 1175–1181.

Melendez, L. V., Hunt, R. D., Daniel, M. D., Fraser, C. E. O., Garcia, F. G., and Williamson, M. D. (1970c). *Int. J. Cancer* **6**, 431–435.

Melendez, L. V., Hunt, R. D., Daniel, M. D., and Trum, B. F. (1970d). *In* "Infections and Immunosuppression in Subhuman Primates" (H. Balner and W. I. B. Beveridge, eds.), pp. 111–117. Williams & Williams, Baltimore, Maryland.

Melendez, L. V., Daniel, M. D., Barahona, H. H., Fraser, C.E.O., Hunt, R. D., and Garcia, F. G. (1971a). *Lab. Anim. Sci.* **21**, 1050–1054.

Melendez, L. V., Hunt, R. D., Daniel, M. D., Blake, B. J., and Garcia, F. G. (1971b). *Science* **171**, 1161–1163.

Melendez, L. V., Hunt, R. D., King, N. W., Barahona, H. H., Daniel, M. D., Fraser, C. E. O., and Garcia, F. G. (1972). *Nature* (*London*), *New Biol.* **235**, 182–184.

Morgan, D. G., Epstein, M. A., Achong, B. G., and Melendez, L. V. (1970). *Nature* (*London*) **228**, 170–172.

Rabin, H. (1971). *Lab. Anim. Sci.* **21**, 1032–1049.

Rabson, A. S., O'Connor, G. T., Lorenz, D. E., Kirschstein, R. L., Legallais, F. G., and Tralka, S. T. (1971). *J. Nat. Cancer Inst.* **46**, 1099–1109.

Tischendorf, P., and Wolfe, L. G. (1970). *Lab. Anim. Care* **20**, 697–702.

Wallen, W. C., Neubauer, R. H., Rabin, H., and Cicmanec, J. L. (1973). *J. Nat. Cancer Inst.* **51**, (to be published).

Wolfe, L. G., Falk, L. A., and Deinhardt, F. (1971). *J. Nat. Cancer Inst.* **47**, 1145–1162.

Chapter 19

The Lucké Renal Carcinoma of the Frog

Allan Granoff

I. Introduction

In recent years herpesviruses have been implicated in the development of a number of animal and human tumors. One of the earliest tumors of suspected virus etiology was the Lucké tumor, a renal adenocarcinoma of the common leopard frog, *Rana pipiens* (Lucké, 1934, 1938). The presence of acidophilic intranuclear inclusions similar in appearance to those found in herpes simplex infections and other virus diseases (Lucké, 1934), the cell-free transmission (Lucké, 1938, 1952), and the finding of "virus particles" similar to herpes simplex virus in certain tumor cells (Fawcett, 1956) provided the earliest evidence that herpesviruses might be oncogenic. This chapter will review the present state of information (of which there is much) and knowledge (of which there is little) of this tumor and the herpesvirus associated with it.

II. The Tumor

A. Geographic Distribution and Incidence

The north central and northeastern parts of the United States and adjacent southern Canada are the major areas where Lucké tumor-bearing frogs are found (Fig. 1). (Lucké, 1952; Lunger *et al.*, 1965; McKinnell, 1965). The frequency of tumor-bearing frogs taken directly from individual collection sites in nature may vary from < 1 to 9% (McKinnell and McKinnell, 1968), a range comparable to that obtained from data on commercially purchased frogs. Lucké reported that tumors were more prevalent in males than females (about 2:1) but he based his calculations on tumor-bearing frogs only, without indicating the total number of frogs of each sex without tumors (Lucké, 1952). McKinnell (1965) has reported an approximate 1:1 ratio between tumor incidence and sex, although in a subsequent study renal tumors were reported more common among female frogs than males (about 2:1) (Mc-

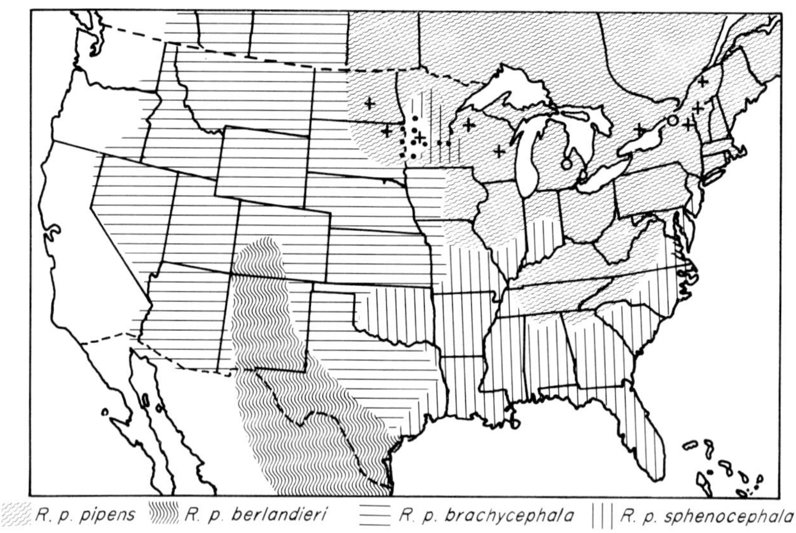

FIG. 1. Map showing the distribution of the major subspecies of *Rana pipiens* in central North America. +, collecting sites populated by frogs susceptible to spontaneous tumor formation. ○, intermediate areas in which collections failed to yield frogs capable of producing tumors spontaneously; numbers collected in these areas were small and the conclusion that those local populations are resistant may not be valid. No reliable reports of renal adenocarcinoma in the other three subspecies are on record. Heavy dots and vertical bars in Minnesota region represent two pigment-pattern mutant varieties of *R. pipiens pipiens*, designated *burnsi* and *kandiyohi*, respectively. Tumors occur in both mutant forms. [Modified from Wright and Wright (1949) and from Rafferty (1967)].

Kinnell and McKinnell, 1968). Both of McKinnell's studies took into account the total population of each sex with or without tumors and may be more reliable than Lucké's. It seems likely that both sexes are equally susceptible to tumor formation. Interestingly, when large adult frogs are held in the laboratory at 25° C for about 8 months, either isolated or under crowded conditions, 25–50% of them may develop tumors (Rafferty and Rafferty, 1961; Rafferty, 1963). A recent study (Marlow and Mizell, 1972) which included histological examination of serial sections of apparently normal frog kidneys suggests a tumor incidence approaching 100%. Confirmation of these results may be of fundamental importance in evaluating the natural history of the disease and its virus etiology.

B. Pathology

1. Gross Pathology

The Lucké tumor can range in size from small single or multicentric early tumors to large masses that have replaced most of the kidney and that may comprise half the body weight of the animal. Simultaneous development of several foci is a likely occurrence. Involvement of kidneys can be unilateral or bilateral, with the liver and lung the most frequent sites of metastases. An example of a typical bilateral tumor *in situ* is shown in Fig. 2, where only tabs of normal kidney remain.

2. Microscopic Pathology

Histologically, tumors are usually well differentiated adenocarcinomas consisting of rather large basophilic cells. Frequently such growths are cystic with pronounced papillary ingrowths (Fig. 3A). In some tumors the component cells are less atypical and are arranged in a more orderly fashion, resembling adenomas rather than adenocarcinomas. Thus, all gradations are found: from the malignant adenocarcinoma to the structurally benign adenoma, cystadenoma, and papillary cystadenoma. It is generally agreed that the tumor cells arise in proximal tubules (Rafferty, 1964), although cells other than those of the proximal tubule (e.g., Wolffian ducts and collecting ducts) may also be sites of malignant transformation (Rafferty, 1972). The frog tumor fulfills all the criteria by which a tumor is recognized as a malignant neoplasm, whether in man or other vertebrates; that is, it invades and destroys the tissue of its origin, and it can metastasize.

An important feature of the Lucké tumor, already alluded to in the Introduction, is the frequent presence of acidophilic intranuclear inclusions. The presence of these inclusions is invariably correlated with the presence of virus as determined by electron microscopy (see below). Al-

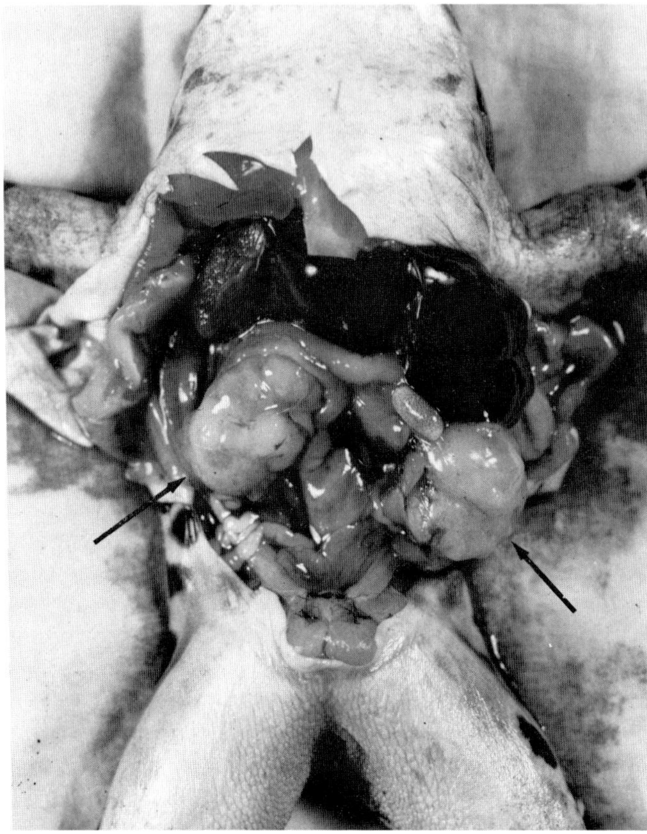

FIG. 2. Bilateral renal adenocarcinomas (Lucké tumor) (arrows) in *R. pipiens*, the leopard frog (From Granoff, 1972a.)

though Lucké (1952) in his early studies recognized that the presence or absence of inclusions had a seasonal variation (more frequent in winter and spring than in summer or autumn), this phenomenon has only recently been firmly established and is discussed more fully in Section II,C. Tumors from frogs captured in the warm summer months or held in the laboratory at 20°–25° C do not contain nuclear inclusions and have a high mitotic index (Fig. 3C). However, cells of tumors in frogs collected while in hibernation or held cold (4°–9° C) in the laboratory have inclusions. The number of inclusion-bearing cells in the neoplastic tissue varies greatly: sometimes relatively few are present; sometimes nearly every cell in some portion of the tumor is affected (Fig. 3B) and such cells appear degenerated.

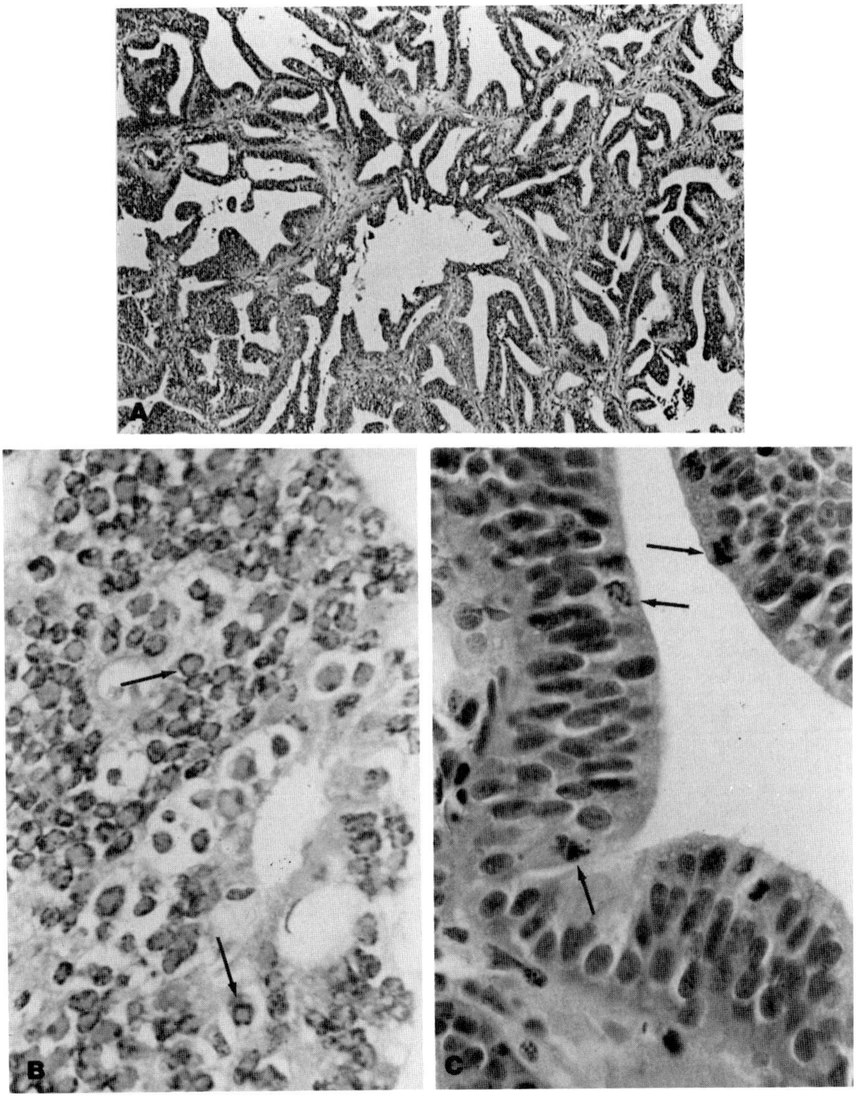

FIG. 3. (A) Low-power photomicrograph of histological section of a Lucké tumor. (B) Tumor cells with virtually all cells containing intranuclear inclusions (arrows). (C) Inclusion-free tumor cells with a number of mitotic figures present (arrows). (From Granoff, 1972a.)

The ultrastructure of tumor cells (Fawcett, 1956; Lunger *et al.*, 1965; Barch *et al.*, 1965; Zambernard and Mizell, 1965) is not relevant to the main issues of this chapter and will only be dealt with as related to the presence of herpesvirus. Fawcett (1956) was the first to describe the presence of "virus particles" similar to herpes simplex virus in cells bearing inclusions, an observation subsequently corroborated (Lunger *et al.*, 1965; Zambernard and Mizell, 1965; Zambernard *et al.*, 1966). Lunger (1964) was able to extract virus particles from inclusion-bearing tumors and showed that their ultrastructure was compatible with known herpesviruses. Figure 4A is an electron micrograph of a tumor cell containing a number of the herpesvirus particles in the nucleus in various stages of development. The cells containing virus are degenerating cells, indicating that the presence of virions is incompatible with cell survival. Figure 4B illustrates extracellular enveloped virus, and Fig. 4C, a negatively stained virus particle (162 capsomeres).

C. *Temperature and Its Relationship to the Presence of Virus*

As noted earlier, the presence of intranuclear inclusions and the presence of herpesvirus are invariably correlated. The first well-documented study on the temperature dependence of inclusion-body formation was made by Roberts (1963), who found that renal tumors of frogs held at 20°–25° C never had intranuclear inclusions whereas those of frogs held at 5° C did. Rafferty (1965) demonstrated, by biopsy, the development of intranuclear inclusions in tumor cells of frogs after 5–7 months at 4° C. Mizell *et al.* (1968) and Skinner and Mizell (1972) placed inclusion-free tumor fragments in the anterior eye chambers of *R. pipiens* as well as other species and followed the development of inclusions (light microscopy) and virus (electron microscopy) in the tumor transplants at various times after the frogs were placed at temperatures ranging from 4° to 26° C. There was a direct correlation between the presence of virus and the time and the temperature of incubation. Replication of herpesvirus was induced up to 11.5° C, with 7.5°–9.5° C the optimal range; above 11.5° C the tumor cells remained virus-free. Under optimal conditions about 30% of cells examined were virus-positive by 3 months.

Urine from tumor-bearing frogs held at 4° C frequently contains large amounts of herpesvirus while urine from tumor-bearing frogs held at 25° C does not (Granoff and Darlington, 1969). Moreover, ascitic fluid from tumor-bearing frogs held at low temperature may also contain herpesvirus (Naegele and Granoff, 1972).

Breidenbach *et al.* (1971) demonstrated that the intact host is not required for induction of virus replication at low temperature. Tissue culture explants of virus-free tumors maintained *in vitro* at 7.5° C produced virus after 3 months.

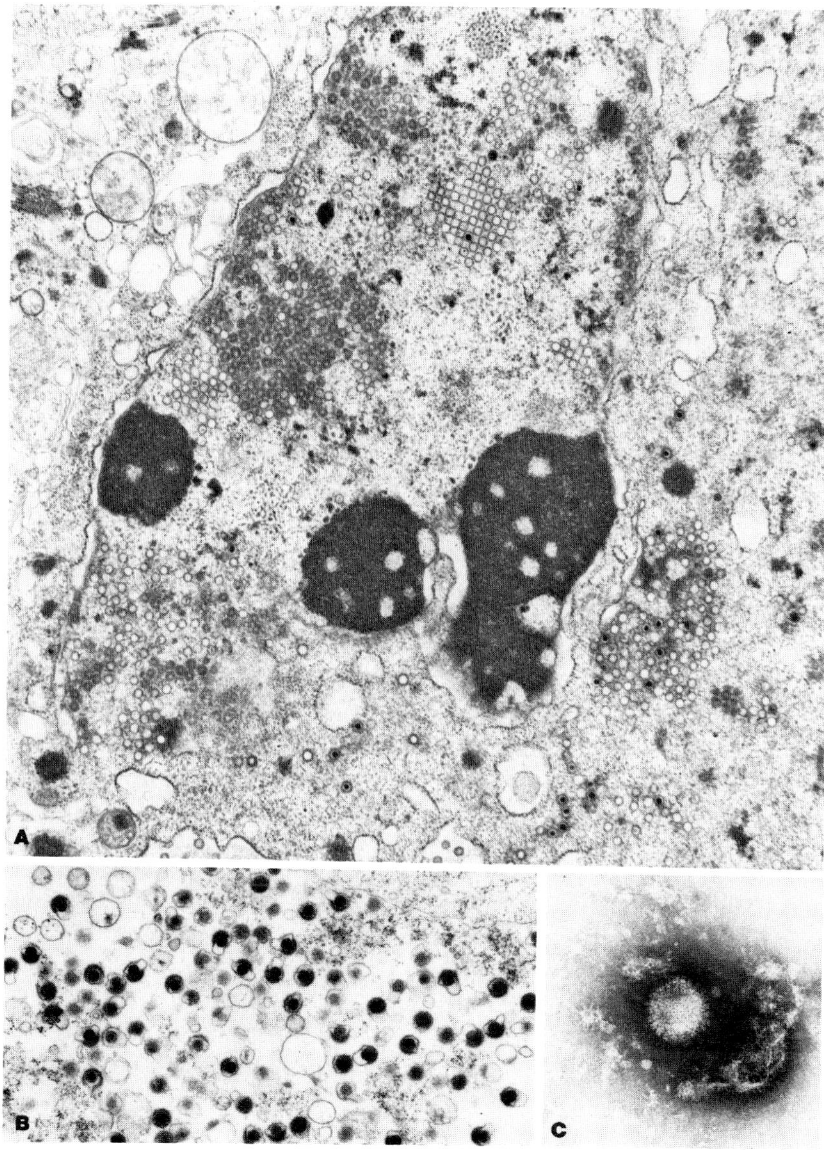

FIG. 4. (A) A thin section of an inclusion-bearing Lucké tumor cell with typical herpesvirus particles in various stages of development in the nucleus. × 12,600 (B) Enveloped virions found extracellularly. × 15,600. (C) A negatively stained nonenveloped particle showing typical herpesvirus morphology. × 72,000. (From Granoff, 1972a.)

The opposite effect can also be demonstrated: Virus-containing tumor cells degenerate and are replaced by virus-free cells at temperatures from 15°–26° C. When frogs bearing virus-positive tumors are moved from 4° C to 20°–22° C, cellular debris and virus are observed in the lumina and no virus-containing inclusions are present by 7 days (Zambernard and Vatter, 1966). Transplantation of fragments of inclusion-positive tumors to the frog anterior eye chamber also results in disappearance of virus within 2–6 weeks at 15°–26° C (Zambernard and Mizell, 1965; Skinner and Mizell, 1972).

Evidence for transcription of viral information in virus-free tumors has been obtained (Collard *et al.*, 1973). Tumor-bearing frogs held at 20°–25° C were given [^{3}H]uridine and [^{3}H]RNA extracted from tumors hybridized with Lucké tumor herpesvirus DNA which had been obtained from herpesvirus particles isolated from the tumor and purified. Normal frog kidney RNA did not bind to viral DNA, and purified virus-specific RNA from tumors did not hybridize to cellular DNA. Thus, virus-free tumors contain herpesvirus genetic information, providing additional evidence for an etiological role of the virus in tumor formation (see Section III,B below). These data also show that the source of virus found at low temperature is the tumor cell and not some other body tissue.

It is clear from the evidence thus far accumulated that replication of the herpesvirus associated with the Lucké tumor is dependent on temperature both *in vivo* and *in vitro*. Neither the mechanism of this dependence nor the significance of the role of temperature in virus replication and Lucké tumor formation is known. Although it is possible that the cell and not the virus is the main temperature-dependent factor, there is no reason to believe that virus and cell are mutually exclusive contributors to the observed temperature effect. Worthy of note are the similarities between induction of the Lucké tumor-associated herpesvirus by cold treatment and induction of other herpesviruses of suspected oncogenicity, such as Epstein-Barr virus by 5-bromodeoxyuridine (Gerber, 1972) and herpes simplex virus type 2 by high pH (Aurelian *et al.*, 1971).

D. *Transplantability*

The Lucké tumor can be transplanted to the anterior chamber of the frog eye and once established can be serially transplanted (Lucké and Schlumberger, 1939; Schlumberger and Lucké, 1949). No significant local tumor growth results if tumor fragments or cell suspensions are implanted in other body sites (Lucké, 1952) even if the frogs are exposed to X-rays or immunosuppressive drugs (R. F. Naegele and A. Granoff, unpublished observations). However, with anterior eye transplants as well as other recipient body sites, the incidence of kidney tumors after 3–6 months has been reported to be higher than in control animals, suggesting that some agent in the transplant specifically induced development of the tumor (Lucké, 1952; Rafferty, 1964). Nevertheless, the only successful transplants of the Lucké tumor have been to the anterior eye chamber.

III. Properties of the Lucké Tumor-Associated Herpesvirus

A. *Physical and Chemical Properties*

Relatively little information is available on the physical and chemical properties of the herpesvirus physically separable from the Lucké tumor. There appears to be nothing distinctive in virus ultrastructure (Lunger, 1964; Toplin *et al.*, 1971) or in development of the virus in tumor cells as reconstructed from electron micrographs (Lunger *et al.*, 1965; Stackpole, 1969). Viral DNA is a linear, double-stranded molecule with a base composition of 45–47% guanine plus cytosine (Wagner *et al.*, 1970; Gravell, 1971).

B. *Oncogenicity*

Although the early transmission experiments of Lucké (1952) with cell-free preparations of tumors suggested a viral etiology, the results of subsequent experiments were generally equivocal (Rafferty, 1964). Experiments with adult frogs were conducted with no apparent regard for the presence or absence of nuclear inclusions in the tumors used to prepare the inoculum. The first significant advance in establishing a virus etiology of the Lucké tumor was made by Tweedell (1967), who demonstrated that as high as 90% of *R. pipiens* embryos or larvae receiving injections of cytoplasmic fractions of inclusion-containing Lucké tumors and held at 20° C developed typical renal tumors as they reached metamorphosis (Fig. 5). The material injected contained herpesvirus as determined by electron microscopy, and filtrates of this material retained activity although it was somewhat diminished. Comparable fractions of normal adult frog kidneys or inclusion-free tumors failed to induce tumors. When froglets bearing induced tumors are moved to 9° C, intranuclear inclusions appear in some tumor cells (Tweedell, 1972) as could be expected based on the information presented in Section II,C. Tumor-inducing activity is destroyed by ether (R. F. Naegele and A. Granoff, unpublished observation) and by protease or by lyophilization, but it is stable to sonication (Tweedell, 1972). Rate zonal centrifugation of cytoplasmic fractions of virus-containing tumors yields oncogenic preparations rich in enveloped herpesvirus (Mizell *et al.*, 1969). Lucké tumors have been induced in embryos of *R. clamitans* and *R. palustris*, and in interspecific

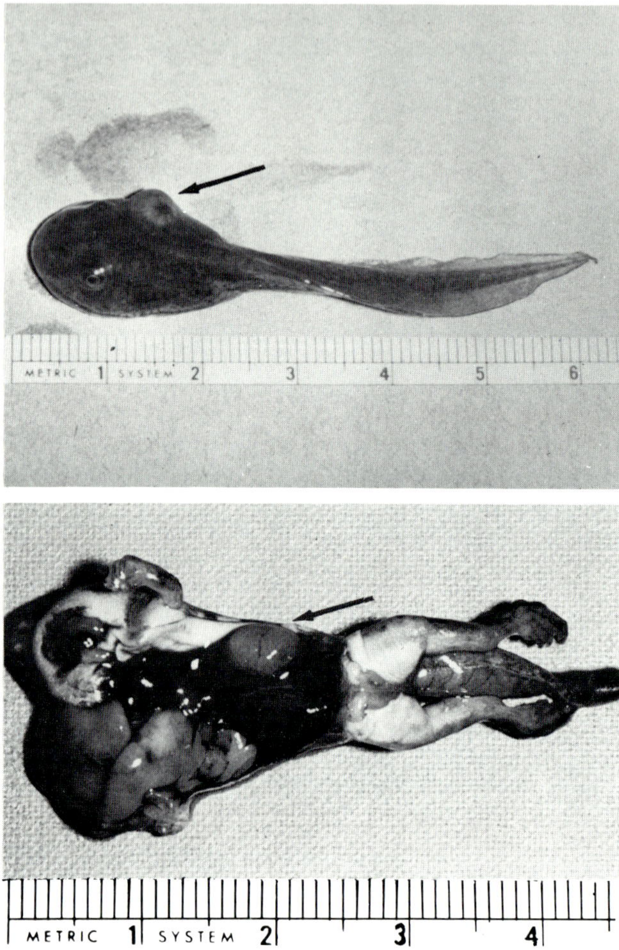

FIG. 5. A renal tumor (arrow) in a tadpole (top) and in a metamorphosing frog (bottom) induced by a cell-free herpesvirus-containing extract of a Lucké tumor. (From Granoff, 1972a.)

hybrids between *R. palustris* and *R. pipiens* (Mulcare, 1969). Transmission of the tumor also has been demonstrated with herpesvirus-containing ascitic fluid obtained from a tumor-bearing frog (Naegele and Granoff, 1972).

C. *The Question of Natural Transmission*

Tweedell (1969) demonstrated that exposure of oocytes to herpesvirus extracted from a Lucké tumor led to tumor development only when oocytes were exposed during ovulation and not when exposed after they had left the animal. He postulated that their vulnerability may be related to the nonelevated vitelline membrane and absence of jelly membranes which are added in the oviduct. Spawning takes place in the spring after frogs have emerged from hibernation, a period when herpesvirus is present in Lucké tumors. In nature the oocytes of an ovulating tumor-bearing frog with ascites (Naegele and Granoff, 1972) would be bathed in virus-containing fluid for several days, offering an ideal situation for infection.

Rafferty (1964) has suggested that contamination of spawning waters with virus-containing urine may play an important role in the life cycle of the Lucké tumor. Although virus has been found in urine of tumor-bearing frogs (Granoff and Darlington, 1969), the oocyte experiment of Tweedell tends to make this possibility less likely.

There have been conflicting reports on the effect of crowded laboratory conditions and its relationship to natural transmission, in the laboratory, of the frog renal adenocarcinoma. Several investigators have found no evidence for natural transmission under laboratory conditions (Lucké, 1952; Rafferty, 1963; Roberts, 1963) while others report that crowded conditions in the laboratory enhance natural transmission among mature frogs (DiBerardino and King, 1965). Since the conditions of each of the experiments differed, it is difficult to draw firm conclusions from them. If infection is a requisite early in frog development, as discussed above, then it is possible, as suggested by DiBerardino and King (1965), that some cofactor such as physiologic stress might promote tumor formation.

It is clear that the cell-free induction of Lucké tumors by herpesvirus-containing fractions of tumors or by ascitic fluid has been conclusively

TABLE I

VIRUSES ISOLATED FROM LUCKÉ TUMORS AND GROWN *IN VITRO*

Virus	Source	Tumor inducer	Reference
Frog virus 4 (FV 4) (herpesvirus)	Pooled urine of tumor-bearing frogs	No	Rafferty (1965), Gravell *et al.* (1968), Granoff *et al.* (1969)
Polyhedral cytoplasmic deoxyribovirus (FV 3)	Normal cultured frog kidneys; homogenates of Lucké tumors and homogenates of livers from normal or Lucké tumor-bearing frogs	No	Granoff *et al.* (1969)
Papova-like virus	Homogenates of Lucké tumors	No	Granoff *et al.* (1969)

TABLE II
CELLS TESTED FOR SUSCEPTIBILITY TO LUCKÉ HERPESVIRUS

Source	Cells
Insect	Mosquito; cabbage looper
Fish	Brown bullhead, fathead minnow, blue gill, rainbow trout (gonad)
Amphibian	African clawed toad (liver or kidney), newt (iris), leopard frog (embryo, adult kidney, Lucké tumor), spring peeper (embryo), toad
Reptile	Lizard (iguana heart, gecko lung), turtle (heart), viper (heart)
Mammalian	Baby hamster (kidney)

demonstrated in the laboratory. Less clear is how transmission and tumor induction take place in nature.

D. Virus Isolation Studies

Attempts to grow tumor-inducing herpesvirus from Lucké tumors in cultured cells have been unsuccessful (Granoff, 1972a). Several viruses have been isolated from Lucké tumors and have been propagated *in vitro* (Table I); they do not induce tumors. The properties of these viruses have been the subject of several reviews (Granoff, 1969, 1972b; Granoff *et al.*, 1969) and will not be dealt with further here. However, it is important to emphasize that one of these isolates, FV 4 (Rafferty, 1965), is a herpesvirus distinct from the one physically separable from the tumor (Gravell *et al.*, 1968; Gravell, 1971). These differences include base composition, base sequence homology, and antigenic composition.

Table II lists cells tested for susceptibility to the Lucké herpesvirus (R. F. Naegele and A. Granoff, unpublished observation). Cells exposed to herpesvirus-containing fractions of Lucké tumors have been held at 7.5° or 25°C for 3–5 months. No evidence of virus replication as determined by cytopathology, cell transformation, or electron microscopy has been obtained.

In view of the fact that several viruses can be found associated with Lucké tumors (Table I) and since the only criterion for purity of tumor-inducing preparations is electron microscopy, some caution is required in evaluating the certainty with which a herpesvirus has been established as the sole etiological agent of this tumor. The relationship of virus to tumor may not be a simple one. Indeed, it may be highly complex, possibly involving an interaction between a defective and helper virus. Isolation and propagation of the etiologic agent in tissue culture remains a high priority task, the accomplishment of which should establish etiology unequivocally and permit studies on the natural history of this tumor not presently possible.

Acknowledgments

The work reported in this chapter was supported by U.S. Public Health Service Research Grant No. CA-07055, National Cancer Institute Virus Cancer Program Contract No. 71-2134 and Childhood Cancer Research Center Grant No. CA-08480, Damon Runyon Memorial Fund for Cancer Research Grant No. DRG-1073 and by ALSAC.

References

Aurelian, L., Standberg, J. D., Melendez, L. V., and Johnson, L. A. (1971). *Science* **174**, 704.
Barch, S. H., Sharer, J. R., and Wilson, G. B. (1965). *Ann. N.Y. Acad. Sci.* **126**, 188.
Breidenbach, G. P., Skinner, M. S., Wallace, J. H., and Mizell, M. (1971). *J. Virol.* **7**, 679.
Collard, W., Thornton, H., Mizell, M., and Green, M. (1973). *Science* **181**, 448.
DiBerardino, M. A., and King, T. J. (1965). *Cancer Res.* **25**, 1910.
Fawcett, D. W. (1956). *J. Biophys. Biochem. Cytol.* **2**, 725.
Gerber, P. (1972). *Proc. Nat. Acad. Sci. U.S.* **69**, 83.
Granoff, A. (1969). *Curr. Top. Microbiol. Immunol.* **50**, 107–137.
Granoff, A. (1972a). *Fed. Proc., Fed. Amer. Soc. Exp. Biol.* **31**, 1626.
Granoff, A. (1972b). *In* "Oncogenesis and Herpesvirus" (P.M. Biggs, G. de-Thé, and L. N. Payne, eds.), pp. 171–182. International Agency for Research on Cancer, Lyon.
Granoff, A., and Darlington, R. W. (1969). *Virology* **38**, 197.
Granoff, A., Gravell, M., and Darlington, R. W. (1969). *In* "Recent Results in Cancer Research." (M. Mizell, ed.), pp. 279–295. Springer-Verlag, New York.
Gravell, M. (1971). *Virology* **43**, 730.
Gravell, M., Granoff, A., and Darlington, R. W. (1968). *Virology* **36**, 467.
Lucké, B. (1934). *Amer. J. Cancer* **20**, 352.
Lucké, B. (1938). *J. Exp. Med.* **68**, 457.
Lucké, B. (1952). *Ann. N.Y. Acad. Sci.* **54**, 1093.
Lucké, B., and Schlumberger, H. (1939). *J. Exp. Med.* **70**, 257.
Lunger, P. D. (1964). *Virology* **24**, 138.
Lunger, P. D., Darlington, R. W., and Granoff, A. (1965). *Ann. N. Y. Acad. Sci.* **126**, 289.
McKinnell, R. G. (1965). *Ann. N.Y. Acad. Sci.* **126**, 85.
McKinnell, R. G., and McKinnell, B. K. (1968). *Cancer Res.* **28**, 440.
Marlow, P., and Mizell, S. (1972). *J. Nat. Cancer Inst.* **48**, 823.
Mizell, M., Stackpole, C. W., and Halperen, S. (1968). *Proc. Soc. Exp. Biol. Med.* **127**, 808.
Mizell, M., Toplin, I., and Isaacs, J. J. (1969). *Science* **165**, 1134.
Mulcare, D. J. (1969). *In* "Recent Results in Cancer Research" (M. Mizell, ed.), pp. 240–253. Springer Verlag, New York.
Naegele, R. F., and Granoff, A. (1972). *J. Nat. Cancer Inst.* **49**, 299.
Rafferty, K. A., Jr. (1963). *Science* **141**, 720.
Rafferty, K. A., Jr. (1964). *Cancer Res.* **24**, 169.
Rafferty, K. A., Jr. (1965). *Ann. N.Y. Acad. Sci.* **126**, 3.
Rafferty, K. A., Jr. (1967). *In* "Renal Neoplasia" (J. S. King, ed.), pp. 301–315. Little, Brown, Boston, Massachusetts.
Rafferty, K. A., Jr. (1972). *In* "Oncogenesis and Herpesviruses" (P. M. Biggs, G. de-Thé, and L. N. Payne, eds.), pp. 159–170. International Agency for Research on Cancer, Lyons.
Rafferty, K. A., Jr., and Rafferty, N. S. (1961). *Science* **133**, 702.
Roberts, M. E. (1963). *Cancer Res.* **23**, 1709.
Schlumberger, H., and Lucké, B. (1949). *Cancer Res.* **9**, 52.

Skinner, M. S., and Mizell, M. (1972). *Lab. Invest.* **26**, 671.

Stackpole, C. W. (1969). *J. Virol.* **4**, 75.

Toplin, I., Mizell, M., Sottong, P., and Monroe, J. (1971). *Appl. Microbiol.* **21**, 132.

Tweedell, K. S. (1967). *Cancer Res.* **27**, 2042.

Tweedell, K. S. (1969). *In* "Recent Results in Cancer Research" (M. Mizell, ed.), pp. 229–239, Springer-Verlag-New-York

Tweedell, K. S. (1972). *Proc. Soc. Exp. Biol. Med.* **140**, 1246.

Wagner, E. K., Roizman, B., Savage, T., Spear, P. G., Mizell, M., Durr, F. E., and Sypowicz, D. (1970). *Virology* **42**, 257.

Wright, A. H., and Wright, A. A. (1949). "Handbook of Frogs and Toads of The United States and Canada." Cornell Univ. Press (Comstock), Ithaca, New York.

Zambernard, J., and Mizell, M. (1965). *Ann. N.Y. Acad. Sci.* **126**, 127.

Zambernard, J. and Vatter, A. E. (1966). *Cancer Res.* **26**, 2148.

Zambernard, J., Vatter, A. E., and McKinnell, R. G. (1966). *Cancer Res.* **26**, 1688.

Chapter 20
Chemotherapy—Molecular Aspects

William H. Prusoff and Barry Goz

A discussion of a "mechanism" of action of an antiviral agent can reach various degrees of sophistication. Do we mean a site of inhibition, such as a herpes simplex virus (HSV) infection of the corneal epithelium, or are we concerned with which enzyme is inhibited or which biopolymer is affected, or are we concerned with the physicochemical basis for such interactions? The latter would be most informative and might afford the opportunity for rational design of antiviral agents with selective toxicity. Although approaches have been made in this direction, for example by Camerman and Trotter (1964), present accomplishments are rather meager indeed.

Several compounds have demonstrated anti-herpesvirus activity in man and hence it may be of value to discuss what is known of the molecular basis for their antiviral action (Fig. 1). Numerous compounds have anti-herpesvirus activity in cell culture but for a variety of reasons have no significant clinical potential and hence will not be discussed.

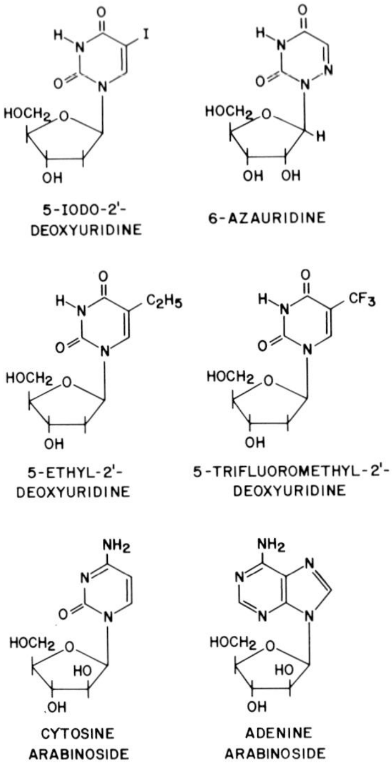

FIG. 1. Molecular structure of several nucleosides with anti-herpesvirus activity.

I. 5-Iodo-2′-Deoxyuridine (IUdR, IdUrd, IDU, Idoxuridine)

Herrmann (1961) made the original observation that IUdR and BUdR inhibit the replication of several DNA viruses *in vitro*, particularly vaccinia and herpes simplex, and Kaufman and his collaborators (references cited in Kaufman, 1965) demonstrated the efficacy of this compound in rabbits and more importantly in man. The studies in rabbit were confirmed and extended to other derivatives of IUdR by a collaborative study by groups at Yale and Johns Hopkins Universities (Perkins *et al.*, 1962). Of particular importance in establishing the specificity of IUdR was the report by Perkins *et al.* (1962) that the *ribo*nucleoside of iodouracil failed to exert any beneficial effect in the control of HSV infection of the rabbit eye under conditions in which IUdR was very efficacious. Similarly, 5-iodouracil neither prevented HSV reproduction nor affected the synthesis of DNA (Hanna, 1966). The problem of whether IUdR is a specific antiviral agent or exerts its effect by producing cell toxicity was investigated by Cramer *et al.* (1963), and they observed inhibition of herpes simplex virus at a concentration one-tenth that required to inhibit cell reproduction. Similarly, IUdR, 3′,5′-

diacetyl IUdR, and BUdR prevented the formation of infectious HSV in rabbit cornea in concentrations that did *not* affect the synthesis of DNA by the normal basal epithelial cells of the cornea (Hanna, 1966). Histological studies by Schumacher and Machemer (1966) revealed that cell regeneration in rabbits of uninfected corneal tissues that were experimentally injured is inhibited by IUdR, but cell regeneration in "normal" tissue infected with a DNA-containing virus is not.

Deoxyribonucleosides with a variety of substituents on carbon-5 of the pyrimidine moiety are of particular interest, not only because of the many biochemical reactions that they affect, but also for their application in areas of genetics, cell biology, radiobiology, and neoplasia, as well as in virology. The presence of a halogen in the 5-position of the pyrimidine moiety markedly affects the physicochemical and biological properties of the nucleoside.

The introduction of an iodine atom in place of the methyl group of thymidine results in an increase in the bulk volume, since the methyl group has a van der Waals atomic radius of 2.00, whereas that of the iodine atom is 2.15. Although the size of the resultant halogenated molecule has been increased, there does not appear to be any hindrance to its capacity to substitute for thymidine in the many enzymic reactions in which the normal metabolite participates, including incorporation into DNA. Indeed, consideration of the composition and structure of the Watson – Crick model of the DNA double helix clearly indicates that steric hindrance, because of the increased van der Waals radius, should not be a detriment to the incorporation of IUdR into DNA in substitution of thymidine. The iodine atom is well removed from the groups required for hydrogen bonding with the adenine moiety of the complementary DNA strand.

However, the replacement of the methyl group of thymidine with the iodine atom markedly affects the electron configuration of the pyrimidine moiety because of the inductive effect of the halogen; this results in more acidic dissociation constants. Because the N-1 position is substituted with the deoxyribose moiety, the proton on the N-3 position must be dissociated. The pK_a of thymidine is 9.8, whereas that of IUdR is 8.25; thus at pH 7.4, the proportion of the ionized or enolic form of IUdR is greater than that of thymidine by a factor of 34. This has obvious implications, not only in the forces binding the two strands of DNA together, but also in regard to influence on DNA replication as well as transcription. This will be discussed later.

An initial approach to understanding the molecular basis for the antiviral activity of IUdR has been described by Prusoff *et al.* (1965). These studies were concerned with the effect of IUdR and its phosphorylated derivatives on those enzymes involved with the formation of precursors of DNA-thymine in a cell-free extract of HSV-infected and noninfected cells. The question posed was whether the enzymes concerned with these biotransformations in the herpesvirus-infected cells are more sensitive to inhibition by IUdR or its phosphorylated derivatives than are the corresponding enzymes of the noninfected cells. That such a difference might exist is supported by a variety of observations. Certain viruses are known to contain specific enzymes within the virion that are introduced into the infected cell, and other viruses are known to induce, via the genome, new enzyme molecules even though the uninfected cell may normally contain the comparable enzyme. In other instances, the increased enzymic activity observed upon viral infection results from an augmentation of the host cell genome producing additional amounts of the preexisting enzyme. In the latter situation, no alteration in susceptibility to inhibition could be anticipated, whereas in the other situations described above the viral enzyme could be more, less, or equally inhibited by the appropriate analogue.

Herpesvirus infection results in a marked increase in the activity of thymidine kinase, thymidylate kinase, DNA polymerase and deoxyribonuclease. Physical differences between enzymes induced by animal viruses and their counterpart in the noninfected cell have been observed. Thus, Nohara and Kaplan (1963) demonstrated that thymidylate kinase induced by infection of rabbit kidney cells with pseudorabies virus has a markedly greater thermostability than the enzyme present in the noninfected cells; however, this may not be due to an alteration in property of the enzyme molecule, but rather to the formation of a protein factor which confers such stability (Kaplan *et al.*, 1967). Differences in heat stability and other properties of DNA polymerase and DNase were observed by Keir and Gold (1963) between the enzymes present in the uninfected host cell and the herpesvirus infected cell.

Prusoff *et al.* (1965) measured thymidine kinase activities in particle-free extracts of African green monkey kidney cells 6 and 7 hours postinfection with HSV and found a threefold increase over that present in the noninfected cells. The activity of both the infected and noninfected cells could be increased threefold by raising the assay incubation temperature from 37° to 51°C, and this procedure enabled the measurement of small changes in the activity present in the noninfected cells. Comparison of the thymidine kinase activities of infected and noninfected cell extracts showed no difference in the effect of raising the incubation temperatures, in their thermal stabilities, or in their sensitivity to the inhibitory effect of IUdR. However, Kit *et al.* (1967) did find altered properties of thymidine kinase (heat stability, response to allosteric effectors, and Michaelis constants) after infection of mouse fibroblasts with HSV.

The thymidylate kinase activities in extracts prepared from African green monkey kidney cells 5, 6, or 7 hours after infection were identical to that of the control, noninfected cells. The relative sensitivity of this activity to inhibition by 5-iodo-2′-deoxyuridylate (IdUMP) was identical (Prusoff *et al.*, 1965).

The triphosphate of IUdR was prepared (Prusoff and Chang, 1968) and shown by Bakhle and Prusoff (1969) to effectively replace on a molar basis the utilization of radioactive deoxythymidine triphosphate (dTTP) for the biosynthesis of DNA by a particulate-free extract of a murine neoplasm. Thus, the utilization of dATP for the formation of DNA was not depressed even by a fourfold excess of iododeoxyuridine triphosphate (IdUTP) over that required to produce 50% inhibition of the utilization of dTTP. In agreement with findings by Russell *et al.* (1964), infection of cells in culture with HSV results in a progressive increase in DNA polymerase activity (Sekely and Prusoff, 1969). No differences were observed by Sekely and Prusoff (1969) in the susceptibility to inhibition by IdUTP of DNA polymerase derived from uninfected cells or cells infected with HSV.

Another site of inhibition investigated is related to dTTP being not only the immediate precursor of DNA thymine, but also a feedback or allosteric inhibitor of thymidine kinase, deoxycytidylate deaminase, and cytidylate reductase, enzymes which regulate the formation of dTTP. It was to be anticipated that IdUTP would mimic deoxythymidine triphosphate in these reactions, since Okazaki and Kornberg (1964) observed BrdUTP to be as inhibitory as dTTP to *E. coli* thymidine kinase. Prusoff and Chang (1969–1970) found IdUTP to be three times more inhibitory than dTTP of thymidine kinase derived from two murine neoplasms; however, IdUTP exerted either an inhibitory or a stimulatory effect on *E. coli* thymidine kinase that was related to the pH of assay incubation (Voytek *et al.*, 1971). In relation to dTTP, IdUTP was also more inhibitory of deoxycytidylate deaminase derived from Ehrlich ascites carcinoma and L5178Y murine lymphoblastic cells (Prusoff and Chang, 1968).

No difference was observed by A. Diwan, B. Goz, and W. H. Prusoff (unpublished experiment) in susceptibility to inhibition of thymidine kinase by dTTP in noninfected cells and cells infected with HSV. However, thymidine kinase specified by HSV (Klemperer *et al.*, 1967) was reported to be significantly less susceptible to inhibition by dTTP than the enzyme present in the uninfected host cell.

A similar comparison was made by Diwan and Prusoff (1968) of the relative susceptibility of deoxycytidylate deaminase to inhibition by IdUTP and by dTTP. Levels of the enzyme present in uninfected cells and cells infected with HSV showed that although the amount of enzymic activity increased almost threefold during infection, there was no alteration in the relative susceptibility to inhibition of the "induced" enzyme by either IdUTP or dTTP.

The binding of the deoxyribonucleoside triphosphates by these allosteric enzymes is believed to depend upon weak secondary forces, such as hydrogen bonding, salt linkage, and van der Waals forces, and to result in conformational changes (allosteric transitions) in the protein. Thus, the inhibition can be removed quickly either by an increase in the normal substrate or a reduction of the concentration of the inhibitor of the enzymic process to a low level. The binding of dCTP by deoxycytidylate deaminase is either stronger or at least more influential than is that of either dTTP or IdUTP, since equimolar amounts of dCTP reverse completely the inhibition exerted by preincubation with the allosteric inhibitor for even 30 minutes (Fiala and Fiala, 1965; Prusoff and Chang, 1968). These effects are summarized in Fig. 2.

Because the above sites of inhibition are of the competitive type or are readily reversible, we believe that the primary inhibitory effect of IUdR resides in an event that is subsequent to incorporation into the viral DNA in substitution of the thymidine moiety. A number of very important biochemical and physical effects result from such incorporation of halogenated deoxyribonucleosides into DNA (Szybalski, 1962; Prusoff *et al.*, 1965) that include (1) increased rate of mutation, (2) increased errors in protein synthesis, (3) inhibition of replication, and (4) increased sensitivity to X, ultraviolet, and near-visible radiations.

Incorporation of halogenated uracil derivatives (BUdR, IUdR) into nucleic acid of animal viruses has been demonstrated (Easterbrook and Davern, 1963; Kaplan and Ben-Porat, 1964, 1966; Prusoff *et al.*, 1963; Kaplan *et al.*,

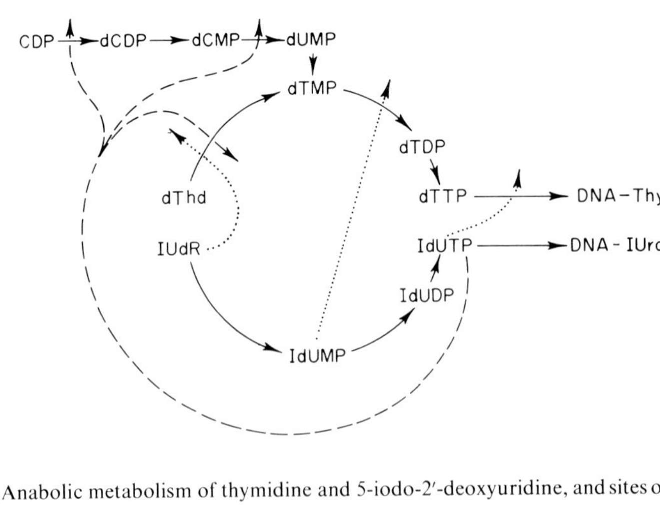

FIG. 2. Anabolic metabolism of thymidine and 5-iodo-2′-deoxyuridine, and sites of inhibition by 5-iodo-2′-deoxyuridine and its phosphorylated derivatives. The intersection of the solid lines by the broken lines depicts a site of inhibition. The dotted lines indicate sites of substrate competitive inhibition, and the dashed lines indicate sites of negative feedback (or allosteric) inhibition.

1965; Kamiya *et al.*, 1965). These halogenated deoxyribonucleosides have no direct effect on extracellular HSV (Ey *et al.*, 1964) and no effect on the adsorption of viruses to cells (Smith, 1963), but they very markedly inhibit the formation of infectious herpesvirus particles, for the ratio of virus particles to infectious virus may be as high as $10^7:1$ (Smith and Dukes, 1964). Schneweis (1965), however, reported that HSV grown in the presence of BUdR lost its ability to be adsorbed. The virus particles formed in the presense of IUdR or BUdR are abnormal in appearance (Smith and Dukes, 1964; Prusoff *et al.*, 1963; Easterbrook and Davern, 1963).

The biochemical basis for the antiviral activity of IUdR and BUdR for pseudorabies virus has been investigated by Kaplan and Ben-Porat (1966) and Kaplan *et al.* (1965). Within 16 hours after infection, BUdR decreased the infectious titer by about 2 logs and IUdR by about 4 logs. The synthesis of viral DNA and of viral antigens were not only not impaired by these analogues, but were formed in greater amounts in drug-treated infected cells relative to untreated infected cells. DNA thymidine was replaced by IUdR to the extent of more than 50%! Furthermore, the DNA formed in the presence of IUdR was sensitive to DNase whereas that formed in the absence of drug was in a form resistant to such enzymic degradation—presumably encapsidated. These investigators posed the question whether halogenated viral DNA was not capable of being encapsidated into a viral particle because of steric reasons or an inability of the halogenated DNA to direct the formation of functional protein required for maturation.

Striking differences were observed between the action of BUdR and IUdR. Whereas the DNA produced in either the BUdR-treated or the control cells is in a form that is insensitive to deoxyribonuclease, only a very small amount of the DNA formed in the presence of IUdR is insensitive to this enzyme. Furthermore, BUdR permits the formation of complete virus particles, even though these are not infectious, but IUdR treatment prevents the formation of significant amounts of either normal or abnormal-appearing virus particles.

The IUdR substituted DNA could be incorporated into virus particles provided thymidine was included during incubation either before or after the formation of this halogenated DNA. Kaplan and Ben-Porat (1966), therefore, concluded that replacement of DNA thymidine by IUdR results in the formation of either no protein coat or an inadequate one. The inclusion of thymidine presumably enabled the synthesis of an adequate amount of functional viral DNA to permit proper protein synthesis resulting in the appropriate assembly of the virus particle. Those complete virus particles that contain DNA substituted with BUdR were postulated to be noninfectious because of either an inability to induce early enzymes or a failure to be adsorbed, to penetrate, or to uncoat because of a faulty protein coat (Kamiya *et al.*, 1965; Kaplan and Ben-Porat, 1966).

The relationship between IUdR, the synthesis of substitued viral DNA, and the formation of the virus particle had been previously investigated. Roizman *et al.* (1963) found IUdR inhibited herpes simplex replication but could not detect incorporation of this analogue into viral DNA, probably because the specific activity of the radioactive analogue used in their experiments was too low. Smith (1963) and Smith and Dukes (1964) found that HSV grown in the presence of IUdR required 10^7 particles to produce the equivalent infectivity produced by a single normal virus particle. Whether these particles contained IUdR in their DNA or even if the defective particles contained DNA per se was not established. These investigators interpreted their results to indicate that the assembly of viral components rather than their production was prevented by IUdR. The interpretation that the virus may produce a faulty protein coat is supported by the observation of Schneweis (1965) who observed that HSV particles formed in the presence of BUdR had lost their ability to be adsorbed to host cells.

Of relevance are the studies in other non-herpesvirus systems since they serve to indicate the varied effect that one may observe with a single drug. Thus, Hirt (1966) found incorporation of BUdR into either one or two strands of polyoma virus DNA had *no* adverse effect on replication; however, the amount incorporated may be a factor. Prusoff *et al.* (1963) found radioactive IUdR to be incorporated into particulate vaccinia virus DNA to the extent of 18% replacement of viral DNA thymidine. McCrea and Lipman (1967) examined the DNA in normal and IUdR-substituted DNA derived from vaccinia virus by a modification of the Kleinschmidt procedure, and they found the IUdR-substituted DNA liberated by osmotic shock extensively fragmented, in contrast to the normal DNA which was consistently relatively long and continuous. McCrea and Lipman (1967) proposed that the decreased pock-forming ability of the IUdR-substituted vaccinia virus particles may be attributed, in part, to the increased fragility of the DNA when released within the host cell by the "uncoating enzyme."

Similarly, Easterbrook and Davern (1963), in a comprehensive study of the effect of BUdR on the replication of vaccinia virus, found a 13% replacement of DNA thymidine by BUdR based on bouyant density gradient analysis of the isolated DNA. They also observed, as did Prusoff *et al.* (1963) and McCrea and Lipman (1967) with IUdR, that the BUdR-substituted DNA was smaller in molecular weight and heterogeneous in density as compared with unsubstituted vaccinia DNA. Joklik (1964) similarly observed that vaccinia virus DNA, in which 13% of the thymidine was replaced by BUdR, was prematurely degraded when uncoated within the host cell.

All these observations may be readily explained if one considers the consequences of incorporation of a halogenated uracil into viral DNA. In those studies which failed to observe incorporation of IUdR or BUdR into viral

DNA one must consider the sensitivity of the analytical methods employed during their investigations. In an attempt to provide understanding of the forces that come into play when a halogenated uracil is present in the herpesvirus DNA, we are forced to consider other systems. Perhaps such consideration will stimulate comparable studies with herpesvirus.

Thus, studies by Goz and Prusoff (1968, 1970a), using phage T4, found a normal yield of viral particles when cells were infected in the presence of IUdR. Infection with IUdR-substituted T4 resulted in the induction of markedly decreased levels of virus-induced enzymes such as deoxycytidylate hydroxymethylase, dihydrofolate reductase, and lysozyme. Immunological studies by Aamodt and Goz (1970) indicated a reduced synthesis of enzyme molecules rather than a normal rate of synthesis of enzyme molecules that were inactive. Furthermore, phenotypic and genotypic rescue experiments by Goz and Prusoff (1970a) revealed that IUdR substitution for thymidine in the phage genome caused a differential inactivation. It has been established by Szybalski *et al.* (1966) that some genes are richer in thymidine residues; therefore the differential inactivation observed by Goz and Prusoff (1970a) may well be related to such differential substitution of IUdR for thymidine in the various genes. Similarly, Stellwagen and Tomkins (1971a,b) showed that incorporation of BUdR into the DNA of a mammalian cell system also caused a selective inhibitory effect of certain genes, as evidenced by a decreased formation of specific enzymes. Thus, they observed an impairment in the synthesis of tyrosine aminotransferase, lactate dehydrogenase, alcohol dehydrogenase, and glucose-6-phosphate dehydrogenase, but *not* of malate dehydrogenase, acid phosphatase, or alanine aminotransferase. Stellwagen and Tomkins (1971a,b) proposed that BUdR exerts its effect by slowing the rate of transcription of certain messenger RNA.

The early studies by Camerman and Trotter (1964) of the crystal and molecular structure of IUdR by X-ray diffraction may have provided a physico-chemical explanation for the observations of Goz and Prusoff (1968, 1970a) and Stellwagen and Tomkins (1971a,b). Camerman and Trotter (1964) found an unusually short intermolecular distance of 2.96 Å between the iodine and the oxygen of the carbonyl group in relation to the calculated distance of 3.55 Å. They postulated that the ability of iodine to form charge transfer bonds may cause an increased interchain attraction that could either prevent or delay the synthesis of viral DNA, thereby permitting normal host defense mechanisms to operate. A logical extension of such an interaction would apply to the process of transcription and hence the observed decreased rate of synthesis of enzymes in the mammalian cell (Stellwagen and Tomkins, 1971a,b) and in the bacterial virus system (Goz and Prusoff, 1968).

The failure of herpesvirus to produce functional protein required for encapsidation of the IUdR-substituted viral DNA may be explained classically by the increased probability of base pair errors caused by the lower pK_a of IUdR ($pK_a = 8.25$) relative to thymidine ($pK_a = 9.8$). Thus the halogenated deoxyribonucleoside, being in the anionic form with a greater probability than that of thymidine, has an increased opportunity to either enter DNA based-paired to guanine rather than adenine or if incorporated appropriately in base pair with adenine may during transcription, when in the enolic form, cause the introduction of a guanine deoxyribonucleotide into mRNA in place of deoxyadenylate. This could subsequently result during translation in the formation of proteins unable to perform their role during virus assembly or maturation.

It is clear that the specific defect incurred by the incorporation of IUdR into herpesvirus DNA has not been elucidated; however, it is also quite apparent that the techniques of protein isolation, such as polyacrylamide gel electrophoresis, electrofocusing, as well as combination of these two techniques with other methods of protein separation, now afford an opportunity to approach this problem with more resolve. The critical observations that have been made are that viral DNA is synthesized (with varying degrees of substitution of DNA thymidine by the halogenated analogues) as are proteins that may be antigenic, concerned with virus coat formation, or involved in cytopathic effects (Siminoff, 1964; Smith and Dukes, 1964; Siminoff and Menefee, 1966; Kaplan *et al.*, 1965; Kaplan and Ben-Porat, 1966; Smith, 1963; Karpas, 1967; Rapp and Vanderslice, 1964; Schneweis, 1965). A key problem remaining is to sort out which protein is either not made, made in an inadequate amount, or is altered in primary structure so that it is nonfunctional or lethal.

The incorporation of IUdR or BUdR into the DNA of mammalian cells, bacteria, phage, and animal viruses increases their sensitivity to the lethal effects of both ultraviolet and ionizing radiations (for appropriate references, see review by Szybalski, 1967). This property of IUdR stimulated the experiments of von Thiele and Wacker (1962) who reported an augmentation of IUdR therapy of herpes simplex keratitis in man when irradiation with light was part of the protocol. Kaplan and Ben-Porat (1966) found that the infectivity of pseudorabies virus formed when IUdR was added 4 hours postinfection was as sensitive to γ-ray inactivation as the virus formed when IUdR was present throughout the infection, and both preparations were about twice as sensitive to radiation as those viruses grown in the absence of IUdR. The enhanced sensitivity of the viruses grown in IUdR supplemented media proved their conclusion that the virus particles did indeed contain IUdR-substituted DNA.

Augmentation of radiation inactivation of herpesvirus has recently been reported by Moore *et al.* (1972) who successfully treated herpetic keratitis in rabbits by a photodynamic inactivation of virus in the presence of a dye.

More important perhaps is their successful application of a combination of a dye and light to patients with recurrent cutaneous herpes infection. Knight (1972) observed marked improvement in patients with recurrent herpes simplex when treated with Grenz rays alone.

A molecular understanding of how halogenated uracil derivatives sensitize DNA to the lethal effects of radiation has been reviewed by Wacker (1963), Elkind and Whitmore (1967), Szybalski (1967), Smith and Hanawalt (1969), Setlow (1968), and Hutchinson and Hales (1970). Mechanistically, Wacker (1963) observed that UV light caused the loss of bromine from bromouracil-substituted DNA with the formation of uracil; Lion (1970) observed the formation of an alkali-labile bond in irradiated bromouracil-labeled DNA. Hotz and Reuschl (1967) observed that bromouracil in DNA increased the amount of the sugar deoxyribose destroyed on UV irradiation, and electron spin data obtained by Koehlein and Hutchinson (1969) are consistent with the appearance of a free radical in the sugar moiety of bromouracil – DNA. Recent studies by Hutchinson and Hales (1970) support an increase in the induction of breaks in bromouracil – DNA compared to normal DNA. These observations are readily explained by the experiments of Rupp and Prusoff (1964, 1965a,b) which proposed and provided evidence that radiation causes the release of the halogen at the 5-position of the uracil moiety with the formation of a uracilyl-free radical. Presumably this uracilyl-free radical, when present in DNA, can abstract a hydrogen from the adjacent deoxyribose of DNA, thereby labilizing the DNA backbone; hence, one observes an increase in the number of breaks in the halogenated uracil-substituted DNA. Such an effect on viral DNA, unless repaired, would obviously result in a lethal event. The photosensitization of viruses to radiation is an area of great promise.

II. 6-Azauracil Ribonucleoside (6-Azauridine)

Azauridine (6-azauracil ribonucleoside) inhibits a variety of RNA and DNA viruses in culture (references cited in Goz and Prusoff, 1970b). Inhibition of HSV replication was reported by Galegov and co-workers (1968) and by Falke and Rada (1970) and of cytomegalovirus by Demidova *et al.* (1969).

Myska and co-workers (1967) reported 6-azauridine to be efficacious in the therapy of herpes simplex infection of the eye in man. This observation is of particular importance because stromal infection was involved, a clinical situation for which 5-iodo-2′-deoxyuridine is not effective. Herpes simplex keratitis in rabbits was similarly affected beneficially by therepy with 6-azauridine (Galegov *et al.*, 1968). The clinical utility of this compound has been extended to include therapy of smallpox (Jaffari and Hussain, 1969), and a 50% reduction in mortality in this dreaded disease was achieved by Rășková and Elis (1971). Although smallpox is not caused by a herpesvirus, its clinical significance merits consideration. The initial observation that 6-azauridine, an analogue of the ribonucleoside, uridine, could inhibit vaccinia virus, a DNA virus, in cell culture was made by Rada *et al.* (1960). Its effectiveness *in vivo* against vaccinia virus was observed by Jasinska *et al.* (1962) and Smějkal and Sorm (1962). A recent review of the clinical use of 6-azauridine in man has been presented by Elis and Rășková (1972).

A molecular basis for the inhibitory activity of this agent has been reviewed and appropriate references cited by Handschumacher and Welch (1960) and by Skoda (1963, 1973). In summary, the mechanism of action involves the phosphorylation of this analogue to the 5′-monophosphate derivative with subsequent inhibition of orotidylate decarboxylase. Thus, one observes an inhibition of the *de novo* formation of uridylate. This inhibition can be reversed by uridine or cytidine which can form uridylate by a metabolic route not affected by 6-azauridine. Although radioactive 6-azauridine has been reported to be incorporated into bacterial RNA, this is not a general observation, and none has been observed in mammalian systems.

Although the probability that the antiviral activity resides in depriving the virus replicating systems of a supply of uridine monophosphate for RNA synthesis, incorporation into viral mRNA or tRNA has not been excluded. However, Lisy and co-workers (1968), in a study of the coding properties of synthetic poly- and oligonucleotides containing 6-azauridine, found them incapable of facilitating the binding of amino acyl–tRNA to ribosomes. Thus, in an excellent review Skoda (1973), concluded that even if "incorporation of 6-azauridine into informational molecules would take place, none of the codons and anticodons containing 6-azapyrimidine nucleoside would possess any coding activity and would thus cause no *errors* in the translation process."

The biosynthesis of herpesvirus RNA is primarily affected by azauridine. This is supported by the observations of Falke and Rada (1970) that uridine or cytidine, but neither thymidine nor orotic acid, could reverse the inhibitory action of this analogue. A similar observation had been made by Rada and Blaskovic (1966) in a comparable study on the effect of 6-azauridine in the replication of vaccinia virus.

6-Azauridine must be phosphorylated to 6-azauridylate before inhibition of orotidylate decarboxylase may occur, and a correlation has been made between the activity of uridine kinase, the enzyme responsible for phosphorylation of the analogue, and the inhibition of viral replication (Rada and Blăškovič, 1961; Rada and Gregusová, 1964; Rada *et al.*, 1964; Kára, 1968).

Critical to the selectivity of action of antimetabolites such as 6-azauridine and 5-iodo-2′-deoxyuridine is the fortunate increase in uridine kinase and thymidine kinase activities in those cells infected with certain susceptible viruses. Thus, these analogues, which are readily transported in and out of cells, are preferentially trapped in their phosphorylated form in those cells that possess such enzymic activity. Hence, viruses that cause an increased uridine kinase activity in the infected cell "prepare" themselves for an early demise by 6-azauridine. Of potential importance are the studies of Rada and Altanerová (1970) and Rada and Hanusovska (1970) who observed that the simultaneous administration of 6-azauridine and a cell-free extract containing uridine kinase to infected cells in culture produced a marked increase in viral inhibition compared with that produced by 6-azauridine alone. Since added 6-azauridylate is not inhibitory because it does not penetrate into the cell, it has been proposed by these investigators that uridine kinase may have entered the cell, presumably by pinocytosis, and may have caused the formation intracellularly of an inhibitory concentration of the phosphorylated analogue.

III. 5-Ethyl-2′-Deoxyuridine

The synthesis of 5-ethyl-2′-deoxyuridine has been reported simultaneously by Swierkowski and Shugar (1969) and Gauri *et al.* (1969), although several biological studies with this compound have been reported since 1966 (Pietrzykowska and Shugar, 1966) as well as a reference to the unpublished synthesis by Swierkowski and Shugar in 1966 (Pietrzykowska and Shugar, (1966).

5-Ethyl-2′-deoxyuridine is an inhibitor of the replication of HSV and of vaccinia virus (Gauri and Malorny, 1967; Heidelberger, cited in Swierkowski and Shugar, 1969) in cell culture and in experimental herpes keratitis in rabbits (Gauri and Malorny, 1967; Gauri, 1968). Of imporatnce is the observation of Gauri *et al.* (1970) who found no inhibition of regeneration of experimentally damaged cornea in rabbits under conditions in which 5-iodo-2′-deoxyuridine was markedly inhibitory. Clinical investigations with 5-ethyl-2′-deoxyuridine by Riehm and Gauri (1969) and by DeDecker (1969) indicated that it has a positive therapeutic effect in the therapy of herpetic keratitis.

Riehm and Gauri (1969) found tritium-labeled 5-ethyl-2′-deoxyuridine, when injected subconjunctivally into the rabbit cornea, to be anabolized to the mono-, di-, and triphosphate derivative, as well as to be incorporated into DNA of the cornea. Although incorporation into the DNA of herpesvirus is highly probable, it has not been investigated or at least not reported as yet. The availability of radioactive 5-ethyl-2′-deoxyuridine (Gauri *et al.*,

1969) should facilitate the answer to this question Pietrzykowska and Shugar (1966, 1967) have indeed demonstrated incorporation of this compound in phage DNA and observed a decrease in the T_m of such DNA by 4.5° relative to unsubstituted DNA which they indicate implies a lower degree of stability. Phage T3 and T7 exhibit no loss of infectivity even though 66% of DNA-thymine has been substituted by 5-ethyluracil. 5-Ethyl-2′-deoxyuridine supported the growth of phage T3 in the absence of thymidine, although the yield was one log higher when grown in the presence of thymidine; this was attributed to a decreased burst size. These results with 5-ethyl-2′-deoxyuridine are in contrast with those observed with 5-iodo-2′-deoxyuridine since although the number of phage particles was not decreased when grown in the presence of IUdR, a marked decrease in infectivity was observed (Goz and Prusoff, 1970a). Thus, the molecular basis for the inhibitory effect of 5-ethyl-2′-deoxyuridine against herpesvirus has yet to be elucidated. Conceivably, the substitution of an ethyl group for the methyl group of DNA thymine could affect the forces concerned with the normal interaction of adjacent bases as well as solvent–polymer organization. This could involve hydrogen bonding or hydrophobic interactions with a resultant effect on DNA replication or transcription.

Of great relevance to its potential clinical use as an antiviral agent is the observation that this compound is nonmutagenic both to phage (Pietrzykowski, cited by Swierkowski and Shugar, 1969) and to *Drosophila melanogaster* (Künkel *et al.*, 1968).

IV. Trifluoromethyl-2′-Deoxyuridine

Although 5-trifluoromethyl-2′-deoxyuridine (F_3TdR) is highly active against HSV (Kaufman and Heidelberger, 1964), studies on the mechanism of antiviral action have largely been done with vaccinia virus. The nucleotide derivative, 5-trifluoromethyl-2′-deoxyuridylate, is known to be an inhibitor of thymidylate synthetase (Reyes and Heidelberger, 1965; Santi and Sakai, 1971) but this is not believed to be the cause of antiviral activity. Rather, as is the case for IUdR, the consequences of incorporation of the analogue into viral DNA are thought to be responsible for viral inhibition.

5-Trifluoromethyl-2′-deoxyuridine is incorporated into the DNA of phage T4 (Gottschling and Heidelberger, 1964) and vaccinia virus (Fujiwara and Heidelberger, 1970). In this regard, Bresnick and Williams (1967) showed that mammalian thymidine kinase was capable of phosphorylating F_3TdR and that F_3TdR inhibited thymidine phosphorylation. Analysis of the DNA of vaccinia grown in the presence of F_3TdR showed a range of F_3TdR substitution for thymidine of 1.4–9.8%. This is a relatively low substitution as compared, for example, to 18% for IUdR replacement of thymidine in vaccinia DNA (Prusoff *et al.*, 1963). The F_3TdR-containing particles, however, with this degree of substitution were noninfective. Fujiwara and Heidelberger (1970) also discerned that the F_3TdR-substituted DNA was smaller than normal DNA, as ascertained by sucrose gradient analysis.

At this writing, the most recent full publication on the mechanism of antiviral activity of F_3TdR is the report of Oki and Heidelberger (1971), again with vaccinia. In this paper, the effects of F_3TdR on viral mRNA and proteins were investigated. Cells infected in the presence of F_3TdR show apparently normal early (30 minutes postinfection) mRNA synthesis as judged by sucrose gradient analysis of a 30-minute [^{3}H]uridine pulse. However, late (4.5 hours postinfection) mRNA was not formed in the drug-treated cells. It was concluded that F_3TdR exerts an effect on late mRNA synthesis because it is incorporated into progeny DNA which is believed to code for the late mRNA synthesis. Early mRNA formation is unaltered because the input DNA, which reputedly codes for the early mRNA, contains no F_3TdR. In keeping with this line of thinking, infection with virions with F_3TdR-substituted DNA results in much reduced early mRNA. Viral protein synthesis was also examined by means of acrylamide gel electrophoresis, and differences were found from normal vaccinia protein patterns when F_3TdR was present during infection. This was true for both early (2 hours postinfection) and late (6 hours postinfection) proteins. Although late mRNA is affected, as is protein synthesis, progeny virus with F_3TdR-substituted DNA appear to adsorb and uncoat similarly to normal virions. The virions formed in the presence of F_3TdR are morphologically abnormal and although infectivity is greatly decreased, the actual yield of particles appears not to be comparably greatly reduced (Fujiwara and Heidelberger, 1970). It remains to be resolved how any significant amount of the late viral proteins or viral particles can be made in light of the almost negligible amount of normal-sized, viral late mRNA synthesized in the presence of F_3TdR.

In a recent abstract Dexter and Heidelberger (1972) report that vaccinia late mRNA synthesized in the presence of F_3TdR lacked 22% of the late and 12% of early sequences when compared to normal late mRNA by DNA–RNA hybridization competition studies.

Why does F_3TdR have a selective chemotherapeutic effect? Perhaps the answer is that not only does increased thymidine kinase activity after vaccinia or herpes infection trap more F_3TdR into viral DNA, but also that viral infection shuts off host DNA synthesis (Joklik, 1966). Indeed, Fujiwara and Heidelberger (1970) demonstrated a significantly greater incorporation of F_3TdR into virion DNA as compared to cellular DNA. In addition, thymidine kinase deficient cells are resistant to F_3TdR (Umeda and Heidelberger, 1968) which is consistent with the above notion.

VI. 1-β-D-Arabinofuranosyl Cystosine (Arabinosyl Cytosine, Cytosine Arabinoside)

Most of the data as well as the controversy as to how 1-β-D-arabinofuranosylcytosine (ara-C) acts, are derived from work with nonviral systems. It was first proposed that ara-CDP arrested cell growth by inhibiting CDP reductase (Chu and Fischer, 1961, 1965). Subsequent studies cast strong doubt on this idea. Isolated CDP reductase is not only poorly inhibited by the phosphorylated forms of ara-C (Moore and Cohen, 1967), but also mouse embryo cells treated with ara-C shows negligible change in dCTP pool size (Skoog and Nordenskjöld, 1971).

It is generally accepted that ara-C must first be phosphorylated in order to be inhibitory. Cells laking the enzyme deoxycytidine kinase which phosphorylates ara-C (Momparler and Fischer, 1968) are resistant to inhibition (Chu and Fischer, 1965). Recently, ara-C resistance was reported also for a mutant HSV which does not induce deoxycytidine kinase activity in a similarly mutated host cell (Hay *et al.*, 1971).

The main point of dispute is whether ara-C or its phosphorylated derivatives inhibit via an effect on DNA or RNA. Ara-C does inhibit DNA synthesis (Chu and Fischer, 1961; Silagi, 1965), and ara-CTP was shown to inhibit a partially purified DNA polymerase (Furth and Cohen, 1968; Momparler, 1969; Graham and Whitmore, 1970b). There is disagreement as to the mode of DNA polymerase inhibition. It is claimed that ara-CTP is only incorporated at the 5′ end of the growing DNA chain and that after such incorporation no other nucleotides are added (Momparler, 1969; Waqar *et al.*, 1971). Contrary evidence demonstrates incorporation within, as well as at the end of, the DNA strand (Graham and Whitmore, 1970b). However, the more crucial issue is whether inhibition of DNA synthesis can account for the lethal effect of ara-C on cells and on viruses.

There is evidence that inhibition of cellular DNA is not the cause of lethality by ara-C. At low ara-C concentrations, which can inhibit DNA synthesis markedly, there is no lethality, and DNA synthesis resumes on drug removal. At higher ara-C concentration, where inhibition of DNA synthesis is only slightly greater, there is a lethal effect. (Graham and Whitmore, 1970a). In another study, after treatment of cells with lethal levels of ara-C, removal of the drug allowed resumption of DNA synthesis even though the cells were still nonviable (Chu and Fischer, 1968). To allow for this evidence and still assume that inhibition of DNA synthesis is the reason for the lethal effect of ara-C, it would be necessary to assume that the slight increase in inhibition of DNA synthesis (Graham and Whitmore, 1970a) affects the synthesis of a critical portion or type of DNA and that the DNA synthesized after removal of lethal levels of ara-C (Chu and Fischer, 1968) is abnormal in nature and nonfunctional.

Alternatively, one may consider that although DNA synthesis is markedly inhibited, the actual site of lethality rests upon an effect on RNA. Ara-C is incorporated into RNA (Silagi, 1965; Creasey *et al.*, 1966; Chu and Fischer, 1968). Chu and Fischer (1968) have presented evidence that ara-C incorporation into RNA, 2 S to 7 S RNA specifically (Chu, 1971), may be the cause of cell death. These workers believe that their data on ara-C incorporation into DNA and RNA show that the rate of incorporation of radioactive ara-C into RNA rather than into DNA correlates with acute cell death. Several observations are not consistent with this basis for lethality. First, ara-C is specifically toxic for the S phase of the cell cycle (Karon and Shirikawa, 1969; Graham and Whitmore, 1970b), the time of DNA synthesis, whereas RNA synthesis occurs in other portions of the cycle as well. Second, the incorporation of ara-C into L cell RNA is not strikingly different at lethal than at nonlethal concentrations of the drug (Graham and Whitmore, 1970b). Lastly, the replication of several RNA-containing viruses is not significantly inhibited by ara-C (Silagi, 1965; Campbell *et al.*, 1968) with the lone exception of rabies virus (Campbell *et al.*, 1968).

Levitt and Becker (1967) and Ben-Porat *et al.* (1968) have investigated the mechanisms of the antiviral activity of ara-C on herpesvirus. Levitt and Becker (1967) ascertained that 20 μg/ml of ara-C would completely inhibit DNA synthesis in HSV-infected cells. If the ara-C was added subsequent to initiation of viral DNA synthesis, the synthesis was immediately and completely inhibited although the DNA synthesized up to that point was encapsidated and DNase resistant. In agreement with these results, ara-C addition at 3 or 6 hours postinfection gave complete inhibition of infectious virus production, but drug addition at 9, 12, or 15 hours postinfection did not significantly reduce virus yield. Ben-Porat *et al.* (1968) reported similar results with pseudorabies virus-infected cells. In this study, there was a correspondence between percent inhibition of DNA synthesis at various ara-C concentrations and the decrease in yield of infectious pseudorabies virus. Both studies indicate inhibition of DNA synthesis as the site of ara-C antiviral activity. In light of the controversy discussed above with regard to the site of lethal inhibition, it would have been of value had these investigators attempted to reverse the ara-C inhibition by either removing the drug or adding deoxycytidine. Had DNA synthesis resumed, and along with it infectious virus production, there would be evidence against the involvement of RNA in the observed inhibition. A contrary finding, resumption of DNA synthesis without increase in infectious virus production, would argue in favor of RNA as a target in ara-C inhibition. In this regard, a recent study by O'Neill *et al.* (1972) with HSV type 2 has shown that ara-C inhibition of infectious virus production is reversible after as long as 22 days of exposing the infected cells to the drug. However, there is a latent period of 5 – 7 days after drug removal before infectious virus appears. The authors speculate that the latent period may be needed to repair defective viral DNA formed in the presence of ara-C. Thus, these recent experiments implicate DNA synthesis as the prime site of ara-C inhibition of herpesvirus.

Another important question which has been raised is whether ara-C is a specific antiviral agent. Ben-Porat *et al.* (1968) argue that it is not. This conclusion is based upon their findings that (a) at comparable ara-C concentrations cellular DNA synthesis in noninfected cells is inhibited more markedly than in cells infected with pseudorabies or herpes simplex virus, (b) infected cells have a lower ability to phosphorylate ara-C as compared to noninfected cells; (c) while in uninfected cells ara-C addition increases deoxycytidine kinase activity, it does not in infected cells; and (d) no increase in deoxycytidine kinase occurs after pseudorabies virus infection. Contrary data has been reported by Hay *et al.* (1971) and Goz (1972) who observed an increase in deoxycytidine kinase activity after HSV infection. The difference in findings may reflect the difference in the virus–host cell systems studied. However, even with the increase of deoxycytidine kinase activity in HSV infected cells (seven- to tenfold over infected cells) the rate of ara-C phosphorylation increases in cell extracts at most by twofold compared to that from uninfected cells. These findings may be related to the observation that the apparent K_m of deoxycytidine kinase in the infected cell extracts is about tenfold higher for ara-C than deoxycytidine (B. Goz, unpublished observations). Thus, it appears likely from the above that ara-C is not a viral-specific inhibitor. Clinical reports of varied success with the drug as an antiviral agent appear to bear this out.

VI. 9-β-D-Arabinofuranosyl Adenine (Adenine Arabinoside)

The compound 9-β-D-arabinofuranosyl adenine (ara-A) has shown great promise as an antiviral agent for a wide variety of DNA viruses including HSV (Privat de Garilhe and de Rudder, 1964; Schabel, 1968; Person *et al.*, 1970). Like ara-C, it is inactive against RNA virus replication (Schabel, 1968). However, in contrast to ara-C whose deaminated metabolite 1-β-D-arabinofuranosyl uracil is inactive against viruses, the hypoxanthine derivative of ara-A is approximately equivalent to the activity of the parent compound (Schabel, 1968).

Although a considerable amount of work has been done on the biochemical effects of ara-A (reviewed by Cohen, 1966; Suhadolnik, 1970), little, if any, investigation has been done, to our knowledge, directly on inhibition of viral replication. Therefore, the following discussion is of work with nonviral systems with the somewhat tenuous assumption that conclusions from such studies can be extended to effects on infected cells.

Ara-A can cause chromosome breaks (Nichols, 1964). Incorporation of labeled adenine or glycine into DNA of TA3 ascites cells was inhibited by ara-A injected into mice. Little if any ara-A is incorporated into RNA or DNA of TA3 ascites tumor cells (LePage, 1970) or L cells (Cohen, 1966).

Ara-ATP did inhibit ribonucleotide reductase and to a greater extent than ara-CTP, but dATP was more effective. Five to eight times more ara-ATP is required to produce inhibition similar to that of dATP (Moore and Cohen, 1967).

Ara-ATP also inhibits DNA polymerase. York and LePage (1965) report the inhibition to be noncompetitive, whereas Furth and Cohen (1968) find competitive inhibition. The latter investigators used a partially purified enzyme from calf thymus while the former group used the 100,000 *g* supernatant fluid of mouse ascites tumor cells. The differences in type of inhibition may be due to variation in degree of purity of the enzyme preparation or to uniqueness of the enzyme source. Again, Furth and Cohen (1968) report that the labeled ara-ATP did not appear to be incorporated into DNA. It has also been reported that ara-ATP like ara-CTP has a chain-terminal effect after incorporation into DNA (Waqar *et al.*, 1971).

Doering *et al.* (1966) studied DNA synthesis and replication of L cells treated with ara-A. The compound inhibited DNA synthesis as well as cell division with negligible effects on RNA or protein synthesis. Cell size increased compared to control, and upon ara-A removal there was not only a decrease in cell size but also a modest increase in cell number. Although DNA synthesis resumed after removal of the drug and was comparable to the control rate, at a later time DNA synthesis ceased while control cells were still synthesizing DNA. Thus, the question of reversibility of ara-A inhibition of DNA synthesis after drug removal is questionable. The evidence linking lethality to inhibition of DNA synthesis is somewhat stronger than for ara-C, particularly since there have been no reports linking ara-A inhibition to RNA synthesis as is the case for ara-C.

VII. Conclusion

We hope that the foregoing has accurately related the present state in the understanding of the molecular mechanisms of antiviral agents used against herpesvirus. We also hope that the vital link between the basic research on viral replication and mechanism of action of antiviral drugs has been made abundantly clear. As we have indicated, finding the mechanism for present drugs sometimes awaits more sophisticated knowledge of the viral replicative process. In addition, the future uncovering of new steps in viral replication, should lead to the design of novel compounds.

It is evident that the molecular basis for the antiviral activity of the several agents discussed is yet to be elucidated. We have acquired a significant amount of biochemical information in regard to specific sites of inhibition; however, such information has been gleaned frequently from a non-herpesvirus system. Direct transfer of such knowledge to the herpesvirus system may be hazardous, since the effect exerted by a compound may be related not only to the specific virus, or even to a strain of virus, under consideration, but also to the type of cell or tissue infected (eye, skin, brain, etc.). Although a biochemical site of inhibition is found, the key question that must be answered is whether a causal relationship does indeed exist between this biochemical event and the observed inhibition of viral replication.

Acknowledgments

We wish to express our sincere appreciation to Mrs. Evelyn Lentz and Miss Jewell McLaughlin for their invaluable assistance in performance of the authors' experimental work cited, and to Miss Lynn Bon Tempo for her cheerful and excellent secretarial service. The authors' research referred to in this review was supported by U.S.P.H.S. Grant CA-05262. One of the authors (B.G) is also supported by U.S.P.H.S. Grant CA-10748.

References

Aamodt, L., and Goz, B. (1970). *Biochem. Pharmacol.* **19**, 2400.
Bakhle, Y. S., and Prusoff, W. H. (1969). *Biochim. Biophys. Acta* **174**, 302.
Ben-Porat, T., Brown, McK., and Kaplan, A. S. (1968). *Mol. Pharmacol.* **4**, 139.
Bresnick, E., and Williams, S. S. (1967). *Biochem. Pharmacol.* **16**, 503.
Camerman, N., and Trotter, J. (1964). *Science* **144**, 1348.
Campbell, J. B., Maes, R. F., Wiktor, T. J., and Koprowski, H. (1968). *Virology* **34**, 701.
Chu, M. Y. (1971). *Biochem. Pharmacol.* **20**, 2057.
Chu, M. Y., and Fischer, G. A. (1962). *Biochem. Pharmacol.* **11**, 423.
Chu, M. Y., and Fischer, G. A. (1965). *Biochem. Pharmacol.* **14**, 333.
Chu, M. Y., and Fischer, G. A. (1968). *Biochem. Pharmacol.* **17**, 753.
Cohen, S. S. (1966). *Prog. Nucl. Acid, Res. Mol. Biol.* **5**, 1.
Cramer, J. W., Wacker, A., and Welch, A. D. (1963). *Biochem. J.* **87**, 26P.
Creasey, W. A., Papac, R. J., Markiw, M. E., Calabresi, P. and Welch, A. D. (1966). *Biochem. Pharmacol.* **15**, 1417.
DeDecker, W. (1969). *Deut. Ophthalmol. Ges.* **69**, 135.
Demidova, S. A., Azadova, N. B., Martynova, V. N., Galegov, G. A., and Zhdanov, V. M. (1969). *Dokl. Akad. Nauks SSR* **186**, 709.
Dexter, D. L., and Heidelberger, C. (1972). *Fed. Proc., Fed. Amer. Soc. Exp. Biol.* **31**, 569.
Diwan, A., and Prusoff, W. H. (1968). *Virology* **34**, 184.
Doering, A., Keller, J., and Cohen, S. S. (1966). *Cancer Res.* **26**, 2444.
Easterbrook, K. B., and Davern, C. I. (1963). *Virology* **19**, 509.
Elis, J., and Rășková, H. (1972). *Eur. J. Clin. Pharmacol.* **4**, 77.
Elkind, M. M., and Whitmore, G. F., eds. (1967). "The Radiobiology of Cultured Mammalian Cells," p. 183. Gordon & Breach, New York.

Ey, R. C., Hughes, W. F., Holmes, A. W., and Deinhardt, F. (1964). *Arch. Ophthalmol.* [N.S.] **71**, 325.
Falke, D., and Rada, B. (1970). *Acta Virol.* (*Prague*) *English Ed.* **14**, 115.
Fiala, S., and Fiala, A. E. (1965). *Cancer Res.* **25**, 922.
Fujiwara, Y., and Heidelberger, C. (1970). *Mol. Pharmacol.* **6**, 281.
Furth, J. J., and Cohen, S. S. (1968). *Cancer Res.* **28**, 2061.
Galegov, G. A., Bikbulatova, R. M., Vanag, K. A., and Shen, R. M. (1968). *Vop. Virusol.* **13**, 18.
Gauri, K. K. (1968). *Klin Monatsbl Augenheilk* **153**, 837.
Gauri, K. K., and Malorny, G. (1967). *Naunynr-Schem; edibergs Arch. Pharmakol. Exp. Pathol.* **257**, 21.
Gauri, K. K., Pflughaupt, K. W., and Müller, R. (1969). *Z. Naturforsch. B* **24**, 834.
Gauri, K. K., Malorny, G., and Riehm, E. (1970). *Arch. Klin. Exp. Ophthalmol. Albrecht von Gractes* **179**, 287.
Gottschling, H., and Heidelberger, C. (1964). *J. Mol. Biol.* **7**, 541.
Goz, B. (1972). *Proc. Amer. Ass. Cancer Res.* **13**, 26.
Goz, B., and Prusoff, W. H. (1968). *J. Biol. Chem.* **243**, 4750.
Goz, B., and Prusoff, W. H. (1970a). *Ann. N.Y. Acad. Sci.* **173**, 379.
Goz, B., and Prusoff, W. H. (1970b). *Annu. Rev. Pharmacol.* **10**, 143.
Graham, F. L., and Whitmore, G. F. (1970a). *Cancer Res.* **30**, 2627.
Graham, F. L., and Whitmore, G. F. (1970b). *Cancer Res.* **30**, 2636.
Handschumacher, R. E., and Welch, A. D. (1960). *In* "The Nucleic Acids" (E. Chargaff and J. N. Davidson, eds.), Vol. 3, p. 453. Academic Press, New York.
Hanna, C. (1966). *Exp. Eye Res.* **5**, 164.
Hay, J., Perera, P. A. J., Morrison, J. M., and Gentry, G. A. (1971). *Strategy Viral Genome, Ciba Found. Symp.* p. 355.
Herrmann, E. C., Jr. (1961). *Proc. Soc. Exp. Biol. Med.* **107**, 142.
Hirt, B. (1966). *Proc. Nat. Acad. Sci. U.S.* **55**, 997.
Hotz, G., and Reuschl, H. (1967). *Mol. Gen Genet.* **99**, 5.
Hutchinson, F., and Hales, H. B. (1970). *J. Mol. Biol.* **50**, 59.
Jaffari, S. M. H., and Hussain, A. (1969). *Indian J. Med. Res.* **57**, 809.
Jasinska, S., Link, F., Blåskovič, D., and Rada, B. (1962). *Acta Virol.* (*Prague*), *English Ed.* **6**, 17.
Joklik, W. K. (1964). *Virology* **22**, 620.
Joklik, W. K. (1966). *Bacteriol. Rev.* **30**, 33.
Kamiya, T., Ben-Porat, T., and Kaplan, A. S. (1965). *Virology* **26**, 577.
Kaplan, A. S., and Ben-Porat, T. (1964). *Virology* **23**, 90.
Kaplan, A. S., and Ben-Porat, T. (1966). *J. Mol. Biol.* **19**, 320.
Kaplan, A. S., Ben-Porat, T., and Kamiya, T. (1965). *Ann. N.Y. Acad. Sci.* **130**, 226.
Kaplan, A. S., Ben-Porat, T., and Coto, C. (1967). *In* "The Molecular Biology of Viruses" (S. J. Colter and W. Paranchych, eds.), p. 527. Academic Press, New York.
Kára, J. (1968). Folio. Biolog. (Praha) **14**, 249.
Karon, M., and Shirakawa, S. (1969). *Cancer Res.* **29**, 687.
Karpas, A. (1967). *Ann. Inst. Pasteur, Paris* **112**, 308.
Kaufman, H. E. (1965). *Progr. med. Virol.* **7**, 116.
Kaufman, H. E., and Heidelberger, C. (1964). *Science* **145**, 585.
Keir, H. M., and Gold, E. (1963). *Biochim. Biophys. Acta* **72**, 263.
Kit, S., Dubbs, D. R., and Anken, M. (1967). *J. Virol.* **1**, 238.
Klemperer, H. G., Haynes, G. R., Shedden, W. I. H., and Watson, D. K. (1967). *Virology* **31**, 120.
Knight, A. G. (1972). *Brit. J. Dermatol.* **86**, 172.

Koehlein, W., and Hutchinson, F. (1969). *Radiat. Res.* **39**, 745.
Künkel, H. A., Gauri, K. K., and Malorny, G. (1968). *Biophysik* **5**, 88.
LePage, G. A. (1970). *Can. J. Biochem.* **48**, 75.
Levitt, J., and Becker, Y. (1967). *Virology* **31**, 129.
Lion, M. B. (1970). *Biochim. Biophys. Acta* **209**, 24.
Lisy, V., Rychlik, I., Smrt, J., Holy, A., and Šorm, F. (1968). *Collect. Czech. Chem. Commun.* **33**, 4111.
McCrea, J. F., and Lipman, M. B. (1967). *J. Virol.* **1**, 1037.
Momparler, R. L. (1969). *Biochem. Biophys. Res. Commun.* **34**, 465.
Momparler, R. L., and Fischer, G. A. (1968). *J. Biol. Chem.* **243**, 4298.
Moore, C., Wallis, C., Melnick, J. L., and Kuns, M. P. (1972). *Infection Immunity* **5**, 169.
Moore, E. C., and Cohen, S. S. (1967). *J. Biol. Chem.* **242**, 2116.
Myška, V., Elis, J., Plevovā, J., and Rāsková, H. (1967). *Lancet* **1**, 1230.
Nichols, W. W. (1964). *Cancer Res.* **24**, 1502.
Nohara, H., and Kaplan, A. S. (1963). *Biochem. Biophys. Res. Commun.* **12**, 189.
Okazaki, T., and Kornberg, A. (1964). *J. Biol. Chem.* **239**, 275.
Oki, T., and Heidelberger, C. (1971). *Mol. Pharmacol.* **7**, 653.
O'Neill, F. J., Goldberg, R. J., and Rapp, F. (1972). *J. Gen. Virol.* **14**, 189.
Perkins, E. S., Wood, R. M., Sears, M. L., Prusoff, W. H., and Welch, A. D. (1962). *Nature (London)* **194**, 985.
Person, J. A., Sheridan, P. J., and Herrmann, E. C., Jr. (1970). *Infection Immunity* **2**, 815.
Pietrzykowska, I., and Shugar, D. (1966). *Biochem. Biophys. Res. Commun.* **25**, 567.
Pietrzykowska, I., and Shugar, D. (1967). *Acta Biochim. Pol.* **14**, 169.
Private de Garilhe, M., and de Rudder, J. (1964). *C. R. Acad. Sci.* **259**, 2725.
Prusoff, W. H., and Chang, P. K. (1968). *J. Biol. Chem.* **243**, 223.
Prusoff, W. H., and Chang, P. K. (1969–1970). *Chem.-Biol. Interact.* **1**, 285.
Prusoff, W. H., Bakhle, Y. S., and McCrea, J. F. (1963). *Nature (London)* **199**, 1310.
Prusoff, W. H. Bakhle, Y. S., and Sekely, L. (1965). *Ann. N.Y. Acad. Sci.* **130**, 135.
Rada, B., and Altanerová, V. (1970). *Acta Virol. (Prague), English Ed.* **4**, 425.
Rada, B., and Blaškovič, D. (1961). *Acta Virol. (Prague), English Ed.* **5**, 308.
Rada, B., and Blaškovič, D. (1966). *Acta Virol. (Prague), English Ed.* **10**, 1.
Rada, B., and Gregusová, V. (1964). *Biochem. Biophys. Res. Commun.* **15**, 324.
Rada, B., and Hanusovska, T. (1970). *Acta Virol. (Prague), English Ed.* **14**, 435.
Rada, B., Šorm, F., and Škoda, J. (1960). *Experientia* **16**, 487.
Rada, B., Smidová, V., and Zavada, J. (1964). *Neoplasma* **11**, 553.
Rapp, F., and Vanderslice, D. (1964). *Virology* **22**, 321.
Rāsková, H., and Elis, J. (1971). cited in Elis, J., and Rāsková, H. (1972).
Reyes, P., and Heidelberger, C. (1965). *Mol. Pharmacol.* **1**, 14.
Riehm, E., and Gauri, K. K. (1969). *Deut. Ophthalmol. Ges.* **69**, 543.
Roizman, B., Aurelian, L., and Roane, P. R. (1963). *Virology* **21**, 482.
Rupp, W. D., and Prusoff, W. H. (1964). *Nature (London)* **202**, 1288.
Rupp, W. D., and Prusoff, W. H. (1965a). *Biochem. Biophys. Res. Commun.* **18**, 145.
Rupp, W. D., and Prusoff, W. H. (1965b). *Biochem. Biophys. Res. Commun.* **18**, 158.
Russell, W. C., Gold, E., Keir, H. M., Omura, H., Wilson, D. H., and Wildy, P. (1964). *Virology* **22**, 103.
Santi, D. V., and Sakai, T. T. (1971). *Biochemistry* **10**, 3598.
Schabel, F. M., Jr. (1968). *Chemotherapy* **13**, 321.
Schneweis, K. E. (1965). *Arch. Gesamte Virusforsch.* **15**, 565.
Schumacher, von H. H., and Machemer, R. (1966). *Ophthalmologica* **152**, 183.
Sekely, L., and Prusoff, W. H. (1969). *Pharmacol. Res. Commun.* **1**, 3.

Setlow, R. B. (1968). *Progr. Nucl. Acid Res. Mol. Biol.* **8**, 257.
Silagi, S. (1965). *Cancer Res.* **25**, 1446.
Siminoff, P. (1964). *Virology* **24**, 1.
Siminoff, P., and Menefee, M. G. (1966). *Exp. Cell Res.* **44**, 241.
Škoda, J. (1963). *Progr. Nucl. Acid Res. Mol. Biol.* **2**, 197.
Škoda, J. (1973). *In* "Handbuch der experimentellen Pharmakologie" (A. Sartorelli and D. Johns, eds.). In press.
Skoog, L., and Nordenskjöld, B. (1971). *Eur. J. Biochem.* **19**, 81.
Šmejkal, F., and Šorm, F. (1962). *Acta Virol. (Prague), English Ed.* **6**, 282.
Smith, K. C., and Hanawalt, P. C., eds. (1969). "Molecular Photobiology: "Inactivation and Recovery." Academic Press, New York.
Smith, K. O. (1963). *J. Immunol.* **91**, 582.
Smith, K. O., and Dukes, C. D. (1964). *J. Immunol.* **92**, 550.
Stellwagen, R. H., and Tomkins, G. M. (1971a). *Proc. Nat. Acad. Sci. U.S.* **68**, 1147.
Stellwagen, R. H., and Tomkins, G. M. (1971b). *J. Mol. Biol.* **56**, 167.
Suhadolnik, R. J. (1970). "Nucleoside Antibiotics." Wiley, New York.
Swierkowski, M., and Shugar, D. (1969). *J. Med. Chem.* **12**, 533.
Szybalski, W. H. (1962). *In* "The Molecular Basis of Neoplasia," pp. 147–171. Univ. of Texas Press, Austin.
Szybalski, W. H. (1967). *Radiat. Res., Suppl.* **7**, 147.
Szybalski, W. H., Kubinski, H., and Sheldrick, P. (1966). *Cold Spring Harbor Symp. Quant. Biol.* **31**, 123.
Umeda, M., and Heidelberger, C. (1968). *Cancer Res.* **28**, 2529.
von Theile, R., and Wacker, A. (1962). *Klin. Monatsbl. Augenheilk.* **141**, 94.
Voytek, P., Chang, P. K., and Prusoff, W. H. (1971). *J. Biol. Chem.* **246**, 1432.
Wacker, A. (1963). *Progr. Nucl. Acid. Res. Mol. Biol.* **1**, 369.
Waqar, M. A., Burgoyne, L. A., and Atkinson, M. R. (1971). *Biochem. J.* **121**, 803.
York, J. L., and LePage, G. A. (1965). *Can. J. Biochem. Physiol.* **44**, 19.

Chapter 21
Chemotherapy of Herpesviruses — Clinical Aspects*

Ernest Jawetz

I. Introduction

Ten years have elapsed since the introduction of idoxuridine (IUdR) for the treatment of herpetic keratitis, the first clinical application of antiviral drug treatment. Other antiviral drugs have, since then been subjected to experimentation, and a few have found acceptance in clinical therapy. It may be appropriate to take stock of the experience of the past 10 years and to assess the validity of antiviral drug treatment of herpetic infections.

* The investigative work done by the author was supported in part by U.S. Public Health Service Grant No. EY 00186.

In this chapter several experimental models for the treatment of herpesvirus infections are first considered briefly. The status of drug treatment of herpetic keratitis in man is then reviewed in some detail. Publications on the use of antiviral drugs in herpes infections involving skin are evaluated with particular reference to recurrent herpes simplex, disseminated herpes simplex, herpes zoster, and varicella in persons with impaired immunologic responses, but other aspects of clinical management are not discussed. Finally, available evidence is summarized on the problem of recognition and treatment of herpes encephalitis, an often fatal disease.

Attempts have been made to summarize and quote important publications in these areas. No claim is made, however, for an exhaustive review of all published literature. At times, review articles (Goz and Prusoff, 1970; McFadzean, 1969; Kaufman, 1963; Gurwith *et al.*, 1971) are quoted, from which individual earlier references can be gleaned.

II. Antiviral Chemotherapy in Experimental Herpes Infections of Laboratory Animals

A. Herpes Simplex Keratitis in Rabbits

The announcement by Kaufman *et al.* (1962a), more than 10 years ago, of a "clinical cure of herpes simplex keratitis by 5-iodo-2-deoxyuridine" provided the first dramatic evidence that an established viral organ lesion could be treated with an antiviral drug. A few months after this announcement striking photographs documented the rapid clinical response to topical IUdR administration (Kaufman *et al.*, 1962b). A double-blind study (Corwin *et al.*, 1963b) and additional reports from other laboratories rapidly confirmed that IUdR was able to modify the course of induced herpetic keratitis in the rabbit, even when treatment was delayed until lesions were fully established, 48 hours after inoculation of the cornea. While temporary clinical improvement followed the intermittent administration of low concentrations (0.1%) of IUdR solutions for just 2 days, such minimal treatment did not greatly reduce the virus content of lesions. More prolonged application of 0.1% IUdR or higher concentrations, e.g., 0.5% IUdR in aqueous solution or ointment, or 0.9% in polyethylene glycol, resulted in more marked and prolonged virus suppression. Even the greater concentrations of IUdR applied to the surface achieved only moderate penetration into the epithelium and only minimal levels in the stroma of the cornea. In addition, there were marked differences in the response of different viral strains. Continued animal passage in a given laboratory might further alter strain characteristics, either toward increased invasiveness, producing deep corneal involvement and encephalitis, or toward loss of pathogenicity (Kaufman, 1963).

The virus concentrations in epithelium of rabbit cornea were estimated at intervals after inoculation. In unimmunized animals the peak virus concentration is usually reached within 48 hours after inoculation when epithelial lesions are fully apparent (Ey *et al.*, 1963; Engle and Stewart, 1964; Jawetz *et al.*, 1965; Underwood *et al.*, 1965). Administration of IUdR begun at that time results in an abrupt fall in virus concentration, so that for the next 2–4 days the treated cornea has only 0.01–1.0% of the virus content of the untreated cornea. Later in the course of infection (herpes simplex virus type 1 keratitis in rabbits runs a natural course of 12–14 days), virus content of the untreated cornea declines more rapidly than that of the treated one. If IUdR administration is stopped about day 7 after infection, the virus content of the treated cornea subsequently may be higher than that of the untreated one (Jawetz *et al.*, 1963, 1965; Engle and Stewart, 1964; Underwood *et al.*, 1965). This suggests that the control of virus replication during a given experimental rabbit infection depends on natural host responses: If the responses are interfered with by virus suppression with an antiviral drug, viral replication may continue longer than in the absence of such drug. The immune response of the experimental animal plays a central role in limiting viral replication (Ey *et al.*, 1963). In the immunized animal the initial viral replication after experimental infection is slower, the peak of virus content of the cornea is reached later (usually at 3–5 days after infection), and IUdR suppression of virus is usually not followed by a secondary rise after the end of 5-day treatment (Jawetz *et al.*, 1965, 1970).

It must be stressed that with most herpes simplex virus (HSV) strains the corneal infection in rabbits (as in man) is a self-limited disease (Underwood *et al.*, 1965; Jawetz *et al.*, 1970). With or without IUdR treatment, keratitis induced by most type 1 HSV strains heals with only fine residual scars in 2–3 weeks. Keratitis induced by most type 2 HSV strains heals within 4–6 weeks (Oh *et al.*, 1972). Virus is not eliminated completely either in IUdR-treated or untreated corneas which have a normal appearance after healing (Engle and Stewart, 1964; Jawetz *et al.*, 1965). Spontaneous recurrences of keratitis or virus shedding can be observed for months or years (Laibson and Kibrick, 1966).

Certain strains of HSV, which are fully susceptible to IUdR in cell culture, produce a keratitis in rabbits that fails to respond adequately to IUdR producing dense stromal opacities irrespective of treatment. The replication of these strains in corneal epithelium is inhibited by IUdR to a similar extent as those other strains which permit a full clinical treatment response (Maloney and Kaufman, 1965). It is probable that the reason for such "treatment resistance" is not the strain's inherent biochemical insusceptibility to IUdR but rather its unusual rapid invasiveness into deeper corneal stroma, perhaps by progression along ciliary nerve fibers (Jawetz *et al.*, 1965).

The selection of IUdR-resistant HSV particles has been observed not only in cell cultures but also in rabbit keratitis treated with IUdR (Laibson *et al.*, 1963; Kobayashi and Nakamura, 1964; Underwood *et al.*, 1965). Such isolates were highly resistant to IUdR both in cell cultures and in infections of rabbit eyes, but they were still susceptible to cytarabine (Underwood *et al.*, 1965). Others have not encountered this selection of IUdR-resistant virus which probably depends on the nature of the HSV strain, originally employed for the production of experimental infections (Coleman *et al.*, 1968).

Early studies explored the possibility that antiviral drug, administered together with corticosteroids in herpetic keratitis of rabbits, might overcome the deleterious effects of the steroids (Kaufman *et al.*, 1962b). Steroids alone enhanced and prolonged viral replication in corneal epithelium, but this effect could be largely overcome by the simultaneous administration of IUdR. The anti-inflammatory effects of the steroid could beneficially influence stromal keratitis in rabbits as long as HSV replication was kept in check by the simultaneous presence of IUdR (Kaufman, 1963; Laibson *et al.*, 1963). While steroids failed to reactivate healed, experimental herpetic keratitis in rabbits (Kibrick *et al.*, 1971), steroids facilitated and enhanced the reinfection of such partially immunized animals with the homologous HSV. This effect was abolished by the simultaneous presence of IUdR in the eye soon after challenge with HSV (Easterbrook *et al.*, 1973).

The initial striking successes of IUdR in experimental herpetic keratitis stimulated a survey of other halogenated pyrimidines and other possible antiviral agents. In his original publication Herrmann (1961) indicated that iodo- and bromodeoxyuridines were active against HSV in cell culture, whereas fluorodeoxyuridine and aminopterin were not. Kaufman *et al.* (1962a) confirmed the therapeutic activity of the iodo and bromo compounds in herpetic keratitis of rabbits, found the chloro compound barely active, and the fluoro compound inactive. Iodo- and fluorouracil were also inactive. Amethopterin also failed to influence rabbit keratitis in the study by Corwin *et al.* (1963a).

Cytarabine, another pyrimidine nucleoside, was shown by Underwood (1962) to be at least as effective as IUdR in herpetic keratitis of rabbits. This activity was confirmed by Kaufman and Maloney (1963) who pointed out that IUdR-resistant rabbits and patients might respond to cytarabine. Further work by Underwood *et al.* (1965) indicated that certain isolates from IUdR-treated eyes were resistant to IUdR but still sensitive to cytarabine. In a comparative study, 0.170 IUdR and an equimolar concentration of cytarabine (0.07%) were both effective in arresting viral lesions in the epithelium of the rabbit eye. However, cytarabine produced some changes in corneal epithelium that were suggestive of greater toxicity than IUdR (Kaufman *et al.*, 1964). This may have discouraged further work with cytarabine in herpetic keratitis. Cytarabine was somewhat effective also in herpetic iritis of rabbits (Kaufman *et al.*, 1970).

Adenine arabinoside, a very insoluble compound, was found relatively ineffective as an 0.06% solution in herpetic keratitis of rabbits by Johnson and Jervey (1964), but when administered as a 3.3% ointment (Kaufman *et al.*, 1970), it was considered comparable to 0.5% IUdR ointment. Subconjunctival injection of 5% adenine arabinoside suspension (but not of 2.5%) markedly suppressed herpetic keratouveitis in rabbits. Some toxic effects of this drug treatment were noted, however.

Trifluorothymidine (trifluoromethyl deoxyuridine) was therapeutically active in a concentration of 0.04 mg/ ml in rabbit keratitis induced by either IUdR-susceptible or IUdR-resistant HSV strains. The drug appeared to be more potent than IUdR and not significantly toxic in the rabbit model (Kaufman and Heidelberger, 1964). Further studies with this compound and clinical trials are in progress.

5-Methylamino-2-deoxyuridine (MAdU) 0.1% was equivalent to 0.1% IUdR in rabbit keratitis, but it was somewhat superior to IUdR as a 0.25% solution and almost free of toxicity for the eye (Nemes and Hilleman, 1965). These compounds are still in the process of being evaluated *in vitro* by plaque inhibition systems which correlate fairly well with several rabbit keratitis models (Laibson, 1970). 5-Ethyl-2-deoxyuridine was injected subconjunctivally as an 0.5% solution to treat stromal corneal changes in late herpetic rabbit keratitis (Gauri, 1968). Some beneficial results were attributed to this form of treatment.

The self-limited course of herpetic keratitis in rabbits (Jawetz *et al.*, 1965; Underwood *et al.*, 1965) suggested a possible role for interferon. Therefore, it was appealing to test the effect of exogenous interferon inducers on the course of herpetic keratitis. Park and Baron (1968) undertook a study of interferon induction with poly I:C administered onto the conjunctiva, into the anterior chamber of the rabbit eye, or intravenously. It was reported that there was rapid clinical healing of all keratitis if the drug was given within 2 or even 3 days of infection. A disturbing aspect of this report is the description of herpetic keratitis which continued at full intensity for at least 13 days in untreated controls and subsided in the treated animals between day 4 and 10 after infection. The latter is the usual course for untreated keratitis in rabbits infected with most strains of HSV type 1 (Ey *et al.*, 1963; Underwood *et al.*, 1965; Jawetz *et al.*, 1970). Another study (Polikoff *et al.*, 1970), with high concentrations of poly I:C (1–2.6 mg/ml) dropped repeatedly into the conjunctival sac from 3 to 72 hours after infection also documented a beneficial effect. In a third study (Kaufman *et al.*, 1969), poly I:C was again shown to have a beneficial effect on herpetic keratitis, but the amount of therapeutic benefit was deemed minimal, far less than that of other available antiviral drugs. A temporary resistance to reinfection or recurrence was also demonstrated. The more recent indication of significant toxicity of some interferon inducers for ocular structures (Ostler *et al.*, 1970) may further diminish the interest in these drugs as potential prophylactic or therapeutic agents in HSV keratitis. A postulated enhancement of topical poly I:C effect with IUdR (Polikoff *et al.*, 1970) was not encountered by Kaufman *et al.* (1969).

Photoinactivation of virus, an unusual approach to the treatment of herpetic keratitis, must be mentioned (Moore *et al.*, 1972). Proflavine sulfate (1%) was applied three times to herpetic keratitis of rabbits and then the eyes were exposed to intense light for 5 minutes on two occasions. This treatment shortened the course of keratitis by comparison with exposure to dye or light alone. Additional studies using this approach are now under way.

B. Skin Infections in Rabbits

A skin infection in rabbits was induced by HSV (Force *et al.*, 1964): The simultaneous intradermal injection of HSV and 1% hyaluronidase resulted in self-limited herpetic vesicles. The subcutaneous injection of 120 mg/kg IUdR 6 hours after infection inhibited viral replication in the skin and aborted lesion formation. Regrettably, no studies on dimethylsulfoxide enhancement of IUdR absorption in this model have been reported. An acetanilide compound with some antiherpes activity in cell culture was strikingly active in this model of rabbit skin infection. However, in an excellent controlled study (Underwood, 1970), this compound was indistinguishable from a placebo in human labial herpes infections.

C. Intracerebral Infection in Laboratory Animals

One of the most severe challenges for any antiviral drug is the test of activity in intracerebral animal infection with HSV. 5-Iodo-2-deoxyuridine has not been effective in such a model. Adenine arabinoside 10% (9-β-D-arabinofuranosyladenine) was first shown to protect hamsters against encephalitic death after infection and treatment in the eye. The drug seemed to be at least 10 times more effective than cytarabine (Sidwell *et al.*, 1968). Intracerebrally infected mice exhibited prolonged survival with HSV encephalitis when adenine arabinoside 500 mg/kg was administered orally twice daily, beginning at the time of infection. With a dose of 2000 mg/kg twice daily by mouth, 40% of animals survived even when treatment was delayed until 24 or 48 hours after intracerebral infection with HSV (Dixon *et al.*, 1968). The virus titer in brain was significantly reduced in these animals (Sloan *et al.*, 1968). When adenine arabinoside was given subcutaneously, even more remarkable survivals were obtained. The increase in the rate of survival varied inversely with the delay in treatment. Upon administration of three doses of the drug, 1000 mg/kg each, during 6-hour periods starting at 48 or at 72 hours after infection, respectively, survival rates of 41 and 22% were obtained. Herpes simplex virus was present in brain suspensions of surviving mice, and it was not resistant to the drug. Brain suspensions from some mice surviving at 21 days did not yield virus. Survivors that were challenged with the homologous HSV exhibited high resistance to rechallenge (Miller *et al.*, 1969). In view of the relative lack of toxicity of adenine arabinoside, this success in saving the life of intracerebrally inoculated mice is remarkable, and clinical trials with this drug seem warranted.

III. Herpetic (HSV) Keratitis in Man

Herpetic keratitis (caused by HSV) is at present probably the leading cause of loss of vision due to external eye disease in the United States. For 35 years the accepted form of treatment has consisted in the mechanical removal of infected corneal cells, often preceded by chemical cauterization (e.g., with iodine, ether, or carbolic acid) (Gundersen, 1936). Such treatment leads to healing of the acute epithelial lesions, dendritic figure, or geographic ulcer in a majority of cases, but the lesions recur in 25–40% of patients within 2 years (Carroll *et al.*, 1967). Repeated attacks of active keratitis tend to lead to opacity of the cornea and impaired vision, particularly if the corneal stroma has become involved.

After Kaufman (1962) established a striking clinical response in experimental keratitis of rabbits with IUdR, he demonstrated a similar effect of IUdR in patients with spontaneous herpetic (HSV) keratitis. The topical application of 1 to 2 drops of a 0.1% solution of IUdR in sterile distilled water (pH 7.4) every 1–2 hours around the clock into the conjunctival sac resulted in regression of epithelial lesions, with healing in 3–8 days in a majority of patients (Kaufman *et al.*, 1962b). Part of the initial report was perhaps overenthusiastic: "Nearly all patients have dramatically improved under therapy and none have become worse. . . . The drug also appears to markedly benefit stromal disease and iritis" (Kaufman *et al.*, 1962a). Other investigators soon provided similar, enthusiastic support for this new form of treatment. Corrigan *et al.* (1962) reported that 15 consecutive patients treated with IUdR exhibited universal rapid relief and healing in 3–4 days without and in 4–6 days with stromal involvement. Furgiuele *et al.* (1962) marveled at the "dramatic improvement . . . in patients with an initial involvement of HSV keratitis. Healing occurred within 72 in all but 1 patient and that one healed in 5 days. No other compound previously used . . . has ever given such dramatic results." Other observers were less vocal in their praise, emphasized the need for double-blind controlled studies (Thygeson *et al.*, 1963; Luntz and MacCallum, 1963) and pointed to some harmful effects of the drug (Corrigan *et al.*, 1962; Sood and Marmion, 1964; Thygeson *et al.*, 1963). Still others strongly rejected IUdR treatment. Thus Ey *et al.* (1963) flatly stated: "IUdR has no effect on herpes virus itself, inhibits virus and cell multiplication to the same extent and has little beneficial effects in rabbits, whereas the immune status governs to a large extent the fate of the virus as well as the course of the disease."

A number of publications during the past 10 years have reviewed and assessed the place of IUdR in the treatment of herpetic keratitis in man (Hughes, 1969; Laibson, 1970; McFadzean, 1969; Jones, 1967; Kaufman, 1965; Jawetz *et al.*, 1970). Many other papers express faith in, or disapproval of, the new form of treatment but supply few specific data for objective evaluation. Rather than list or describe each of those reports, I propose to present the points which appear to be crucial for the evaluation of any drug in herpetic keratitis of man and then to summarize the results of all available controlled drug treatment trials.

First, HSV epithelial keratitis in man tends to be self-limited, as it is in the rabbit. Although this infection is notoriously prone to relapses (Carroll *et al.*, 1967; Hughes, 1969), each episode of epithelial activity tends to subside within 1–4 weeks (Thygeson *et al.*, 1963; Ey *et al.*, 1963). Therefore, any evaluation must consider the speed of recovery, as well as the number of patients "cured" by a given drug or procedure.

Second, in an attack of epithelial keratitis, the earlier a patient begins to improve the greater the chance that uncomplicated healing will take place. This makes it probable that IUdR treatment will most frequently lead to improvement if the drug is applied very early in the disease. Any evaluation of treatment response must, therefore, consider the age of lesions at the beginning of treatment as well as the time from start of treatment to healing (Thygeson *et al.*, 1963).

Third, in herpetic keratitis, HSV replicates mainly in epithelium of the cornea, and virus can often be isolated from epithelial cells. If the corneal stroma becomes involved, cultures from the stroma rarely yield HSV isolates. The traditional treatment of epithelial keratitis by removing infected epithelial cells can logically be compared with the application of antiviral drugs to epithelium. The absence of significant virus concentrations in stroma militates against any likelihood of antiviral drugs being effective in stromal involvement through direct suppression of virus there.

Fourth, deep stromal lesions may be in part a manifestation of hypersensitivity but may also be due to viral action on keratocytes, inflammatory changes, or necrosis. Stromal lesions can be alleviated by the topical administration of anti-inflammatory drugs, particularly corticosteroids. These, in turn, promote virus proliferation in epithelium and thus lead to enlarged epithelial lesions (Patterson and Jones, 1967), enhanced structural damage to the cornea, and the risk of perforation. While IUdR probably cannot influence deep stromal lesions which are not primarily caused by virus replication, it could prevent the secondary virus-induced epithelial damage which is promoted by steroids. Thus the simultaneous use of corticosteroids and antiviral drugs must be evaluated.

Fifth, many antiviral drugs also affect uninfected cells, and particularly affect actively regenerating epithelial cells. These untoward side effects may parallel in intensity the antiviral efficacy of the drug. Thus any evaluation of an antiviral drug must consider the need to maintain an adequate drug concentration for a sufficient time in order to produce a beneficial antiviral effect, yet minimize the drug's harmful aspects. The transparency of the cornea is essential to its function. Thus even limited damage to corneal structures by a drug may vitiate its antiviral benefits.

Sixth, herpetic keratitis has a striking predilection toward clinical recurrence (Carroll *et al.*, 1967). Repeated administration of antiviral drugs may lead to the selection of drug-resistant viral mutants. The ease and rapidity with which such mutants emerge during the treatment may determine the usefulness of the drug.

Within this framework, the results of comparative and controlled clinical trials on IUdR can be considered. There are significant variations in the criteria of evaluation, time of treatment, and nature of controls. Thus no two studies are strictly comparable among those listed in Table I. Five studies employing inert placebo controls document an advantage of IUdR treatment over placebo (Jawetz *et al.*, 1970). By contrast, the two studies which compared topical IUdR administration to cauterization revealed that, in dendritic epithelial keratitis not treated with steroids, healing occurred as regularly after removal of infected cells following cauterization as after IUdR treatment (Davidson and Evans, 1964; Patterson and Jones, 1967). In dendritic keratitis aggravated by steroids, however, cure followed cauterization in only 3 of 9 cases, whereas cure followed IUdR treatment in 11 of 15 cases—a significant difference. It is probable that in large herpetic epithelial ("geographic") ulcers IUdR treatment is preferable to cauterization even when corticosteroids have not been administered. Instead of 0.1% IUdR solutions which require frequent administration, 0.5% IUdR ointment can be applied four times daily with a similar therapeutic effect (Thomas *et al.*, 1965).

Can administration of IUdR during acute herpetic keratitis influence the frequency of recurrences by "eradicating" the virus infection? Although it has been suggested that IUdR "specifically eradicates virus from the cornea

TABLE I

RESULTS OF CONTROLLED STUDIES ON THE TREATMENT OF HERPETIC KERATITIS WITH IODOXURIDINE (IUdR)

Reference	IUdR			Control		
	Days administered	Estimate of Success (No. total)	Estimate of Success (%)	Material or procedure	Estimate of success (No. total)	Estimate of success (%)
Burns (1963)	5–9	15/23	65	Placebo	5/15	33
Patterson *et al.* (1963)	5	24/33	74	Placebo	2/29	7
Davidson and Evans (1964)	7	8/17	47	Gamma globulin	7/14	50
				Cauterization	15/20	75
Jepson (1964)	7	11/12	92	Placebo	7/12	58
Laibson and Leopold (1964)	8	15/22	68	Placebo	7/26	27
Hart *et al.* (1965)	7	14/19	74	Placebo	2/13	15
Patterson and Jones (1967)	7	32/38	84	Cauterization	34/39	87

under some circumstances" (Kaufman, 1963), at least three studies (Davidson and Evans, 1964; Carroll *et al.*, 1967; Patterson and Jones, 1967) indicated that recurrences occurred with the same frequency in patients who had been treated with IUdR and in those who had not. Kaufman and Maloney (1963) had proposed that the simultaneous administration of IUdR to stromal keratitis treated with corticosteriods might diminish the risk of activating epithelial replication of HSV. This drug "cover" has found only limited acceptance (Hughes, 1969) in spite of early endorsements (Thomas *et al.*, 1965). Corticosteroids can enhance bacterial and fungal as well as viral infections in the eye and may inhibit healing of the corneal stroma. Although topical corticosteroids apparently do not increase the frequency of HSV shedding of epithelial lesions following initial experimental infection in rabbits (Kibrick *et al.*, 1971), they do prolong virus production in the cornea (Jawetz *et al.*, 1963) and enlarge epithelial defects (Patterson and Jones, 1967). A controlled trial by Patterson and Jones (1967) proved the benefit of adding IUdR when steroids were employed for the treatment of stromal HSV keratitis. Ten of 24 (42%) patients on placebo and steroid developed an epithelial ulcer, but only 4 of 26 (15%) receiving IUdR steroid developed this complication. This statistically significant difference support the desirability of employing the antiviral drug together with the steroid in stromal keratitis, but the study also acknowledges that the "cover" provided by the antiviral drug is far from complete.

The role of drug resistance of HSV strains in the failure of IUdR treatment is not clearly established. Since the inception of clinical IUdR treatment, some patients have been encountered who failed to respond to the drug. Isolates of HSV from some of these patients were markedly more resistant to IUdR in cell culture than were the majority of isolates (Laibson *et al.*, 1963; Kobayashi and Nakamura, 1964). However, other isolates from nonresponding patients seemed to be fully susceptible to IUdR *in vitro* but had the ability to penetrate rapidly into corneal stroma of experimental animals (Jawetz *et al.*, 1965). The incidence of truly drug-resistant isolates does not seem to have changed greatly in the 10 years since IUdR came into widespread clinical use. In 1967–1968 only 2 drug-resistant strains were found among isolates from 12 patients who appeared to be "treatment-resistant" to IUdR (Coleman *et al.*, 1968). There is no good evidence that the widespread use of IUdR in herpetic keratitis has exerted sufficient selection pressure to favor IUdR-resistant HSV on a large scale. In part, this might be attributed to the peculiar transmission pattern of HSV. The source of HSV infecting an eye is commonly the respiratory tract or the skin, but very rarely another human eye. Thus far IUdR has been applied principally to eye lesions and to mucous membranes or skin. Thus, there has been only limited opportunity for the spread of IUdR-resistant mutants which might emerge in the course of IUdR treatment. Even in patients whose keratitis fails to respond to IUdR treatment, HSV is often difficult to isolate while the drug is being administered at frequent intervals. In such cases, HSV isolation can again be accomplished 48 hours after topical IUdR had been discontinued (Coleman *et al.*, 1969).

A number of untoward reactions to IUdR are commonly observed. True hypersensitivity can occur which may manifest itself as contact dermatitis of eyelids. Treatment with IUdR may produce follicular conjunctivitis, superficial punctate erosions of the epithelium, or subepithelial ghost opacities in areas of earlier herpetic epithelial lesions. These and other manifestations of toxicity increase in frequency and severity with the duration of IUdR application (Thygeson *et al.*, 1963; Hughes, 1969). For this reason, treatment should probably not exceed 7–10 days. If a response to IUdR occurs, it is seen within 4–7 days of treatment.

Since IUdR is incapable of "eradicating" HSV from herpetic keratitis, or diminishing the recurrence rate (Carroll *et al.*, 1967), and since the possibility of increased resistance to IUdR must be considered, other antiviral drugs have been sought. 5-Methylamino-2-deoxyuridine (Nemes and Hilleman, 1965), 5-ethyl-2-deoxyuridine (Gauri, 1968; Laibson, 1970), and several biguanidines have been tested in experimental herpetic keratitis but have not yet been used in clinical ophthalmology. Cytosine arabinoside (cytarabine) penetrates better and is more effective than IUdR *in vitro* and in experimental keratitis, but it seems to be significantly more toxic (Kaufman *et al.*, 1964). In man cytarabine administered topically is toxic for basal layers of the corneal epithelium, which may result in ulcers or corneal edema (Kaufman, 1963). No publication has appeared on a comprehensive series of patients with herpetic keratitis treated with cytarabine. Trifluorothymidine may have significant advantages over IUdR in cell culture and experimental keratitis (Kaufman and Heidelberger, 1964). Studies on the treatment of human herpetic keratitis with this drug are in progress.*

Two drugs called oxolin and florenal (the nature of these drugs in unknown to me) have been employed in patients in the U.S.S.R. Florenal is said to be comparable to IUdR in cell culture and in herpetic keratitis of rabbits and to have exerted "a positive therapeutic effect . . . in 35 of 36 patients with superficial forms of herpetic keratitis." It was also said to be effective in "severe stromal forms of herpetic keratitis" and in zoster keratouveitis as well as in adenovirus infection. The study was uncontrolled but the effects "appeared dramatic" (Maichuck, 1971).

p-Fluorophenylalanine (*p*-FPA) 0.2% ointment was believed to be ther-

* *Amer. J. Ophthal.* **73**, 932, 1972.

apeutically equivalent to IUdR 0.1% ointment in the treatment of herpetic keratitis. An ointment incorporating both *p*-FPA and IUdR was claimed to be even more effective. A "synergistic" action was postulated between these inhibitors of viral protein synthesis and of viral DNA synthesis, respectively. The average time to healing with the mixture was 3 days in 20 patients, with *p*-FPA it was 3–4 days in 14 of 15 patients, and with IUdR it was 5 days in 17 of 18 patients. These differences were believed to be significant (Graupner *et al.*, 1969).

An attempt has been made to treat human herpetic keratitis with an "interferon inducer" poly I:C. A solution of 1 mg/ml was used topically, introducing 1 drop into the conjunctival sac every hour from 9 a.m. to 10 p.m. Of 21 patients receiving this regimen, 81% are said to have good results, meaning that all corneal staining disappeared in 12 days or less. By comparison 12 patients receiving a 0.2% IUdR solution in the same schedule had good results in only 42% of the patients (Guerra *et al.*, 1970). Insufficient details were presented for a critical evaluation of this uncontrolled trial. In view of the ocular toxicity of poly I:C demonstrated in rabbits (Ostler *et al.*, 1970), one must anticipate further cautions trials before forming an opinion on this therapeutic approach. However, Centifanto *et al.* 1970) found that in humans the topical administration of poly I:C to the conjunctival sac induces only very small amounts of interferon in tear fluids. When poly I:C was administered four times daily, minimal amounts of interferon were produced for the first 2 days, and none could be detected thereafter. This suggested that topical interferon inducers might be even less effective in man than in the rabbit with herpetic keratitis. These same investigators (Kaufman *et al.*, 1971) added another sobering experience: Interferon inducers have markedly different efficacy in different species. Thus, tilorone HCl appears to be a safe and effective interferon inducer in mice, but in man it is neither safe nor effective by either the systemic or the topical route of administration.

Cryotherapy has been proposed as an effective treatment for herpetic keratitis (Fulhorst *et al.*, 1972), but no controlled comparison with antirival drugs is available. It may be concluded that the topical application of IUdR in epithelial herpetic keratitis undoubtedly can have a beneficial effect, and that IUdR, used together with steroids in stromal herpetic keratitis, can definitely counteract (partially or completely) the enhancement of herpes multiplication attributable to steroids. However, many aspects of herpetic keratitis can be treated with conventional methods (cauterization plus mechanical removal of cells) as effectively as with IUdR. The position of other drugs (trifluorothymidine and cytosine or adenine arabinosides) is not yet clearly established.

IV. Herpesvirus Infections with Prominent Skin Lesions (Simplex, Zoster, Varicella)

A. Disseminated Herpes Simplex Infections

The initial successes with treatment of ocular HSV herpetic keratitis encouraged attempts to influence HSV lesions of skin and mucous membranes by topical drugs. Several anecdotal, uncontrolled observations suggested a beneficial effect of the application of 0.5% IUdR ointment to early herpetic lesions. Schofield (1964) reported that 50 patients with herpes progenitalis all responded to 0.5% IUdR ointment applied three times daily for 2–7 days. Twenty patients believed that their previous, untreated course of herpetic lesions lasted 10 days on the average, whereas with IUdR ointment lesions cleared in 7 days. No ointment controls were mentioned. Four patients with lymphatic leukemia and extensive mucocutaneous herpes at the Mayo Clinic showed a beneficial response to 0.5% IUdR ointment as compared to 4 similar untreated patients (Muller *et al.*, 1972). However, other studies which compared this drug ointment to a placebo ointment failed to reveal any benefit (Burnett and Katz, 1963; Ive, 1964; Juel-Jensen and MacCallum, 1965; McCallum, 1964). Hutfield (1964) found no differences between IUdR and phenyl mercuric dinaphthyl methane disulfonate in genital herpes.

It seems possible that the low solubility of IUdR did not permit it to reach sites in the skin where herpesviruses replicated. To circumvent this difficulty the drug might be mechanically injected into the lower layers of the epidermis where virus replicates, or it might be brought there by a suitable vehicle which could greatly increase its absorption and diffusion. Both of these approaches have been tried. Juel-Jensen and MacCallum (1965) used a Dermojet gun to administer aqueous 0.1% IUdR to HSV lesions of the face. In a controlled trial the average duration of lesions in the drug group (12 patients) was 2.17 days, whereas in the placebo group (11 patients) it was 4.09 days. This shortening of the lesion time by 1.92 days was considered significant. Some pain was associated with the gun blast, but the pain of herpes may have been relieved, and later recurrences of herpetic lesions did not occur at the treated site.

Corbett *et al.* (1966) reported that in a controlled study 0.1% IUdR in 1.4% polyvinyl alcohol resulted in a marked acceleration of healing of cutaneous HSV lesion, if the remedy was applied within 12 hours of onset. A careful, double-blind repetition of this study employing 0.1% IUdR in 1.4% polyvinyl alcohol, or 0.5% IUdR ointment revealed no beneficial effect whatever of the drug over the placebo (Kibrick and Katz, 1970). Furthermore, the placement of drug or placebo on alternate squares of skin in the preeruptive phase of varicella also showed no difference. These are disturbing discrepancies in results of controlled trials with the same drug on comparable patients.

Dimethylsulfoxide (DMSO) was employed as a vehicle for IUdR in several treatment trials. The purpose of this approach was to facilitate the penetration of IUdR and to have the drug dissolved in DMSO and deposited at lower levels of the epidermis when water replaced DMSO. MacCallum and Juel-Jensen (1966) performed a controlled trial with 5% IUdR in DMSO in HSV lesions of the face. The solution was painted on lesions with a brush three times daily for 3 days, to a total of 1 ml. Ten patients receiving IUdR in DMSO had an average shortening of 6.3 days in the duration of lesions, compared to untreated lesions, and an average shortening of 2 days compared to DMSO alone. Evidently DMSO by itself was an effective form of local therapy. The belief was also expressed that local recurrences at the same site were markedly reduced after drug treatment. The uncontrolled treatment of 20 patients with HSV lesions by the hourly application of 1% IUdR in DMSO was uniformly beneficial by shortening the "expected" duration of the lesions (Turnbull *et al.*, 1969). In view of the marked variability of herpetic skin lesions, this "confirmatory" report unfortunately adds little. Because of the possible toxicity of DMSO, its investigational use in the United States has been curtailed, and no controlled studies of topical IUdR in DMSO have been reported.

A compound which exhibited marked activity in a model of cutaneous infection of rabbits, 4-[2-nitro-1-(*p*-tolylthio)ethyl]-acetanilide, was submitted to a carefully controlled clinical trial. In clinical labial herpes this drug could not be distinguished from placebo. A marked "beneficial" effect of placebo was observed, again stressing the need for double-blind studies (Underwood, 1970). Another compound, 3-ethoxy-2-oxobutyraldehyde, also effective in rabbit herpes, could not be distinguished from placebo cream when it was applied to human skin herpes as 2.5% cream. The difference in activity between experimental and clinical lesions may be the large amount of virus already present in human skin lesions prior to the development of symptoms (Underwood and Nichol, 1971). Juel-Jensen (1970) treated 6 patients with severe generalized herpes simplex with intravenous cytarabine 0.3–2.0 mg/kg/day for 5 days. All patients were said to have had a "dramatic recovery." The drug induced only transient depression of the bone marrow in some patients, none in others. Several other patients with disseminated herpes simplex treated with cytarabine are included in a summary by Chow *et al.* (1970).

Severe, generalized herpes simplex with prominent lesions of skin and mucous membranes occurs most commonly in infants as part of infection acquired at birth or *in utero* or in immunodeficient persons subject to other disease or treatment. The extreme variability of clinical disease and the difficulty of predicting the outcome of HSV infection in infants have been stressed (Torphy *et al.*, 1970; Nahmias, 1970). In spite of the often serious prognosis, some infants recover completely with only symptomatic treatment. This makes any evaluation of antiviral drug treatment difficult until a large, randomized, controlled series has been accumulated.

B. Herpes Zoster Infections

The lesions of herpes zoster are exceedingly variable, ranging from limited vesicular eruption along part of a single sensory nerve with minor pain to a widespread massive eruption with severe systemic symptoms and intense and lasting local pain.

Juel-Jensen *et al.* (1970) have applied IUdR in DMSO to the topical treatment of localized herpes zoster in Britain. In one double-blind trial, patients with comparable painful zoster lesions painted 5% IUdR in DMSO, DMSO alone, or scented saline onto their lesions with a brush four times daily for 4 days. The group receiving IUdR lost their pain in 3 days; those receiving DMSO lost the pain after 13.5 days; and those receiving saline, after 30 days.

In a second trial the same authors applied 40% IUdR in purified 100% DMSO to gauze covering the area of zoster lesions, keeping the gauze moist for 4 days. This resulted in a statistically significant shortening of the period of pain and the time to complete healing of vesicles. The median time for healing with IUdR in DMSO was 3 days, with 100% DMSO alone 65 days, and with saline 14.5 days, indicating that IUdR alone was harmful. No new lesions occurred during the continuous application of 40% IUdR in DMSO, whereas this "often" happened in placebo groups. The time for healing of vesicular lesions was not significantly altered. While this report gives good evidence for a beneficial effect of 40% IUdR in DMSO for the suppression of pain in shingles, the nature of the antiviral chemotherapeutic effect in man is not clear, and the potential harmful effects of DMSO and the 0.5–0.75 gm IUdR absorbed systemically each day will require more extensive careful trials before such topical therapy can be accepted for general use.

During the past several years, many patients with generalized herpes zoster or with severe varicella were treated with antiviral drugs in medical centers all over the world. Most of these patients also suffered from leukemia or immunodeficiency or had been treated with immunosuppressive drugs. There is a prevailing belief that a proportion of these patients showed some improvement attributable to antiviral drug treatment. However, no controlled series of patients has been reported. As all other herpesvirus infections, herpes zoster presents a broad spectrum of disease severity which makes evaluation of treatment in single cases virtually impossible.

Hall *et al.* (1969) treated 7 patients with disseminated herpes zoster with cytarabine (cytosine arabinoside) 100 mg/m^2 body surface/day. Six of these patients improved. One similar successfully treated patient was reported by Prager *et al.* (1971). Chow *et al.* (1970) summarized 17 cytarabine-treated patients reported until mid-1970: In 17 infections it was claimed that only 2 failed to respond to treatment. The more severely ill patients with herpes zoster received cytarabine 40–100 mg / m^2 body surface daily for 6 – 7 days by intravenous infusion. The less severe, localized zoster lesions were treated with cytarabine 20 mg / m^2 body surface day for 1 – 3 days. All zoster lesions in Chow's series were said to be arrested within 2 days after beginning cytarabine infusions, whereas in 70% of untreated patients comparable lesions were believed to continue for more than 2 weeks. All zoster pain was said to have disappeared within 2 days, whereas it may persist in some untreated persons for weeks. The lack of a controlled, randomized study made it impossible to evaluate these reports beyond quoting them. Early results in a carefully planned, randomized, double-blind study on cytarabine treatment of disseminated herpes zoster do not support such an enthusiastic view (T. Merigan, personal communication).

C. Cytomegalovirus (CMV) Infections

Antiviral treatment has been attempted in newborns with congenital cytomegalovirus infection. 5-Iodo-2-deoxyuridine 100 mg / kg body weight/day was given intravenously for 5 days to three severely damaged, CMV-infected infants (Conchie *et al.*, 1968; Barton and Tobin, 1970). There was some reduction in viruria but no apparent change in clinical status or outlook.

Cangir *et al.* (1967) treated 5 leukemic children, suspected of having cytomegalovirus pneumonia with 5-fluoro-2-deoxyuridine in full antileukemic doses. There was some questionable clinical improvement, but the diagnosis was not fully substantiated by virologic means.

Cytarabine has been employed in several hospitals to treat small groups of infants with congenital CMV infection. Plotkin and Steller (1969) treated three infants with 10 –15 mg / kg body weight/day cytarabine for 5 days. There was no great clinical improvement, but CMV excretion was reduced temporarily in one and eliminated altogether in another infant. Kraybill *et al.* (1972) gave 3– 5 mg / kg body weight cytarabine as a single intramuscular dose daily for 15 days to two infants. Marked toxicity occurred, with vomiting, neutrapenia, and thrombocytopenia, and there was no unequivocal influence on the presence or excretion of CMV virus. McCracken and Luby (1972) treated four infants with congenital, disseminated CMV infection with cytarabine by giving 8 mg / kg / day or 25 gm / kg / day by rapid intravenous infusion. The drug depressed virus excretion only transiently and had no definite beneficial effect on the clinical course of the infection. There was significant hematologic and hepatic toxicity. It is probable that serum levels sufficient to inhibit the virus markedly were not maintained for any length of time because cytarabine is very quickly cleared from the blood.

On the whole, it appears that the response of infants with disseminated CMV infection to antiviral therapy has been fairly unsuccessful. In part this may be attributable to the impaired immune mechanism of CMV-infected children. Only a controlled, multi-institutional study may have the opportunity to assess treatment results in the wide spectrum of disease associated with CMV infections.

Until April 1972, there have been no reports on controlled studies of interferon inducers or of exogenous interferon made in human leukocytes in the treatment of disseminated herpesvirus infections or congenital CMV infections.

V. Herpesvirus Encephalitis

Herpes simplex virus is a common cause of sporadic, fatal encephalitis. Although known for 30 years, the specific diagnosis has been made much more frequently during the last 5 years when the possibility of antiviral treatment was first proposed (Breeden *et al.*, 1966). Herpes simplex virus central nervous system involvement may occur in disseminated HSV infection in neonatal life (Nahmias, 1970; Golden *et al.*, 1969), as part of a symptomatic or asymptomatic primary infection in children or adults, or as recurrence in a previously infected person. It most commonly produces a form of aseptic meningitis, but may manifest itself as acute necrotizing encephalitis, an intracranial mass lesion, or the "temporal lobe" syndrome (Gurwith *et al.*, 1971). While aseptic meningitis is often self-limited and leaves no sequelae, the outlook for HSV encephalitis is grave.

The specific diagnosis of HSV encephalitis is increasingly based on early brain biopsy which permits the isolation of the virus in cell culture or the identification of its antigens by immunofluorescence. A serologic diagnosis of HSV encephalitis by the demonstration of complement-requiring neutralizing antibody has been proposed (Lerner *et al.*, 1970). Early antibody has been proposed (Lerner *et al.*, 1970). Early antibody responses in the cerebrospinal fluid measured by passive hemagglutination or immunofluorescence are under study (A. J. Nahmias, personal communication). The results with IUdR treatment have been carefully compiled and analyzed by Gurwith *et al.* (1971). In order to evaluate the possible success of antiviral treatment, the natural history of HSV encephalitis must be considered. As in all other forms of HSV infection, the clinical spectrum is broad and the outcome quite variable. Among a small number of untreated, noncomatose patients, mortality varied from 0 – 50% (total of 4 deaths in 26 patients, or 15%), whereas among untreated, comatose patients the mortality varied from 33 – 80% (total 41 deaths in 58 patients, or 71%). The overall mortality of untreated patients was 51% (55 deaths in 108 patients).

By contrast, the overall mortality of patients receiving IUdR was 30% (6 deaths in 20 patients) reported until mid-1971. The mortality among IUdR-treated patients with coma was 29% (strikingly different from the 71% among untreated patients with coma). However, an additional 7 of 20 treated patients (35%) survived with severe and debilitating neurological or mental impairments, which raise doubts regarding the "therapeutic triumph" of an antiviral treatment which possibly changed a fatal outcome to survival with massive brain damage.

Most published reports deal with 1 or 2 cases, each treated intravenously with 300–500 mg/kg IUdR over a 5-day period, provided the patient survived that long. The largest experience reported to date is that of Nolan *et al.* (1970) and Meyer *et al.* (1970). Six of 13 patients with diagnosed herpesvirus encephalitis were treated with IUdR—an average of 430 mg/kg in a period of 5 days. Two patients who yielded virus on brain biopsy died before the 5-day treatment could be completed. All four, fully treated patients recovered without residua. However, these four surviving patients were diagnosed only by serologic means, not virus isolation. Of the seven untreated patients (in earlier years), three died and four survived with significant neurological defects.

Tomlinson and MacCallum (1970) reviewed part of the British experience with IUdR treatment of herpetic encephalitis. No beneficial effect was observed in three patients given 100 mg/kg/day IUdR for 2–5 days, and large amounts of virus were recovered from the brains at autopsy. In five other patients, treatment results were indeterminate.

With slow, continuous intravenous infusion of IUdR in the above doses, concentrations of 2.5 μg/ml microbiologically active IUdR are not regularly found in serum or cerebrospinal fluid of treated patients and only occasionally, are found in their urine. Most type 1 HSV strains required 5 – 15 μg / ml IUdR for inhibition in cell culture, and most type 2 strains required 5 times higher concentrations, or more (Lerner and Bailey, 1972).

In most microbial infections, effective chemotherapy requires the presence of meaningful concentrations of the antimicrobial drug in body fluids or tissues. By analogy it seems unlikely that IUdR could have a pronounced antiviral effect in the absence of measurable inhibitory levels, unless one were to postulate preferential accumulation of drug in infected cells. Good antiviral levels of IUdR in tissues or central nervous system could probably be achieved only if the drug were to be administered in high doses by repeated, rapid intravenous infusion.

Nevertheless there are alluring possibilities that the encouraging results reported by Nolan *et al.* (1970) and summarized by Gurwith *et al.* (1971) might be attributed not to accident but to early diagnosis and transient presence of slightly inhibitory amounts of drug in tissues and body fluids—just sufficient to tip the balance in favor of the host. Until the completion of a controlled trial, this possibility cannot be entirely discarded.

The results of IUdR treatment (200–580 mg/kg total dose) in herpetic encephalitis of newborns—part of disseminated HSV infection—are even less encouraging in terms of the ultimate outcome.

Treatment with IUdR may have produced temporary improvement in a newborn infant with systemic HSV infection, but the child died with widespread organ damage (Partridge and Millis, 1968). Another neonate with disseminated HSV and encephalitis, treated with IUdR (Golden *et al.*, 1969) in the same dose, showed clinical improvement with diminished seizure activity. However, 15 days after completion of the 5-day course, seizures recurred, and HSV was again isolated from spinal fluid. A second course of IUdR was followed by apparent recovery from infection but exceedingly severe brain damage. Heroic treatment resulted in an anencephalic child. The infant treated by Charnock and Cramblett (1970) with 410 mg/kg IUdR survived but with significant neurological impairment. Of six treated infants reported only one appears to be well; the others died or are severely retarded (Gurwith *et al.*, 1971). However, observations are recorded of sudden and dramatic improvement after the institution of IUdR treatment (Partridge and Millis, 1968; Golden *et al.*, 1969), followed by relapse. Cerebral decompression may significantly contribute to the survival of patients with necrotizing encephalitis. Thus single or repeated brain biopsy procedures may be indirectly helpful in such patients. This factor has not been controlled in any published study.

In all trials of intravenous treatment with IUdR, toxic effects were encountered in varying degrees. Stomatitis, leukopenia, and alopicia were prominent, and bacterial superinfections presented difficulties during the period of leukopenia.

A single case of HSV aseptic meningitis and encephalitis was treated with a double-stranded synthetic ribonucleic acid poly I:C as an interferon inducer (Bellanti *et al.*, 1971). Interferon levels were elevated in the patient prior to administration of the inducer, and it was not possible to establish that further interferon induction occurred after administration of the inducer. The benefits of treatment, if any, could not be assessed, and there was extensive cerebral cortical necrosis.

A cautious review of all published evidence up to March, 1972 suggests to me that no unequivocal recommendations can be made for the treatment of HSV encephalitis. It is not possible to conclude that this disorder—even if diagnosed very early—should be treated with cytotoxic drugs in high dosage. Only unbiased, controlled, double-blind studies can provide the answer. The current fashion of intensive treatment at all cost may well be more damaging than helpful.

VI. Conclusions

Diseases caused by herpesviruses were the first disorders in which antiviral drug therapy was attempted on a large scale. Of the many chemicals capable of inhibiting viral replication in cell culture, only a few have significant therapeutic efficacy in the treatment of established infections in animal models, and still fewer seem to provide any possible benefit in human disease. Even in herpetic keratitis, the disease most definitely influenced by antiviral drug treatment, there are only relatively rare patients whose large epithelial lesions unequivocally benefit more from antiviral drugs than from other available conventional forms of management.

In disseminated forms of herpesvirus infections, the severe toxicity of available antiviral drugs has limited the dose which could be tolerated, and consequently insufficient concentrations of drug have reached the involved tissues. This may be partly responsible for the lack of conclusive evidence of therapeutic benefit from antiviral drugs in these disseminated infections and in encephalitis. Improved modes of administration (e.g., brief intravenous infusions of very high doses or use of penetrating vehicles) may improve this discouraging outlook in the future. It is possible that new drugs of striking antiviral efficacy will become available with only mild systemic or local toxicity for the host's tissue. At present this is a hope rather than a reasoned expectation.

Acknowledgments

I am grateful to Dr. Stephen N. Cohen for his critical review and thoughtful comments on this manuscript.

References

Barton, B. W., and Tobin, J. O'H. (1970). *Ann. N. Y. Acad. Sci.* **173**, 90–95.

Bellanti, J. A., Catalano, L. W., Jr., and Chambers, R. W. (1971). *J. Pediat.* **78**, 136.

Breeden, C. J., Hall, T. C., and Tyler, H. R. (1966). *Ann. Intern. Med.* **65**, 1050.

Burnett, J. W., and Katz, S. I. (1963). *J. Invest. Dermatol.* **40**, 7.

Burns, R. P. (1963). *Arch. Ophthalmol.* [N.S.] **70**, 381.

Cangir, A., Sullivan, M. P., Sutow, W. W., and Taylor, G. (1967). *J. Amer. Med. Ass.* **201**, 612.

Carroll, J. M., Martola, E. L., Laibson, P. R., and Dohlman, C. H. (1967). *Amer. J. Ophthalmol.* [3] **63**, 103.

Centifanto, Y. M., Goorha, R. M., and Kaufman, H. E. (1970). *Amer. J. Ophthalmol.* [3] **70**, 1006.

Charnock, E. L., and Cramblett, H. G. (1970). *J. Pediat.* **76**, 459.

Chow, A. W., Foerster, J., and Hryniuk, W. (1970). *Antimicrob. Ag. Chemother.* pp. 214–217.

Coleman, V. R., Tsu, E., and Jawetz, E. (1968). *Proc. Soc. Exp. Biol. Med.* **129**, 761.

Coleman, V. R., Thygeson, P., Dawson, C. R., and Jawetz, E. (1969). *Arch. Ophthalmol.* [N.S.] **81**, 22.

Conchie, A. F., Barton, B. W., and Tobin, J. O'H. (1968). *Brit. Med. J.* **4**, 162.

Corbett, M. B., Sidell, C. M., and Zimmerman, M. (1966). *J. Amer. Med. Ass.* **196**, 441.

Corrigan, M. J., Gilkes, M. J., and Roberts, D.S.C. (1962). *Brit. Med. J.* **2**, 304.

Corwin, M. E., Coleman, V. R., Riegelman, S., Okumoto, M., Jawetz, E., and Thygeson, P. (1963a). *Invest. Ophthalmol.* **2**, 578.

Corwin, M. E., Okumoto, M., Thygeson, P., and Jawetz, E. (1963b). *Amer. J. Ophthalmol.* **55**, 225.

Davidson, S. I., and Evans, P. J. (1964). *Brit. J. Ophthalmol.* **48**, 678.

Dixon, G. J., Sidwell, R. W., Miller, F. A., and Sloan, B. J. (1968). *Antimicrob. Ag. Chemother.* pp. 172–179.

Easterbrook, M. *et al.* (1973). *Invest. Ophthalmol.* **12**, 181.

Engle, C. G., and Stewart, R. C. (1964). *J. Immunol.* **92**, 730.

Ey, R. C., Hughes, W. F., Holmes, A. W., and Deinhardt, F. (1963). *Trans. Amer. Ophthalmol. Soc.* **61**, 100.

Force, E. E., Stewart, R. C., and Haff, R. F. (1964). *Virology* **23**, 363.

Fulhorst, H. W., Richards, A. B., Bowbyes, J., and Jones, B. R. (1972). *Amer. J. Ophthalmol.* [3] **73**, 46.

Furgiuele, F. B., Pentecost, G. F., Klein, M., and McGavic, J. S. (1962). *Trans. Amer. Ophthalmol. Soc.* **60**, 243.

Gauri, V. K. K. (1968). *Klin. Monatsbl. Augenheilk.* **153**, 837.

Golden, B., Bell, W. E., and McKee, A. P. (1969). *J. Amer. Med. Ass.* **209**, 1219.

Goz, B., and Prusoff, W. H. (1970). *Annu. Rev. Pharmacol.* **10**, 143.

Graupner, K., Klein, S., and Müller, F. (1969). *Albrecht von Graefes Arch. Klin. Exp. Ophthalmol.* **177**, 89.

Guerra, R., Frezzotti, R., Bonanni, R., Dianzani, F., and Rita, G. (1970). *Ann. N.Y. Acad. Sci.* **173**, 823–830.

Gundersen, T. (1936). *Arch. Ophthalmol.* **15**, 225.

Gurwith, M. J., Harman, C. E., and Merigan, T. C. (1971). *Calif Med.* **115**, 63.

Hall, T. C., Wilfter, C., Jaffe, N., Traggis, D., Lux, S., Rompf, P., and Katz, S. (1969). *Trans. Ass. Amer. Physicians* **82**, 201.

Hart, D. R. L., Brightman, V. J. F., Readshaw, G. G., Porter, G. T. J., and Tully, M. J. (1965). *Arch. Ophthalmol* [N.S.]. **73**, 623.

Herrmann, E. C. (1961). *Proc. Soc. Exp. Biol. Med.* **107**, 142.

Hughes, W. F. (1969). *Amer. J. Ophthalmol.* [3] **67**, 313.

Hutfield, D. C. (1964). *Brit. J. Vener. Dis.* **40**, 210.

Ive, F. A. (1964). Brit. J. Dermatol. **76**, 463.

Jawetz, E., Schultz, R., Coleman, V. R., Okumoto, M., and Tong, M. (1963). *Antimicrob. Ag. Chemother.* pp. 693–698.

Jawetz, E., Schultz, R., Coleman, V., R., and Okumoto, M. (1965). *J. Immunol.* **95**, 635.

Jawetz, E., Coleman, V. R., Dawson, C. R., and Thygeson, P. (1970). *Ann. N.Y. Acad. Sci.* **173**, 282–291.

Jepson, C. N. (1964). *Amer. J. Ophthalmol.* [3] **57**, 213.
Johnson, A. W., and Jervey, E. D. (1964). *Arch. Ophthalmol.* [N.S.] **72**, 826.
Jones, B. R. (1967). *Trans. Ophthalmol. Soc. U.K.* **87**, 537.
Juel-Jensen, B. E. (1970). *Brit. Med. J.* **2**, 154.
Juel-Jensen, B. E., and MacCallum, F. O. (1965). *Brit. Med. J.* **1**, 901.
Juel-Jensen, B. E., MacCallum, F. O., Mackenzie, M. R., and Pike, M. C. (1970). *Brit. Med. J.* **4**, 776.
Kaufman, H. E. (1962). *Proc. Soc. Exp. Biol. Med.* **109**, 251.
Kaufman, H. E. (1965). *Progr. Med. Virol.* **7**, 116–159.
Kaufman, H. E. (1963). *Invest. Ophthalmol.* **2**, 504.
Kaufman, H. E., and Heildelberger, C. (1964). *Science* **145**, 585.
Kaufman, H. E., and Maloney, E. D. (1963). *Arch. Ophthalmol.* [N.S.] **69**, 626.
Kaufman, H. E., Nesburn, A. B., and Maloney, E. D. (1962a). *Arch. Ophthalmol.* [N.S.] **67**, 583.
Kaufman, H. E., Martola, E. L., and Dohlman, C. (1962b). *Arch. Ophthalmol.* [N.S.] **68**, 235.
Kaufman, H. E., Capella, J. A., and Maloney, E. D. (1964). *Arch. Ophthalmol.* [N.S.] **72**, 535.
Kaufman, H. E., Ellison, E. D., and Waltman, S. R. (1969). *Amer. J. Ophthalmol.* [3] **68**, 486.
Kaufman, H. E., Ellison, E. D., and Townsend, W. M. (1970). *Arch. Ophthalmol.* [N.S.] **84**, 783.
Kaufman, H. E., Centifanto, Y. M., Ellison, E. D., and Brown, D. C. (1971). *Proc. Soc. Exp. Biol. Med.* **137**, 357.
Kibrick, S., and Katz, A. S. (1970). *Ann. N.Y. Acad. Sci.* **173**, 83–89.
Kibrick, S., Takahashi, G. H., Leibowitz, H. M., and Laibson, P. R. (1971). *Arch. Opthalmol.* [N.S.] **86**, 694.
Kobayashi, S., and Nakamura, T. (1964). *Jap. J. Ophthalmol.* **8**, 14.
Kraybill, E. N., Sever, J. L., Avery, G. B., and Movassaghi, N. (1972). *J. Pediat.* **80**, 485.
Laibson, P. R. (1970). *Arch. Ophthalmol.* [N.S.] **83**, 637.
Laibson, P. R., and Kibrick, S. (1966). *Arch. Ophthalmol.* [N.S.] **75**, 254.
Laibson, P. R., and Leopold, I. H. (1964). *Trans. Amer. Acad. Ophthalmol. Otolaryngol.* **68**, 22.
Laibson, P. R., Sery, T. W., and Leopold, I. H. (1963). *Arch. Ophthalmol.* [N.S.] **70**, 52.
Lerner, A. M., and Bailey, E. J., (1972). *J. Clin. Invest.* **51**, 45.
Lerner, A. M., Bailey, E. J., and Nolan, D. C. (1970). *J. Immunol.* **104**, 607.
Luntz, M. H., and MacCallum, F. O. (1963). *Brit. J. Ophthalmol.* **47**, 449.
McCallum, D. I. (1964). *Brit. J. Dermatol.* **76**, 459.
MacCallum, F. O., and Juel-Jensen, B. E. (1966). *Brit. Med. J.* **2**, 805.
McCracken, G. H., and Luby, J. P. (1972). *J. Pediat.* **80**, 488.
McFadzean, J. A. (1969). *Advan. Pharmacol. Chemother.* **7**, 309.
Maichuk, Y. F. (1971). *Invest. Ophthalmol.* **10**, 408.
Maloney, E. D., and Kaufman, H. E. (1965). *Invest. Ophthalmol.* **4**, 872.
Meyer, J. S., Bauer, R. B., River-Olmos, V. M., Nolan, D. C., and Lerner, A. M. (1970). *Arch. Neurol.* (*Chicago*) **23**, 438.
Miller, F. A., Sloan, B. J., and Silverman, C. A. (1969). *Antimicrob. Ag. Chemother.* pp. 192–195.
Moore, C., Wallis, C., Melnick, J. L., and Kuns, M. D. (1972). *Infection Immunity* **5**, 169.
Muller, S. A., Herrmann, E. C., and Winkelmann, R. K. (1972). *Amer. J. Med.* **52**, 102.
Nahmias, A. J. (1970). *N. Engl. J. Med.* **282**, 684.
Nemes, M. M., and Hilleman, M. R. (1965). *Proc. Soc. Exp. Biol. Med.* **119**, 515.
Nolan, D. C., Carruthers, M. M., and Lerner, A. M. (1970). *N. Engl. J. Med.* **282**, 10.
Oh, J. O., Moschini, G. B., and Stevens, T. (1972). *Infection Immunity* **5**, 412.

Ostler, H. B., Oh, J. O., Dawson, C., and Burt, W. L. (1970). *Nature (London)* **228**, 362.
Park, J. H., and Baron, S. (1968). Science **162**, 811.
Partridge, J. W., and Millis, R. R. (1968). *Arch. Dis. Childhood* **43**, 377.
Patterson, A., and Jones, B. R. (1967). *Trans. Ophthalmol. Soc. U.K.* **87**, 59.
Patterson, A., Fox, A. D., Davies, G., Maguire, C., Sellers, P. W. H., Wright, P., Rice, N.S.C., Cobb, B., and Jones, B. R. (1963). *Trans. Ophthalmol. Soc. U.K.* **83**, 583.
Plotkin, S.A., and Steller, H. (1969). *Antimicrob. Ag. Chemother.* pp. 372–379.
Polikoff, R., Cannavale, P., Dixon, P., and Dipuppo, A. (1970). *Amer. J. Opthalmol.* [3] **69**, 650.
Prager, D., Bruder, M., and Sawitsky, A. (1971). *J. Pediat.* **78**, 321.
Schofield, C. B. S. (1964). *Brit. J. Dermatol.* **76**, 465.
Sidwell, R. W., Dixon, G. J., Schabel, F. M., and Kaump, D. H. (1968). *Antimicrob. Ag. Chemother.* pp. 148–154.
Sloan, B. J., Miller, F. A., Ehrlich, J., McLean, I. W., and Machamer, H. E. (1968). *Antimicrob. Ag. Chemother.* pp. 161–171.
Sood, N. N., and Marmion, V. J. (1964). *Brit. J. Ophthalmol.* **48**, 609.
Thomas, C. I., Purnell, E., and Rosenthal, M. S. (1965). *Amer. J. Ophthalmol.* [3] **60**, 207.
Thygeson, P., Sexton, R. R., and Corwin, M. E. (1963). *Trans. Pac. Coast Oto-Ophthalmol. Soc.* p. 81.
Tomlinson, A. H., and MacCallum, F. O. (1970). *Ann. N.Y. Acad. Sci.* **173**, 20–28.
Torphy, D. E., Ray, C. G., McAlister, R., and Du, J. N. H. (1970). *J. Pediat.* **76**, 405.
Turnbull, B. C., MacGregor, I., and Stringer, H. C. W. (1969). *N.Z. Med. J.* **70**, 317.
Underwood, G. E. (1962). *Proc. Soc. Exp. Biol. Med.* **111**, 660.
Underwood, G. E. (1970). *Ann. N.Y. Acad. Sci.* **173**, 782–793.
Underwood, G. E., and Nichol, F. R. (1971). *Appl. Microbiol.* **22**, 588.
Underwood, G. E., Elliott, G. A., and Buthala, D. A. (1965). *Ann. N.Y. Acad. Sci.* **130**, 151–167.

Author Index

Numbers in italics refer to the pages on which the complete references are listed.

B

C

D

E

F

G

H

I

J

K

L

M

Q

R

S

T

W

Subject Index

F

R

S

B 5
C 6
D 7
E 8
F 9
G 0
H 1
I 2
J 3